The Handbook of Fatigue Management in Transportation

In the world of transportation, fatigue is a silent killer that can affect us all. Understanding fatigue, including how to manage it to minimise safety risk, is of great importance. However, while it is one thing to recognise that fatigue is a critical safety issue, it is quite another to set up a successful, scientifically informed fatigue risk management programme. This book is here to help. It has been carefully designed as a comprehensive reference point, bringing together international expertise from leaders in fatigue science, and showcasing valuable insights from transportation industry practitioners.

The 40 authored chapters are divided into six sections, to better understand fatigue science, the consequences of fatigue in transportation, contributors to fatigue, managing fatigue and promoting alertness, real-world case studies of fatigue management in practice, and future perspectives. While it is possible to read each chapter in isolation, most will be gained by reading the book as a whole. Each chapter starts with an abstract overview and concludes with summary bullet points, creating a handy "quick check" for key points.

This accessible text is for those who are interested in supporting alert and safe transportation operations. It is suitable for professionals, transport managers, government advisors, policy makers, students, academics, and anyone who wants to learn more. All transport modes (road, rail, maritime and aviation) are considered. For anyone waking up to the complex challenge of fatigue management, this handbook is a must.

The Handbook of Fatigue Management in Transportation

Waking Up to the Challenge

Edited by
Christina M. Rudin-Brown
and Ashleigh J. Filtness

CRC Press
Taylor & Francis Group
Boca Raton London New York

CRC Press is an imprint of the
Taylor & Francis Group, an **informa** business

Cover Design: Laurence Filtness

First edition published 2023
by CRC Press
6000 Broken Sound Parkway NW, Suite 300, Boca Raton, FL 33487-2742

and by CRC Press
4 Park Square, Milton Park, Abingdon, Oxon, OX14 4RN

CRC Press is an imprint of Taylor & Francis Group, LLC

© 2024 selection and editorial matter, Christina M. Rudin-Brown and Ashleigh J. Filtness; individual
chapters, the contributors

Library of Congress Cataloging-in-Publication Data
Names: Rudin-Brown, Christina, editor. | Filtness, Ashleigh J., editor.
Title: The handbook of fatigue management in transportation : waking up to the challenge /
edited by Christina M. Rudin-Brown and Ashleigh J. Filtness.
Description: First edition. | Boca Raton, FL : CRC Press, 2023. |
Includes bibliographical references and index.
Identifiers: LCCN 2022061595 | ISBN 9781032081397 (hardback) |
ISBN 9781032081441 (paperback) | ISBN 9781003213154 (ebook)
Subjects: LCSH: Fatigue–Prevention. | Transportation–Physiological aspects. |
Transportation–Safety measures. | Sleep deprivation–Prevention. | Fatigue in the workplace.
Classification: LCC RC1045.F37 H36 2023 | DDC 616/.0478–dc23/eng/20230202
LC record available at https://lccn.loc.gov/2022061595

ISBN: 978-1-032-08139-7 (hbk)
ISBN: 978-1-032-08144-1 (pbk)
ISBN: 978-1-003-21315-4 (ebk)

DOI: 10.1201/9781003213154

Typeset in Times
by Newgen Publishing UK

Contents

SECTION 1   Fatigue Science and Transportation

SECTION 2   Fatigue-Related Consequences in Transportation

SECTION 3   *Factors that Contribute to Fatigue and Sleepiness in Transportation*

SECTION 4 *Managing Fatigue and Promoting Alertness in Transportation*

SECTION 5   Transportation Fatigue Risk Management in Practice

SECTION 6   Fatigue Risk Management of the Future

Contributors

Christer Ahlström
Swedish National Road and Transport
  Research Institute (VTI), and
  Department of Biomedical
  Engineering, Linköping University,
  Linköping, Sweden

Torbjörn Åkerstedt
Karolinska Institute and Stockholm
  University, Stockholm, Sweden

Anna Anund
Swedish National Road and
  Transport Research
  Institute, and Linköping University,
  Linköping, Sweden

Nora Balfe
Iarnród Eireann Irish Rail, Dublin,
  Ireland

Thomas J. Balkin
Walter Reed Army Institute of Research,
  Silver Spring, USA

Dan Basacik
Rail Safety and Standards Board,
  London, UK

Nicholas G. Bathurst
Fatigue Countermeasures Laboratory,
  NASA Ames Research Center,
  Moffett Field, USA

Laura Bienenfeld
Metropolitan Transportation Authority,
  Brooklyn, USA

Verna Blewett
Appleton Institute for Behavioural
  Science, Central Queensland
  University, Wayville, Australia

Janine Chapman
Appleton Institute for Behavioural
  Science, Central Queensland
  University, Wayville, Australia

Anna Sjörs Dahlman
Swedish National Road and
  Transport Research Institute,
  Linköping, Sweden and Chalmers
  University of Technology,
  Gothenburg, Sweden

Ragnhild Davidse
SWOV Institute for Road Safety
  Research, The Hague, Netherlands

Drew Dawson
Appleton Institute, Central Queensland
  University, Wayville, Australia

Jaime K. Devine
Institutes for Behavior Resources, Inc.,
  Baltimore, USA

Frederik Diederichs
Fraunhofer Institute of Optronics,
  System Technologies and Image
  Exploitation (IOSB), Karlsruhe,
  Germany

Geneviève Dubé
Transportation Safety Board of Canada,
  Gatineau, Canada

Tamara Dumanovsky
Joslyn Levy & Associates,
    New York, USA

Ashleigh J. Filtness
Transport Safety Research Centre,
    Loughborough University,
    Loughborough, UK

Dorothee Fischer
Institute for Aerospace Medicine,
    German Aerospace Center, Cologne,
    Germany

Erin E. Flynn-Evans
Fatigue Countermeasures Laboratory,
    NASA Ames Research Center,
    Moffett Field, USA

Simon Folkard
Department of Psychology, Swansea
    University, Swansea, UK

Clémentine François
Tobii AB, Liège, Belgium

Karl E. Friedl
US Army Research Institute of
    Environmental Medicine,
    Frederick, USA

Michelle S. Gauthier
Transportation Safety Board
    of Canada, Gatineau,
    Canada

Zachary L. Glaros
Fatigue Countermeasures Laboratory,
    NASA Ames Research Center,
    Moffett Field, USA

Charles Goldenbeld
SWOV Institute for Road
    Safety Research, The Hague,
    Netherlands

Nelson Gonzalez
Metropolitan Transportation Authority,
    Brooklyn, USA

Michelle Grech
The University of Queensland, Brisbane,
    Australia

Kevin B. Gregory
Fatigue Countermeasures Laboratory,
    NASA Ames Research Center,
    Moffett Field, USA

Ben Groome
Tram Operations Limited, Croydon, UK

Sarah Harris
Transportation Safety Board of Canada,
    Gatineau, Canada

Cassie J. Hilditch
Fatigue Countermeasures Laboratory,
    Department of Psychology,
    San José State University,
San José, USA

Lily Hirsch
Appleton Institute for Behavioural
    Science, Central Queensland
    University, Wayville, Australia

Kimberly A. Honn
Sleep and Performance Research Center
    & Department of Translational
    Medicine and Physiology,
    Washington State University,
    Spokane, USA

Steven R. Hursh
Institutes for Behavior Resources, Inc.,
    Baltimore, USA

Muataz Jaber
Metropolitan Transportation Authority,
    Brooklyn, USA

Bradley Jennings
Tram Operations Limited,
Croydon, UK

Göran Kecklund
Stockholm University, Stockholm,
Sweden

Crystal L. Kirkley
Fatigue Countermeasures Laboratory,
NASA Ames Research Center,
Moffett Field, USA

Anastasi Kosmadopoulos
Central Queensland University,
Wayville, Australia

Darian Lawrence-Sidebottom
Operations Research Department,
Naval Postgraduate School,
Monterey, USA

Mikael Ljung Aust
Volvo Cars Safety Centre,
Volvo Car Corporation,
Gothenburg, Sweden

Daria Luisi
Metropolitan Transportation Authority,
Brooklyn, USA

Ishbel Macgregor-Curtin
Iarnród Eireann Irish Rail, Dublin,
Ireland

Clinton Marquardt
PMI Inc. /
www.SleepandDreams.com,
Ottawa, Canada

Elaine C. Marqueze
Department of Epidemiology, School of
Public Health, Catholic University of
Santos, Santos, Brazil

Panagiotis Matsangas
Operations Research Department,
Naval Postgraduate School,
Monterey, USA

Sally Maynard
Transport Safety Research Centre,
Loughborough University,
Loughborough, UK

Walter T. McNicholas
Department of Respiratory and Sleep
Medicine, University College Dublin,
Dublin, Ireland

Ann Mills
Rail Safety and Standards Board,
London, UK

David Mohan
Transportation Safety Board of Canada,
Gatineau, Canada

Claudia R.C. Moreno
Department of Health, Life Cycles, and
Society, School of Public Health,
University of São Paulo, São Paulo,
Brazil and Stress Research Institute,
Psychology Department, Stockholm
University, Stockholm, Sweden

Emily M. Moslener
Sleep and Performance Research Center
& Department of Translational
Medicine and Physiology,
Washington State University,
Spokane, USA

Anjum Naweed
Appleton Institute for
Behavioural Science, Central
Queensland University, Wayville,
Australia

Matthew Nicholson
Operations Research Department, Naval
  Postgraduate School, Monterey, USA

Evita Papazikou
Transport Safety Research Centre,
  Loughborough University,
  Loughborough, UK

Ross O. Phillips
Norwegian Centre for Transport
  Research (TØI), Oslo, Norway

Fran Pilkington-Cheney
Psychology Department, School of
  Social Sciences, Nottingham Trent
  University, Nottingham, UK

Jana Price
National Transportation Safety Board,
  Washington, DC, USA

Claire Quigley
Transport Safety Research Centre,
  Loughborough University,
  Loughborough, UK

Arnaud Rabat
Armed Forces Biomedical Research
  Institute, Brétigny sur Orge, France

Amy C. Reynolds
Adelaide Institute for Sleep Health,
  Flinders University, Adelaide,
  Australia

Samantha M. Riedy
Walter Reed Army Institute of
  Research, Silver Spring, USA

Bart Roets
Faculty of Economics and Business
  Administration, Ghent University, and
  On Track Lab Research Centre and
  Performance Data Division, Infrabel
  Belgian Railways, Brussels, Belgium

Ari Rosberg
Transportation Safety Board of Canada,
  Gatineau, Canada

Mark R. Rosekind
Department of Health Policy and
  Management, Johns Hopkins
  University, Baltimore, USA

Christina M. Rudin-Brown
Human Factors North, Inc., Toronto,
  Canada and Transportation Safety
  Board of Canada, Gatineau,
  Canada

Mikael Sallinen
Finnish Institute of Occupational
  Health, Helsinki, Finland

Nita Lewis Shattuck
Operations Research Department,
  Naval Postgraduate School,
  Monterey, USA

Shamsi Shekari Soleimanloo
Institute for Social Science Research
  (ISSR), The University of
  Queensland, Brisbane, Australia

Simon Smith
Institute for Social Science Research
  (ISSR), The University of
  Queensland, Brisbane, Australia

Cynthia Spencer
Tram Operations Limited,
  Croydon, UK

Madeline Sprajcer
Appleton Institute, Central Queensland
  University, Wayville, Australia

Rachel Talbot
Transport Safety Research Centre,
  Loughborough University,
  Loughborough, UK

Yvonne Taylor
National Police Wellbeing Service,
    College of Policing, Ryton-on-
    Dunsmore, Warwickshire, UK

Pierre Thiffault
Transport Canada, Ottawa, Canada

Matthew J.W. Thomas
Appleton Institute, Central Queensland
    University, Wayville, Australia

Jackie Townsend
Tram Operations Limited, Croydon, UK

Melissa A. Ulhôa
Faculty of Medicine, Educational
    Union of Vale do Aço, Ipatinga,
    Brazil

Hans P.A. Van Dongen
Sleep and Performance Research Center
    & Department of Translational
    Medicine and Physiology,
    Washington State University,
    Spokane, USA

Ingrid van Schagen
SWOV Institute for Road Safety
    Research, The Hague,
    Netherlands

Lea Sophie Vink
Human Performance, Austro Control,
    Vienna, Austria

Andy Wallace
Tram Operations Limited,
    Croydon, UK

Patrick Warren
Metropolitan Transportation Authority,
    Brooklyn, USA

Jérôme Wertz
Tobii AB, Liège, Belgium

Ann Williamson
Transport and Road Safety (TARS)
    Research Group, UNSW, Sydney,
    Australia

Katherine Wilson
National Transportation Safety Board,
    Washington, DC, USA

Johanna Wörle
Würzburg Institute for Traffic Sciences
    (WIVW), Veitshöchheim, Germany

Mark Young
University of Southampton,
    Southampton, UK

Foreword

Fatigue comes in many forms, illustrated by its numerous synonyms as can be seen by simply consulting any thesaurus and, especially, Google. Interestingly, it is not a term one commonly uses for oneself, but rather, we personally use feelings such as "worn out", sleepy, tired, exhausted, or weary. Instead, it is usually the common term used by physicians, physiologists, psychologists, and occupational health investigators in their assessment of those under study. Hence "fatigue" has been a subject of numerous studies over the last hundred or so years, studies of which many were laboratory focused rather than of an occupational nature. Like those being conducted today, these past studies of fatigue have largely been linked to cognitive rather than to physical fatigue. Moreover, until the last 20 years or so, relatively few have been directed towards transport in its various forms, where fatigue is increasingly becoming a critical factor for our contemporary 24/7 society—hence, the need for this unique handbook on fatigue management in transportation-a major focus of which covers so many aspects of transportation.

With other wider aspects of tiredness-cum-sleepiness, this book considers the impact of fatigue not only on road and train drivers, pilots, seafarers, and machine operators, but also takes a much wider operational perspective applicable to managers and transportation overseers, including strategic approaches that can result in critical review of overall company transport policies. This handbook provides insights applicable and most useful to top managers as well as to those directly in actual control of their forms of transport. Neglect of this aspect can also result in considerable financial costs to organisations apart from the adverse impact on the health and well-being of the human operator, and to their families.

Despite claims and apparent alarms that, today, we live in a "sleepless society", this situation is probably no worse than it ever was (Horne, 2016) as sleep loss and even "fatigue from overwork" were then largely seen as merely the consequences of everyday working life. Fortunately, today, we have become much more enlightened and willing to address fatigue management, as can be seen in the following chapters.

Arguably, the most important aspect of fatigue, here, is sleeplessness, particularly when it leads to falling asleep during vehicle operation, which arguably causes most transportation deaths in the western world. For example, driving whilst sleepy on dull monotonous roads, in the early morning, at a time when one is normally asleep, is especially hazardous. Sleepiness within these conditions also has less obvious, much understated (neurocognitive) effects, as a driver or other vehicle operator can easily become more distracted from focusing on the road or task ahead, with unduly lengthy and dangerous distractions. Fatigued drivers in these conditions also often experience subtle mood changes, particularly in having greater optimism and the belief in being able to continue in this knowingly sleepy state (Horne, 2016).

These more subtle, neurocognitive effects of fatigue provide further illustration of how wider aspects of cognitive fatigue may well impact decisions made by transport managers, for example, when needing to focus on operator schedules. This would especially be the case when managers deal with unexpected events during adverse ongoing situations, avoiding irrelevant distractions (and maybe an unwitting, untimely adherence to company policy), and in so doing be less able to maintain a flexible approach and adopt a greater overview to such a challenging situation. Moreover, fatigue would make it challenging to be aware of one's potential for adverse "heightened emotionality", particularly under work pressures.

This impressive and unique *Handbook of Fatigue Management in Transportation: Waking Up to the Challenge* contains many novel aspects of fatigue in transportation and comprises a variety of comprehensive, up-to-date accounts by many renowned experts from different countries. The editors bring two complementary perspectives to the book. Dr Christina M. Rudin-Brown, an experienced transportation safety and human factors researcher and investigator, provides expert insight into operator behaviour, crash causation, and broader fatigue management perspectives. Ashleigh Filtness, Professor in Transport Human Factors and Sleep Science, has fundamental sleep science training and a human biology background, which she applies to the transportation context. Through their networks, they have brought together academic and industry thought leaders on fatigue management to produce this comprehensive text. In summary, the book's contents will provide for greater transport safety and the healthier well-being for those in the transport industry, and no doubt, financial savings of one sort or another for the organisations concerned.

Professor Jim Horne
Sleep Research
Loughborough University
UK

REFERENCE

Horne J. (2016). *Sleeplessness–assessing sleep need in society today.* Palgrave Macmillan.

Acknowledgements

The editors gratefully acknowledge the assistance and contribution of the following organisations and people:

- Loughborough University's Transport Safety Research Centre and School of Design and Creative Arts, for providing Professor Filtness the academic freedom to work on the handbook.
- The Transportation Safety Board of Canada (TSB), for giving Dr Rudin-Brown leave to work on the book in her spare time.
- Mr. Laurence Filtness for his creative ideas and talents in designing the book cover.
- Ms. Kirsty Hardwick and colleagues at Taylor & Francis, CRC Press, for their guidance and responsiveness throughout the book development process.
- Our families, for their words of encouragement and understanding despite the many hours we devoted to the book.

Christina M. Rudin-Brown has been a transportation safety and human factors enthusiast since 1999. She has investigated the existence, influence, and management of human fatigue in incidents and occurrences across all modes of transportation and taught modal accident investigators the principles of investigating for human fatigue since 2012. She has been a Senior Human Factors Investigator with the Transportation Safety Board of Canada (TSB) since joining the organisation in 2012 and, since 2017, has managed the TSB's Human Factors and Macro Analysis division. She is also a part-time consultant with Toronto-based human factors engineering company, Human Factors North, Inc.

Dr Rudin-Brown holds PhD and Master of Arts degrees in Experimental Psychology from the University of Toronto (Canada), a BA (Hons) in Psychology from the University of Ottawa (Canada), and was a past board member of the Canadian College for Certified Professional Ergonomists (CCCPE). She was previously a Senior Research Fellow with the Human Factors team at the Monash University Accident Research Centre (MUARC) in Melbourne (Australia; 2009–2012) and spent over 10 years prior to that as a Human Factors specialist with the Canadian federal department of transport's (Transport Canada's) Road Safety Directorate. Dr Rudin-Brown has published over 100 peer-reviewed papers across a number of transportation safety areas, including operator fatigue, behaviour and adaptation, driver speed choice, operator distraction, road infrastructure and rail level crossing safety, transportation safety policy, child and adult occupant protection, and operator impairment from drugs and alcohol. She is or has acted as an expert member of several international transportation working groups and safety committees, including those of the International Organisation for Standardisation (ISO) and the US Transportation Research Board (TRB). She is co-editor, with Dr. Samantha Jamson, of the book *Road Safety and Behavioural Adaptation: Theory, Evidence, and Action*, published by Taylor & Francis (CRC Press).

Ashleigh J. Filtness is a Professor of Transport Human Factors and Sleep Science at Loughborough University Transport Safety Research Centre (UK). She is fascinated by sleepiness and fatigue and their impact on safety, and has over 15 years' experience in transportation safety research. She is a Fellow of the Higher Education Academy (FHEA) and a Chartered Biologist (C.Biol). Over her career Professor Filtness has authored over 90 peer-reviewed publications and attracted research funding of more than £3.3 million from government, industry, and competitive grant schemes.

Professor Filtness holds a BSc (Hons) degree in Human Biology from Loughborough University. She was awarded her PhD from Loughborough University in 2011 for her thesis entitled "Obstructive Sleep Apnoea and Daytime Driver Sleepiness". Following the completion of her PhD, she moved to Australia where she worked first at Monash University Accident Research Centre (MUARC) from 2011 to 2013, and then at Queensland University of Technology, Centre for Accident Research and Road Safety–Queensland (CARRS-Q) from 2013 to 2016. Whilst at MUARC and CARRS-Q, Professor Filtness worked on a variety of road safety research projects funded by both industry and competitive grant schemes. She gained experience in a range of research methodologies extending her knowledge of driving simulators and developed expertise in various road safety topics, including driver sleepiness, systems thinking, driver distraction, situation awareness, alcohol impairment, the management of heavy vehicle drivers working hours, driver behaviour at rail level crossings, and hot air ballooning incident analysis.

Professor Filtness returned to Loughborough University as a Senior Research Associate working on the EU H2020 funded SafetyCube project from 2016 to 2018. Following completion of SafetyCube, she became a lecturer (2018–2020), then a senior lecturer (2020–2022), and finally a professor (2022–present). She currently leads a team of researchers across several projects seeking to better understand driver sleepiness, driver fatigue, and any aspects of impairment and safety. Details of her work are available at https://ashleighfiltness.net/.

Professor Filtness balances her busy part-time work schedule with being mum to daughter Elysia and son Xavier. She and her husband, Edd, enjoy walking and share a passion for hot air ballooning. Ashleigh is an advocate for transportation safety, women in academia, dyslexia awareness, and support for "first in family" to university.

Introduction

*Christina M. Rudin-Brown[1] and
Ashleigh J. Filtness[2]*

[1]Human Factors North, Inc., Toronto, Canada
[2]Loughborough University, Loughborough, UK

Fatigue is a normal physiological and behavioural state. It is a daily experience for all people. Normal fatigue lets us know that it is time to sleep—everybody sleeps; therefore, everyone gets sleepy. Fatigue in and of itself is not a safety concern—feeling tired while sat at home in a comfy armchair watching a favourite show is not likely to cause harm. However, for drivers, pilots, mariners, and other operators of the many vehicles within and across the transport sector, experiencing fatigue while operating a vehicle can have catastrophic consequences. And it is not only in operators that fatigue can increase the risk of an occurrence—for those who support transport operations, such as shift schedulers, supervisors, and managers, fatigue can also contribute to heightened, though less-direct, risk.

The role of normal fatigue is homeostatic in nature, reliably and rhythmically leading to periods of reduced alertness while optimising conditions for good-quality, restorative sleep. Fatigue becomes problematic when opportunities for good-quality sleep are limited, do not coincide with the homeostatic rhythm, or are not prioritised. Nowhere are these conditions more prevalent than in today's 24/7 transportation industries. While falling asleep at the controls is the most obvious symptom of fatigue in transportation operations, less extreme and apparent fatigue levels are reliably associated with performance impairments and are risk factors to occupational and transportation safety. Crash and incident statistics provide some evidence for these effects, yet because its symptoms are not always observable, fatigue is not always documented in crash databases, making the prevalence of fatigue in transportation difficult to estimate. Regardless, the US National Highway Traffic Safety Administration (NHTSA, undated) estimates that annually in the US about 100,000 police-reported crashes involve drivers who are experiencing fatigue. These crashes injure nearly 50,000 people and cause about 800 deaths. Fatigue is similarly involved in crashes and occurrences in other transport modes. Statistical research by the US National Transportation Safety Board (NTSB) (Marcus & Rosekind, 2017) has found that, on average, 20% of their air, rail, highway, and marine investigations cited fatigue as a probable cause, contributing factor, or finding.

Globally, transportation workers are concerned about these statistics and the health and safety consequences of fatigue (ITF, undated). Survey data have revealed that many transportation workers report not getting enough sleep because of their work schedules (NSF, 2012). In this National Sleep Foundation poll, compared to non-transportation workers, train operators and airline pilots were most likely to report sleep-related job performance problems. One in five pilots (20%) admitted that they have made a serious error and one in six train operators (18%) and truck drivers (14%) said that they have had a "near miss" due to sleepiness. The multi-continent 'E-Survey of Road users' Attitudes' (ESRA) reports that 20% of European, 22% of North American, 23.5% of Asian/Oceanian, and 24.5% of African drivers had driven at least once in the previous month while they were so sleepy that they had trouble keeping their eyes open (ESRA, undated).

As experienced transportation safety and human factors researchers, we the editors are similarly concerned with the impact of fatigue in transport and how to best address its management. Discussions over many years, first as colleagues at the Monash University Accident Research Centre (MUARC) in Australia, and later at various transportation safety and fatigue management conferences and symposia, inspired and motivated us to do something about what we consider to be a solvable problem. We wanted to do something that was both creative and practical, while at the same time something that was personally and professionally fulfilling. We knew that our collective networks of like-minded colleagues, who were similarly passionate about improving safety and the greater society, would make an edited book a feasible and attractive option.

Welcome to *The Handbook of Fatigue Management in Transportation: Waking Up to the Challenge*! This is the book that helps readers to "wake up to the challenge" of this highly dangerous and complex issue. The book considers all aspects of fatigue and fatigue management in transportation, bringing together a wealth of experience from thought leaders in transportation fatigue research and industry experts from around the world. The content covers road, rail, maritime, and aviation safety. While the book can be read as a whole, individual chapters in isolation can also help readers find and understand those aspects which are most relevant.

The book is timely because fatigue in transportation is an ever-emerging and evolving issue. The constantly increasing vehicle operation taking place, in developing and more developed nations alike, spurs and sustains an ongoing risk related to fatigue that at times appears to be—at least at the moment—tacitly accepted by our society. However, the greater the emergence and acceptance of a "24-h society", the greater the chance that vehicle operators in all modes of transport will control their vehicles during natural daily low points in alertness and following periods of inadequate sleep. Alongside this increase in fatigue risk, positive signs are emerging that we are or will be able to effectively mitigate and manage it. These include more and better research on the causes and consequences of fatigue and on what is most effective in terms of managing it and its associated challenges. We are also fortunate to be working at a time when more and more effective means of quickly and effectively communicating research results and strategies to mitigate fatigue are evolving. For example, internet and social media availability create a wider reach for those wishing to learn about fatigue and effect positive change. This convergence of research and communication acts as a catalyst for improvement. This book is intended to inspire and assist in this regard.

The problem of fatigue management in transport is not tackled in isolation; instead, the globally shared knowledge and lessons learnt make it relevant to all. Similarly, the benefits of fatigue management in transportation are not limited to safety and to those who directly operate within the transport system. Indirect benefits of fatigue management in transport range from improved physical and mental health of those who work in the transport domain, as well as of those who travel as paying passengers or who interact with commercial drivers as members of the road transport system, to more effective and efficient supply chains, more satisfied customers, a more positive corporate culture, and increased consumer trust.

This book brings together a broad range of chapter authors with diverse backgrounds, including researchers, practitioners, industry, policymakers, and administrators. All are active in their fields of research or industries and share a passion for fatigue management. Through the words of these world experts, the difficulties and challenges associated with fatigue and its management are described and analysed, while inspiration is offered on how to best effect change.

The book is divided into six sections, following a loosely historical order, beginning with a review of some of the more theoretical and historically challenging issues surrounding fatigue management in transportation. Section 1, 'Fatigue science and transportation', includes chapters focused on fatigue science, research, and evaluation, and on challenges faced by fatigue scientists and practitioners. For example, in Chapter 1.1, Thomas Balkin and colleagues Samantha Riedy, Arnaud Rabat, and Karl Friedl review the challenges associated with defining and measuring fatigue, and propose a definition that they believe is more concise and clear, and that does not conflate fatigue with the related construct of sleepiness. Chapter 1.2 sees Mikael Sallinen and Göran Kecklund contemplate the challenges associated with measuring fatigue and provide advice for how researchers can minimise potentially confounding variables and maximise analysis and interpretation of results. Then in Chapter 1.3, Anna Anund and Anna Sjörs Dahlman tackle the challenges that are common in fatigue research and evaluation and in efforts to enforce fatigue countermeasures. Matthew Thomas, Madeline Sprajcer, and Drew Dawson elaborate in Chapter 1.4 on the wide-ranging effects of fatigue, not only on operator performance, but also on neurobehavioural performance, higher order cognitive functioning, and shifts in psychosocial performance. Section 1 concludes with Chapter 1.5 by Ashleigh Filtness and Anna Anund, who describe a practical method to approach and evaluate an organisation's fatigue situation, understand problem areas, and propose countermeasures that are most likely to succeed.

Section 2, 'Fatigue-related consequences in transportation', provides content on the most objective, measurable consequences of—ineffectively managed—fatigue in transportation, that is, crashes and occurrences. Chapters in this section cover all modes of transport, including road (Chapter 2.1 by Charles Goldenbeld, Ingrid van Schagen, and Ragnhild Davidse), rail (Chapter 2.2 by Dan Basacik, Ann Mills, Mark Young, Ishbel Macgregor-Curtin, and Nora Balfe), marine (Chapter 2.3 by Nita Lewis Shattuck, Darian Lawrence-Sidebottom, Panagiotis Matsangas, and Matthew Nicholson), air (Chapter 2.4 by Katherine Wilson and Jana Price), and multi-modal (Chapter 2.5 by Christina Rudin-Brown, Geneviève Dubé, Michelle Gauthier, David

Mohan, and Ari Rosberg). Once they have digested these chapters, readers will, no doubt, be better placed to understand the sometimes subtle and unexpected effects of fatigue in their own transport industry or domain. In Chapter 2.6, Sarah Harris describes evidence suggesting the role of fatigue in an aspect of transportation that is not often considered: That of occurrence survivability. She concludes that integrating fatigue management with emergency management and increasing passenger awareness can help mitigate the risk of pre-emergency fatigue and improve the overall probability of survival during an emergency scenario. Rounding out the section is Chapter 2.7 on legal and regulatory frameworks for managing fatigue in transportation by Drew Dawson, Madeline Sprajcer, and Matthew Thomas. These authors describe changes that have happened in recent years, as well as future challenges that are likely in terms of the implementation of more flexible approaches to fatigue management.

It is the universal experience of fatigue that makes it an interesting and challenging area of focus. For example, in the workplace, it is a common though unusual risk factor because both work and home factors can contribute to fatigue. Section 3, 'Factors that contribute to fatigue and sleepiness in transportation', turns to identifying and describing these contributing and causal variables. In Chapter 3.1, Anastasi Kosmadopoulos provides a clear and concise explanation of the human circadian system and describes how disruption of sleep-wake and circadian regulatory processes can exacerbate the accumulation of fatigue and impair the quality of subsequent sleep. In Chapter 3.2, Cassie Hilditch and Dorothee Fischer provide a comprehensive explanation of the causes, consequences, and countermeasures for jet lag, sleep timing, and sleep inertia, and their effects on fatigue and related performance impairments. They conclude that, for each of these fatigue risks, strategic exposure to bright light can be used to help realign sleep timing and promote alertness. Chapter 3.3 by Walter McNicholas reviews the potential impact on driving of behavioural sleep disturbance, medical disorders associated with excessive daytime sleepiness, and insomnia, including management considerations. In Chapter 3.4, Ann Williamson describes the evidence showing that task-related factors alone, and not necessarily physiological factors, can cause problems of fatigue management and performance deterioration in transportation tasks. She explains how passive monitoring tasks that require sustained attention are common in transportation and should be of concern. Effective strategies to overcome task-related fatigue effects include providing breaks from the task and/or making the primary monitoring task more engaging and interesting. Finishing off Section 3 is Chapter 3.5 on the importance of lifestyle as a mediator of fatigue and sleepiness in those professionals working in the transportation sector. Melissa Ulhôa, Elaine Cristina Marqueze, and Claudia Moreno conclude that, while some lifestyle factors like mild physical activity and good nutrition can decrease fatigue, other factors—like tobacco and alcohol use and sleep problems—can exacerbate it, so understanding of these factors is important to manage fatigue symptoms effectively.

Once the contributing factors to fatigue are identified and explained, the question then is "how can these contributors to fatigue best be managed to reduce the associated risk?" Because fatigue has many contributing factors, and not all solutions will work for all people and situations, a multi-faceted approach to fatigue management is likely to be the most successful. Section 4, 'Managing fatigue and promoting alertness in transportation', showcases some of the latest developments and recent research in managing fatigue and promoting alertness in transportation, and aims to address the challenge of how to mitigate the effects of fatigue. Chapter 4.1 provides an overview of current key fatigue management strategies and gives insight into future novel options to manage fatigue. Authors Madeline Sprajcer, Matthew Thomas, and Drew Dawson describe traditional prescriptive and risk-based approaches to fatigue management and explain the more recent trend towards implementation of "hybrid" models. In Chapter 4.2, Clinton Marquardt explains why transportation shift workers tend to resist rules that dictate when they can work and when they can rest, and how fatigue managers can improve workers' acceptance of work and rest rules by building awareness about fatigue and sharing information about personal benefits that can result from better fatigue management. In Chapter 4.3, Steven Hursh and Jaime Devine discuss the history, implementation, limitations, and proper use of biomathematical models of fatigue for fatigue risk management in transportation, and conclude that these models are one technological tool to be used as part of a successful fatigue risk management system. The concept of "fatigue risk thresholds" is presented next in Chapter 4.4, wherein authors Emily Moslener, Hans Van Dongen, and Kimberly Honn provide guidance for establishing and applying fatigue risk thresholds in one's given domain. They conclude that, while the appropriate level for a fatigue risk threshold is context-dependent, comparison with pre-established standards, historical records, or previously collected evidence of acceptable risk levels under similar circumstances can provide a basis for setting a threshold level for a given transportation industry or domain. In a similar vein, in Chapter 4.5 Ross Phillips describes how established measures can be used to build so-called "fatigue profiles" allowing people operating different forms of vehicles and vessels in the road, rail, and sea transport sectors to be compared on the occurrence, causes, and effects of fatigue. Next, Chapter 4.6 examines the many challenges associated with the development, adoption, and use of fatigue detection technologies. Authors Clémentine François and Jérôme Wertz present a practical methodology to be used to assess the performance and reliability of fatigue detection technologies. In Chapter 4.7, Fran Pilkington-Cheney describes some individual countermeasures to fatigue for vehicle operators, and stresses that, before deciding on an appropriate countermeasure, it is vital to understand the cause of fatigue, be it sleep- and/or task-related. Chapter 4.8 by Shamsi Shekari Soleimanloo and Simon Smith presents the benefits of using bright light to improve alertness in vehicle operators, and concludes that large-scale naturalistic driving studies are required to validate the alerting effects of light in the real world and to explore its potential side effects like visual/eye discomfort and distraction. In Chapter 4.9, authors Anjum Naweed, Janine Chapman, and Amy Reynolds explain, using three key transport industries (rail, road, and maritime [reef tourism]), how fatigue in transportation is closely linked to health conditions and the poor health of drivers/vehicle operators. Torbjörn Åkerstedt and Mikael Sallinen then turn to flight time limitations and scheduling in airline pilots in Chapter 4.10, and explain how the results of a series of recent studies of long- and short-haul operations conclude that encroachment on the window of circadian low (WOCL; 0200-0559h) and early morning flights are key factors contributing to fatigue in this operational group. Finally in Chapter 4.11, Ashleigh Filtness, Sally Maynard, Rachel Talbot, Claire Quigley, and Evita Papazikou consider the important topic of fatigue among a group of at-risk drivers: Those who are young and novice. A practical method for how young novice drivers could best be engaged in a driver education programme on driver fatigue is described. Such a method, when implemented, would likely be brief, use a mix of theoretical and practical exercises/examples, and require repeat exposure to materials by participants.

Historically, one of the many barriers to effective fatigue management has been an unwillingness to discuss fatigue. This reluctance can be found with individual vehicle operators who are unwilling to admit to experiencing fatigue and companies that may overlook fatigue management because it is a difficult, almost impossible, task. This lack of dialogue limits learning from the shared experience of others, something this book tries to address by including a section (Section 5, 'Transportation fatigue risk management in practice') dedicated to personal experiences, or case studies, within workplaces of fatigue management approaches. Chapters in this section cover a range of industries and domains in transport. For example, Chapter 5.1 by Jackie Townsend, Cynthia Spencer, Andy Wallace, Bradley Jennings, and Ben Groome describes a real-world case study based on the experience of London's Tram Operations Limited (TOL) in implementing their fatigue management and wellness programme, which has received several rail industry awards. Chapter 5.2 by Bart Roets and Simon Folkard presents a real-world case study based on Belgium's railway traffic control centres, and describes the "Hourly Risk Index", a new risk-based model for the evaluation of staff rosters that is freely available now as an open-source package. Lessons learnt in implementing an obstructive sleep apnoea assessment programme in the US rail transportation industry are described in Chapter 5.3 by co-authors Daria Luisi, Tamara Dumanovsky, Laura Bienenfeld, Muataz Jaber, Nelson Gonzalez, and Patrick Warren, highlighting the areas that a federally mandated programme could address to ensure successful implementation across the industry. In Chapter 5.4, Michelle Grech provides an overview of work-related challenges that can lead to fatigue in seafarers engaged on international commercial ships, and introduces fatigue-related technologies that objectively predict or detect seafarer fatigue and the role these can play to support fatigue risk management systems at sea. Yvonne Taylor next applies her in-depth knowledge of the UK policing domain in Chapter 5.5 to review transportation-related challenges faced by this group. She explains how favourable shift patterns and fatigue risk management practices are likely to improve morale, welfare, and overall safety, including road safety, and will ultimately lead to better quality of service being delivered to the public. In Chapter 5.6, Pierre Thiffault introduces the notion of driver fatigue in the motor carrier industry and describes the Canadian federal transport regulator's efforts to address it through both prescriptive and non-prescriptive approaches. Chapter 5.7 by Lea Sophie Vink concludes the section with an interesting take on managing fatigue in the air traffic management (ATM) sector, and the benefits of using digital devices to off-set monotony, skill-fade and fatigue, and other means of combating prolonged periods of reduced workload. She concludes that, as systems become more automated and the job becomes more "monitoring" focused in future, ATM systems must keep operators engaged to reduce fatigue risk.

The problem of fatigue in transportation has existed for as long as transportation has existed. The basic biological human need for sleep and natural variation in alertness across the day have always been there. However, the transportation landscape is changing—for example, through automation—so it becomes vital to consider fatigue risk management of the future. Section 6, 'Fatigue risk management of the future', does just that. Chapters in this section include the current and future consequences of road vehicle automation, described in Chapter 6.1 by Christer Ahlström, Johanna Wörle, Mikael Ljung Aust, and Frederik Diederichs, as well as the current and more distant effects on fatigue of space transport and travel, described in Chapter 6.3 by Crystal Kirkley, Zachary Glaros, Nicholas Bathurst, Cassie Hilditch, and Erin Flynn-Evans. In Chapter 6.2, Anjum Naweed, Verna Blewett, Lily Hirsch, and Ashleigh Filtness describe an interesting and "cautionary tale" of a research exercise that began in 2013. Ten years on, this chapter revisits the results and explores how futures free of fatigue-related risk were envisioned at the time, the ways rail organisations believed this would be achieved, and whether their ideals matched a future that is all but realised. The section and the book finishes with hope and inspiration for the future of fatigue management, delivered by authors of Chapter 6.4, Mark Rosekind, Erin Flynn-Evans and Kevin Gregory. They explain that there is significant opportunity to improve on current fatigue risk management system approaches, and a need to expand fatigue management for all modes of transportation at the policy and societal levels. A roadmap of 16 specific opportunities and/or actions is proposed to improve future fatigue management by enhancing strategies, policies, and societal expectations.

In creating this book, we have come to recognise the importance of challenging beliefs and norms within ourselves, our society, and the workplace. What has become clear throughout the process is that one person's—or one organisation's—experience of fatigue is not necessarily the same as another's. Likewise, for any one individual, their experience of fatigue may vary from day to day. Recognising these differences is helpful when planning for fatigue risk management. What *is* universal is that the human brain needs sleep——when pushed to its limits the need to sleep is stronger than the will to stay awake. Therefore, a goal in fatigue management is to challenge. Challenge beliefs that the performance impairing effects of fatigue can be overcome. Challenge the acceptance that fatigue risk is normal and cannot be avoided. Challenge misunderstandings regarding the reciprocal relationship between fatigue and mental/physical health. Challenge the perception that fatigue is the responsibility of the vehicle operator, alone. We must accept the challenge that employers, policymakers, industry bodies, regulators, trainers/educators, vehicle manufacturers, and vehicle operators *all* have a role to play in reducing the risks of fatigue by each claiming responsibility for their own impact. As you embark on this challenge, we hope you find this Handbook useful and would love to hear about your experiences. Please get in touch with us at A.J.Filtness@lboro.ac.uk and crudinbrown@hfn.ca.

Compared to when they are tired, alert people are more attentive, react more quickly, are less distractible, make clearer decisions, take fewer risks, are less stressed and aggressive, and are healthier and happier—all of which can lead to safer transportation. Transportation safety has improved dramatically over the years; however, in recent times there has been a reduction in the rate of road safety improvement.

For example, the downward trend seen in the number of road traffic fatalities in the European Union between 2010 and 2020 was much more gradual than the downward trend between 2000 and 2010 (European Commission, 2021). While we should take inspiration from the progress made in other transportation safety-related areas (e.g., increased use of seat belts, decreased drinking and driving), now is the time to take action in terms of fatigue management. It is time to harvest the high-hanging fruit—the harder to address, more complex issues that need tackling. Fatigue management will never be easy, but it is a worthy endeavour that demands our attention. It is time to wake up to the challenge!

REFERENCES

ESRA (E-Survey of Road users' Attitudes) (undated). E-Survey of road users' attitudes. Accessed January 9, 2023. www.esranet.eu/en/.

European Commission (2021). 2021 road safety statistics: What is behind the figures? Accessed January 7, 2023. https://transport.ec.europa.eu/2021-road-safety-statistics-what-behind-figures_en.

ITF (International Transport Workers' Federation) (undated). Fatigue and road safety: Keeping road transport workers safe. Accessed December 31, 2022. www.itfglobal.org/en/sector/road-transport/fatigue-and-road-safety.

Marcus, J. H., & Rosekind, M. R. (2017). Fatigue in transportation: NTSB investigations and safety recommendations. *Injury Prevention*, *23*(4), 232–238.

NHTSA (National Highway Traffic Safety Administration) (undated). Drowsy driving. Accessed January 3, 2023. www.nhtsa.gov/risky-driving/drowsy-driving.

NSF (National Sleep Foundation) (2012). Sleepy pilots, train operators and drivers. *Science Daily* (March). Accessed 31 December 2022. www.sciencedaily.com/releases/2012/03/120304141858.htm.

Section 1

Fatigue Science and Transportation

1.1 Toward a More Precise Definition of Fatigue

*Thomas J. Balkin,[1] Samantha M. Riedy,[1]
Arnaud Rabat,[2] and Karl E. Friedl[3]*

[1]Walter Reed Army Institute of Research,
Silver Spring, MD, USA
[2]Institut de Recherche Biomédicale des Armées,
Brétigny-sur-Orge, France
[3]US Army Research Institute of Environmental
Medicine, Frederick, MD, USA

CONTENTS

There is no term in current scientific usage more in need of clarification than fatigue.

Bartley and Chute, 1945

1.1.1   INTRODUCTION

It is more than a little ironic that of the many disciplines that include the word "fatigue" in their lexicons (e.g., metallurgical engineering, medicine, and weight-lifting), the one most lacking a widely accepted, reasonably precise, and nominally coherent definition of this word is ours—the field of "fatigue risk management".

For anyone who even casually follows the scientific fatigue risk management literature, it is hard to miss the fact that inclusion of the word "fatigue" in the title of one of our published papers provides the potential reader with only the vaguest notion of what to expect in the ensuing text. Elucidation requires perusal of both the paper's Introduction (where we generally feel compelled to provide a working definition of

DOI: 10.1201/9781003213154-3

fatigue) and the Methods section (where the operationalisation of that working definition is described).

The decision by the editors of this book to lead with the present chapter constitutes an (at least implicit) acknowledgement that our field currently lacks a consistent, widely accepted definition of fatigue—a fact that has been pointed out repeatedly over many decades (e.g., see Bartley & Chute, 1945, 1947; Balkin & Wesensten, 2011; Hockey, 2013; and Pattyn et al., 2018). Mirroring what we do in our scientific papers, one goal of the present chapter is to provide the reader with an understanding of what is being described and discussed under the label of "fatigue" in the subsequent chapters of this volume.

In this chapter, the definitions of "fatigue" from Phillips (2015) and Gurubhagavatula et al. (2021) are analysed and discussed. Both definitions are broad and generally consistent with how we in the fatigue management field currently conceptualise "fatigue". They can therefore be considered an appropriate "anchor" for all of the chapters of the present volume. Indeed, their broadness constitutes a significant virtue: The definitions comfortably encompass the wide variety of factors that individually and collectively constitute threats to operational performance and safety. And for those of us familiar with the relevant scientific literature, they are also reassuringly familiar in terms of both their scope and particulars.

However, despite their consistency with current thinking, these types of definitions of "fatigue" are becoming increasingly problematic for the fatigue management field. This is because they include some logical incongruities and ambiguities that obfuscate the concept of fatigue and conflate it with "sleepiness" and, to a lesser extent, "alertness".

Lastly, an example of a more precise definition of fatigue—one that was developed in 2020 by North Atlantic Treaty Organization (NATO) working group *"Biomedical Bases of Mental Fatigue and Military Fatigue Countermeasures"*[1]—is presented and discussed in terms of its potential to clarify the concept of fatigue and to facilitate progress in our field because of its clarity, orthogonality from "sleepiness" and other related concepts, potential for generating testable hypotheses, and its straightforward relevance to both military and civilian operations.

1.1.2 DIFFERENTIATING FATIGUE FROM OTHER CONCEPTS

One effort to comprehensively define "fatigue" was produced by Phillips (2015), who performed an exhaustive review of the relevant literature and distilled his resulting insights into what he called a "whole definition" of fatigue:

Fatigue is a suboptimal psychophysiological condition caused by exertion. The degree and dimensional character of the condition depends on the form, dynamics and context of exertion. The context of exertion is described by the value and meaning of performance to the individual; rest and sleep history; circadian effects; psychosocial factors spanning work and home life; individual traits; diet; health, fitness and other individual states; and environmental conditions. The fatigue condition results in changes in strategies or resource use such that original levels of mental processing or physical activity are maintained or reduced.

This definition has three significant virtues: First, it emphasises the role of "exertion"—specifically, the idea that fatigue is always the result of some sort of effortful activity. Second, it characterises fatigue as a subjective experience with an underlying physiological basis. And third, it mostly avoids conflation with the concept of "sleepiness" (although "rest and sleep history" are lumped together in the long list of contextual factors that determine the "form, dynamics and context of exertion"). Together, these aspects of the definition make it potentially useful (e.g., testable and implementable) while maintaining its consistency with the broadly construed notions of fatigue as understood by both the professional and lay communities. However, the utility of this definition is, in the final analysis, vitiated by including that long list of contextual factors that ultimately determine how, and the extent to which, "exertion" is experienced and manifested. The useful precision that was potentially gained by defining "fatigue" as a state that arises solely from application of "exertion" is lost when the latter is conceptualised as a state that is influenced by such a wide and diverse variety of (sometimes nebulous and impossible to quantify) contextual factors (e.g., psychosocial states and traits, diet, and the physical environment). Thus, based on this definition, each time fatigue is experienced it is potentially a product of a completely unique combination of diverse and fluid factors. This makes the concept of "exertion" impossible to operationalise and study scientifically. To be clear, we are not suggesting that this conceptualisation of "exertion" is necessarily incorrect—only that it is not especially useful for informing the design of scientific studies of fatigue, nor, as a practical matter, for determining the appropriate countermeasures to apply in specific instances of fatigue in the operational environment (other than the obvious one of allowing operators to stop exerting themselves).

In a position paper authored by several luminaries in our field under the auspices of the American Academy of Sleep Medicine and Sleep Research Society, Gurubhagavatula et al. (2021) provided guiding principles for devising optimal work shift durations. Recognising that we in the fatigue management field often conflate the concepts of "fatigue" and "sleepiness", the authors begin with an attempt to deconflict these concepts by suggesting working definitions for three constructs: alertness, sleepiness, and fatigue:

(1) Alertness: The ability to direct and sustain attention, which is influenced by prior sleep and sleep loss, circadian rhythmicity, time on task (duration of continuous work), and other factors. Alertness manifests as the ability to maintain the attention necessary to perform a task at a specified level. Sleepiness is associated with reduced alertness.

Parts of this definition of alertness are concise, coherent, and useful, specifically: *"The ability to direct and sustain attention…"* and *"Alertness manifests as the ability to maintain the attention necessary to perform a task at a specified level"*. These statements can be operationalised in a straightforward way. However, this clarity and usefulness is undermined by the phrase *"…which is influenced by prior sleep and sleep loss, circadian rhythmicity, time on task (duration of continuous work), and other factors"*. This is because (a) the term "influenced by" is nebulous—suggesting a mediating effect of these factors without ruling out a cause–effect relationship; (b) the addition of *"and other* [unspecified] *factors"* to this list does

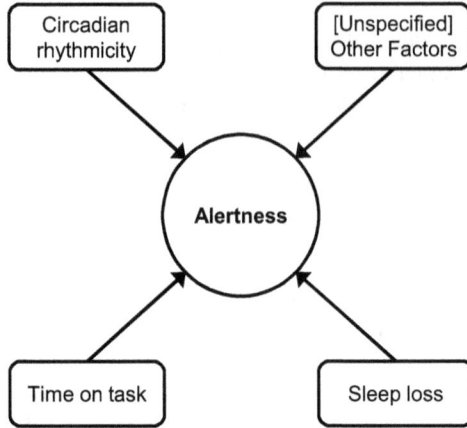

FIGURE 1.1.1 Factors that "influence" alertness according to the definition by Gurubhagavatula et al. (2021).

not increase clarity—in fact, it does the opposite (as described below); and (c) the statement that "*Sleepiness is associated with reduced alertness... .*" obscures the concept of "alertness" as they have described it, since the term "associated with" is so vague that it can mean anything from "causes" to "correlated with" to "antonymous with". See Figure 1.1.1 for a graphic representation of the concept of "alertness" as defined by Gurubhagavatula et al. (2021).

Similarly, Gurubhagavatula et al.'s (2021) definition of sleepiness is fairly standard, at least until the final sentence in which a relationship between sleepiness and fatigue is suggested:

> (2) Sleepiness: A state of increased tendency to fall sleep (sic), resulting from sleep loss or extended wakefulness, circadian rhythmicity, medications, or various sleep disorders. Sleepiness manifests objectively as an increased likelihood to fall asleep rapidly, and subjectively as an increased need or desire to sleep. Sleepiness is a contributor to mental fatigue.

It is not clear what is meant by "a contributor to" although this phrase is more suggestive of a cause–effect relationship than "associated with." See Figure 1.1.2 for a graphic representation of the concept of "sleepiness" as defined by Gurubhagavatula et al. (2021).

Lastly, Gurubhagavatula et al. (2021) provide the following working definition of fatigue:

> (3) Fatigue: A state of reduced mental or physical performance capability, resulting from sleep loss or extended wakefulness, circadian rhythmicity, workload, or other factors. As used in operational settings, fatigue manifests as performance impairment when engaging in a task. Mental fatigue implies decreased or degraded cognitive performance; physical fatigue implies decreased or degraded physical performance.

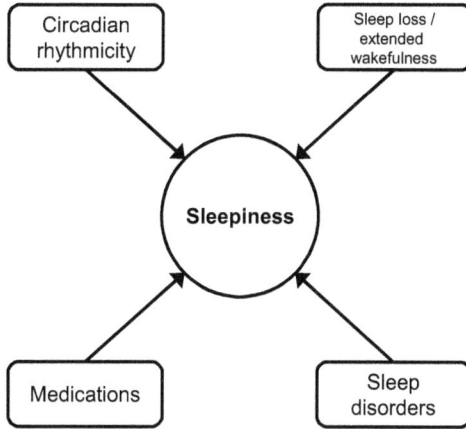

FIGURE 1.1.2 Factors that "result" in sleepiness according to the definition by Gurubhagavatula et al. (2021).

This definition of fatigue has two virtues: (a) It is largely consistent with the current conceptualisations of fatigue held by the scientific and professional communities as well as the lay public (i.e., it conveys the "general idea" of fatigue as it is widely understood). In fact, except for the addition of unspecified "other factors" as possible antecedent conditions, it closely adheres to the definition found in the fatigue management guidelines published by the International Civil Aviation Organisation (ICAO) in which fatigue results from "sleep loss or extended wakefulness, circadian phase, or workload (mental and/or physical activity)". And (b) it is broad enough to encompass whatever variations in the definition may be employed by most individuals or subgroups within the scientific, professional, and lay communities.

However, this definition also has some weaknesses: (a) it is actually so broad and imprecise that its utility as an explanation for observed behaviour—much less its utility for identifying an appropriate "fatigue"' countermeasure in an operational setting—is vitiated. If fatigue results from *"sleep loss or extended wakefulness, circadian rhythmicity, workload, or other factors"*, then labelling a worker as "fatigued" is essentially equivalent to labelling that worker as "potentially impaired for several possible and unspecified reasons". This is, in part, because appending *"... or other* [unspecified] *factors"* onto the list of antecedent conditions opens up such a wide universe of possibilities that the nature of any specific instance of fatigue becomes opaque.

And, because sleep loss and circadian rhythmicity are included in the short list of antecedent conditions for each construct, the distinction among alertness [*"The ability to direct and sustain attention"*], sleepiness [*"A state of increased tendency to fall sleep (sic)"*], and fatigue [*"A state of reduced mental or physical performance capability"*] is significantly diminished. See Figure 1.1.3 for a graphic representation of the antecedent conditions for alertness, sleepiness, and fatigue as defined by Gurubhagavatula et al. (2021).

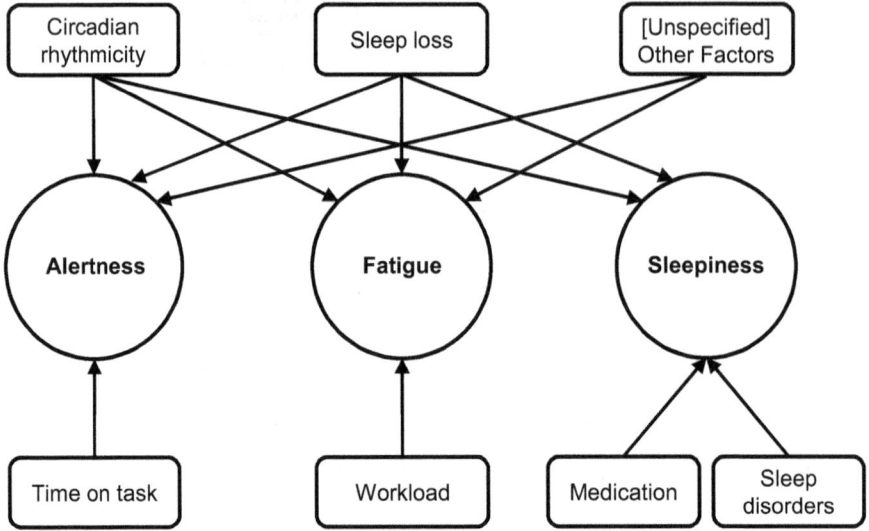

FIGURE 1.1.3 Overlap of factors that are antecedents to alertness, fatigue, and sleepiness according to the definitions by Gurubhagavatula et al. (2021).

By providing working definitions of alertness, sleepiness, and fatigue, Gurubhagavatula et al. (2021) were clearly attempting to delineate these concepts in a meaningful and useful way. However, as illustrated in Figure 1.1.3, the demarcations between the three concepts become indistinct (and, it is here argued, problematic) when overlapping antecedent conditions are included in their definitions. To help understand why this is a problem, it is useful to harken back to the classic paper by MacCorquodale and Meehl (1948).

1.1.3 HYPOTHETICAL CONSTRUCTS AND INTERVENING VARIABLES

In their classic paper, "On a distinction between hypothetical constructs and intervening variables", MacCorquodale and Meehl (1948) suggest that there are two ways to conceptualise the unseen but hypothesised "entities, processes, or events" that help describe and explain observed behaviours.

As they conceived of it, a *hypothetical construct* is something that cannot be seen or measured directly, but which is conjectured to exist, and is invoked to explain observable behaviour. Hypothetical constructs have broad ("surplus") meaning that cannot be derived by combining *"the variables that underlie the concept"* (Doleys, 2017). In other words, hypothetical constructs are broad, gestalt-like concepts with meanings that are not derived from antecedent conditions in any straightforward manner.

In sharp contrast, an *intervening variable* is a concept that is "systematically defined in terms of its antecedents and is dependent upon these [antecedents] for its meaning" (Doleys, 2017). Thus, intervening variables constitute an efficient way of abstracting empirical, cause–effect relationships but, unlike hypothetical constructs, they lack emergent meaning that extends beyond those specified relationships.

Gurubhagavatula et al. (2021) clearly sought to disentangle and deconflict the concepts of fatigue, alertness, and sleepiness for the operational community. However, it appears that their effort was tempered by a parallel (and understandable) desire to do so in a way that does not render the concept of "fatigue" unrecognisable to those members of both the general public and the professional community who use it as a synonym for "sleepiness". In short, it appears that they undertook the tricky task of orthogonalising the definitions of "fatigue" and "sleepiness" without explicitly rejecting the notion that these two words are at least partly synonymous.

They did this by providing a very broad definition of fatigue, starting with the words, *"A state of reduced mental or physical performance capability... ."* In the parlance of MacCorquodale and Meehl (1948), this initial portion of the definition is hypothetical construct-like. But they also include in their definition a partial list of antecedent conditions: *"... .sleep loss or extended wakefulness, circadian rhythmicity, workload..."* that makes the definition more intervening variable-like. (Remember that intervening variables are defined by their cause–effect relationships). Then, however, a semblance of a hypothetical construct-like broadness was restored by ending the list of antecedents with *"...or other* [unspecified] *factors."* Likewise, the definition of alertness is structured as an intervening variable except for the inclusion of *"...and other* [unspecified] *factors"* in the list of antecedent conditions.

In contrast, sleepiness is more strictly conceptualised by Gurubhagavatula et al. (2021) as what MacCorquodale and Meehl (1948) would call an intervening variable. To wit, sleepiness is conceptualised as an easily quantifiable construct ("tendency to fall asleep") with a non-infinite list of antecedent conditions (*"...sleep loss or extended wakefulness, circadian rhythmicity, medications, or various sleep disorders"*).

Although Gurubhagavatula et al. (2021) do not employ the terminology of MaCorquodale and Meehl (1948), it appears that their intention was to broadly frame "fatigue" (reduced performance capability) as a hypothetical construct that subsumes the more narrowly defined intervening variables of "sleepiness" (tendency to fall asleep) and "alertness" (the ability to direct and sustain attention). This is not illogical: it makes sense that an increased tendency to fall asleep and/or an inability to attend to a task would be antithetical to performance of that task. However, specifying in its definition that *"sleep loss"* and *"circadian rhythmicity"* are antecedent conditions of fatigue as well as sleepiness and alertness does more to obscure any intended distinctions among these concepts than it does to distinguish them. This is because (a) including antecedent conditions in the definition of "fatigue" undermines its utility as an over-arching hypothetical construct. Indeed, it is likely that it was, at least partly, recognition of this fact that prompted MacCorquodale and Meehl (1948) to write their classic paper in which they differentiate, and explain the logical need for differentiating, hypothetical constructs from intervening variables. And (b) overlap in the lists of antecedent conditions included across the definitions of "fatigue", "sleepiness", and "alertness" (as depicted in Figure 1.1.3) blurs the distinctions among these concepts and legitimises (in fact, reinforces) the practice of using these words interchangeably.

1.1.4   SO WHAT?

How important is it to our scientific and professional community to have a clear defin-ition of fatigue that is orthogonal to the definitions of sleepiness and alertness? Some might argue that the answer to this question is "not very". And again, the paper by Gurubhagavatula et al. (2021) can be used to illustrate the point. The express purpose of that paper was to provide "guiding principles" for devising shift durations in oper-ational environments. Nine such "guiding principles" are described, based on consid-erations such as workload, commute time, spacing of breaks, workers' chronotypes, the circadian phase(s) during which shifts occur and the "impact of the shift on workers' ability to obtain adequate sleep between shifts". The guiding principles effectively and accurately reflect and summarise much of the current knowledge on work shift schedules. They are thoughtful and evidence-based and, to the extent that they are followed by industry, can help optimise the productivity, safety, and well-being of workers. So, from an industry standpoint (i.e., those concerned about the performance and safety of their employees), the utilitarian value of these guiding principles is not diminished by the non-orthogonality of the definitions of "sleepi-ness", "alertness", and "fatigue". In fact, these definitions probably could have been omitted from the paper without impacting its practical utility in the least.

1.1.5   SO, WHY BOTHER TIGHTENING UP THE DEFINITION OF FATIGUE?

The answer is, in part, that our lack of a clear definition of fatigue, and especially one that is orthogonal to the definition of sleepiness, hinders scientific progress. It is becoming increasingly clear that the physiological basis of sleep loss-induced per-formance deficits does not overlap completely with the physiological basis of time-on-task-induced performance deficits. For example, Quiquempoix et al. (2022) recently showed that although a moderate dose of caffeine was effective for improving some aspects of performance (i.e., sustained attention) in human subjects during 27 hours of continuous wakefulness, it had no beneficial effect on the rate at which performance (both for sustained attention and executive processes) declined as a function of time-on-task (TOT). From an operational standpoint, this finding has clear implications for predicting the duration of beneficial caffeine effects on the performance of operators. From a scientific standpoint, it indicates that the search for an effective TOT counter-measure is unlikely to involve the adenosinergic receptor system.

A clear, concise, agreed-upon definition of fatigue—e.g., one in which task diffi-culty and TOT are recognised as the cause of fatigue—would facilitate our collective ability to conduct research and make discoveries that have the potential to advance the field of fatigue management on an accelerated timeline. For example, determining the biological basis of fatigue could revolutionise the practice of fatigue management, potentially resulting in development of fieldable fatigue biomarkers (which could be implemented as fitness-for-duty tests before and/or during work shifts), identifica-tion of individual differences in fatiguability as a stable, and possibly heritable, trait (which could be used to individualise work shift parameters and/or inform decisions regarding the administration of fatigue-specific countermeasures on an individual basis) or even guide development of interventions that prophylactically prevent accrual of fatigue for use in operational environments (e.g., during military combat operations or emergency operations following natural disasters). However, the speed with which these and other fatigue management-relevant basic and applied scientific accomplishments can be achieved depends on the extent to which researchers share a common definition of fatigue from which testable hypotheses can be generated. And the faster that such discoveries are made, the faster they can and will be implemented to improve performance and safety in operational settings.

Although efforts have been undertaken to determine and characterise the physiological basis of fatigue (e.g., see Meeusen et al., 2021, who suggest that fatigue is a specific brain state that is determined, at least in part, by alterations in adenosinergic and dopaminergic neurotransmission in anterior cortical brain regions), such efforts, by necessity, reflect relatively narrow operational definitions of "fatigue" (e.g., "time on task" *or* "sleep loss" *or* "circadian desynchrony" *or* "workload"). Of course, it is hypothetically possible to conduct a series of studies in which the neurophysiological effects of each of the specific antecedent conditions listed by Gurubhagavatula et al. (2021) (see Figure 1.1.3) is assessed individually. This would allow identification of any neurophysiological changes common to each which would suggest, albeit not unequivocally, a neurophysiological basis of broadly defined fatigue. However, inclusion of unspecified "other" antecedent conditions in this definition effectively precludes even this difficult approach. Clearly, it will not be possible to design scientific studies aimed at determining the biological basis of fatigue until we settle upon a conceptualisation of fatigue that is orthogonal to sleepiness and alertness, and for which the list of antecedents is finite and clearly delimited.

1.1.6 THE NATO DEFINITION OF FATIGUE

The NATO working group HFM-331 *"Biomedical Bases of Mental Fatigue and Military Fatigue Countermeasures"* was formed in 2020 to address the question of how best to sustain military operational performance. Naturally, the first order of business for this group (of which three of the current authors—TB, AR, and KF—are members) was to determine the scope of effort—i.e., to produce a working definition of "fatigue". After extensive discussion (also within a previous Exploratory Team in 2019) and more than a little debate, the group's consensus was that fatigue would be defined as *"a psychobiological state induced by prolonged exertion that has the potential to reduce performance."*

First, it should be noted that the NATO definition is not inconsistent with those provided by Gurubhagavatula et al. (2021) and Phillips (2015), except that it is narrower and thus clearer. As many have repeatedly suggested or implied in the past, fatigue can be usefully conceptualised as an intervening variable that results exclusively from continuous performance on a task (e.g., see Gergelyfi et al., 2021; Blain et al., 2016; Hockey, 2013; Boksem & Tops, 2008; Van Cutsem et al., 2017; and Meeusen et al., 2021). The definition focuses on aspects of military and civilian operational environments that, by any definition, can produce a state of fatigue: task difficulty and time on task. This definition does not suggest that performance is *not* decremented by additional factors such as sleep loss, illness, circadian desynchrony, mental and/or physical load, etc. But it does imply that such factors do not directly produce (or constitute) fatigue, *per se*. Rather, they are conceptualised as *mediators and/or additional factors* that interact with and/or accelerate, rather than actually cause, fatigue (e.g., see Balkin & Wesensten, 2011; Muck et al., 2020).

In the NATO definition, fatigue is also characterised as *"psychobiological"*—a subjective state that has a physiological basis. Although the physiological underpinnings of the psychobiological state described by the NATO definition have not been determined definitively, studies showing changes in brain activity that track TOT effects resulting from performance of a demanding cognitive task (e.g., Gergelyfi et al., 2021; Kamzanova et al., 2020; Lim et al., 2010; Boksem & Tops, 2008) indicate that a unique neurophysiological basis to the subjective/objective experience of fatigue exists—and this state can be induced in the absence of sleep loss, circadian desynchrony, etc.

Another important aspect of the NATO definition is that it specifically defines fatigue as a state that has the *"potential"* to reduce performance. In this respect, it is consistent with several prior conceptualisations of fatigue by the scientific community (e.g., Gergelyfi et al., 2021; Blain et al., 2016; Hockey, 2013; Boksem & Tops, 2008; Van Cutsem et al., 2017; Meeusen et al., 2021), and with current usage by the lay public—i.e., as a subjective state in which performance deficits can be avoided, at least temporarily, by exerting increased effort. This is consistent with several previously proposed models of fatigue, including one proposed by Hockey (2013), depicted in Figure 1.1.4. This "Motivational control model of executive control, effort and fatigue" in which attainment of (or a decision to modify) performance goals is determined by the operator's motivation level relative to his/her ongoing assessment of the costs and benefits of applying increasing effort to sustain performance as fatigue accrues over time. Specifically, in this model, effort is expended (either mental or

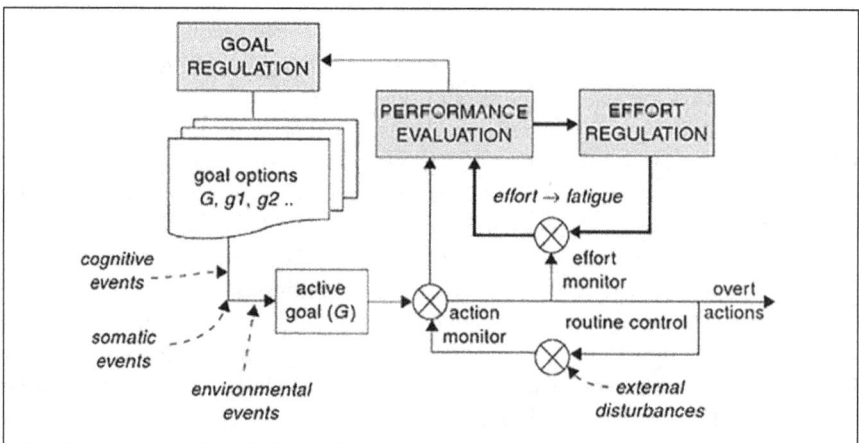

FIGURE 1.1.4 Robert Hockey's (2013) "Motivational control model of executive control, effort and fatigue". Reprinted with permission.

physical work) to achieve a specific goal (G). An "action monitor" tracks the actions being applied toward achievement of the goal, and an "effort monitor" tracks the amount of effort being expended to perform those actions. At the "performance evaluation" node, an assessment is made regarding the likelihood that the current actions will result in attainment of the desired goal. Fatigue accrues with TOT, so the "effort regulation" node, based on input from the "performance evaluation" node, increases effort as fatigue accrues in order to maintain nominally adequate progress toward achievement of the goal. As fatigue continues to accrue, the "goal regulation" node weighs options to determine whether continued action toward achievement of the original goal is worth the increased effort, or if an alternative, more easily achieved goal should be substituted for the original goal.

1.1.7 CONCLUSIONS

Although it can be argued that up to this point our field has managed to survive, and even thrive, despite our fuzzy and occasionally disparate conceptualisations of "fatigue" (and perhaps, in some instances *because* of this fuzziness), the premise of the present chapter is twofold: (a) that the field of fatigue management currently lacks a reasonably specific and coherent definition of "fatigue" and (b) that we stand to gain more than we would lose by adopting a definition of fatigue that more narrowly, concisely, and coherently reflects the unique goals of the fatigue management community: Enhancement and sustainment of performance and safety in operational environments.

What would we gain? First, the adoption of a more coherent definition would facilitate scientific discoveries that could be rapidly translated into the field. Advancements might include, for example, discovery of the physiological basis of operationally relevant mental fatigue and subsequent development of individualised countermeasures, improved fitness-for-duty tests, and advanced fatigue monitoring technologies. Such advancements are currently hindered, if not precluded, by the fuzziness of current conceptualisations of fatigue. (For example, it would be difficult to design a functional brain imaging study of fatigue using "*a state of reduced mental or physical performance capability, resulting from sleep loss or extended wakefulness, circadian rhythmicity, workload, or other factors*" as the definition.) Second, it would help to appropriately characterise the profession of "fatigue management" as a specialty that subsumes "sleep management" rather than one that is conflated with it.

What would be lost are whatever benefits accrue to our discipline by virtue of its indistinctness and conflation with other fields (especially the field of sleep management). To the extent that fatigue is defined broadly and vaguely, and to the extent that this definition suggests multiple (if not limitless) antecedent causal factors, then so is the range of potential opportunities for both fatigue management practitioners and scientists seemingly broadened. However, this broadness is a double-edged sword: We, as a discipline, risk becoming increasingly viewed as the proverbial "*jack of all trades, master of none*", while specialists in allied disciplines encroach upon these opportunities. One example of this is the birth (at least within the United States [US]) of commercial entities that, for a fee, provide seminars and training on "sleep health" to employees of private firms and government. Of course, such information can be useful to employees. But the impact of such programmes appears to be modest (Redeker et al., 2019)—an outcome that would likely be improved if this information was presented within the context of (i.e., as a component of) a comprehensive fatigue management system.

It is suggested that meaningful progress in the field of fatigue management will increasingly depend upon development and wide acceptance within our community of a clearer definition of fatigue—one that conceptualises it as an operationally relevant and unique psychobiological state that is clearly differentiated from other psychobiological states like "sleepiness" and "circadian desynchrony" (which would more usefully be considered mediators, rather than components, of fatigue).

This is more easily said than done. There currently exists no single entity that exerts enough authority and influence over the scientific and professional fatigue management communities to decide upon and declare an official definition of fatigue. It is more likely that a more coherent definition of fatigue will evolve via the incremental accrual of scientific advancements and publications in which the advantages of such conceptualisations become increasingly apparent.

SUMMARY POINTS FOR PRACTITIONERS

- Current conceptualisations of fatigue tend to be nebulous and confusing, primarily because they frequently blur and conflate the concepts of "fatigue" and "sleepiness". The scientific and professional fatigue management communities would benefit from adoption of a clear, operationally relevant definition of "fatigue" that does not overlap with that of "sleepiness", and that facilitates the generation of testable hypotheses.
- As an example, the definition of fatigue devised by a NATO research group, "a psychobiological state induced by prolonged exertion that has the potential to reduce performance", has distinct advantages over current broader definitions. (Prolonged exertion is defined as the application of effortful, goal-directed behaviour over time.)
- The NATO definition improves clarity (it is simple and concise) and specificity (fatigue arises as a function of task difficulty and TOT). It also tacitly relegates factors such as "sleep loss" and "circadian desynchrony" to the status of "moderating variables" while elevating the status of "fatigue" to that of a distinct, meaningful, central determinant of operational performance and safety.
- Without a more coherent, precise, and widely accepted definition of fatigue, recognition of "fatigue management" as a legitimate, distinct scientific and professional entity is in danger of eroding.

ACKNOWLEDGEMENTS

This material has been reviewed by the Walter Reed Army Institute of Research, and there is no objection to its presentation and/or publication. The opinions or assertions contained herein are the private views of the authors and are not to be construed as official or as reflecting the position of the US Department of the Army or the Department of Defense.

NOTE

1   All conceptualisations of fatigue include, either explicitly or implicitly, a "mental" component because fatigue is ultimately a subjective state that reflects extant mental activity. The title of NATO working group HFM-331 was selected to make it clear that its focus is on the fatigue that results solely from exertion of mental effort.

REFERENCES

Balkin, T. J., & Wesensten, N. J. (2011). Differentiation of sleepiness and mental fatigue effects. In P. L. Ackerman (Ed.), *Cognitive fatigue: Multidisciplinary perspectives on current research and future applications* (pp. 47–66). American Psychological Association. https://doi.org/10.1037/12343-002

Bartley, S. H., & Chute, E. (1945). A preliminary clarification of the concept of fatigue. *Psychological Review, 52*(3), 169–174. https://doi.org/10.1037/h0059244

Bartley, S. H., & Chute, E. (1947). *Fatigue and impairment in man.* McGraw-Hill Book Company. https://doi.org/10.1037/11772-000

Blain, B., Hollard, G., & Pessiglione, M. (2016). Neural mechanisms underlying the impact of daylong cognitive work on economic decisions. *Proceedings of the National Academy of Sciences of the United States of America, 113*(25), 6967–6972. https://doi.org/10.1073/pnas.1520527113

Boksem, M. A., & Tops, M. (2008). Mental fatigue: Costs and benefits. *Brain Research Reviews, 59*(1), 125–139. https://doi.org/10.1016/j.brainresrev.2008.07.001

Doleys, D. M. (2017). Chronic pain as a hypothetical construct: A practical and philosophical consideration. *Frontiers in Psychology, 8,* 664. https://doi.org/10.3389/fpsyg.2017.00664

Gergelyfi, M., Sanz-Arigita, E. J., Solopchuk, O., Dricot, L., Jacob, B., & Zénon, A. (2021). Mental fatigue correlates with depression of task-related network and augmented DMN activity but spares the reward circuit. *Neuroimage, 243,* 118532. https://doi.org/10.1016/j.neuroimage.2021.118532

Gurubhagavatula, I., Barger, L. K., Barnes, C. M., Basner, M., Boivin, D. B., Dawson, D., Drake, C. L., Flynn-Evans, E. E., Mysliwiec, V., Patterson, P. D., Reid, K. J., Samuels, C., Shattuck, N. L., Kazmi, U., Carandang, G., Heald, J. L., & Van Dongen, H. P. A. (2021). Guiding principles for determining work shift duration and addressing the effects of work shift duration on performance, safety, and health: Guidance from the American Academy of Sleep Medicine and the Sleep Research Society. *Journal of Clinical Sleep Medicine: Official publication of the American Academy of Sleep Medicine,* 10.5664/jcsm.9512. Advance online publication. https://doi.org/10.5664/jcsm.9512

Hockey, R. (2013). *The psychology of fatigue: Work, effort and control.* Cambridge: Cambridge University Press. https://doi.org/10.1017/CBO9781139015394

International Civil Aviation Organisation. (2015). *Fatigue management guide for airline operators, 2nd edition.* Montreal, Canada: International Civil Aviation Organisation. www.icao.int/safety/fatiguemanagement/FRMS%20Tools/FMG%20for%20Airline%20Operators%202nd%20Ed%20(Final)%20EN.pdf

Kamzanova, A., Matthews, G., & Kustubayeva, A. (2020). EEG coherence metrics for vigilance: Sensitivity to workload, time-on-task, and individual differences. *Applied Psychophysiology and Biofeedback, 45*(3), 183–194. https://doi.org/10.1007/s10484-020-09461-4

Lim, J., Wu, W. C., Wang, J., Detre, J. A., Dinges, D. F., & Rao, H. (2010). Imaging brain fatigue from sustained mental workload: An ASL perfusion study of the time-on-task effect. *Neuroimage, 49*(4), 3426–3435. https://doi.org/10.1016/j.neuroimage.2009.11.020

MacCorquodale, K., & Meehl, P. E. (1948). On a distinction between hypothetical constructs and intervening variables. *Psychological Review, 55*(2), 95–107. https://doi.org/10.1037/h0056029

Meeusen, R., Van Cutsem, J., & Roelands, B. (2021). Endurance exercise-induced and mental fatigue and the brain. *Experimental Physiology, 106*(12), 2294–2298. https://doi.org/10.1113/EP088186

Muck, R. A., Van Dongen, H. P. A., Schmidt, M. A., Wisor, J. P., Layton, M. E., DePriest, D. M., Honn, K. A., & Satterfield, B. C. (2020). *DRD2* C957T genotype modulates the time-on-task effect during total sleep deprivation. *Chronobiology International, 37*(9–10), 1457–1460. https://doi.org/10.1080/07420528.2020.1804925

Pattyn, N., Van Cutsem, J., Dessy, E., & Mairesse, O. (2018). Bridging exercise science, cognitive psychology, and medical practice: Is "cognitive fatigue" a remake of "the emperor's new clothes"?. *Frontiers in Psychology, 9*, 1246. https://doi.org/10.3389/fpsyg.2018.01246

Phillips, R. O. (2015). A review of definitions of fatigue—And a step towards a whole definition. *Transportation Research Part F: Traffic Psychology and Behaviour, 29*, 48–56. https://doi.org/10.1016/j.trf.2015.01.003

Quiquempoix, M., Sauvet, F., Erblang, M., Van Beers, P., Guillard, M., Drogou, C., Trignol, A., Vergez, A., Léger, D., Chennaoui, M., Gomez-Merino, D., & Rabat, A. (2022). Effects of caffeine intake on cognitive performance related to total sleep deprivation and time on task: A randomized cross-over double-blind study. *Nature and Science of Sleep, 14*, 457–473. https://doi.org/10.2147/NSS.S342922

Redeker, N. S., Caruso, C. C., Hashmi, S. D, Mullington, J. M., Grandner, M., & Morgenthaler, T. I. (2019). Workplace interventions to promote sleep health and an alert, healthy workforce. *Journal of Clinical Sleep Medicine: JCSM: Official Publication of the American Academy of Sleep Medicine, 15*(4), 649–657. https://doi.org/10.5664/jcsm.7734

Van Cutsem, J., Marcora, S., De Pauw, K., Bailey, S., Meeusen, R., & Roelands, B. (2017). The effects of mental fatigue on physical performance: A systematic review. *Sports Medicine (Auckland, N.Z.), 47*(8), 1569–1588. https://doi.org/10.1007/s40279-016-0672-0

1.2 Measuring Operator Fatigue and Sleepiness

Mikael Sallinen[1] and Göran Kecklund[2]

[1]Finnish Institute of Occupational Health,
Helsinki, Finland
[2]Stockholm University, Stockholm, Sweden

CONTENTS

1.2.1   WHY MEASUREMENT OF FATIGUE IN TRANSPORT IS IMPORTANT

Vehicle operator fatigue is a largely acknowledged safety hazard in all transport modes (Sallinen & Hublin, 2015) and thus, measuring this hazard has been the focus of numerous studies (Dawson et al., 2014). This chapter especially addresses the practical aspects of measuring operator fatigue, such as why and how to measure it and what to take into account when interpreting the results. In addition, a few examples of measuring operator fatigue in various transport modes are given to concretise the topic.

The main idea behind measuring operator fatigue is to be able to quantify the hazard. This kind of data can be used in at least three ways to promote safety in transport. First, it provides an avenue for researchers to acquire generalisable knowledge of conditions and factors that affect operator fatigue. This knowledge can be used to develop, for example, duty and rest time regulations and rules at a societal and company level. Second, operator fatigue may be collected at a company level for an overall risk assessment. This kind of company-specific data makes it possible to take into account just those conditions and factors that are typical of the operators of that company. Third, operator fatigue may be measured at the individual level to identify and treat clinically significant impairments in fatigue.

Risk assessment at the company level includes many components under which data on operator fatigue can be utilised, such as identification of hazards and risks

DOI: 10.1201/9781003213154-4

- principles and goals
- organisational structures
- roles and responsibilities
- processes

- hazard recognition
- risk analysis
- risk assessment
- risk mitigation

FRMS policy and documentation

FR management

FRM assurance

FRM promotion

- inspections and auditions
- case investigations
- fatigue reporting
- fatigue data collection and analyses

- safety culture
- education
- communication

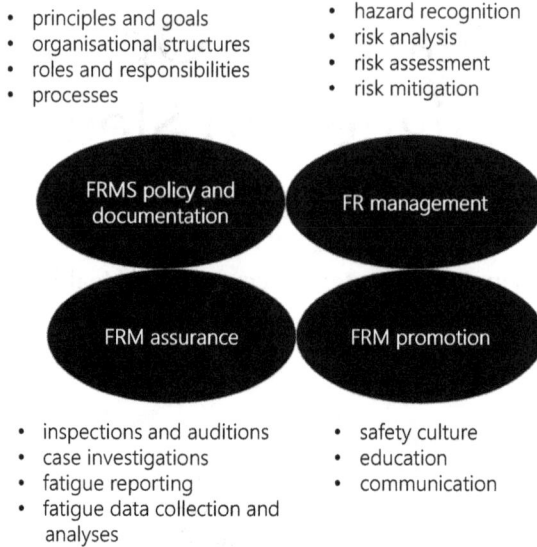

FIGURE 1.2.1 Components of fatigue risk management systems (FRMS) in civil aviation (adapted from IATA, ICAO, IFALPA, 2011; 2015).

related to operator fatigue, controlling the identified risks, and monitoring these risks in the long run. Figure 1.2.1 shows an example of the components of fatigue risk management in aviation. Of these components, data on operator fatigue can be utilised when (i) managing risks associated with fatigue, (ii) assuring the fatigue risk management system, and (iii) promoting safety through, for example, training and communication. Figure 1.2.2 shows measures a company may take to mitigate operator fatigue. As can be seen, fitness-for-duty monitoring (number 9) and identification of fatigue symptoms (number 10)—the areas where measurement of operator fatigue happens—are mentioned as ways to prevent on-duty fatigue and related errors from occurring.

A pitfall of measuring operator fatigue is to consider this step as a sufficient measure to manage related risks. For this reason, it is of utmost importance to first have a comprehensive risk assessment model in which the measurement component can be embedded. Measuring fatigue without the proper utilisation of the collected data may even demotivate operators to consider fatigue as a safety hazard and make them less likely to report it when they otherwise would, thereby negating any potential safety benefit of reporting.

In addition to the safety aspect, the proper utilisation of data on operator fatigue may promote operators health in the long run, especially if the utilisation leads to better sleep and recovery. This is a significantly less considered topic than safety-related questions, but based on population studies, shortened sleep increases a person's chance of getting a chronic disease (Itani et al., 2017).

In all, measuring operator fatigue provides at best a solid basis to assess the related risks and effectively mitigate them, whereas, at worst, it may demotivate operators

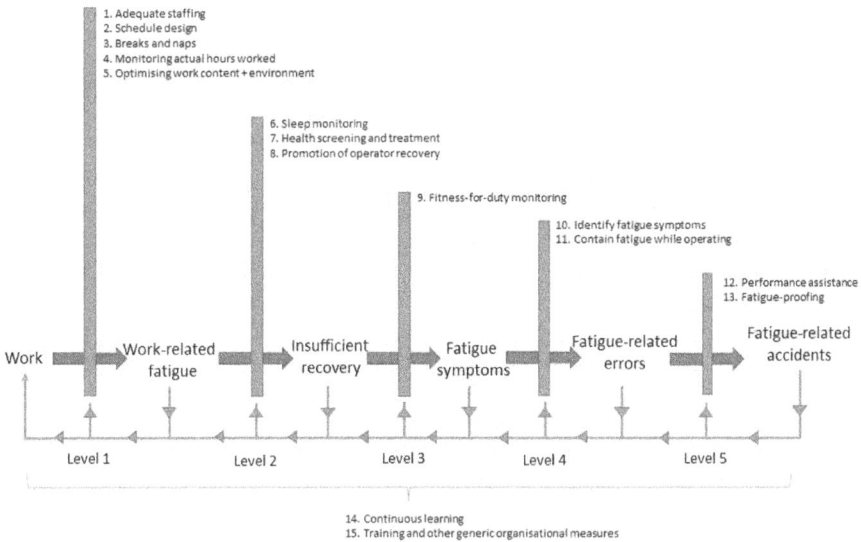

FIGURE 1.2.2 Measures to mitigate risks associated with driver fatigue within a company fatigue risk management system (FRMS) (reproduced from Phillips (2016), with permission).

from actively collaborating with the employer to tackle this safety issue. Which of these options is realised depends largely on how well cooperation from fatigue reporting to fatigue management efforts works between all parties involved.

1.2.2 HOW VEHICLE OPERATOR FATIGUE CAN BE MEASURED

There are many methods to measure vehicle operator fatigue. Generally, it is recommended that more than one method is used for this purpose. This recommendation is based on the multidimensionality of fatigue itself. Fatigue can manifest itself on a mental, physical/physiological, and on a performance level. It is also important to note that there is no method, yet, to measure fatigue directly and comprehensively. In other words, all measures, independent of the method, provide us with only an indirect estimation of fatigue.

The methods developed to measure vehicle operator fatigue can be divided into physiological (e.g., brain activity such as brief intrusions of sleep into wakefulness present in the electroencephalography (EEG) and ocular measures such as blink duration), performance (vigilance, driving performance), behavioural ones (overt behaviour), and self-reports (Sparrow et al., 2019). To be able to select adequate methods for one's own purposes, it is also important to consider the setting (context), operator target group, and purpose of measurements. An attempt to categorise the methods based on these factors is presented in Table 1.2.1.

The measurement of operator fatigue in the workplace is usually conducted to assess how fatiguing certain shifts and combinations thereof are. There are multiple methodological choices for this purpose. A common prerequisite for obtaining valid data is a "just/open culture"—"the way we do things around here" to maximise safety—as most of the feasible methods rely on vehicle operators self-reporting. Examples of such methods are fatigue reporting forms (for an example, see IATA, ICAO, IFALPA, 2015) and shift-specific questionnaires (e.g., Bergen Shift Work Questionnaire by Flo et al. 2012). For the latter, one may also use well-validated fatigue scales developed for field settings, such as the Karolinska Sleepiness Scale (KSS) (Åkerstedt et al., 2014) and the Samn–Perelli Fatigue Scale (SPS) (Samn & Perelli, 1982). These scales can be completed by an operator either retrospectively after vehicle operation has finished or while "sitting behind the wheel" (i.e., during vehicle operation).

Operator fatigue can also be estimated by collecting data on vehicle movements, such as accelerations, decelerations, lane position, and speed (Stern et al., 2019). This kind of data collection technique is most advanced for road transportation. It requires instrumentation of vehicles with suitable technology and makes it possible to objectively evaluate, for example, driving style in general and even more importantly the occurrence of safety-critical events. Of course, it is important to bear in mind that both driving style and safety-critical events may be explained by reasons other than driver fatigue. Thus, there is a need for combining this kind of data with data that more directly measure fatigue. In addition to the above-mentioned self-reporting methods, one may use, for example, bio-mathematical models of fatigue for this purpose.

At the core of bio-mathematical models of fatigue is an algorithm through which imported data—usually working hour and sleep-wake data—are processed (Civil Aviation Safety Authority, 2014; Dawson et al., 2011). The algorithm is usually validated against empirical data at least to some extent and uses the components of either the two- or three-process model of alertness as its determinants. The processes are: (1) time since awakening (homeostatic process/sleep pressure), (2) time of day (circadian process), and—for the three-process model—sleep inertia (waking process) (for more on bio-mathematical models of fatigue, see Chapter 4.3 and for more information about the two process model, see Chapter 3.1). Some models also include job characteristics, such as rest breaks and the level and nature of activity required, among the determinants. The so-called one-step models require both actual working hours and sleep-wake data to be imported, whereas the so-called two-step models require only the former because they predict sleep periods based on the imported working hours (step 1) and only then predict fatigue (step 2). To employ a model appropriately, it is important to understand its limitations. Typically, these models do not, for example, (a) incorporate inter-individual variability in fatigue, (b) take into account the psychological and social determinants of sleep-wake behaviours, or (c) convert the predicted fatigue levels into a risk of human error or of a safety incident (Dawson et al., 2011). Neither of these models is suitable for predicting fatigue for an individual vehicle operator.

In the laboratory setting, fatigue is usually measured to identify clinically significant fatigue on an individual level. Examples of measures developed for this purpose are the Multiple Sleep Latency Test, the Maintenance of Wakefulness Test, and the Oxford Sleep Resistance Test (Penzel et al., 2019; Huang et al., 2020). In the laboratory setting, methods are also used to identify possible sleep disorders, such as obstructive sleep apnoea, shift work disorder, and primary insomnia. Examples of such methods are the Epworth Sleepiness Scale (ESS) (Johns, 1991), the Stop Bang Questionnaire (Chung et al., 2016), and polysomnography.

A laboratory examination may also include a vehicle simulator study and a field study (see Table 1.2.1). The latter can be conducted under either completely naturalistic or somewhat controlled conditions, such as using conditions designed to compare differences between shifts of standard and extended duration in operator fatigue during the day and at night. In both, the measurement of fatigue covers operator-related data such as fatigue self-ratings and vehicle-related data, including, for example, lane drifting. In fact, the same rule of measurement applies to the measurement of fatigue in the workplace, the main difference lying in the precision with which fatigue can be measured.

In summary, before measuring vehicle operator fatigue, it is essential to crystallise the main purpose for collecting data and the target group of operators, and to select the data collection methods accordingly. Usually, it is recommended to use more than one method of data collection to get a reliable overall picture of operator fatigue. To estimate the risks related to operator fatigue, it is important to measure not just operators themselves but to also measure vehicle dynamics. When interpretating the results, it is important to bear in mind both the strengths and weaknesses of each data collection method (see below sub-section 1.2.3). Finally, it is essential to develop and maintain a "just/open" safety culture and especially the no-punitive aspect of it to be able to reliably measure operator fatigue. Almost all related measurement methods are, at least to some extent, susceptible to distortion and thus the results may easily be skewed towards the desired goal if all parties do not share the same aim of managing operator fatigue as effectively as possible.

1.2.3 MOST COMMONLY USED SUBJECTIVE FATIGUE RATING SCALES

A recent paper systematically reviewed the literature to examine whether drivers are aware of their level of fatigue while driving (Cai et al., 2021). The systematic review identified 34 studies, of which 32 (94%) utilised the KSS. The KSS is a nine-point Likert-type scale, ranging from 1 = "extremely alert" to 9 = "very sleepy, great effort to keep awake, fighting sleep" (Åkerstedt et al, 2014). A KSS rating of 6 ("some signs of sleepiness") or higher represents increased levels of fatigue; however, severe consequences in terms of driving impairment are usually not observed until KSS rating of 8 ("sleepy, some effort to keep awake").

The KSS is a measure of state-related, or situational, fatigue and the operator is asked to rate the level of fatigue they experienced during the previous 5-minute period. The reason for the retrospective 5-minute approach is to avoid the situation where the act of asking about sleepiness itself inadvertently acts as an alertness-increasing event and reduces KSS scores.

During a normal (not longer than 8 to 9 hours) night drive, a driver's KSS rating often starts at step 3 or 4 and ends at step 6 or 7 (Åkerstedt et al., 2014). If driving duration exceeds 9 hours, higher KSS ratings (7 or 8) can be found at the end of the drive. However, vulnerable drivers may have KSS ratings of 8 and sometimes even 9 at the end of a night drive even if driving duration is not extended (Åkerstedt et al., 2014). Validation studies have shown that the KSS is as sensitive an indicator of fatigue as are objective measures like long eye closure and prolonged reaction times measured with the Psychomotor Vigilance

TABLE 1.2.1

Categorisation of Methods to Measure Operator Fatigue

Setting	Target Group	Purpose	Method Categories	Examples of Methods/Measures
Company	All/selected group of operators	To assess fatigue-related risks at a company/group level	a) Subjective reports b) In-vehicle data recorders c) Bio-mathematical modelling of fatigue	a) Fatigue reporting forms, shift-specific questionnaires, fatigue scales b) Lane position, speed, accelerations, decelerations c) FAID, BAM, CAS, SAFTE, SWP
Lab/clinic	Operators with suspected excessive fatigue	To make a clinical examination on work ability at an individual level	a) Clinical interview b) Clinical questionnaires c) Sleep recording d) Lab-based fatigue tests	a) Structured Clinical Interview for Diagnosis of Sleep Disorders (SCIDS) b) ESS, Fatigue Severity Scale, STOP Bang, Berlin Questionnaire c) Sleep diary, PSG (at lab/home) d) MSLT, MWT, Osler
Lab/clinic + field study	Operator with suspected excessive fatigue	To make a clinical examination on work ability at an individual level	a) Sleep measurement b) Self-rating scales c) Performance tests d) Driver behaviour e) In-vehicle data recorders	a) Sleep diary, activity monitor b) KSS, SPS c) PVT d) ORD (video data) e) Lane position, speed, accelerations, decelerations
Lab/clinic + vehicle simulator	Operators with suspected excessive fatigue	To make a clinical examination on work ability at an individual level	a) Operator-related methods b) In-vehicle data recorders	a) Physiology (EEG, EOG, HRV), self-ratings (KSS, SPS), behaviour (eye closures, limb movements, steering wheel movements) b) lane position, accelerations, decelerations, speed

FAID—the Fatigue Assessment Tool by InterDynamics; BAM—the Boeing Alertness Model; CAS—The Circadian Alertness Simulator; SAFTE—Sleep, Activity, Fatigue, and Task Effectiveness; SWP—the Sleep Wake Predictor; ESS—the Epworth Sleepiness Scale; PSG—polysomnography; MSLT—Multiple Sleep Latency Test; MWT—Maintenance of Wakefulness Test; OSLER—Oxford Sleep Resistance Test; KSS—the Karolinska Sleepiness Scale; SPS—the Samn-Perelli Fatigue Scale; PVT—the Psychomotor Vigilance Task; ORD—the Observer Rating of Drowsiness; EEG—electroencephalography; EOG—electrooculography; HRV—heart rate variability.

Task (PVT), a reaction time task where participants are required to press a button in response to a stimuli presented on a screen as soon as it is observed (Åkerstedt et al., 2014). Therefore, KSS is particularly useful for naturalistic driving studies, where drivers rate their fatigue at pre-determined times and/or locations (Hallvig et al., 2014). The review by Cai et al. (2021) showed that the KSS—and subjective ratings of fatigue in general—was more strongly correlated with physiological markers of sleepiness, such as long eye blink duration and increased alpha and theta EEG activity (micro-sleep episodes), than were driving outcomes. Still, subjective fatigue ratings do predict driving impairment; for example, lane variability and crash events (Cai et al., 2021). Yet, the correlations with objective measures of fatigue were stronger in driving simulator studies than in naturalistic studies, indicating that the measurement situation needs to be well-controlled (e.g., exclude the influence of workload and other factors that may influence the fatigue level) to obtain accurate associations between objective and subjective markers of fatigue.

It should be emphasised that the correlations between subjective and objective measures of fatigue can become weaker if one takes individual differences into account. For instance, a study by Ingre et al. (2006a) showed large differences among drivers, in terms of overall driving performance and blink duration, that were independent of subjective fatigue level.

Other subjective instruments measuring situational fatigue that were identified in the systematic review were the Stanford Sleepiness Scale (SSS), the Samn–Perelli Checklist, and the Likelihood of Falling Asleep (LFA) scale. However, only a handful of driving studies used these instruments, although it should be stressed that the SSS is widely used in experimental sleep research, and the Samn–Perelli checklist is common in studies of fatigue in aviation (Gawron, 2016).

The most common rating scale that measures trait-like fatigue (related to excessive daytime sleepiness) in relation to driving is the ESS. The ESS is a global measure of sleepiness (or sleep-related fatigue complaints) based on eight common situations in most people's life, such as watching television and "in a car, while stopped for a few minutes in the traffic" (Johns, 1991). Each situation is rated on a four-grade scale, ranging from 0 "would never doze" to 3 "high chance of dozing". The ESS score varies from 0 to 24, with 10 or higher representing critical fatigue. Validation studies of the ESS have shown mixed findings (see Johns, 1998; Chervin, 2000) and several studies have failed to observe significant correlations between EES score and crash involvement (Connor et al. 2002; Drake et al. 2010). These findings suggest that situational sleepiness may be a better predictor of crash events than trait-like measures of sleepiness, such as the ESS.

The benefits of using subjective rating instruments to measure vehicle operator fatigue include that they are easy to use and are low-cost, and often the only feasible alternative for monitoring fatigue in naturalistic situations. Operators' awareness of fatigue is also important by itself, as lack of awareness may indicate that the consequences of fatigue risks are not fully understood.

The most important limitations associated with subjective fatigue measures are a driver's desires to please or their opinions about the topic being investigated, and their expectations or mindset regarding the study topic, both can lead to biased fatigue reports, resulting in either underestimation or overestimation of the "true" fatigue level (Åkerstedt et al., 2014; Gawron, 2016). Another limitation is that it may not always be possible to collect frequent reports of situational fatigue in naturalistic studies. To only collect ratings at the beginning and at the end of a work period (or drive) may not always capture sufficiently representative assessments of drivers' fatigue level. One should also be aware that other driver states, for example, acute stress, can mask the underlying fatigue level. Finally, it is a much-debated question whether all drivers can accurately rate their own level of fatigue, making this method less than ideal and illustrating the importance of using multiple measures of fatigue data collection wherever possible.

To sum up, subjective rating scales such as the KSS represent a reliable and accurate method to monitor and collect driver fatigue data, but precision will improve if other, more objective, indicators of fatigue, such as those related to driver physiology and driving performance, are also collected simultaneously.

1.2.4   EXAMPLES OF MEASURING FATIGUE IN TRANSPORTION

In field settings, self-rating scales and short performance tasks are often sufficient to measure operator fatigue. In addition, bio-mathematical models of fatigue can be used as a kind of objective reference, or validity check, for self-rating scales and short performance tasks.

There are some key guidelines for how to use self-ratings and task performance in field settings. First, it is good to have more than one measurement point per duty period. A minimum is to measure fatigue at the beginning and end of the duty period but preferably also, for example, in the beginning and end of each rest break or at certain critical phases, such as in phases of flight in air transport. Second, it is recommended to apply more than one measurement method to get a reliable picture of the situation. Third, it is important to have a sufficient number of vehicle operators (e.g., 10 at a minimum) and data points per condition. Fourth, it is good to include a control (i.e., well-rested) condition and to have the same drivers measured in both (i.e., a repeated measures study design). Following these guidelines will make it easier to interpret obtained results and to draw valid conclusions from them. Below are some examples of field studies conducted by the authors that were based on these four guidelines.

1.2.4.1   Examples of Field Studies

We have conducted a series of three field studies to examine on-duty fatigue in long-haul truck drivers (Pylkkönen et al., 2015), commercial airline pilots (Sallinen et al., 2017), and tram drivers (Onninen et al., 2020). The set of measurements used in these studies consisted of self-rated fatigue using the KSS, predicted fatigue using the Sleep-Wake Predictor (SWP), and actual sleep using a sleep diary and a wrist-worn activity monitor. All SWP results are based on importing the measured work shift and sleep-wake data of each participant into the model. In addition, airline pilots' performance-based fatigue was measured by the PVT. In all of these studies, the

TABLE 1.2.2

Mean Self-ratings and Mean SWP Fatigue Model Predictions on the KSS in Three Field Studies on Long-Haul Airline Pilots (Example 1), Long-Haul Truck Drivers (Example 2), and Tram Drivers (Example 3)

	Duty Start		Duty Middle		Duty End	
	Self-rating	Prediction	Self-rating	Prediction	Self-rating	Prediction
Example 1						
Non-night flights	3.1	4.1	4.3	4.3	4.2	5.4
Night flights	4.1	4.8	5.7	6.0	5.3	7.0
Example 2						
Non-night trips	3.0	4.4	3.2	4.5	3.8	5.3
Night trips	3.3	4.6	4.5	5.8	5.0	7.1
Example 3						
Morning shifts	4.0	5.0	4.2	4.9	4.2	4.8
Evening shifts	2.8	4.0	3.5	4.4	4.6	5.9

measurement period per participant was quite long, varying from 2 weeks (truck drivers) to 2 months (airline pilots).

Example 1

Table 1.2.2 shows the mean KSS ratings of long-haul airline pilots and the corresponding SWP predictions for the beginning, middle and end of non-night and night flights. The self-ratings were, on average, 0.8 to 0.9 units lower than the SWP predictions. In addition, the two data collection methods agreed that the highest level of fatigue was reached during night-time flights but disagreed on the flight phase where this peak in fatigue occurred. The discrepancy is probably due to a so-called masking effect, meaning that the heightened workload and activity needed by pilots during the landing phase of flight masks the pilots' perception of fatigue accumulated in the body (so-called latent fatigue). Less work-related activity is required while cruising and, thus, the accumulated physiological fatigue may surface, making pilots rate themselves as more fatigued during this phase.

Example 2

Table 1.2.2 shows the mean KSS ratings of long-haul truck drivers and the corresponding SWP predictions for the beginning, middle, and end of non-night and night trips. Both the self-ratings and the predictions showed an increasing trend toward the end of the trip, independent of trip type. In addition, the predictions consistently showed higher fatigue levels than the self-ratings during both trip types (1.3 to 2.1 KSS unit difference, depending on the phase and type of the trip). As with the airline pilot data, the masking effect may at least partly explain this finding, in that fatigue self-ratings may be attenuated by high workload that is experienced during the work shift. However, it is also possible that the truck drivers simply underestimated their fatigue levels. This is suggested by a rather large and consistent difference between the self-ratings and the predictions, despite the fact that driving on highways is usually rather monotonous, making it more likely for the accumulated physiological fatigue to manifest itself in self-ratings.

Example 3

Table 1.2.2 shows the mean KSS ratings of tram drivers and the corresponding SWP predictions for the beginning, middle, and end of morning and evening shifts. Again, the predicted levels were higher than the self-rated ones (morning shift: 0.8 KSS units; evening shift: 1.3 KSS units). However, both methods show the highest level of fatigue at the end of the evening shift, which can be explained by the fatiguing effects of both the homeostatic and circadian processes. Outside Table 1.2.2, it can be mentioned that the self-ratings showed small but quite consistent beneficial effects of rest breaks on fatigue (morning shift: 0.8 KSS units; evening shift: 0.4 KSS units), whereas the predicted results showed no such benefit.

Example 4

Figure 1.2.3 shows airline pilots' self-rated fatigue (KSS) and PVT perform-ance during Helsinki–New York evening outbound flights and, after two local nights, during New York–Helsinki night-time inbound flights. The measure-ment points were (a) the top of climb (point at which cruising altitude has been reached after takeoff) and (b) the top of descent (point at which the descent to final approach altitude is initiated). As with the previous examples, the self-ratings showed higher fatigue levels for the night-time shift than for the non-night-time one. In addition, there seemed to be a trend of increasing self-rated fatigue towards the end of flight regardless of the time of day. Interestingly, the results did not show an impairment in PVT performance during the night-time inbound flights as compared to the non-night-time outbound flights. This some-what unexpected result may be due to the relatively short duration of the task (5 min) and/or situational factors that may have interfered with the pilots' ability to stay focused on task performance.

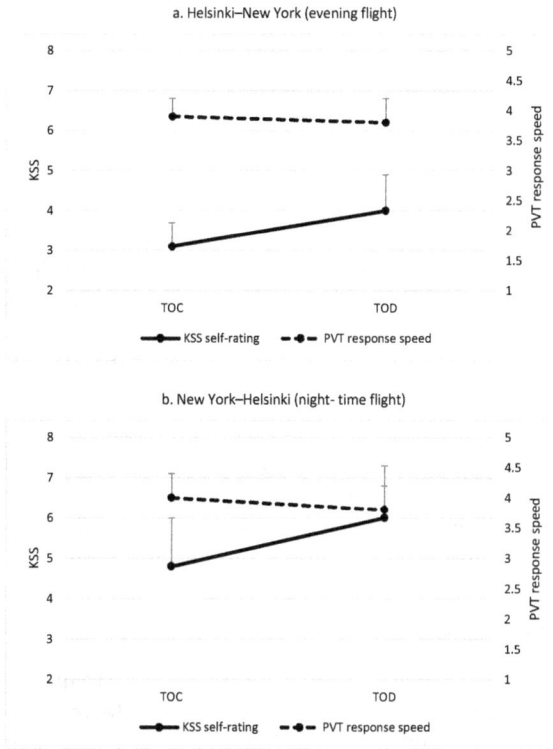

FIGURE 1.2.3 Self-rated (mean KSS score, solid line) and PVT performance (mean response speed (1/response time (ms) x 1000), dotted line) defined fatigue among civil airline pilots during (a) Helsinki–New York outbound flight (start time 13:00h, end time 23:40h in Helsinki time) and (b) New York–Helsinki inbound flight after two local nights (start time 23:30h and end time 09:30h in Helsinki time). N= 29. Unpublished data.

1.2.5 KNOWLEDGE GAPS

When applying methods to measure operator fatigue, it is important to be aware of some gaps in our current knowledge. One of these gaps is related to the level at which self-rated fatigue can be said to be accompanied by microsleeps and near-crash events in real-world settings. In addition to the level of fatigue, we also need to know more about the association between the accumulated time with fatigue and crash risk. Is it possible to have a moderate level of fatigue, such as KSS 6, for a long time and still maintain safe driving performance? There is convincing evidence that subjective fatigue scales are associated with physiological signs of fatigue and sleepiness, and with driving impairment such as lane departures. Thus, it seems fair to conclude that vehicle operators are aware of on-the-job fatigue. However, the correlations are stronger in driving simulator studies than under actual driving conditions (Cai et al., 2021). The level of both subjective and objective fatigue indicators is usually lower in field studies than in simulator studies, and is normally lower during alert (e.g., daytime), as opposed to during sleep-deprived (e.g., night-time), driving (Hallvig et al., 2013). There are a few well-controlled field studies showing that, despite the generally low subjective fatigue level in real-life driving, the association of these ratings with impaired driving performance is statistically significant (Hallvig et al., 2014). Nevertheless, the relationship between indicators of fatigue and their association with driving impairment is complex, especially in real-world settings. Further research is needed on this topic.

Another important knowledge gap is individual differences in operator fatigue. On a group level, subjective ratings, physiological indicators, and behavioural measures of fatigue often show substantial correlations; however, it is much more difficult to make precise predictions on the individual level. For example, the propensity of poor driving performance is much higher in some drivers despite not showing severe fatigue levels (Ingre et al., 2006b). Thus, more research is needed on determinants of between-driver individual (trait) differences (e.g., age, sex, health, personality traits related to tolerance of insufficient sleep, and extended time awake) and within-individual (state) differences (e.g., day-to-day variations in sleep quality, sleep duration, workload, mood, and time urgency) in driver fatigue and the associated driving impairment.

1.2.6 CONCLUSIONS

Before starting to measure operator fatigue, it is important to understand the setting (context), the operator target group, and the purpose of the measurement. It is also equally important to have a plan for how the collected data will be utilised. Also, in order to obtain as "truthful" results as possible, it is important to invest in the development and maintenance of a "just/open" safety culture in the workplace. For the measurement of vehicle operator fatigue, this means, among other things, open communication about the measurements themselves and their purpose. In the long run, it is also essential that employees are aware of how the results of the measurements are and will be utilised.

With regard to the methodological aspects, there is a large variety of methods for measurement of fatigue in transport, ranging from questionnaire-based instruments, to rating scales of situational fatigue, standardised tests such as the MSLT, and monitoring of physiological, behavioural, and vehicle motion indicators. In real-world settings, measurement of electrophysiological indicators and eye movements can be challenging, and the recorded data normally need a lot of processing. This is a costly measurement approach that may only be feasible in research studies, wherein the aim is to gain detailed knowledge of fatigue process itself and its determinants.

Another disadvantage with physiological and driving performance-based fatigue indicators is that they are relative. Hence, it is difficult to conclude if an operator is experiencing high fatigue levels without comparing the data with data collected during a period of alert working for the same individual. Thus, the optimal method for measurement of fatigue in transport operations seems to be self-rating scales such as the KSS. The KSS measures situational fatigue, is easy to use, and is a low-cost method, and available data suggests that the ratings can predict objective fatigue indicators, including impaired driving such as lane departures. Furthermore, operators' awareness of fatigue is often a key parameter in fatigue risk management and, compared with other methods, subjective ratings can provide relatively robust information of the absolute level of fatigue. It should be stressed, though, that subjective rating instruments such as the KSS also have methodological limitations and the raters' expectations and mindset may sometimes lead to biased reports. For this reason, it is worth considering also collecting objective data, for example, that which is based on bio-mathematical modelling. Finally, it is essential to understand the strengths and limitations of the different methods. The importance of this caveat is emphasised, especially when selecting methods and when interpreting the obtained results.

SUMMARY POINTS FOR PRACTITIONERS

- To benefit from measuring vehicle operator fatigue, it is important to have a clear plan and framework for how the collected data will be used.
- For a transport company to obtain reliable data from their employees, it is essential to first develop and maintain a safety culture where reporting on fatigue is considered as safety-promoting activity and thus encouraged.
- To select adequate methods, it is crucial to carefully consider the setting (context), target group, and purpose of measurements.
- To correctly interpret the results obtained, it is good to know the strengths and limitations of the methods used.
- For now, methods based on self-reporting seem to be the first choice to measure fatigue in real-world settings. It is important to bear in mind that there is no single method to collect data relating to all dimensions of fatigue.

REFERENCES

Åkerstedt, T., Anund, A., Axelsson, J., & Kecklund, G. (2014). Subjective sleepiness is a sensitive indicator of insufficient sleep and impaired waking function. *Journal of Sleep Research*, *23*, 240–252.

Cai, A.W.T., Manousakis, J.E., Lo, T.Y.T., et al. (2021). I think I'm sleepy, therefore I am– Awareness of sleepiness while driving: A systematic review. *Sleep Medicine Review*, *60*. https://doi.org/10.1016/j.smrev.2021.101533

Chervin, R.D. (2000). The multiple sleep latency test and Epworth sleepiness scale in the assessment of daytime sleepiness. *Journal of Sleep Research*, *9*, 399–401.

Chung, F., Abdullah, H.R., & Liao, P. (2016). STOP-Bang questionnaire: A practical approach to screen for obstructive sleep apnea. *Chest*, *149*, 631–638.

Civil Aviation Safety Authority. (2014). Biomathematical fatigue models–Guidance document. www.icao.int/safety/fatiguemanagement/ArticlesPublications/ biomathematical_fatigue_models.pdf

Connor, J., Norton, R., Ameratunga, S., et al. (2002). Driver sleepiness and risk of serious injury to car occupants: Population based case control study. *British Medical Journal*, *324*, 1125.

Dawson, D., Ian Noy, Y., Härmä, M., Akerstedt, T., & Belenky, G. (2011). Modelling fatigue and the use of fatigue models in work settings. *Accident Analysis and Prevention, 43,* 549–564.

Dawson, D., Searle, A.K., & Paterson, J.L. (2014). Look before you (s)leep: Evaluating the use of fatigue detection technologies within a fatigue risk management system for the road transport industry. *Sleep Medicine Review, 18,* 141–152.

Drake, C., Roehrs, T., Breslau, N., et al. (2010). The 10-year risk of verified motor vehicle crashes in relation to physiologic sleepiness. *Sleep, 33,* 745–752.

Flo, E., Bjorvatn, B., Folkard, S., et al. (2012). A reliability and validity study of the Bergen Shift Work Sleep questionnaire in nurses working three-shift rotations. *Chronobiology International, 29,* 937–946.

Gawron, V.J. (2016). Overview of self-reported measures of fatigue. *International Journal of Aviation Psychology, 26,* 120–131.

Hallvig, D., Anund, A., Fors, C., et al. (2013). Sleepy driving on real road and in the simulator–a comparison. *Accident Analysis and Prevention, 50,* 44–50.

Hallvig, D., Anund, A., Fors, C., Kecklund, G., & Åkerstedt, T. (2014). Real driving at night–predicting lane departures from physiological and subjective sleepiness. *Biological Psychology, 101,* 18–23.

Huang, Y., Aumüller, P., Fietze, I., Penzel, T., & Veauthier, C. (2020). Comparison of the Oxford sleep resistance test and the multiple sleep latency test. *Physiological Measurement, 6,* 41:104005. http://doi.org/10.1088/1361-6579/ab9feb.

IATA, ICAO, IFALPA. (2011). Fatigue risk management systems–Implementation guide for operators. 1st Edition. www.icao.int/safety/fatiguemanagement/FRMS%20Tools/FRMS%20Implementation%20Guide%20for%20Operators%20July%202011.pdf

IATA, ICAO, IFALPA. (2015). Fatigue management guide for operators. Second Edition. www.icao.int/safety/fatiguemanagement/FRMS%20Tools/FMG%20for%20Airline%20Operators%202nd%20Ed%20(Final)%20EN.pdf

Ingre, M., Åkerstedt, T., Peters, B., Anund, A., & Kecklund G. (2006a). Subjective sleepiness, simulated driving performance and blink duration: Examining individual differences. *Journal of Sleep Research, 15,* 47–53.

Ingre, M., Åkerstedt, T., Peters, B., et al. (2006b). Subjective sleepiness and accident risk avoiding the ecological fallacy. *Journal of Sleep Research, 15,* 142–148.

Itani, O., Jike, M., Watanabe, N., Kaneita, Y. (2017). Short sleep duration and health outcomes: A systematic review, meta-analysis, and meta-regression. *Sleep Medicine, 32,* 246–256.

Johns, M.W. (1991). A new method for measuring daytime sleepiness: The Epworth sleepiness scale. *Sleep, 14,* 540–545.

Johns, M.W. (1998). Rethinking the assessment of sleepiness. *Sleep Medicine Review, 2,* 3–15.

Onninen, J., Hakola, T., Puttonen, S., et al. (2020). Sleep and sleepiness in shift-working tram drivers. *Applied Ergonomics, 88,* 103153. http://doi.org 10.1016/j.apergo.2020.103153.

Penzel, T., Fietze, I., Schöbel, C., & Veauthier, C. (2019). Technology to Detect Driver Sleepiness. *Sleep Medicine Clinics, 14,* 463–468.

Phillips, R.O. (2016). Countermeasures for use in fatigue risk management. TØI Report 1488/2016. Oslo: Norwegian Centre for Transport Research (TØI). www.toi.no/getfile.php?mmfileid=43284

Pylkkönen, M., Sihvola, M., Hyvärinen, H.K., et al. (2015). Sleepiness, sleep, and use of sleepiness countermeasures in shift-working long-haul truck drivers. *Accident Analysis and Prevention, 80,* 201–210.

Sallinen, M., & Hublin, C. (2015). Fatigue-inducing factors in transportation operators. In S. M. Popkin (Ed.), *Worker Fatigue and Transportations Safety* (pp. 138–173). Sage Publications. Reviews of Human Factors and Ergonomics, 10.

Sallinen, M., Pylkkönen, M., Puttonen, S., Sihvola, M., & Åkerstedt, T. (2020). Are long-haul truck drivers unusually alert? A comparison with long-haul airline pilots. *Accident Analysis and Prevention*, *137*, 105442. http://doi.org/10.1016/j.aap.2020.

Sallinen, M., Sihvola, M., Puttonen, S., et al. (2017). Sleep, alertness and alertness management among commercial airline pilots on short-haul and long-haul flights. *Accident Analysis and Prevention*, *98*, 320–329.

Samn, S., and Perelli, L. (1982). Estimating aircrew fatigue: A technique with implications to airlift operations. Technical Report No. SAM-TR-82-21. Brooks AFB, TX: USAF School of Aerospace Medicine.

Sparrow, A.R., LaJambe, C.M., & Van Dongen, H.P.A. (2019). Drowsiness measures for commercial motor vehicle operations. *Accident Analysis and Prevention*, *126*, 146–159.

Stern, H.S., Blower, D., Cohen, M.L., et al. (2019). Data and methods for studying commercial motor vehicle driver fatigue, highway safety and long-term driver health. *Accident Analysis and Prevention*, *126*, 37–42.

1.3 Challenges in Fatigue Research and Enforcement

Anna Anund[1,2] and Anna Sjörs Dahlman[1,4]

[1]Swedish National Road and Transport Research Institute, Linköping, Sweden
[2]Linköping University, Linköping, Sweden
[4]SAFER Vehicle and Traffic Safety Centre and Department of Electrical Engineering at Chalmers University of Technology, Gothenburg, Sweden

CONTENTS

1.3.1 FATIGUE OR SLEEPINESS AND ITS RELATIONSHIP WITH COUNTERMEASURE EFFECTIVENESS

Driver fatigue is a state that is involved in between 15% and 30% of all road crashes, and sleepy drivers have between 2.5 and 3.5 times higher risk of being involved in a crash than drivers who are well rested (Bioulac et al., 2017; Connor et al., 2002). The reasons behind this increased crash risk among fatigued drivers are numerous and not only due to sleepiness caused by time-of-day effects and lack of sleep (Åkerstedt, Folkard, & Portin, 2004). Task-related underload or overload (Williamson et al., 2011) also contributes to the risk of incidents and crashes (see also Chapter 3.4). The combination of factors, for example, night driving under task-related underload, is even more problematic. To identify the most effective countermeasure for a given situation, there is a need to understand the reasons behind driver fatigue (May & Baldwin, 2009). A fatigued driver who is sleep deprived needs sleep to recuperate, but a driver experiencing fatigue due to underload needs a change of task to remain alert, whereas fatigue due to cognitive overload can be mitigated by a reduction of workload.

A challenge in fatigue research that makes it difficult to select and implement effective countermeasures is isolating sleep-related fatigue and task-related fatigue as these often develop simultaneously. Likewise, it is difficult to manipulate the type of fatigue to be studied, especially in driver fatigue research as there will always be a fatiguing effect of the driving task itself. It is also very difficult for an individual to determine whether the feeling of fatigue is due to sleep loss or due to engaging in the same task for too long, or both. It is not always possible for a driver to acknowledge the feeling of fatigue. Most drivers who have been involved in fatigue-related crashes are aware of having been fatigued before the crash; however, the criticality is that drivers cannot foresee when it impairs their driving behaviour, or when they are close to sleep onset (Anund & Åkerstedt, 2010). A challenge is therefore to know how to convince drivers who experience fatigue to take action before it is too late.

1.3.1.1 Use of Crash Data to Inform Countermeasure Selection and Implementation

Looking into the crash statistics and also at self-reported sleepiness, underreporting of fatigue-related crashes is well known to be high (Horne & Reyner, 1999; Åkerstedt, 2000). The reasons are varied. First, driving in a fatigued condition is illegal in many countries. In Sweden, for example, it is regulated in the same legalisation as drunk driving (Regeringskansliet, 1998). While fatigue regulations may be enacted with best intentions, the consequence for crash statistics can be negative since drivers are not very keen on reporting being sleepy after having caused a crash. Second, professional drivers may not want to admit to themselves (or to others) that they are unable to stay alert while driving, which can contribute to underreporting. It is well known that professional drivers must often fight to stay awake during their work shifts. For instance, about 20% of city bus drivers and coach drivers report fighting to stay awake at least two to four times a week (Kecklund et al., 2014; Miller, Filtness, Anund, Maynard, & Pilkington-Cheney, 2020). Finally, when a crash happens it is most often due to multiple factors. Because it is difficult to isolate fatigue as a singular main causal factor, and because the proof needed to cite fatigue as a main cause is essentially unattainable within current policing resources, crash causation is usually assigned to more measurable factors, such as driver impairment and/or driver error.

1.3.1.2 Choosing Effective Countermeasures

Most police officers do not have routines and tools to measure and determine if the reason for a crash is driver fatigue directly or indirectly. If a driver is injured or killed, then it is even more difficult. However, there are other ways to understand the magnitude of the problem. For example, we know that the introduction of milled rumble strips on roadway shoulders reduces the number of severe crashes (seriously injured and killed persons) on motorways by almost 24% (Anund & Vadeby, 2021). These strips are placed outside the lane marking. For a driver to experience the audible and vibratory warnings of rumble strips, a vehicle's wheel needs to first cross the profiled edge line. There is reason to believe that lane exceedances and crossing a rumble strip are often due to driver fatigue, and the reduction in crashes is thus a clear indication of the magnitude of fatigue's negative effects on driving performance. A challenge here is to ensure that the feedback drivers receive from rumble strips or from any type of fatigue warning system motivates them to take a break, rather than allows them to keep on driving when they are fatigued. There are studies that support positive effects not only from infrastructure rumble strips, but also from in-vehicle system like lane departure warnings (Sternlund, Strandroth, Rizzi, Lie, & Tingvall, 2016).

From the operator or company perspective, there is a need to manage problems related to driver fatigue. An open/just culture is essential, where input, cooperation, and open discussions from various stakeholders (e.g., employers, workers, occupational health and safety professionals, and policymakers) are vital components of establishing an effective fatigue management system (Phillips, Kecklund, Anund, & Sallinen, 2017). A strategy used by most companies has been to provide workers with education on fatigue. It is reasonable to assume that education is an effective countermeasure. However, up to now there is limited evidence that clearly supports this conclusion (Pylkkönen et al., 2018).

In recent years a lot of effort has gone into the development of driver support systems to detect driver fatigue in order to inform or warn drivers (Dawson, Searle, & Paterson, 2014) but no system is perfect. It has been shown that a fusion of sensors and algorithms is needed, and that time on task and time of the day are important factors to consider to achieve high sensitivity and specificity (Nilsson et al., 2017). Most research and development efforts are focused on the detection and less on the countermeasures and their effectiveness, despite the fact that most drivers are aware of being fatigued (Anund & Åkerstedt, 2010). A challenge in future research will be to select the most promising countermeasures and evaluate any effect(s) related to observed behavioural changes. The understanding of a fatigue warning system's effectiveness is highly dependent not only on its detection sensitivity/specificity, but also on the effectiveness of the activated countermeasure.

1.3.2 INTER– AND INTRA-INDIVIDUAL DIFFERENCES IN SENSITIVITY TO FATIGUE

One of the major challenges in fatigue research and, consequently, in developing, selecting, and implementing effective countermeasures, is accounting for individual differences in sensitivity to fatigue. Individual differences are related to how easily one becomes fatigued, one's ability to handle fatigue when it occurs, and the consequences of fatigue in terms of, for instance, driving performance and well-being. Individual differences are also important in relation to one's capacity to resist falling asleep (Caldwell et al., 2005; Van Dongen, Vitellaro, & Dinges, 2005) and to one's reaction and response to a given warning (Anund, Kecklund, Peters, & Åkerstedt, 2008; Anund, Kecklund, Vadeby, Hjalmdahl, & Åkerstedt, 2008; May & Baldwin, 2009). These individual differences should be taken into consideration in fatigue research.

Not only do they influence the detection and prediction of fatigue, but they are also of great importance in terms of identifying effective countermeasures.

There are both inter-individual differences (differences between individuals) and intra-individual differences (day-to-day variation within the same individual) in sensitivity to fatigue. Intra-individual differences can be related to poor sleep, stressful life events, lifestyle choices, diet, temporary illness, physical activity, alcohol intake, and many other things that can influence sensitivity to fatigue from one day to another. Some of the most impactful inter-individual factors are described below.

How much sleep one needs to feel rested varies considerably between individuals. A consensus report of sleep experts suggested that adults should sleep on average 7 or more hours per night on a regular basis to promote optimal health (Watson et al., 2015). However, young adults, individuals recovering from sleep debt, and individuals with illnesses may require more sleep—even 9 or more hours per night. Insufficient sleep affects humans in various ways, degrading both cognitive and physical performance and increasing the need for sleep and the propensity to fall asleep. Of great importance is how well a driver can continue to perform the driving task despite being fatigued. Laboratory-based sleep deprivation studies have found substantial inter-individual differences in performance impairment from sleep loss (Van Dongen, Baynard, Maislin, & Dinges, 2004). These inter-individual differences are so important (explaining more than 50% of the total variance in performance impairment) that it is not reasonable to consider all individuals to be equal in their responses to sleep loss.

One of the most impactful factors on sensitivity to fatigue is chronotype, which represents the individual preference to be active early or late in the day and to sleep early or late at night (Kerkhof, 1985). Chronotype is partially biologically mediated and determines the optimal timing of sleep for the individual. The two extremes are called eveningness ("night owls") and morningness ("larks" or "early birds") but most individuals have some flexibility in the timing of their sleep period. Night owls feel especially sleepy during the initial hours after awakening from night-time sleep and larks prefer to retire early to bed and to awaken quite early in the morning feeling well-rested. There is considerable variation in how well different individuals tolerate work hours that are poorly aligned with their chronotype (Härmä, 1993). It has been shown that individuals drive less safely outside their optimal time of day, which could contribute to the increased number of road crashes during certain times of day (Del Rio-Bermudez, Diaz-Piedra, Catena, Buela-Casal, & Di Stasi, 2014).

Several personality traits have been identified as important for driver fatigue, including extraversion, sensation seeking, and conscientiousness (Thiffault & Bergeron, 2003). Individuals who are extroverts and sensation seekers may be more sensitive to driver fatigue especially in less demanding road environments where road monotony can lead to task-related fatigue. High sensation seeking is also a common personality trait among individuals that have reported falling asleep at the wheel (Thiffault & Bergeron, 2003). Conscientiousness, on the other hand, can be regarded as an inter-individual protective factor against driver fatigue. Conscientious individuals are better able to activate resources to stay on task compared to individuals who are less conscientious (Hidalgo-Gadea, Kreuder, Krajewski, & Vorstius, 2021).

There are considerable individual differences in the degree to which stress exposure disrupts sleep, resulting in difficulty falling and staying asleep. Some individuals experience drastic deterioration of sleep when stressed, whereas others do not, or are less affected by stress (Kalmbach, Anderson, & Drake, 2018). Sensitivity to stress will therefore also indirectly influence sensitivity to fatigue in individuals that experience poor sleep due to stress. Research has shown that genetics, familial history of insomnia, gender, and environmental stress are some of the factors that influence how one's sleep system responds to stress (Kalmbach et al., 2018).

Females in general seem to be at greater risk of experiencing fatigue than males, especially when working night shifts (Di Milia et al., 2011). It is unknown whether this difference between men and women has a biological cause (i.e., a sex difference) or whether it is due to gender aspects as females may more easily recognise and admit feeling fatigued than males.

Ageing seems to result in a gradual deterioration of the mechanisms that support the physiological, circadian, and sleep systems, suggesting a relationship between age and fatigue (Di Milia et al., 2011). Older adults appear to better tolerate sleep deprivation (Lowden, Anund, Kecklund, Peters, & Åkerstedt, 2009). It is, however, important to note that they are still impaired by sleep loss, and can be at high risk of fatigue-related crashes relative to their performance when well rested (Cai et al., 2021). Looking into the prevalence of fatigue while driving as well as into crashes caused by sleepy drivers, young drivers are clearly overrepresented (Connor et al., 2002). A greater vulnerability to the effects of sleep deprivation and slowing of their ability to anticipate traffic hazards may contribute to the increased risk of fatigue-related road crashes in younger drivers (Cai et al., 2021; Smith, Horswill, Chambers, & Wetton, 2009).

Chronic medical conditions can affect sleep quality and quantity and cause excessive daytime fatigue. Sleep disorders such as insomnia and obstructive sleep apnoea (OSA) significantly increase daytime fatigue and risk of fatigue-related crashes (Smolensky, Di Milia, Ohayon, & Philip, 2011). Several other medical conditions, such as asthma, chronic obstructive pulmonary disease (COPD), and rheumatoid arthritis, as well as certain classes of medications, can also contribute to excessive daytime fatigue and are increasingly being recognised as risk factors for driving incidents.

Individual differences are also important in relation to countermeasures for fatigue. For example, two of the most effective countermeasures are napping and caffeine intake. There are considerable individual differences in the usefulness of these countermeasures, both when it comes to the effectiveness of the countermeasure and the willingness and ability to take the countermeasure. For instance, taking a nap is not possible for everyone as some individuals find it difficult to sleep during the daytime. Regarding caffeine, there are large differences in sensitivity to caffeine and how long lasting the effect is (Lorist & Tops, 2003).

Inter-individual differences imply a great challenge in standardising testing conditions in fatigue research. Fatigue researchers need to balance between studying a homogeneous group of participants who are expected to react similarly to the test conditions and a heterogeneous sample that might show great variation in the results but, on the other hand, will also better reflect the general population. Individuals that represent the extremes, e.g., the very old and very young, or larks and night owls, are often those who exhibit the largest problems with fatigue when the circumstances are not favourable for them.

1.3.3 FATIGUE STUDY CHALLENGES

A clear view of the magnitude of driver fatigue is needed to understand when, how, and where mitigation strategies are needed. There is also a need to understand the factors that are main contributors to driver fatigue, as well as an understanding of the effectiveness of different countermeasures.

The balance between ecological validity (how similar something is to the real world) and a high degree of control is important to consider when setting up a fatigue study (Anund & Kircher, 2009). If the aim is to understand the effect of a specific countermeasure, then it is important to control the development of fatigue using a fixed environment and instead vary the countermeasure. If the aim is to understand how fatigue develops during, for example, night-time driving, then it is better to per-form the test on real roads, at night. One limitation will, however, be that even though the way of inducing driver fatigue is done in the same way, there is no guarantee that you will collect enough data covering both daytime and night-time fatigue, as well as alert driving during daytime and night-time. A challenge is that the development of driver fatigue, as well as the effectiveness of a given countermeasure, is highly individual.

The test situation itself can also influence the development of fatigue. In driving studies, the nature of the driving task (monotonous or complex) and environmental conditions (traffic density, type of road, weather, etc.) can either accelerate or slow the development of fatigue. The use of driving simulators is common in fatigue research and drivers often become fatigued more easily in simulators, partly due to motion sickness (Fors, Ahlström, & Anund, 2018). Wearing measurement equipment and performing research-related secondary tasks are other influential factors. If the research also includes sleep tracking, wearing measurement equipment during sleeping or napping can disturb normal sleep. Finally, the mere fact that the individual is aware that sleep is being tracked can influence sleep patterns.

When evaluating, for example, a driver fatigue system sensitivity/specificity there is a need for a reliable measure of fatigue to compare with (see Chapter 1.2). This could be determined either with objective or with subjective measures. An objective measure that is often referred to is brain activity (electroencephalography [EEG]); however, such an analysis is mainly focused on being a sleep and less is known about sleepiness and fatigue. One way to look at sleepiness is to consider where in the brain sleep occurs. Recent studies have indicated that localised sleep in certain brain areas is more prevalent the closer the driver is to sleep onset (Ahlström, Jansson, & Anund, 2017). The exact point of sleep onset is something that drivers are not able to recognise themselves and it would require a set of obtrusive sensors to measure physiologically.

The most common objective measurements of driver fatigue rely on blink parameters such as blink duration, frequency of long blinks, or percentage of eye closure (PERCLOS). Blink parameters can be measured both obtrusively (electrodes) or unobtrusively (camera). If the data will be used only offline, then brain activity measures (EEG) can be used. However, this method is time-consuming methodologically and, just as for blink-related measures, there are individual differences in EEG patterns during sleepiness. An alternative is to use subjective measures of fatigue. This means that the drivers are asked to report their level of sleepiness. One of the most common scales is the Karolinska Sleepiness Scale (KSS) (Åkerstedt & Gillberg, 1990). To make sure that subjective measures are measuring what they are designed to measure, drivers need to be trained beforehand. One challenge is that this type of scale does not discriminate between sleep-related fatigue and task-related fatigue. There are results showing that this scale does not work optimally for reporting fatigue during tasks with high cognitive load. Regardless of whether the fatigue data are objective or subjective, it is important to define the resolution of the measurements as this defines the possibility of accurately measuring potentially subtle differences in levels of fatigue.

When performing fatigue studies, it is important to keep track of external, potentially confounding factors that can influence participants' sleep and fatigue. Before starting data collection, the researchers should track the drivers' sleep the night before, what they have been eating, and if they have been drinking caffeine or energy drinks, etc., as these factors will influence their behaviour and sensitivity to fatigue.

1.3.4 ENFORCEMENT CHALLENGES

The law regarding driving impairment varies by countries and jurisdictions. In many countries, driving in a fatigued state is regulated for professional drivers through 'Hours of Service' regulations or by national regulations connected to negligence in traffic. Since driver fatigue is a significant contributor to death and serious injury on our roads (Bioulac et al., 2017), enforcement strategies of existing fatigue and/or related legislation are important tools to increase road safety. However, the difficulties in identifying a fatigued driver on the road and difficulties in detecting and measuring fatigue can limit the effectiveness of enforcement strategies. There are major differences in enforcement that targets alcohol intoxication compared to driver fatigue, even though it has been demonstrated that these have similar negative effects on safe driving performance (Williamson & Feyer, 2000). The main difference is that, for alcohol, there is usually a defined limit of blood alcohol content (BAC) that can be measured via a blood test or by a breathalyser. For fatigue on the other hand, there are no similar thresholds that can be measured objectively. In addition, an individual's BAC remains even after a crash or if a driver is stopped by police, whereas signs of fatigue can change rapidly depending on the situation.

There have been attempts to develop tools for roadside fatigue assessment. For example, in Canada and Australia, the police work with checklists in two steps. A first set of questions are asked and if any of them indicate a risk of fatigue, a second more detailed set of questions are administered. The most common type of protocol is based on a Canadian police tool that uses a two-step investigation checklist. Initially, four questions are administered that assess time of day, deviation(s) from normal circadian rhythm, hours awake, and sleep/wake history (Gertler, Popkin, Nelson, & O'Neil, 2002). If the answer to any of these questions points to an elevated risk of fatigue, the investigator conducts a more thorough and focused examination of fatigue.

To be able to prove that a crash is due to fatigue, an investigator must be able to show that a driver was in a state of fatigue, and that actions taken, or decisions made, by the driver are consistent with known changes in behaviour that are expected when a person is fatigued. The burden of proof is a clear limitation to being able to correctly hold someone accountable for being fatigued after a crash or at a police roadside check.

The number of fatigue-related crashes is likely to be underestimated given the difficulty in identifying crash causation. Under-reporting of fatigue in crash statistics can mislead policymakers to think that there is no need to address fatigue because it causes only a small number of crashes. Similarly, on an individual level, not all drivers recognise fatigue as a traffic safety problem. This can be due to failure to recognise signs and symptoms of fatigue in themselves, and due to an unwillingness to acknowledge or report being sleepy. In fact, research has shown that sleep-deprived individuals commonly fail to accurately assess their level of sleepiness as compared to objective measures of their alertness (Horne, 2010). This implies that they are largely unaware of their increasing performance impairments (Van Dongen, Maislin, Mullington, & Dinges, 2003). Sleep-deprived individuals may overestimate their ability to overcome the negative effects of fatigue. It is also very difficult for an observer to judge another driver's level of fatigue by simply looking at them (Ahlström, Fors, Anund, & Hallvig, 2015). Therefore, objective measures of fatigue are important for enforcement.

Driver monitoring systems in vehicles provide the possibility to mitigate risks associated with driver fatigue. The fatigue countermeasures could be various types of warnings to the driver or activation of automated driving functions in the vehicle, such as safe stop manoeuvres or advanced driver assistance systems (ADAS). The European Union (EU) general safety regulations for motor vehicles (2019/2144) require that all new vehicles of category M (cars and buses) and N (trucks) be equipped with driver drowsiness and attention warning systems. Driver monitoring developments are also being incorporated into the European New Car Assessment Programme (Euro NCAP) Safety Assist protocols. From 2023 onwards, direct driver monitoring will be required for a vehicle model to get a full score in the Euro NCAP rating (Fredriksson, Lenné, van Montfort, & Grover, 2021).

Current driver monitoring systems for fatigue detection face various challenges including difficulty in accurately detecting and differentiating between different driver states, such as fatigue, distraction, and illness. The systems are often camera-based and therefore require certain light conditions and driver postures for accurate detection. Consequently, while driver monitoring systems might perform well in controlled laboratory environments, it is much more challenging to reliably detect driver states in real-world on-road driving where the environmental conditions vary greatly and there might be "noise factors" such as sunglasses, hats, and face masks, for example. There is also a risk of bias in the monitoring systems' detection algorithms if they perform differently depending on, for example, a driver's gender, race, facial features, or other characteristics. Reliable and accurate detection of driver state is crucial to be able to not only trigger the right type of warning or action from the vehicle, but also to identify effective countermeasures.

It is possible that, in the future, driver monitoring systems could be used for enforcement purposes. The challenge is to promote the legislation to make it mandatory for vehicle manufacturers to install the systems, and to allow investigators and law enforcement officers to get access to the data. Theoretically, the driver state detection output from such a unit could also be downloaded and/or stored. One of the main challenges would be to ensure data privacy and make sure that users (e.g., drivers) do not manipulate such a system.

There is no doubt that there are a lot of challenges in identifying the causes and consequences of fatigue. With careful planning it is possible to get the best possible data to inform our understanding, but this must always be interpreted with an awareness of limitations. Just because it is difficult does not mean we should not try.

SUMMARY POINTS FOR PRACTITIONERS

- The causes and consequences of fatigue in drivers need to be considered to identify and implement the most effective countermeasures.
- There are major individual differences both in fatigue development and in the effect of countermeasures. Age, gender, chronotype, and personality are some of the factors to be considered.
- There is no exact measure of fatigue in individual drivers, and the evidence needed for enforcement of a minimal level of driver alertness does not currently exist.

REFERENCES

Ahlström, C., Fors, C., Anund, A., & Hallvig, D. (2015). Video-based observer rated sleepiness versus self-reported subjective sleepiness in real road driving. *European Transport Research Review, 7*(38). https://doi.org/10.1007/s12544-015-0188-y

Ahlström, C., Jansson, S., & Anund, A. (2017). Local changes in the wake electroencephalogram precedes lane departures. *Journal of Sleep Research, 26*(6), 816–819. doi:10.1111/jsr.12527

Åkerstedt, T. (2000). Consensus statement: Fatigue and accidents in transport operations. *Journal of Sleep Research, 9*(4), 395.

Åkerstedt, T., Folkard, S., & Portin, C. (2004). Predictions from the three-process model of alertness. *Aviation, Space, and Environmental Medicine, 75*, A75–A83.

Åkerstedt, T., & Gillberg, M. (1990). Subjective and objective sleepiness in the active individual. *International Journal of Neuroscience, 52*, 29–37.

Anund, A., & Åkerstedt, T. (2010). Perception of sleepiness before falling asleep. *Sleep Medicine, 11*(8), 743–744. doi:10.1016/j.sleep.2010.06.001

Anund, A., Kecklund, G., Peters, B., & Åkerstedt, T. (2008). Driver sleepiness and individual differences in preferences for countermeasures. *Journal of Sleep Research, 17*(1), 16–22. doi:10.1111/j.1365-2869.2008.00633.x

Anund, A., Kecklund, G., Vadeby, A., Hjalmdahl, M., & Åkerstedt, T. (2008). The alerting effect of hitting a rumble strip—A simulator study with sleepy drivers. *Accident Analysis and Prevention, 40*(6), 1970–1976. doi:10.1016/j.aap.2008.08.017

Anund, A., & Kircher, K. (2009). *Advantages and disadvantages of different methods to evaluate sleepiness warning systems* (VTI report 664A). Linköping, Sweden. Retrieved from www. diva-portal.org/smash/get/diva2:675399/FULLTEXT02.pdf.

Anund, A., & Vadeby, A. (2021). Rumble strips, continuous shoulder and centerline. In R. Vickerman (Ed.), *International encyclopeida of transport* (vol. 2, pp. 549–553). Elsevier Ltd.

Bioulac, S., Franchi, M., Arnaud, M., Sagaspe, P., Moore, N., Salvo, F., & Philip, P. (2017). Risk of motor vehicle accidents related to sleepiness at the wheel: A systematic review and meta-analysis. *Sleep, 40*(10). doi:http://dx.doi.org/10.1093/sleep/zsx134

Cai, A. W. T., Manousakis, J. E., Singh, B., Kuo, J., Jeppe, K. J., Francis-Pester, E.,... . Anderson, C. (2021). On-road driving impairment following sleep deprivation differs according to age. *Scientific Reports, 11*(1), 21561. doi:10.1038/s41598-021-99133-y

Caldwell, J. A., Mu, Q., Smith, J. K., Mishory, A., Caldwell, J. L., Peters, G.,... . George, M. S. (2005). Are individual differences in fatigue vulnerability related to baseline differences in cortical activation? *Behavioral Neuroscience, 119*(3), 694–707. doi:10.1037/0735-7044.119.3.694

Connor, J., Norton, R., Ameratunga, S., Robinson, E., Civil, I., Dunn, R.,.... Jackson, R. (2002). Driver sleepiness and risk of serious injury to car occupants: Population based case control study. *British Medical Journal, 324*, 1–5.

Dawson, D., Searle, A., & Paterson, J. (2014). Look before you (s)leep: Evaluating the use of fatigue detection technologies within a fatigue risk management system for the road transport industry. *Medicine Reviews, 18*, 141–152.

Del Rio-Bermudez, C., Diaz-Piedra, C., Catena, A., Buela-Casal, G., & Di Stasi, L. L. (2014). Chronotype-dependent circadian rhythmicity of driving safety. *Chronobiology International, 31*(4), 532–541. doi:10.3109/07420528.2013.876427

Di Milia, L., Smolensky, M. H., Costa, G., Howarth, H. D., Ohayon, M. M., & Philip, P. (2011). Demographic factors, fatigue, and driving accidents: An examination of the published literature. *Accident Analysis and Prevention, 43*(2), 516–532. https://doi.org/10.1016/j.aap.2009.12.018

Fors, C., Ahlström, C., & Anund, A. (2018). A comparison of driver sleepiness in the simulator and on the real road. *Journal of Transportation Safety & Security, 10*(1–2), 72–87. doi:10.1080/19439962.2016.1228092

Fredriksson, R., Lenné, M. G., van Montfort, S., & Grover, C. (2021). European NCAP program developments to address driver distraction, drowsiness and sudden sickness. *Frontiers in Neuroergonomics, 2*(33). doi:10.3389/fnrgo.2021.786674

Gertler, J., Popkin, S., Nelson, D., & O'Neil, K. (2002). *Toolbox for Transit Operator Fatigue* (TCRP Report 81). Retrieved from TCRP Report 81: Toolbox for Transit Operator Fatigue (trb.org).

Härmä, M. (1993). Individual differences in tolerance to shiftwork: A review. *Ergonomics, 36*(1–3), 101–109. doi:10.1080/00140139308967860

Hidalgo-Gadea, G., Kreuder, A., Krajewski, J., & Vorstius, C. (2021). Towards better microsleep predictions in fatigued drivers: Exploring benefits of personality traits and IQ. *Ergonomics, 64*(6), 778–792. doi:10.1080/00140139.2021.1882707

Horne, J. (2010). Sleepiness as a need for sleep: When is enough, enough? *Neuroscience and Biobehavioral Reviews, 34*(1), 108–118. doi:10.1016/j.neubiorev.2009.07.009

Horne, J., & Reyner, L. (1999). Vehicle accidents related to sleep: A review. *Occupational and Environmental Medicine, 56*(5), 289–294.

Kalmbach, D. A., Anderson, J. R., & Drake, C. L. (2018). The impact of stress on sleep: Pathogenic sleep reactivity as a vulnerability to insomnia and circadian disorders. *Journal of Sleep Research, 27*(6), e12710. doi:https://doi.org/10.1111/jsr.12710

Kecklund, G., Radun, I., Ingre, M., Fors, C., Ihstrom, J., & Anund, A. (2014). Bus drivers' working hours and their effects on sleep and fatigue. *Journal of Sleep Research, 23*, 286–287.

Kerkhof, G. A. (1985). Inter-individual differences in the human circadian system: A review. *Biological Psychology, 20*(2), 83–112.

Lorist, M. M., & Tops, M. (2003). Caffeine, fatigue, and cognition. *Brain and Cognition, 53*(1), 82–94. https://doi.org/10.1016/S0278-2626(03)00206-9

Lowden, A., Anund, A., Kecklund, G., Peters, B., & Åkerstedt, T. (2009). Wakefulness in young and elderly subjects driving at night in a car simulator. *Accident Analysis and Prevention, 41*(5), 1001–1007. doi:10.1016/j.aap.2009.05.014

May, J. F., & Baldwin, C. L. (2009). Driver fatigue: The importance of identifying causal factors of fatigue when considering detection and countermeasure technologies. *Transportation Research Part F: Psychology and Behaviour, 12*(3), 218–224. doi:10.1016/j.trf.2008.11.005

Miller, K. A., Filtness, A. J., Anund, A., Maynard, S. E., & Pilkington-Cheney, F. (2020). Contributory factors to sleepiness amongst London bus drivers. *Transportation Research Part F-Traffic Psychology and Behaviour, 73*, 415–424. doi:10.1016/j.trf.2020.07.012

Nilsson, E., Ahlström, C., Barua, S., Fors, C., Lindén, P., Svanberg, B.,.... Anund, A. (2017). *Vehicle Driver Monitoring–Sleepiness and Cognitive load* (VTI report 937A). Retrieved from http://vti.diva-portal.org/smash/get/diva2:1096341/FULLTEXT01.pdf

Phillips, R. O., Kecklund, G., Anund, A., & Sallinen, M. (2017). Fatigue in transport: A review of exposure, risks, checks and controls. *Transport Reviews, 37*(6), 742–766. doi:10.1080/01441647.2017.1349844

Pylkkönen, M., Tolvanen, A., Hublin, C., Kaartinen, J., Karhula, K., Puttonen, S., & Sallinen, M. (2018). Effects of alertness management training on sleepiness among long-haul truck drivers: A randomized controlled trial. *Accident Analysis and Prevention, 121*, 301–313.

Regeringskansliet. (1998). Traffic Ordinance 1276. In Government (Ed.), 1276 (vol. 3). Stockholm, Sweden.

Smith, S. S., Horswill, M. S., Chambers, B., & Wetton, M. (2009). Hazard perception in novice and experienced drivers: The effects of sleepiness. *Accident Analysis and Prevention, 41*(4), 729–733. doi:10.1016/j.aap.2009.03.016

Smolensky, M. H., Di Milia, L., Ohayon, M. M., & Philip, P. (2011). Sleep disorders, medical conditions, and road accident risk. *Accident Analysis and Prevention, 43*(2), 533–548. doi:https://doi.org/10.1016/j.aap.2009.12.004

Sternlund, S., Strandroth, J., Rizzi, M., Lie, A., & Tingvall, C. (2016). The effectiveness of lane departure warning systems–A reduction in real-world passenger car injury crashes. *Traffic Injury Prevention.* doi:http://dx.doi.org/10.1080/15389588.2016.1230672

Thiffault, P., & Bergeron, J. (2003). Fatigue and individual differences in monotonous simulated driving. *Personality and Individual Differences, 34*(1), 159–176. https://doi.org/10.1016/S0191-8869(02)00119-8

Van Dongen, H., Baynard, M., Maislin, G., & Dinges, D. (2004). Systematic interindividual differences in neurobehavioral impairment from sleep loss: Evidence of trait-like differential vulnerability. *Sleep, 27*(3), 423–433.

Van Dongen, H., Maislin, G., Mullington, J., & Dinges, D. (2003). The cumulative cost of additional wakefulness: Dose-response effects on neurobehavioral functions and sleep physiology from chronic sleep restriction and total sleep deprivation. *Sleep, 15*(26), 117–126. doi:10.1093/sleep/26.2.117

Van Dongen, H., Vitellaro, K., & Dinges, D. (2005). Individual differences in adult human sleep and wakefulness: Leitmotif for a research agenda. *Sleep, 28*(4), 479–496.

Watson, N. F., Badr, M. S., Belenky, G., Bliwise, D. L., Buxton, O. M., Buysse, D. J.,... . Tasali, E. (2015). Recommended amount of sleep for a healthy adult: A joint consensus statement of the American Academy of Sleep Medicine and Sleep Research Society. *Sleep, 38*(6), 843–844.

Williamson, A., & Feyer, A. (2000). Moderate sleep deprivation produces impairments in cognitive and motor performance equivalent to legally prescribed levels of alcohol intoxication. *Occupational and Environmental Medicine, 57*, 649–655.

Williamson, A., Lombardi, D. A., Folkard, S., Stutts, J., Courtney, T. K., & Connor, J. L. (2011). The link between fatigue and safety. *Accident Analysis and Prevention, 43*(2), 498–515. doi:10.1016/j.aap.2009.11.011

1.4 The Effects of Fatigue on Performance in Transportation Operations

Matthew J.W. Thomas, Madeline Sprajcer, and Drew Dawson

Appleton Institute, Central Queensland University, Wayville, SA, Australia

CONTENTS

1.4.1 INTRODUCTION AND CONTEXT

By their very nature, transport operations occur 24 hours per day, 365 days per year, across the globe. In the vast majority of instances, workers are responsible for the operation of the vehicle, and are therefore critical in the maintenance of safety. In this context, fatigue presents a tangible risk, given the wide range of impacts fatigue has on human performance. Internationally, fatigue has been implicated in between 10 and 20% of all road crashes, and has been identified as a significant source of risk in other transport industries (Horne & Reyner, 1995).

The major causes of fatigue in transport operations are (1) the time of day (with higher risk associated with operations at night/during the window of circadian low); (2) extended wakefulness; (3) inadequate sleep (both acute and

DOI: 10.1201/9781003213154-6

cumulative); (4) pathological sleepiness (caused by disorders such as sleep apnoea); and (5) prolonged work hours (Åkerstedt, 2000).

Humans are a diurnal species, with a long evolutionary predisposition to be awake during the day and asleep during the night (Duffy & Czeisler, 2002). Significant relationships have been identified between time of day and fatigue-related crash risk, especially in road transport. These time of day effects are largely seen as a product of our circadian rhythms of performance and alertness, with increased crash prevalence during the primary window of circadian low during the late night and early morning hours (02:00 to 06:00) and a lesser peak during the afternoon secondary window of circadian low (Pack et al., 1995; Summala, Hakkanen, Mikkola, & Sinkkonen, 1999).

Likely compounding these daily rhythms of alertness and performance, factors such as restricted sleep and extended wakefulness are also significant contributors to fatigue-related incidents and crashes. A recent review article has highlighted that even a moderate amount of sleep restriction in the 24 hours prior to operations in transport industries is associated with significant increase in crash risk, with the suggestion that less than 5 hours sleep should be seen as demonstrative of likely impairment (Dawson, Sprajcer, & Thomas, 2021). Similarly, continuous wakefulness greater than 16 hours has been shown to be associated with performance impairment, with only moderately extended wakefulness of 17 to 19 hours associated with levels of performance impairment similar to those seen with a blood alcohol concentration of 0.05% (50 mg/dL), a level typically used to demonstrate culpable impairment (Dawson & Reid, 1997; Williamson & Feyer, 2000).

Finally, the nature of the work is seen to contribute to fatigue in and of itself, as well as exacerbate the effects of fatigue from other sources, for instance, workload, the type of task being worked, or other issues such as sleep disorders. In the road transport industry, fatigue has been found to be directly associated with long periods of work at a monotonous task (Feyer & Williamson, 1995). Similarly, a longer duty period and a greater number of take-offs and landings in a given duty period have been shown to be associated with pilot fatigue in air transport operations (Powell, Spencer, Holland, Broadbent, & Petrie, 2007).

While the factors that contribute to the occurrence of fatigue are relatively well understood, the precise mechanisms by which fatigue leads to changes in human performance, and in turn impacts on transport operations, introduce an additional level of complexity. Fatigue is a multi-dimensional construct, with a range of effects on operator performance that begins with basic changes at a physiological and neurobiological level. These changes are manifested in degraded cognitive performance at primary levels of cognitive processing, such as perception, attention, memory and reaction time (Dinges et al., 1997), and higher-order levels of cognitive processing such as decision-making (Harrison & Horne, 2000). In turn, fatigue is also manifested in a range of psychosocial impacts from changes in emotional regulation, mood and communication that have their own flow-on effects in terms of interpersonal interaction and teamwork (Banks & Dinges, 2007).

Fatigue's effects on performance are, in and of themselves, not the causes of incidents and crashes in transport operations. Rather, these effects result in changes in operational performance that are highly context and task specific. While in many transport settings, operators are able to modify their behaviour to minimise the risks

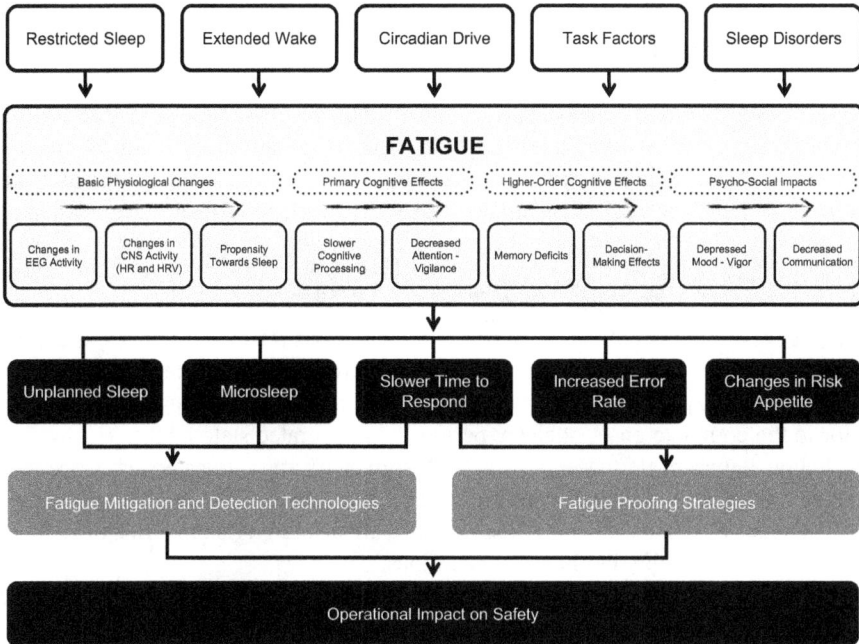

FIGURE 1.4.1 A functional model of the complex relationship between sources of fatigue and safety in transport operations.

associated with fatigue, our traditional view has been that of fatigue causing performance *deficits* and fatigue is often constructed simply in terms of impairment. These changes to operational performance are further moderated by formal and informal risk mitigation strategies at the organisational, team, and individual levels. Two key risk management strategies implemented to manage potential performance decrements are technological solutions and fatigue-proofing strategies. Fatigue detection technology is increasingly being used by transport operators to detect operator state (i.e., to detect when an individual has fallen asleep or is likely to fall asleep). Fatigue proofing instead refers to strategies that can be implemented by individuals or teams to prevent fatigue-related performance decrements from leading to poor safety outcomes (i.e., incidents, near misses). This combination of operator performance and risk mitigation strategies leads to the level of safety achieved by a transport system as a whole, as illustrated in Figure 1.4.1.

This chapter will provide an overview of the wide range of performance decrements associated with fatigue that can negatively impact the safety of transport operations.

1.4.2 EFFECTS OF FATIGUE ON PERFORMANCE

Fatigue is typically defined as a state of impaired performance, or in terms of reduced capability to perform both physical and mental work (Brown, 1994). The various forms of performance impairment associated with fatigue in turn have considerable impacts on the safety of transport operations. These impacts range from the extreme impacts where operators are unable to maintain wakefulness through to more subtle implications for decision-making and team performance.

There is ample research that has examined the range of impacts fatigue has on human performance, as they relate to transportation operations. We now turn to focus on research from the laboratory and provide a concise overview of the extant literature that has examined the ways in which fatigue is associated with performance degradation.

1.4.2.1 MICROSLEEPS AND MAINTAINING WAKEFULNESS

The most obvious risks of fatigue in transport operations relate to instances where the operator is unable to sustain wakefulness and inadvertently falls asleep. This may be in the context of a microsleep, or a longer period of sleep occurring while on duty. Prior to the complete onset of sleep, periods of accelerated state lability (increasing oscillation between alertness and lowered vigilance) are associated with operator drowsiness and very short sleep episodes called microsleeps (Binks, Waters, & Hurry, 1999; Dinges & Kribbs, 1991). These episodes are also high risk in terms of fatigue-related impact on safety in transport operations.

In transportation settings in which there are no robust forms of protection offered through automation, such as auto-pilot (aviation) or forms of automatic train protection (rail), even microsleeps can lead to incidents and crashes caused by loss of control and/ or collision. Specifically, localised microsleeps can occur without conscious awareness and if they occur in regions of the brain essential for driving, they will in turn have an impact on safety (Ahlstrom, Jansson, & Anund, 2017). Unfortunately, given the 24-hour nature of transport operations, the history of fatigue-related accidents is riddled with instances where an operator has fallen asleep, leading to catastrophic outcomes (Horne & Reyner, 1999) (see also Chapters 2.4 and 2.5 of this book).

Our drive for sleep is influenced by two main factors—circadian processes and homeostasis. The circadian process reflects changes in alertness across the 24-hour day as a function of our circadian rhythms (Ferguson et al., 2012). This effect occurs in combination with homeostatic processes—where the pressure for sleep builds as a function of time awake and the amount of prior sleep an individual has obtained (Åkerstedt & Folkard, 1997; Borbély, 1982). Accordingly, in transport operations the risk of an unintended sleep episode can be quantified in terms of the combined influence of circadian and homeostatic sleep drives.

1.4.2.2 NEUROBEHAVIOURAL PERFORMANCE

Beyond simply falling asleep "at the wheel", the negative impacts of fatigue on neurobehavioural performance have been well established in the scientific literature, and have given rise to a range of performance decrements relevant to transport operations.

Operator fatigue has been clearly associated with changes in activity within the central nervous system (CNS). Electroencephalography (EEG) studies have demonstrated that the decreased arousal, slowed sensorimotor functions, and impaired information processing associated with fatigue are linked to consistent changes in an individual's EEG measures. These changes include increased delta, theta, and alpha activity as well as cortical deactivation (Kecklund & Åkerstedt, 1993; Lal & Craig, 2002). Similarly, other CNS changes such as decreased heart rate and increased heart-rate variability are associated with fatigue (Mascord & Heath, 1992). These changes primarily reflect changes in an operator's level of physiological arousal, with lower arousal levels symptomatic of fatigue-related impairment.

With respect to cognitive processes more broadly, there have been a range of theories put forward to explain the association between fatigue and various cognitive outcomes. Some of these theories favour a primary impact on lower-order cognitive processes, such as vigilance and attention (Durmer & Dinges, 2005), with flow-on effects to higher-order forms of cognitive processing. Other research has focussed on the neurobiological impacts of fatigue on specific regions of the brain, such as the thalamus, which is responsible for processes such as attention and arousal, and the prefrontal cortex (PFC), which is responsible for a range of higher-order cognitive executive functions (Thomas, et al., 2000).

The effects of fatigue on both arousal and information processing are associated with significant changes in many areas of neurobehavioural performance relevant to transport operations. These changes can include impaired reaction time, decreased vigilance, and a propensity towards distraction.

Allocation of attention and distractibility, both critical in terms of risk in transport operations, have consistently been shown to be negatively influenced by fatigue. For instance, studies of sleep restriction have found that the voluntary allocation of attention is impaired, whereas the involuntary allocation of attention is enhanced (Lee, Manousakis, Fielding, & Anderson, 2015). This means we become less in control over where we focus our attention when fatigued. Specifically in the context of transport operations, it has been shown that fatigue increases predisposition to distraction (Anderson & Horne, 2013). Increased distraction can negatively impact safety in terms of missed cues, and failures to respond to critical situations across all forms of transport.

Compounding the effects of fatigue, there are clear "dose–response" relationships between key fatigue-related variables such as restricted sleep and extended wakefulness on neurobehavioural performance. With respect to restricted sleep, even a modest amount of sleep restriction (~6 hours of sleep per night) is associated with a decline in performance across a week, with decreasing amounts of sleep associated with increasing amounts of performance impairment (Belenky et al., 2003; Van Dongen, Maislin, Mullington, & Dinges, 2003). Similarly, with respect to extended wakefulness, performance impairment continues to increase in magnitude alongside extended wakefulness (Williamson & Feyer, 2000). Further, there are strong interactions between these variables and the circadian drive of alertness, meaning that, during the windows of circadian low, the effects of factors such as time awake or restricted sleep are amplified (Dawson & Reid, 1997).

1.4.2.3 Decision-Making Performance

Fatigue has also been shown to be associated with negative impacts on the decision-making process, again with specific implications for transport operations.

Firstly, fatigue has been shown to be associated with impairment of innovative thinking and flexible decision-making (Harrison & Horne, 1999). These forms of impairment have significant implications for transport operations where operators must respond, often under considerable time pressure, to novel situations, especially those relating to unexpected failures in technology. Recent research has highlighted the possible influence of fatigue on self-monitoring and self-regulatory processes, such as maintaining attention and avoiding distraction, suggesting a putative role of metacognitive processing in fatigue-related decision-making deficits (Aidman, Jackson, & Kleitman, 2019).

Fatigue is also associated with more subtle changes in decision-making, including shifts in risk perception and risk "appetite". Several studies have demonstrated an increase in risk taking and risky decision-making under conditions of sleep deprivation (Hockey, John Maule, Clough, & Bdzola, 2000; Killgore, Balkin, & Wesensten, 2006; Venkatraman, Chuah, Huettel, & Chee, 2007). However, research from simulator studies using real-world tasks, such as commercial aviation, suggests that this relationship might not be transferable to real-world settings where operators have been found to make more conservative decisions in the face of fatigue (Petrilli, Thomas, Lamond, Dawson, & Roach, 2007).

1.4.2.4 PSYCHOSOCIAL PERFORMANCE

Research has found a range of effects of fatigue on psychosocial domains such as mood, communication, and teamwork. These effects of fatigue on affective and interpersonal domains demonstrate both the true multi-dimensional impacts of fatigue on performance and the cascading effects from lower-order cognitive processes, such as response speed, through to the higher-order cognitive processes involved in the coordination of complex team activities in transportation operations.

With respect to mood in general, fatigue has been shown to have a range of negative effects, such as decreases in happiness and activation and increases in depressive mood (Paterson et al., 2011). Further, fatigue is associated with decreases in the ability of individuals to effectively regulate their emotions (Watling, Pawlik, Scott, Booth, & Short, 2017). Fatigue is also associated with amplified reactions to negative stimuli (Zohar, Tzischinsky, Epstein, & Lavie, 2005), and fatigued individuals may be more influenced by emotion in their collaborative decision-making processes than people who are well rested (Anderson & Dickinson, 2010). In the operational context of aviation, it has been demonstrated that fatigue is associated with an increased prevalence of negative affective states, including confusion, stress, and frustration (Drury, Ferguson, & Thomas, 2012).

Fatigue also has deleterious effects on speech and communication. From changes in speech intonation and speed (Harrison & Horne, 1997) to an increase in communication errors (Neville, Bisson, French, Boll, & Storm, 1994), fatigue has significant potential to impact effective information transfer, communication, and teamwork (Harrison & Horne, 2000). For transport operations, this has significant implications for all situations where communication and teamwork are critical, from maintaining normal crew coordination on the bridge of a cargo vessel during berthing operations to the identification of systems malfunctions and the generation of optimal solutions in emergency situations on the flight-deck.

1.4.3 REAL-WORLD JOB PERFORMANCE, RISK, AND SAFETY

The relationship between fatigue and performance in real-world transport operations is not simply one of performance impairment, and the relationship between fatigue, risk and safety outcomes is not nearly as straightforward as seen in the laboratory. Indeed, there are inherent limitations of the traditional deficit model of safety, and considerable scientific evidence relating to compensatory control, performance protection, and fatigue proofing strategies.

1.4.3.1 Association between Fatigue and Poor Safety Outcomes

Across all modes of transport, the acute effects of fatigue, resulting in unintended sleep episodes or microsleeps, are the most obvious and potentially most catastrophic of impacts. In the case of an unintended sleep episode or microsleep there is a clear and evident relationship between performance impairment and poor safety outcomes.

In the context of road transport, the impacts of fatigue on driver performance are well documented. For example, drivers are slower to react, pay less attention to other traffic and traffic signs, and are poorer in changing gears (Feyer & Williamson, 1995). In studies of train drivers, an association has been demonstrated between fatigue and poorer speed control (Dorrian, Roach, Fletcher, & Dawson, 2006), and increased fuel use (Dorrian, Hussey, & Dawson, 2007). Further, studies examining the operational impact of fatigue in commercial aviation have highlighted an overall increase in crew error rates, with fatigued crews making approximately twice as many errors per flight as non-fatigued crews (Thomas and Ferguson, 2010).

The more subtle impacts on individual and team performance relating to complex impacts of fatigue on, for example, situation awareness, problem identification, decision-making and teamwork are somewhat more difficult to establish definitively. However, the analysis of incidents and accidents across various modes of transport has established associations between fatigue and dynamic team performance in a number of instances (Strauch, 2015).

1.4.3.2 Compensatory Control, Performance Protection, and Fatigue Proofing

So far, this chapter has presented fatigue in the context of a *deficit* model of safety, whereby fatigue is seen in terms of deleterious effects including degraded performance and increased risk. However, in recent years, a more ecologically valid approach to fatigue in transport operations has highlighted a range of informal strategies used by operators when fatigued that in turn can be seen to enhance safety of operations. (For more on fatigue countermeasures, see Section 4 of this book.)

First, a set of countermeasures is often used by operators to combat the potential negative impacts of fatigue (and other factors such as low workload) on performance and safety. For instance, rest breaks and short naps are frequently utilised to mitigate the impacts of fatigue in transport operations (Hayashi, Motoyoshi, & Hori, 2005; Tucker, Folkard, & Macdonald, 2003). Similarly, and especially in the context of road transport, common countermeasures to fatigue include activities such as drinking coffee or other caffeinated drinks, adjusting the ventilation, eating sweets, and listening to the radio or music (Feyer & Williamson, 1995). While there is substantial evidence supporting the utility of caffeine use, the evidence supporting other alerting strategies such as opening windows and using loud music is equivocal at best (Schwarz et al., 2012).

Second, beyond the use of simple countermeasures, individuals and teams have also been shown to deploy processes of compensatory control, which involves the (re) allocation of resources dynamically (Hockey, 1997). In the face of fatigue, operators are able to conserve resources in times of low work demands, and conversely increase effort when required. In this way, the negative impacts of fatigue on performance are minimised through the dynamic allocation of effort. For instance, even in the face of considerable fatigue associated with long-haul airline operations, flight crew engage in activities to increase alertness and concentration for critical phases of flight such as approach and landing.

A range of other processes have been shown in studies of real-world operator performance to counteract the potentially negative influence of fatigue on performance and safety. For instance, even though fatigue has been shown to increase the rate at which pilots make errors during commercial aviation operations, fatigued pilots also increase the detection and management of error, ensuring no overall impact on operational safety (Thomas & Ferguson, 2010). Similarly, fatigued pilots, when faced with complex operational decisions, have been found to be more thorough in their decision-making processes, taking more factors into consideration and deliberating on potential solutions for longer periods of time than when not fatigued (Petrilli et al., 2007).

A range of other informal strategies have been observed across a range of transport operations that either reduce the likelihood of a fatigue-related error occurring, or facilitate the detection of a fatigue-related error happening. These so-called "fatigue proofing strategies" ensure that, even in the face of fatigue, safe operations are able to be maintained (Dawson, Chapman, & Thomas, 2012). Although often informal in their initial adoption, many of these strategies are able to be captured, and subsequently integrated into training programmes, such as Bridge Resource Management (maritime) or Crew Resource Management (aviation) (Dawson & Thomas, 2019).

1.4.4   SUMMARY AND CONCLUSIONS

In transport operations, fatigue poses a significant risk to safety, through a wide range of negative impacts on operator performance. When one is fatigued, basic physiological changes in central nervous system activity give rise to a considerable array of impacts on neurobehavioural performance, higher order cognitive functioning, and shifts in psychosocial performance that both individually and in combination pose a threat to safe and efficient performance.

Although fatigue is implicated in a significant proportion of incidents and accidents across all modes of transport, recent research has begun to underscore the ways in which both individuals and teams in transport operations actively respond to the ubiquitous threat of fatigue. From compensatory effort, performance protection strategies, and other fatigue proofing processes, the story of the impacts of fatigue on safety is significantly tempered by an emergent understanding of resilient and adaptive performance. Across all transportation modes, non-technical skills training programmes that formally develop competencies in fatigue proofing strategies offer a new focus for fatigue management beyond simply reducing the occurrence of fatigue or technological solutions to fatigue detection.

To this end, the future of safer transport systems must not only seek to mitigate the deficits in performance brought about by fatigue, but also to better understand and harness the mechanisms by which operators respond to and proactively mitigate the risks associated with fatigue in day-to-day transport operations.

SUMMARY POINTS FOR PRACTITIONERS

- Fatigue has wide-ranging effects on performance, ranging to difficulty maintaining wakefulness and microsleeps through to more subtle impacts on attention, reaction-time, and distractibility.
- The impacts of fatigue on performance not only affect the individual, but also influence teamwork through changes in mood, communication, and interpersonal interaction.
- In real-world contexts, the impacts of fatigue on performance are often mitigated through fatigue proofing strategies, whereby individuals and teams are able to deploy strategies to ensure their fatigue state does not impact their real-world task performance in a way that is a detriment to safety.

REFERENCES

Ahlstrom, C., Jansson, S., & Anund, A. (2017). Local changes in the wake electroencephalogram precedes lane departures. *Journal of Sleep Research, 26*(6), 816–819.

Aidman, E., Jackson, S. A., & Kleitman, S. (2019). Effects of sleep deprivation on executive functioning, cognitive abilities, metacognitive confidence, and decision making. *Applied Cognitive Psychology, 33*(2), 188–200.

Åkerstedt, T. (2000). Consensus statement: Fatigue and accidents in transport operations. *Journal of Sleep Research, 9*(4), 395–395.

Åkerstedt, T., & Folkard, S. (1997). The three-process model of alertness and its extension to performance, sleep latency, and sleep length. *Chronobiology International, 14*(2), 115–123.

Anderson, C., & Dickinson, D. L. (2010). Bargaining and trust: The effects of 36-h total sleep deprivation on socially interactive decisions. *Journal of Sleep Research, 19*(1-Part-I), 54–63. https://doi.org/10.1111/j.1365-2869.2009.00767.x

Anderson, C., & Horne, J. A. (2013). Driving drowsy also worsens driver distraction. *Sleep Medicine, 14*(5), 466–468. https://doi.org/10.1016/j.sleep.2012.11.014

Banks, S., & Dinges, D. F. (2007). Behavioral and physiological consequences of sleep restriction. *Journal of Clinical Sleep Medicine, 03*(05), 519–528. doi:10.5664/jcsm.26918

Belenky, G., Wesensten, N. J., Thorne, D. R., Thomas, M. L., Sing, H., Redmond, D. P.,.... Balkin, T. J. (2003). Patterns of performance degradation and restoration during sleep restriction and subsequent recovery: A sleep dose-response study. *Journal of Sleep Research, 12*, 1–12.

Binks, P. G., Waters, W. F., & Hurry, M. (1999). Short-term total sleep deprivations does not selectively impair higher cortical functioning. *Sleep, 22*(3), 328–334.

Borbély, A. A. (1982). A two-process model of sleep regulation. *Neurobiology, 1*,195–204.

Brown, I. D. (1994). Driver fatigue. *Human Factors, 36*(2), 298–314.

Dawson, D., Chapman, J., & Thomas, M. J. W. (2012). Fatigue proofing: A new approach to reducing fatigue-related risk using the principles of error management. *Sleep Medicine Reviews, 16*(2), 167–175.

Dawson, D., & Reid, K. (1997). Fatigue, alcohol and performance impairment. *Nature, 388*, 235.

Dawson, D., Sprajcer, M., & Thomas, M. (2021). How much sleep do you need? A comprehensive review of fatigue related impairment and the capacity to work or drive safely. *Accident Analysis and Prevention, 151*, 105955. doi:https://doi.org/10.1016/j.aap.2020.105955

Dawson, D., & Thomas, M. J. W. (2019). Fatigue management in practice–It's just good teamwork. *Sleep Medicine Reviews, 48*.

Dinges, D. F., & Kribbs, N. B. (1991). Performing while sleepy: Effects of experimentally-induced sleepiness. In T. H. Monk (Ed.), *Sleep, Sleepiness and Performance* (pp. 97–128). Oxford, England: John Wiley & Sons.

Dinges, D. F., Pack, F., Williams, K. B., Gillen, K. A., Powell, J. W., Ott, G. E.,... . Pack, A. I. (1997). Cumulative sleepiness, mood disturbance, and psychomotor vigilance performance decrements during a week of sleep restricted to 4–5 hours per night. *Sleep, 20*(4), 267–277.

Dorrian, J., Hussey, F., & Dawson, D. (2007). Train driving efficiency and safety: Examining the cost of fatigue. *Journal of Sleep Research, 16*(1), 1–11.

Dorrian, J., Roach, G. D., Fletcher, A., & Dawson, D. (2006). The effects of fatigue on train handling during speed restrictions. *Transportation Research Part F: Traffic Psychology and Behaviour, 9*(4), 243–257.

Drury, D. A., Ferguson, S. A., & Thomas, M. J. W. (2012). Restricted sleep and negative affective states in commercial pilots during short haul operations. *Accident Analysis and Prevention, 45S*, 80–84.

Duffy, J. F., & Czeisler, C. A. (2002). Age-related change in the relationship between circadian period, circadian phase, and diurnal preference in humans. *Neuroscience Letters, 318*(3), 117–120.

Durmer, J. S., & Dinges, D. F. (2005). Neurocognitive consequences of sleep deprivation. *Seminars in Neurology, 25*(1), 117–129. doi:10.1055/s-2005-867080

Ferguson, S. A., Paech, G. M., Sargent, C., Darwent, D., Kennaway, D. J., & Roach, G. D. (2012). The influence of circadian time and sleep dose on subjective fatigue ratings. *Accident Analysis and Prevention, 45*, 50–54.

Feyer, A.-M., & Williamson, A. M. (1995). The influence of operational conditions on driver fatigue in the long distance road transport industry in Australia. *International Journal of Industrial Ergonomics, 15*(4), 229–235.

Harrison, Y., & Horne, J. A. (1997). Sleep deprivation affects speech. *Sleep, 20*(10), 871–877.

Harrison, Y., & Horne, J. A. (1999). One night of sleep loss impairs innovative thinking and flexible decision making. *Organizational Behavior and Human Decision Processes, 78*(2), 128–145. doi:10.1006/obhd.1999.2827

Harrison, Y., & Horne, J. A. (2000). The impact of sleep deprivation on decision-making: A review. *Journal of Experimental Psychology: Applied, 6*, 236–249.

Hayashi, M., Motoyoshi, N., & Hori, T. (2005). Recuperative power of a short daytime nap with or without stage 2 sleep. *Sleep, 28*(7), 829–836.

Hockey, G. R. J. (1997). Compensatory control in the regulation of human performance under stress and high workload: A cognitive-energetical framework. *Biological Psychology, 45*, 73–93.

Hockey, G. R. J., John Maule, A., Clough, P. J., & Bdzola, L. (2000). Effects of negative mood states on risk in everyday decision making. *Cognition and Emotion, 14*(6), 823–855. doi:10.1080/02699930050156654

Horne, J. A., & Reyner, L. A. (1995). Sleep related vehicle accidents. *BMJ, 310*(6979), 565–567. doi:10.1136/bmj.310.6979.565

Horne, J. A., & Reyner, L. A. (1999). Vehicle accidents related to sleep: A review. *Occupational and Environmental Medicine, 56*(5), 289. http://dx.doi.org/10.1136/oem.56.5.289

Kecklund, G., & Åkerstedt, T. (1993). Sleepiness in long distance truck driving: An ambulatory EEG study of night driving. *Ergonomics, 36*(9), 1007–1017. doi:10.1080/00140139308967973

Killgore, W. D., Balkin, T. J., & Wesensten, N. J. (2006). Impaired decision making following 49 h of sleep deprivation. *Journal of Sleep Research, 15*(1), 7–13.

Lal, S. K., & Craig, A. (2002). Driver fatigue: Electroencephalography and psychological assessment. *Psychophysiology, 39*(3), 313–321.

Lee, J., Manousakis, J., Fielding, J., & Anderson, C. (2015). Alcohol and sleep restriction combined reduces vigilant attention, whereas sleep restriction alone enhances distractibility. *Sleep, 38*(5), 765–775.

Mascord, D. J., & Heath, R. A. (1992). Behavioral and physiological indices of fatigue in a visual tracking task. *Journal of Safety Research, 23*, 19–25.

Neville, K. J., Bisson, R. U., French, J., Boll, P. A., & Storm, W. F. (1994). Subjective fatigue of C-141 aircrews during Operation Desert Storm. *Human Factors, 36*(2), 339–349.

Pack, A. I., Pack, A. M., Rodgman, E., Cucchiara, A., Dinges, D. F., & Schwab, C. W. (1995). Characteristics of crashes attributed to the driver having fallen asleep. *Accident Analysis and Prevention, 27*(6), 769–775.

Paterson, J. L., Dorrian, J., Ferguson, S. A., Jay, S. M., Lamond, N., Murphy, P. J., Philip, P., & Dawson, D. (2011). Changes in structural aspects of mood during 39–66h of sleep loss using matched controls. *Applied Ergonomics, 42*(2), 196–201. https://doi.org/10.1016/j.apergo.2010.06.014

Petrilli, R. M., Thomas, M. J. W., Lamond, N., Dawson, D., & Roach, G. D. (2007). Effects of flight duty and sleep on the decision-making of commercial airline pilots. In J. M. Anca (Ed.), *Multimodal Safety Management and Human Factors* (pp. 259–270). Aldershot, UK: Ashgate.

Powell, D., Spencer, M. B., Holland, D., Broadbent, E., & Petrie, K. J. (2007). Pilot fatigue in short-haul operations: Effects of number of sectors, duty length, and time of day. *Aviation, Space, and Environmental Medicine, 78*(7), 698–701.

Schwarz, J. F., Ingre, M., Fors, C., Anund, A., Kecklund, G., Taillard, J., Philip, P., & Åkerstedt, T. (2012). In-car countermeasures open window and music revisited on the real road: Popular but hardly effective against driver sleepiness. *Journal of Sleep Research, 21*(5), 595–599.

Strauch, B. (2015). Investigating fatigue in marine accident investigations. *Procedia Manufacturing, 3*, 3115–3122. doi:https://doi.org/10.1016/j.promfg.2015.07.859

Summala, H., Hakkanen, H., Mikkola, T., & Sinkkonen, J. (1999). Task effects on fatigue symptoms in overnight driving. *Ergonomics, 42*(6), 798–806.

Thomas, M., Sing, H., Belenky, G., Holcomb, H., Mayberg, H., Dannals, R., Wagner Jr, H., Thorne, D., Popp, K., & Rowland, L. (2000). Neural basis of alertness and cognitive performance impairments during sleepiness. I. Effects of 24 h of sleep deprivation on waking human regional brain activity. *Journal of Sleep Research, 9*(4), 335–352.

Thomas, M. J. W., & Ferguson, S. A. (2010). Prior sleep, prior wake, and crew performance during normal flight operations. *Aviation, Space and Environmental Medicine, 81*, 665–670.

Tucker, P., Folkard, S., & Macdonald, I. (2003). Rest breaks and accident risk. *Lancet, 361*, 680.

Van Dongen, H. P., Maislin, G., Mullington, J. M., & Dinges, D. F. (2003). The cumulative cost of additional wakefulness: Dose-response effects on neurobehavioral functions and sleep physiology from chronic sleep restriction and total sleep deprivation. *Sleep, 26*(2), 117–126.

Venkatraman, V., Chuah, Y. L., Huettel, S. A., & Chee, M. W. (2007). Sleep deprivation elevates expectation of gains and attenuates response to losses following risky decisions. *Sleep, 30*(5), 603–609.

Watling, J., Pawlik, B., Scott, K., Booth, S., & Short, M. A. (2017). Sleep loss and affective functioning: More than just mood. *Behavioral Sleep Medicine, 15*(5), 394–409. doi:10.1080/15402002.2016.1141770

Williamson, A. M., & Feyer, A. M. (2000). Moderate sleep deprivation produces impairments in cognitive and motor performance equivalent to legally presribed levels of alcohol intoxication. *Occupational and Environmental Medicine, 57*(10), 649–655.

Zohar, D., Tzischinsky, O., Epstein, R., & Lavie, P. (2005). The effects of sleep loss on medical residents' emotional reactions to work events: A cognitive-energy model. *Sleep, 28*(1), 47–54. doi:10.1093/sleep/28.1.47

1.5 A Practical Human Factors Method for Developing Successful Fatigue Countermeasures

Ashleigh J. Filtness[1] and Anna Anund[2–4]

[1]Transport Safety Research Centre, Loughborough University, Loughborough, Leicestershire, UK
[2]Swedish National Road and Transport Research Institute, Linköping, Sweden
[3]Linköping University, Linköping, Sweden
[4]Stockholm University, Stockholm, Sweden

CONTENTS

This chapter provides an easy-to-follow method to evaluate a company's fatigue situation, understand the problem areas, and propose countermeasures that are targeted to be most likely to succeed. A case study example of London bus drivers is used to illustrate this approach. Countermeasures are any actions taken to counteract, minimise, or manage fatigue in the workplace.

DOI: 10.1201/9781003213154-7

1.5.1 FATIGUE AND SLEEPINESS: TWO INTERACTING COMPONENTS

In order to manage driver fatigue in transportation it is important to understand the underlying reasons behind fatigue and to recognise that most often fatigue is caused by multiple factors. When designing countermeasures, it is vital that the proposed approach is targeted at the specific problem (cause of fatigue). Defining fatigue itself is difficult with definitions encompassing a broad range of elements. In this chapter we consider fatigue and sleepiness to be two related and interacting concepts and argue that effective countermeasures can only be introduced if their distinction is recognised in order to apply the most appropriate countermeasure for the problem.

Sleepiness: Every person will get sleepy during a 24-hour period because sleep is an everyday biological need. As such, there is potential for all employees within the transport industry to experience sleepiness at some point. This is different from other transportation-related impairments, for example, alcohol, which are directly within the drivers' control through choice whether to engage or not. The feeling of sleepiness is influenced by how long it has been since a person last slept (homeostatic pressure) and their body clock (circadian rhythm) (Åkerstedt, Ingre, Kecklund, Folkard, & Axelsson, 2008). Sleepiness is therefore very specific and can only be mitigated by sleep itself or influencing biology such as with products containing the chemical compound caffeine which acts on the brain.

Fatigue: This is a much broader concept with many causes. Sleepiness itself may increase fatigue. Other causes include task-related factors such as highly demanding situations (active fatigue), for example, completing a secondary task at the same time as the primary task, as well as low demanding task situations (passive fatigue). For example, undertaking an activity for a long period of time or monotony (May and Baldwin, 2009).

In their model of fatigue (Figure 1.5.1), May and Baldwin (2009) recognise two types of fatigue: fatigue induced by the task itself and sleep-related fatigue.

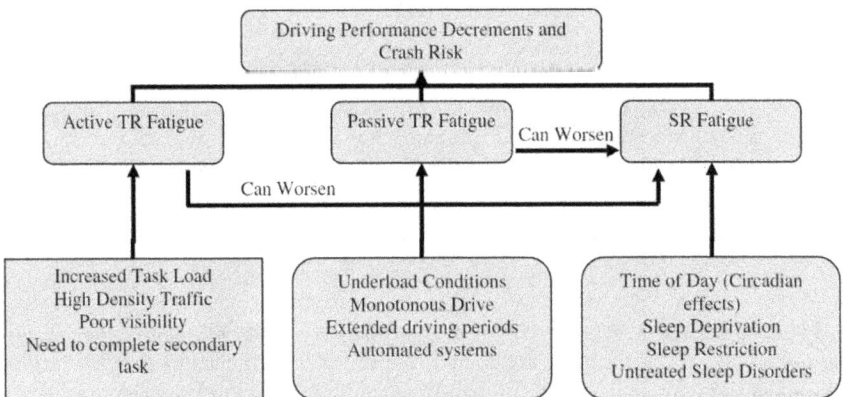

FIGURE 1.5.1 A model of fatigue (May and Baldwin, 2009, reproduced with permission). 'TR' = task-related; 'SR' = sleep-related.

May and Baldwin (2009) go on to note that although performance decrements may be similar for each type of fatigue it is important to determine the source of the fatigue as appropriate countermeasures will differ depending on the underlying causation. For example, taking a break when feeling fatigued can be beneficial because it allows space to rest and recover. However, if a person is sleepy, they will retain this sleepiness through a period of rest because rest alone is not enough to mitigate sleepiness; in this case, a nap or caffeine would be more beneficial. To go further still, it is necessary to also understand the sleep structure within a nap in order to most effectively reduce sleepiness. That is, either a nap should be short (10 to 15 minutes) in order to avoid entering deep sleep, or most optimal is to sleep for approximately 90 minutes corresponding to a full sleep cycle, thereby reducing the likelihood of sleep inertia on waking in both cases. Ultimately, the aim of any countermeasures should be to increase alertness and appropriately minimise the relevant underlying causes of the impairment.

1.5.2　SAFETY CRITICAL SITUATIONS

The important issue is not fatigue itself, but rather when and where fatigue occurs. Feeling fatigued is a natural part of human life. If a person is fatigued while watching TV at home in the evening, then that is not necessarily a problem; in contrast, feeling fatigued while driving a truck on the motorway can have catastrophic consequences.

Sleepiness can be particularly devastating within the driving context. It is widely reported that individuals are able to recognise their own increasing sleepiness (Cai et al., 2021), even if they are unable to detect an exact moment of "falling asleep" (Anund & Åkerstedt, 2010). Experiencing any signs of sleepiness should be enough for a driver to take action (Anund & Åkerstedt, 2010); however, many drivers continue their journey despite feeling sleepy. For example, it has been reported that nearly 70% of people continue to drive when they know they are sleepy (Watling et al., 2016), although their reasons for doing so might differ. Unfortunately, because sleep is a biological need, when it reaches critical level, the brain will sleep regardless of any effort to remain awake. This is often described as a microsleep. Considering a microsleep of 2 seconds travelling on a motorway at 70 miles per hour, a vehicle can travel approximately 205 feet or 62 m in that time without a driver being in full control. During this time if a driver is unresponsive, they will take no evasive action to avoid a crash; as such, collision with any object will be at the original travel speed with no effort to apply the brakes. This is why sleep-related crashes are often at high speed and of high severity (Filtness et al., 2017).

The frequency of microsleeps increases the sleepier a person gets. Microsleeps are not uniform across the brain's structures; rather, they can appear in local parts of the brain, such as the visual cortex, where an overload is prevalent. This means that a person can have localised microsleeps in parts of the brain that are essential for driving without knowing it (Ahlstrom, Jansson, & Anund, 2017).

Lack of sleep impacts a wide range of performance and attention processes, such as response accuracy and speed (Dorrian & Dinges, 2006), reaction time (Bougard et al., 2016), difficulty remaining focused, keeping up to date and grasping fast changing information (Horne, 2012), and lapses in attention (Durmer & Dinges, 2005). An interesting feature of sleep loss is its impact on reaction time. Fast reaction times are important for safe driving. Taken on an average, reaction time is something that slows with increasing sleepiness; however, looking in detail, it is apparent that this relationship is not linear. The true influence of sleepiness is an increase in response performance variability, which leads to a mean slowing of reactions. While an alert person may have consistent fast reactions, the same person when sleepy will have some reactions that are equivalent to those when they were alert, but they will also have other reaction times that are much slower. It is not that every reaction is slowed, but rather that some specific reactions may be significantly slowed. Figure 1.5.2 shows an individual's reaction times to a Psychomotor Vigilance Task (PVT). The PVT is a 10-minute-long reaction time task that requires the participant to respond by pressing a button as soon as they see a stimulus on-screen. The dark grey line shows reaction times when the participant was alert after a normal 7- to 8-hour sleep; the light grey line shows the same individual's performance after sleep restriction to 5 hours. It is apparent that even when sleepy some of the participant's responses are within a similar duration to those when the participant is alert; however, there is an increasing number of reaction times that are noticeably slower, including nine occurrences of reaction time slower than 500 ms, which would be considered a "lapse".

When designing countermeasures, it is important to recognise that fatigue-related impairment is not uniform. Rather, the more fatigue an individual experiences, the greater the variability in their responses. Therefore, within the context of driving,

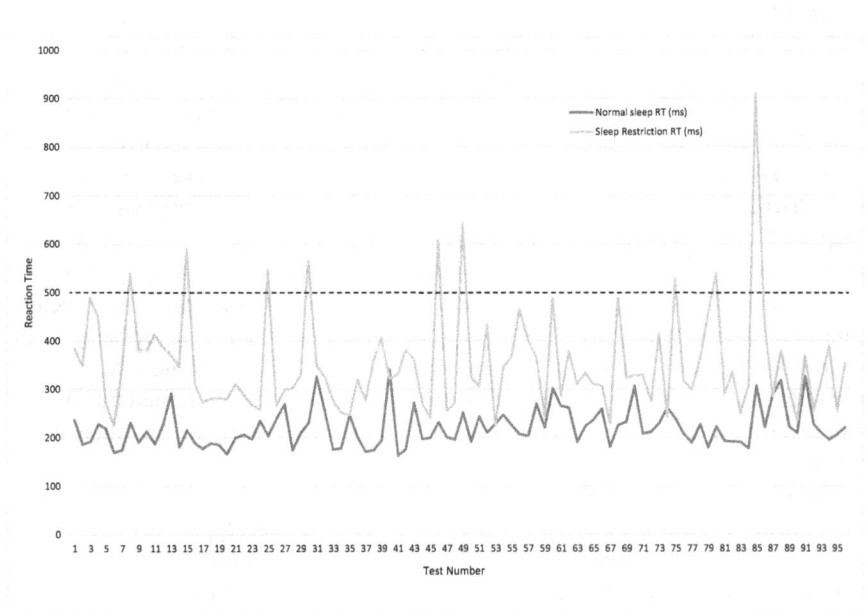

FIGURE 1.5.2 Psychomotor vigilance task reactions over 10 minutes for one participant following normal sleep (dark grey line) and following sleep restriction to 5 hours (light grey line). Duration of 500 ms is indicated by dotted line to show lapses. (Source: a single participant's PVT reaction time from Shenfield et al., 2020.)

the most effective countermeasures will always be those that prevent fatigue from occurring at all (Haddon, 1972).

1.5.3 SUCCESSFUL COUNTERMEASURE SELECTION

Workplace-related fatigue is a unique occupational risk. While most workplace hazards are confined within a work setting, the causes of fatigue are not (Gander et al., 2011). As both work-related and non-work-related factors influence fatigue, the remit for potential countermeasures is broad. There is also a balance that some countermeasures may be considered as potential to influence non-work-related factors rather than control that might be apparent towards work-related factors. In order to invoke a successful countermeasure, it is necessary to recognise who a countermeasure might be best targeted towards and for what duration of time that countermeasure should be deployed. It is the responsibility of an individual driver to turn up fit for work, but the employer also has a responsibility to ensure that their occupational setting is established in a way that best promotes alertness. As such, some countermeasures may be targeted towards the driver, while others may be targeted towards the manager or broader workplace setting. In either case, for the countermeasure to be successful it must be effective at changing existing behaviour. At the same time, it is important to be aware of individual differences, and not to expect that drivers or managers will be identical. Their knowledge, motivation, and possibility to act to avoid fatigue differ.

One approach to categorising countermeasures is to consider the timeframe from detecting the fatigue that the countermeasure should be deployed in. Taking timeframe as the basis of definition, strategic, tactical, and operational, countermeasure deployment can be equated to long, mid, and short timeframes (see Table 1.5.1). It is likely that the most effective approach to fatigue management will include countermeasures at each level and some countermeasures targeting aspects across multiple levels. For example, establishing a system that allows the possibility to substitute a well-rested driver, if needed, is a strategic countermeasure. But if a driver is detected as being fatigued during a shift and an alternative driver is sent out to replace them, this would be an operational countermeasure at the point of enactment.

TABLE 1.5.1

Timeframe of Deployment for Strategic, Tactical, and Operational Countermeasures Informed by the Work of EC Commissioned Project PANACEA (Grant Agreement 953426)

	Strategic	Tactical	Operational
Timeframe from impairment that countermeasure is deployed	Long term—requiring ongoing engagement for prolonged period after the shift impairment is detected	Mid term—soon after but not during the shift impairment is detected	Short term—occurring during the shift when impairment is detected

Strategic countermeasures are those concerned with long-term behavioural change. This may be a behaviour change at a driver or a company level and will usually require ongoing engagement. The behaviour to be influenced by the counter-measure can occur at any point: on-shift, during driving, or between shifts. Examples include lifestyle coaching (advice on changing lifestyle to minimise fatigue), hours of service (HoS) regulations, and fatigue risk management systems (FRMS).

Tactical countermeasures are those concerned with the short- to mid-term coun-termeasure requirement, but not requiring the deployment of the countermeasure on the shift where the impairment was detected. Often tactical countermeasures will seek to reduce the chance that a driver will arrive, or become, impaired on-shift. Examples include shift scheduling that is informed by a biomathematical model, advice on man-aging fatigue while commuting to work, and occupational health/medical assessment.

Operational countermeasures are those concerned with the here and now. They are actions that need to take place during a shift (between clocking on and clocking off for shift, break times within a shift included), within a short timeframe of the impairment being detected. Examples include in-vehicle fatigue alerts, napping, and use of caffeine.

Any selected countermeasures should target a specific cause of fatigue. However, it is not enough to make a recommendation for a particular countermeasure without also ensuring that the countermeasure is usable and acceptable to the target audience. As such, stakeholder engagement throughout any process to develop countermeasures is essential. For example, a commonly identified countermeasure is education for drivers. However, in practice education alone will not have a desired impact unless drivers are able to recognise when they are fatigued, feel motivated to do

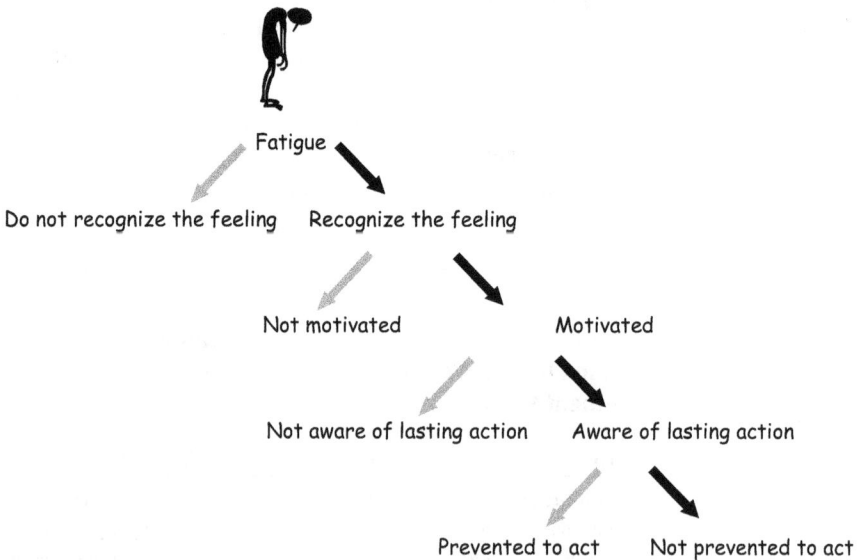

FIGURE 1.5.3 The chain of decisions relating to countermeasure use and driver fatigue (Anund, Fors, Kecklund, Leeuwen & Åkerstedt, 2015).

something, and are not prevented from applying what they have learnt (Figure 1.5.3). Continued stakeholder engagement will help to identify any potential barriers so that recommended countermeasures can be adapted to best suit the needs of the industry under consideration.

A major limitation of selecting successful countermeasures is a lack of randomised control trials (RCTs). RCTs use a method for evaluating an intervention in which participants are randomly allocated to a group receiving an intervention, or to a control group not receiving an intervention. Randomisation ensures that the allocation of groups is unbiased, allowing scientific control over external influences of outcome in order to remove confounding factors. However, RCTs are costly to achieve, practically difficult in a workplace setting, and are rarely undertaken in driver fatigue research. Without this type of investigation, there will always be limitations in understanding how effective driver fatigue countermeasures truly are. This is a limitation of the research field that is yet to be overcome.

1.5.4   A HUMAN FACTORS APPROACH TO DEVELOPING COUNTERMEASURES TO FATIGUE/SLEEPINESS

We have conducted multiple investigations that have ended in recommendations of countermeasures for fatigue. Each time we have approached the situation using a systematic human factors approach. We share the approach here, as it may be useful to others embarking on similar investigations.

A central consideration is the perspective of "the user in the loop". This is a term which has origins in technology solutions, but here we use it more broadly, in that user engagement is necessary in developing countermeasures. This should ideally include target users at all levels of a workplace that may interact with the countermeasures, for example, drivers, driver managers, shift schedulers, and health and safety managers.

Step 1: Take time to understand the situation. It is important to distinguish between written practice and what is happening day to day. For example, there may be a situation where a company has a suitable documented fatigue management policy, but in reality, employees may not be aware of or follow this. To get a full picture of the situation, multiple data collection activities are needed. Each data collection exercise should be planned around appropriate research questions designed to achieve the ultimate aim of understanding the current fatigue situation. Data collection activities may include:

- review of policy documents;
- talking to drivers (focus groups or interviews);
- examining shift patterns (could run shifts through different biomathematical models);
- shadowing (accompanying) a driver at work;
- observing driver training;
- talking to managers (focus groups or interviews);
- conducting an anonymous survey of drivers (separate to talking to drivers as anonymity increases honesty in response).

From each data collection activity, a set of key findings should be identified.

Step 2: Synthesise findings into key insights. Insights are the elements that provide new information about the fatigue situation, indicating where countermeasures may be beneficial. Insights are often combinations of several findings across the different data collection activities. For example, identifying what key issues came up in each data collection activity, then what this means to the management of fatigue and why this matters. The process of translating findings into insights should identify all of the fatigue-related problems and what is contributing to these problems.

Step 3: Map potential solutions onto identified problems. For each identified problem/contributor to fatigue, identify a potential solution. The potential solutions should be informed by current research literature and existing best practice. They could be generated through discussion with fatigue management experts. Countermeasure solutions need to match the cause of fatigue. For example, a countermeasure appropriate for task-related fatigue will not be beneficial if the problem is caused by a lack of sleep. We find that this step works best through group discussion of all those involved in the data collection, as a group dynamic can reveal varied perspectives. Once a full list of potential solutions is generated, it is important to review and combine where appropriate. For example, it may be that some countermeasure solutions are appropriate for multiple problems. Consider the strengths and weaknesses of each countermeasure solution, and discount those with little or no potential to reduce driver fatigue. Group similar types of countermeasures under a common theme. Consider the feasibility of implementing each countermeasure. Difficult to implement countermeasures should not be excluded, but this process will likely help prioritise the countermeasures that should be implemented first. Recommended countermeasures should have a multi-level approach that is in line with the consensus statement from the Working Time Society on managing sleep-related fatigue associated with non-standard working hours (Wong, Popkin & Folkard, 2019).

Step 4: Implement countermeasures and review. Ideally, this is a continuous process in which the recommended countermeasures are implemented, more data are collected, the delivery of these countermeasures is reviewed, and finally the countermeasures are enhanced.

1.5.5 CASE STUDY: LONDON BUS DRIVER FATIGUE

This case study is a real-world example of the steps outlined in sub-section 1.5.4 for London city bus drivers. Full details of the outcome of this work can be found in Filtness et al. (2019).

1.5.5.1 CONTEXT

This work was funded by Transport for London (TfL), which sought independent research services to understand the situation in terms of the extent and nature of fatigue, contributing factors to fatigue, and identification of countermeasure solutions to address fatigue in London city bus drivers. There are over 9 000 buses operating in London on approximately 700 different routes. Over a year this equates to approximately 2.5 billion passengers transported, by approximately 25 000 bus drivers (TfL n.d.). The bus network is provided by ten independent operating companies, which are all contracted to provide their service to TfL. The network operates 24 hours per day, meaning that bus drivers are shift workers, which increases vulnerability to fatigue due to sleep disturbance (Åkerstedt, 1991).

1.5.5.2 Understand the Situation (Step 1)

A targeted literature review focusing on bus driver fatigue and best practice in fatigue countermeasures was conducted alongside five data collection activities: review of policy documents, focus groups with bus drivers, interviews with bus driver managers, anonymous survey of bus drivers, and on-road observation study. However, at the time of the data collection, none of the operating companies had a specific fatigue management policy that could be included in the review. Data collection took place in 2018.

Focus groups were conducted with a total of 65 drivers. One group was held at each company. The main research questions were: Is fatigue a problem for bus drivers? If so, what causes fatigue? And how do drivers manage their fatigue?

Interviews with 11 bus driver managers were also completed, at least one per company. The main research questions were: Do managers believe that fatigue is a problem? If so, how is it being managed (by drivers and operators)?

The anonymous survey was completed by 1 353 drivers. It was open to all bus drivers from all bus operating companies. The main research questions were: What is the prevalence of fatigue? What are the key contributing factors to fatigue?

The on-road observation included 16 drivers from one company. Each driver was observed twice while driving the same route at different times of day. The main research questions were: Does time of day (early vs. day shift) influence sleep prior to shift, self-reported sleepiness and stress during shift, and physiological indicators of sleepiness?

1.5.5.3 Key Insights (Step 2)

The first key finding was that London bus drivers do experience driver fatigue. Until this data collection, there were some people in the industry who believed that the active task of regularly stopping and starting a city bus promoted alertness and therefore fatigue would not be prevalent. In all focus groups, drivers discussed experiences of fatigue (Maynard et al., 2021). From the survey, 21% of participants stated that they have had to fight sleepiness at least two to three times every week, with 36% of participants reporting having had a "close call" due to fatigue in the previous 12 months (Miller et al., 2020).

Other key findings related to identifying the contributors to fatigue. Overall, a wide range of factors were identified as contributing to fatigue, summarised under five themes. Not every driver reported experiencing every contributing factor, and the impact of any particular factor varied among drivers and for the same driver at different times.

Management of sleep, particularly prior to early shifts, was reported to be a problem in the survey, and was recorded prior to the on-road observation, where the average amount of sleep that drivers reported getting prior to an early shift was only 4 hours and 50 minutes. Linked to this factor, *scheduling issues*, such as shift irregularity and duration of time off between shifts, was also a reported problem. Shifts did not start at a uniform time (varying on a minute-by-minute basis), and it was difficult for drivers to adjust their bedtime to a similar level of detail to obtain sufficient seep. *Facilities for rest* at work were identified as a potential problem, for instance, because the lack of access to a toilet impacted how drivers chose to manage their fatigue (or not) (i.e., by avoiding drinking beverages containing caffeine). The *disciplinary culture* of many workplaces led to drivers not reporting fatigue. Of those survey participants who had had a sleep-related road crash while driving a bus, 77% said that their employer would not know that fatigue had contributed to the crash. Finally, *work stress and overall health* were reported by drivers as contributing to their fatigue. Several stressors were reported in the focus groups, including interactions with passengers and with service controllers over the radio.

1.5.5.4 MAP SOLUTIONS TO PROBLEMS (STEP 3)

As a result of step 3, five main areas for potential countermeasures were identified aligning with the five key findings of data collection.

Education: To limit fatigue, a major focus should be on education of drivers around the importance of good quality sleep and their responsibility to manage their own sleep; however, education should extend beyond this to also include families, managers, shift schedulers, and company personnel more broadly. This countermeasure addresses the key findings of management of sleep. This is an example of a tactical countermeasure that may become strategic, if it becomes an embedded element of workplace practices which translates into lifestyle changes. A one-time education programme may be considered to be a tactical countermeasure, but if it is further developed into lifestyle coaching, then it would become strategic.

Working conditions: To manage fatigue in drivers, it was recommended to provide suitable facilities for drivers to eat and rest—for example, providing a place for drivers to rest during shifts, rather than requiring them to take breaks in a bus stop. This countermeasure addresses the key finding of facilities for rest. From the drivers' point of view, using a rest facility during a shift is an example of an operational countermeasure. From the company point of view, changing the workplace culture so that drivers have access to and are willing to use rest facilities would be considered a strategic countermeasure as it is related to long-term behavioural change.

Schedules and rosters: To minimise fatigue and maximise drivers' opportunities for sleep, incorporating fatigue considerations when designing shift schedules was recommended. At the time of data collection, the majority of schedules were being designed based on the most cost-efficient delivery of the service and did not take fatigue into account. Scheduling should follow best practice in shift design, for example, using forward shift rotations (those that change from, e.g., morning, to afternoon, to evening shifts) and allowing a minimum of 11 hours off between shifts. It is also recommended to consider individual needs in relation to commuting time as well as other factors like childcare and family situation. These countermeasures address the key findings related to scheduling. Changes to scheduling are considered a tactical countermeasure that is instigated by the company.

Open culture: One of the biggest barriers to fatigue management is a lack of recognition that fatigue is a problem. This was the case for London bus drivers. It is not surprising that some companies were unaware that fatigue was a problem for their drivers, as drivers were not comfortable in telling their employer when they were struggling with fatigue. If fatigue is not talked about, then it will be impossible to effectively manage. Developing an open culture will allow drivers to report fatigue so that they and their companies can work together to reduce fatigue. Part of this culture should include a reporting system whereby drivers are able to easily report when they are feeling fatigued, so that this information can be used for strategic and operational countermeasures. At an operational level, managers could respond by deploying a countermeasure; at a strategic level, ongoing, long term examination of these reports could identify common causes of fatigue and monitor the impact of countermeasures. This countermeasure addresses the findings around disciplinary culture. Changing a disciplinary culture to an open one is a strategic countermeasure.

Health: Improving driver health is an important goal that comprises several sub-countermeasures. For example, a tactical countermeasure would be to provide health screening, particularly for obstructive sleep apnoea as this sleep disorder is commonly experienced and when untreated reduces daytime alertness (see Chapter 3.3). Driver stress and general health are also associated with fatigue at work. A tactical solution for a company could be to provide opportunities for drivers to buy healthy food options at the depot. However, to maintain long-term driver health mitigations for fatigue, they would need to be addressed with a strategic countermeasure such as lifestyle coaching.

1.5.5.5 Implement Countermeasures and Review (Step 4)

Ultimately, the final decision on what countermeasures to implement is made by senior managers. But that decision should be informed by research. In the case of London bus driving, the following commitments were made after the work was completed:

- TfL will introduce a requirement for fatigue risk management systems for any company that operates London buses under new contracts.
- TfL will ensure that all managers have undertaken fatigue training.
- TfL will make £500,000 available to help bus operating companies undertake further work to establish the most effective interventions to reduce fatigue.
- All rosters will be reviewed by bus operating companies against best practice to reduce the risk of fatigue.
- TfL and bus operating companies will ensure that driver representatives are given the opportunity to be trained in fatigue management.

- There will be a greater focus among senior TfL executives on the health and well-being of drivers.
- TfL will foster a more open and honest culture across the industry.

As a research team we have continued to share our findings and share our experiences.

1.5.6   CONCLUSION

For any approach to fatigue management to be effective there is a need for shared responsibility. A wide range of involved parties will be most influential, including drivers (and their families), managers, companies, regulators, unions, and enforcement agencies. Within fatigue management there can be a tendency to put all the onus on the driver without putting in place the support systems to empower the drivers to manage their own alertness. It is therefore especially important to consider all parties when designing and implementing fatigue countermeasures.

Different drivers will experience differing causes of fatigue, and within fatigue management, not all solutions will work for all people. Therefore, a multi-countermeasure holistic approach will yield best results. There is no quick fix for reducing fatigue; a long-term commitment is needed. If a countermeasure is to be successful, it is important to not give up too early. All countermeasures should be periodically reviewed and adjusted, as needed. The ideal evaluation would be to undertake an RCT during the implementation of countermeasures. If this is not possible, then monitoring of change over time can also be beneficial. As a research area there is a current lack of robust evidence supporting the effectiveness of many countermeasures.

Open company culture is essential to successful fatigue management. Fatigue is a personal experience and there is currently no 100% accurate way to measure it. As such, management of fatigue relies on open and honest discussions between drivers and their employers. These discussions cannot take place unless there is trust and openness within the company. For industries coming from a discipline culture, transition to open culture can be difficult to achieve and often takes considerable time. A step-by-step approach is likely to be most beneficial.

SUMMARY POINTS FOR PRACTITIONERS

- Taking a systematic approach to understand the situation, synthesise findings into key insights, map solutions to problems, implement countermeasures and review is the most effective way to introduce fatigue countermeasures.
- To be effective, countermeasures must be targeted towards the specific cause(s) of fatigue.
- Knowing the difference between sleepiness and fatigue will help in developing appropriate countermeasures.
- Fatigue management is everyone's responsibility; countermeasures should be targeted across all parties, for example, drivers, companies, and regulators.
- There is no single solution to fatigue; instead, a range of countermeasures should be put forward, including strategic (long-term), tactical (medium-term), and operational (short-term) options.

REFERENCES

Ahlstrom, C., Jansson, S., & Anund, A. (2017). Local changes in the wake electroencephalogram precedes lane departures. *Journal of Sleep Research*, *26*(6), 816–819.

Åkerstedt, T. (1991). Shift work and sleep disturbances. *Sleep and Health Risk* (pp. 265–278). Springer.

Åkerstedt, T., Ingre, M., Kecklund, G., Folkard, S., & Axelsson, J. (2008). Accounting for partial sleep deprivation and cumulative sleepiness in the three-process model of alertness regulation. *Chronobiology International*, *25*(2–3), 309–319.

Anund, A., & Akerstedt, T. (2010). Perception of sleepiness before falling asleep. *Sleep Medicine*, *8*(11), 743–744.

Anund, A., Fors, C., Kecklund, G., Leeuwen, W. V., & Åkerstedt, T. (2015). *Countermeasures for fatigue in transportation: A review of existing methods for drivers on road, rail, sea and in aviation.* Linköping: Swedish National Road and Transport Research Institute (VTI).

Bougard, C., Moussay, S., Espié, S., & Davenne, D. (2016). The effects of sleep deprivation and time of day on cognitive performance. *Biological Rhythm Research*, *47*(3), 401–415.

Cai, A. W., Manousakis, J. E., Lo, T., Horne, J. A., Howard, M. E., & Anderson, C. (2021). I think I'm sleepy, therefore I am–Awareness of sleepiness while driving: A systematic review. *Sleep Medicine Reviews*, 101533.

Dorrian, J., & Dinges, D. F. (2006). Sleep deprivation and its effects on cognitive performance. In T. Lee-Chiong (Ed). *Encyclopedia of Sleep Medicine* (pp. 139–143). NJ: John Wiley & Sons.

Durmer, J. S., & Dinges, D. F. (2005, March). Neurocognitive consequences of sleep deprivation. *Seminars in Neurology*, *25*(01), 117–129.

Filtness, A. J., Anund, A., Maynard, S., Miller, K., Pilkington-Cheney, F., Dahlman, A., & Ihlström, J. (2019). Bus driver fatigue final report. http://content.tfl.gov.uk/bus-driver-fatigue-report.pdf

Filtness, A. J., Armstrong, K. A., Watson, A., & Smith, S. S. (2017). Sleep-related vehicle crashes on low speed roads. *Accident Analysis & Prevention*, *99*, 279–286.

Gander, P., Hartley, L., Powell, D., Cabon, P., Hitchcock, E., Mills, A., & Popkin, S. (2011). Fatigue risk management: Organizational factors at the regulatory and industry/company level. *Accident Analysis & Prevention*, *43*(2), 573–590.

Haddon Jr, W. (1972). A logical framework for categorizing highway safety phenomena and activity. *Journal of Trauma and Acute Care Surgery*, *12*(3), 193–207.

Horne, J. (2012). Working throughout the night: Beyond 'sleepiness'–impairments to critical decision making. *Neuroscience & Biobehavioral Reviews*, *36*(10), 2226–2231.

May, J. F., & Baldwin, C. L. (2009). Driver fatigue: The importance of identifying causal factors of fatigue when considering detection and countermeasure technologies. *Transportation Research, Part F: Traffic Psychology and Behaviour*, *12*(3), 218–224.

Maynard, S., Filtness, A., Miller, K., & Pilkington-Cheney, F. (2021). Bus driver fatigue: A qualitative study of drivers in London. *Applied Ergonomics*, *92*, 103309.

Miller, K. A., Filtness, A. J., Anund, A., Maynard, S. E., & Pilkington-Cheney, F. (2020). Contributory factors to sleepiness amongst London bus drivers. *Transportation Research, Part F: Traffic Psychology and Behaviour*, *73*, 415–424.

Shenfield, L., Beanland, V., Filtness, A., & Apthorp, D. (2020). The impact of sleep loss on sustained and transient attention: An EEG study. *PeerJ*, *8*, e8960v.

Transport for London [TfL]. (n.d.). Buses. Retrieved June 04, 2019 from https://tfl.gov.uk/corporate/about-tfl/what-we-do/buses

Watling, C. N., Armstrong, K. A., Smith, S. S., & Wilson, A. (2016). The on-road experiences and awareness of sleepiness in a sample of Australian highway drivers: A roadside driver sleepiness study. *Traffic Injury Prevention*, *17*(1), 24–30.

Wong, I. S., Popkin, S., & Folkard, S. (2019). Working time society consensus statements: A multi-level approach to managing occupational sleep-related fatigue. *Industrial Health*, SW-6.

Section 2

Fatigue-Related Consequences in Transportation

2.1 Fatigue-Related Consequences on Road Crashes

Charles Goldenbeld, Ingrid van Schagen, and Ragnhild Davidse

SWOV Institute for Road Safety Research, The Hague, Netherlands

CONTENTS

DOI: 10.1201/9781003213154-9

2.1.1   INTRODUCTION

Fatigue in road traffic is a common problem. Almost everybody drives[1], at times, while seriously fatigued. Among other things, this has to do with the fact that fatigue has many different origins. Fatigue can be sleep-related or task-related. Sleep-related fatigue stems from, for example, insufficient or low-quality sleep or being awake while your biological clock urges you to sleep. Task-related fatigue can arise when you have been behind the wheel for a long time or when you have to perform too many, or very complicated, driving tasks for too long, but also when there are too few, or when tasks are too simple. Section 3 of this book provides more details about the origins of fatigue. The next paragraphs discuss the prevalence of fatigued driving, the size of the problem in terms of road safety, the characteristics of fatigue-related road crashes, and the characteristics of drivers involved in fatigue-related crashes. The chapter begins with a short description of how to determine whether a driver is fatigued or whether a road crash is fatigue-related.

2.1.2   HOW TO QUANTIFY THE ROLE OF FATIGUE IN ROAD CRASHES?

It is not at all straightforward to quantify the role of fatigue in road crashes. This would require constant measurements of the brain activity of drivers, which is technically possible, but unfeasible in practice. Unlike for alcohol or drugs, there is no easy applicable blood or breath test to directly measure the presence of fatigue of a driver, let alone the level of fatigue of a crash-involved road user. Moreover, the involvement in a crash itself is likely to have made symptoms of fatigue disappear, as it is likely to give an adrenaline rush. Neither is it likely that the driver involved will admit having been fatigued or having fallen asleep. Whether fatigue has played a role in the occurrence of a crash can only be assessed indirectly by the subjective judgement of the (police) investigators, or by applying proxy or surrogate measures of fatigue in a post hoc analysis of an accident database (Dawson et al., 2018). As a result, fatigue-related crashes are easily misclassified; consequently, the role of fatigue in road safety is likely to be underestimated (Armstrong et al., 2013; Filtness et al., 2017; Jackson et al., 2011; Radun et al., 2013).

The most common methods to establish a possible role of fatigue in road crashes are police assessments, in-depth crash investigations, naturalistic driving (ND) studies, and surveys. In-vehicle monitoring devices can also give an indication of fatigued driving. Each of these methods is briefly presented next.

2.1.2.1   POLICE ASSESSMENTS

Broadly speaking, the police have two tasks related to fatigued driving: (1) proactively identifying drivers who are too fatigued to participate safely in traffic or who violate driving and rest time regulations and (2) reactively identifying the potential role of fatigued driving in a road crash that has already happened. The first task gives some insight into the prevalence of fatigue in road traffic, and the second provides insights into the share of road crashes that are fatigue related.

Regarding the first task, there are few, if any, police enforcement actions targeted directly at identifying fatigued driving in everyday traffic, as there are actions focusing on drink-driving, using mobile phones or on the correct use of seatbelts. Fatigued driving is sometimes identified because the police stop drivers who are wrongly suspected of drink or drug driving. Some countries offer or have offered training to policemen to help recognising fatigued driving, for example, in Australia, Canada, and Finland, as set out by Radun et al. (2013). A Finnish survey (Radun et al., 2013) showed that a large majority of the police officers who received a training course (95%) considered such a training useful and a majority of those without such a training (80%) had indicated to believe that such a training would be beneficial for them. However, there is no objective evidence that training and education improve correct detection of fatigue in drivers in practice. There are also police actions to check violations of the driving and rest time regulations/hours of service regulations for commercial drivers (Goldenbeld, 2017). Violations of these regulations, however, are not a direct proof of fatigue, but they give indication of the possible presence of fatigue.

As indicated, for the second police task, assessing the role of fatigue in road crashes, there is little objective information that can help the police identify the role of fatigue in a crash. Some countries have developed criteria for identifying fatigue-related road crashes, but these criteria differ between countries or even between police forces within a country, and there is no guarantee that police officers apply the criteria correctly. For example, Dawson et al. (2018) observed that different Australian jurisdictions use different criteria for identifying fatigue-related crashes and that police officers in these jurisdictions received no formal training in the application of these criteria.

2.1.2.2 In-depth Crash Investigations

In-depth crash investigations collect much more data about a crash than standard police investigations (Davidse, 2019; Otte, Pund & Jänsch, 2009; Salo et al., 2006; Wundersitz & Baldock, 2011). In general, a multidisciplinary team including traffic engineers, vehicle engineers, and behavioural scientists visits the crash site, inspects the vehicle and the road, and interviews witnesses to get an in-depth insight into the crash causation process and the (combination of) causal factors. To assess whether a crash is (also) caused by driver fatigue, the crash characteristics must fulfil a set of predefined criteria—for example, the car ran off the road without any driver steering manoeuvres or braking, or bumped into a car or object in front, while the driver had a clear view of the road in front and had not used alcohol or drugs. The exact criteria differ between studies (Dawson et al., 2018). In-depth crash investigations give information about the proportion of fatigue-related crashes within the studied crash types.

2.1.2.3 Naturalistic Driving Studies

ND studies provide insight into driver behaviour in everyday trips by continuously recording details of the driver, the vehicle, and the surroundings using small cameras and sensors mounted to the vehicle, without experimental control (Van Schagen

& Sagberg, 2012). Comparison of the number of crashes and near crashes in situations where the driver shows observable signs of fatigue (e.g., yawning, frequent eye blinking) with similar situations without signs of fatigue gives an indication of the risk of fatigue in road traffic.

2.1.2.4 SURVEYS

The role of fatigue in road safety is also studied by means of surveys in which drivers report about fatigued driving and, if they have been involved in a crash, whether fatigue had contributed to its occurrence. Questionnaire surveys are usually anonymous, meaning that there is probably no strong bias due to answering in a socially acceptable way. In interviews, however, respondents may be less inclined to admit socially undesirable answers, such as fatigued driving. Surveys provide information about the prevalence of fatigued driving and about the share of crashes related to fatigue.

2.1.2.5 IN-VEHICLE MONITORING DEVICES

Many studies have looked into the (technical) possibilities of automatically detecting whether a driver is fatigued (Matthews et al., 2019). Two main approaches can be distinguished. The first approach monitors driving behaviour and compares the drivers' current driving behaviour with their normal (baseline) behaviour to identify deviations that may result from fatigued driving, for example, swerving and frequent speed variations. The second approach monitors the faces of drivers to identify signs of fatigue like eyelid closures and yawning, as in the ND studies discussed before. Fatigue monitoring devices are generally meant to warn a fatigued driver (see Chapter 4.6). In theory, they can also give an indication of the prevalence of fatigued driving, for example, when they are implemented in fleet or company vehicles and where warning data are collected, and of whether fatigue played a role in a crash. Currently, however, the penetration of these devices in cars is far too low, and systems are not yet sufficiently validated to be reliably used for these purposes.

2.1.3 WHAT IS THE PREVALENCE OF FATIGUED DRIVING?

Almost everyone is tired sometimes, due to a short or poor night's sleep, for instance. Consequently, fatigued driving can be expected to be a widespread phenomenon not only in large countries or for long-distance truck drivers, but also in small countries and for ordinary car drivers.

In the international ESRA[2] survey (the E-Survey of Road users' Attitudes) among 35,000 road users from 32 countries worldwide, car drivers were asked about driving while fatigued. On average, around 20% of the European car drivers reported that, during the last one month, they had driven at least once while they were so sleepy that they had trouble keeping their eyes open. In North America, this was around 22%; in Asian/Oceanian countries, it was around 23.5%, and in African countries it was around 24.5% (Goldenbeld & Nikolaou, 2019 —see Figure 2.1.1).

SELF-DECLARED BEHAVIOUR AS A CAR DRIVER
Drive when you were so sleepy that you had trouble
keeping your eyes open

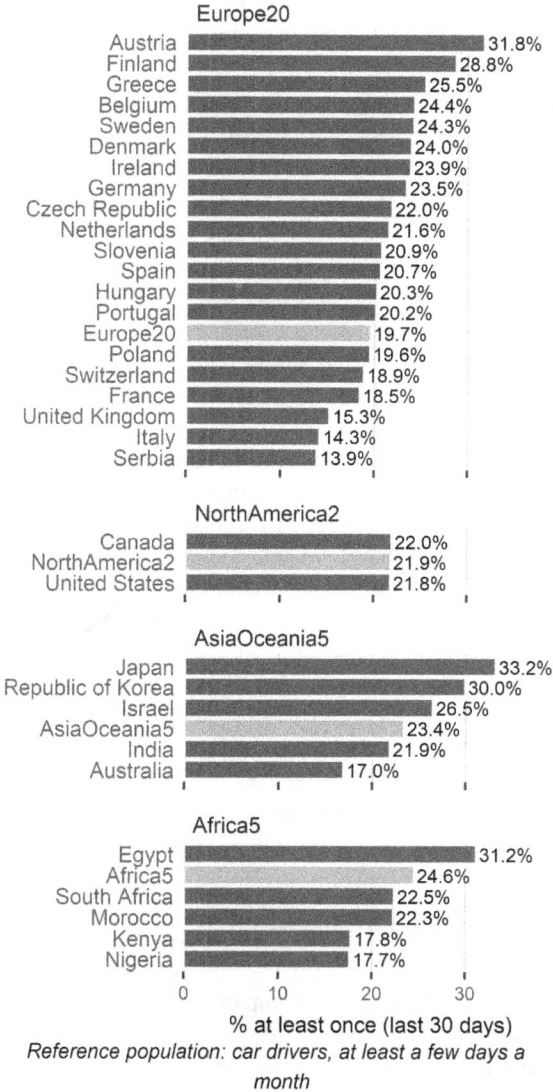

Europe20

Country	%
Austria	31.8%
Finland	28.8%
Greece	25.5%
Belgium	24.4%
Sweden	24.3%
Denmark	24.0%
Ireland	23.9%
Germany	23.5%
Czech Republic	22.0%
Netherlands	21.6%
Slovenia	20.9%
Spain	20.7%
Hungary	20.3%
Portugal	20.2%
Europe20	19.7%
Poland	19.6%
Switzerland	18.9%
France	18.5%
United Kingdom	15.3%
Italy	14.3%
Serbia	13.9%

NorthAmerica2

Country	%
Canada	22.0%
NorthAmerica2	21.9%
United States	21.8%

AsiaOceania5

Country	%
Japan	33.2%
Republic of Korea	30.0%
Israel	26.5%
AsiaOceania5	23.4%
India	21.9%
Australia	17.0%

Africa5

Country	%
Egypt	31.2%
Africa5	24.6%
South Africa	22.5%
Morocco	22.3%
Kenya	17.8%
Nigeria	17.7%

% at least once (last 30 days)
Reference population: car drivers, at least a few days a month

FIGURE 2.1.1   Self-declared prevalence of fatigued driving.

Based on a large-scale ND study in the USA among passenger car drivers, Dingus et al. (2016) estimated that around 1.5% of the total distance driven was driven while fatigued.

Various studies have attested to the fact that commercial drivers and, in particular, long-distance drivers are specifically vulnerable to fatigued driving (Craft, 2007; ETSC, 2011; Thiffault, 2011; Wise, Heaton & Patrician, 2019). A recent European survey among nearly 2,800 truck, bus, and coach drivers (Vitols & Voss, 2021) reported that:

- 60% of the truck drivers and 66% of the bus and coach drivers said they regularly feel tired when driving;
- nearly one-third of the truck drivers and a quarter of the bus and coach drivers said they had fallen asleep at the wheel while driving at least once in the previous 12 months, and
- a quarter of the truck drivers and almost one-third of the bus and coach drivers said they nearly crashed due to fatigue in the previous 12 months.

Commercial drivers have to comply with the driving and rest time regulations or hours of service regulations (among others) to prevent fatigued driving. In the European Union, based on reports from Member States, almost 2 million offences were detected in the period 2017 to 2018 (European Commission, 2021b). This could also be an indication of fatigued driving in the commercial sector. Figure 2.1.2 shows the development of the types of driving offences over the last decade (2007 to 2018). It seems that the share of offences related to breaks and driving time (e.g., too few or too long breaks, or too long driving time within a certain time frame) has been declining, but the share of faulty driving time records offences almost doubled in this period. Corrected for enforcement effort, there was a slight decrease in offences detected at the roadside: from 2.17 in 2015/2016 to 2.11 in 2017/2018 per 100 working days checked as the EU average. The EU average detection rate of offences at the premises slightly increased in this period: from 4.19 to 4.35 per 100 working days checked.

2.1.4   HOW BIG IS THE PROBLEM OF FATIGUE-RELATED ROAD CRASHES?

This section describes the size of the problem of fatigue-related road crashes in three ways: the share of fatigue-related crashes in all crashes, the chance of getting involved in a crash when fatigued compared to being well-rested (i.e., the crash risk), and the economic impact of fatigue-related crashes.

2.1.4.1   SHARE OF FATIGUE-RELATED ROAD CRASHES

Estimates of the share of fatigue-related crashes differ widely between individual studies—from as low as 5% up to 50%, but, overall, it can be assumed that driver fatigue is a contributing factor in 15 to 20% of road crashes (SWOV, 2019). Differences between individual studies are mainly due to differences in definitions and research

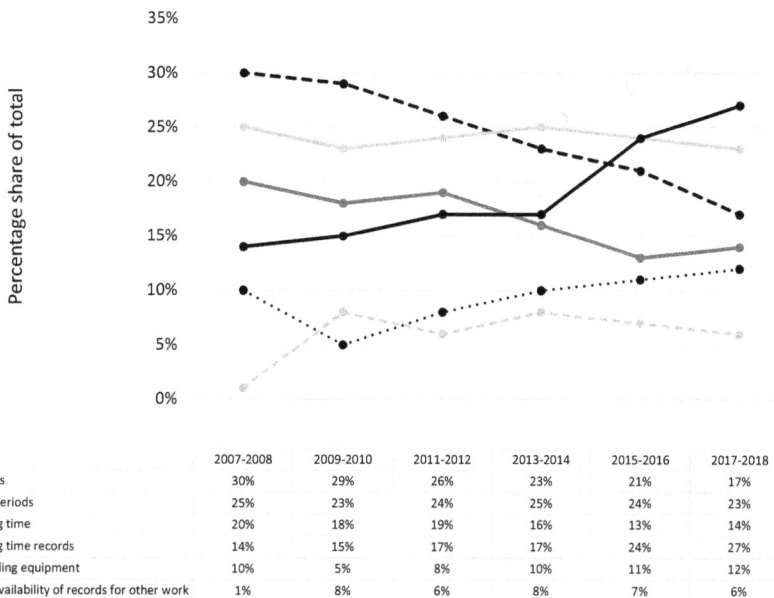

	2007-2008	2009-2010	2011-2012	2013-2014	2015-2016	2017-2018
breaks	30%	29%	26%	23%	21%	17%
rest periods	25%	23%	24%	25%	24%	23%
driving time	20%	18%	19%	16%	13%	14%
driving time records	14%	15%	17%	17%	24%	27%
recording equipment	10%	5%	8%	10%	11%	12%
lack/availability of records for other work	1%	8%	6%	8%	7%	6%

FIGURE 2.1.2 Types of driving and rest time offences in the EU for the decade 2007/8 to 2017/18.

Reprinted from European Commission (2021b) with permission from: http://eur-lex.eur opa.eu, © European Union, 1998–2022.

methodology used to determine whether a crash-involved driver was fatigued (Dawson et al., 2018; Shinar, 2017; SWOV, 2019). The lowest percentages originate from analyses of police-registered crash circumstances, and the highest percentages originate from in-depth crash investigations (European Commission, 2021a). In general, shares are greater for crashes involving trucks (ETSC, 2001; Goldenbeld et al., 2011; McKernon, 2009) and for fatal and motorway crashes (Moradi, Nazari & Rahmani, 2019; Shinar, 2017).

2.1.4.2 CRASH RISK WHEN DRIVING FATIGUED

In general, the risk of getting involved in a crash increases considerably when a driver is fatigued. Again, methodologies to determine the risk, and thus the individual study results, vary widely (Talbot & Filtness, 2017). After having jointly analysed the results of 14 different studies, Moradi, Nazari, and Rahmani (2019) report an odds ratio (OR) of 1.29, meaning that the crash risk when driving while fatigued is 1.29 times the crash risk when driving without being fatigued. This is a best estimate: with 95% certainty the OR is between 1.24 and 1.34. A ND study in the USA (Dingus et al., 2016) that was not yet included in the meta-analysis reported a substantially higher risk: an OR of 3.4 with a 95% confidence interval of between 2.3 and 5.1.

2.1.4.3 ECONOMIC IMPACT

Road crashes in general are associated with considerable socio-economic costs, consisting of immaterial human costs and material costs related to production loss, medical treatment, property damage, and administration. There are wide differences between countries in terms of exact method and cost items included in the calculation. Based on information from countries that use the internationally recommended methodology, Wijnen and Stipdonk (2016) estimated the costs of all road crashes to amount to 3.3% of the gross domestic product (GDP) for high-income countries and between 1.1 and 2.9% for low–and middle-income countries. As 15 to 20% of the road crashes can be assumed to be fatigue-related (SWOV, 2019), the economic impact of fatigue-related crashes amounts to up to one fifth of these costs, i.e., 0.66% of the GDP of a high-income country. For example, for the USA, with a GDP of around $20.9 trillion in 2020, this would mean an amount of $138 billion annually. This comes close to the more advanced estimates of Léger, Pepin, and Caetano (2019), who estimated the direct socio-economic costs of fatigued driving to be between $139.4 billion and $152 billion per year.

Because fatigue-related crashes are particularly common for commercial drivers, there are huge direct costs for employers as well. For the USA, the cost of road crashes for employers is estimated to be $72.2 billion, around 60% of which is for crashes occurring on the job (NETS, 2021). If it is conservatively assumed that one-fifth of the on- and off-the-job crashes of employed drivers are fatigue related, this would mean that fatigued driving costs USA employers around almost $15 billion annually. This is more than the cost of alcohol- and speed-related crashes (reported by NETS, 2021, to cost $8.0 billion and $9.8 billion, respectively) and close to the cost of distracted driving ($18.8 billion, also reported by NETS, 2021).

2.1.5 WHAT ARE THE MAIN CHARACTERISTICS OF FATIGUE-RELATED ROAD CRASHES?

In general, a crash is likely to be fatigue related if it has some of the following characteristics (Dawson et al., 2018; Horne & Reyner, 2001):

- The crash occurred on a high-speed road.
- The crash occurred between midnight and dawn.
- The vehicle ran off the road or bumped into a (stationary) car/object in front.
- The driver had a clear view of the road.
- There were no skid marks.
- There were no passengers in the vehicle.
- There were no other plausible explanations (such as alcohol use or indisposition).

2.1.5.1 Crash Location

Fatigue-related crashes occur relatively often on motorways or on other high-speed inter-urban roads, especially in rural environments with a monotonous character (Filtness et al., 2017; Thiffault, 2011). But fatigue-related crashes also occur at other locations. For example, Filtness et al. (2017) reported that in Queensland, Australia, around 40% of fatigue-related crashes occur on low-speed roads, including roads inside urban areas.

2.1.5.2 Time of Day

Various studies from different countries worldwide (listed in Jackson et al., 2011) identified two daily peaks for fatigue-related crash risk: one large peak in the early hours of the morning, with a second, smaller peak mid-afternoon. These peaks are most likely related to the human biological clock, which makes people more prone to fatigue at times when the human body is programmed to sleep.

2.1.5.3 Type of Crash

The typical fatigue crash is a single vehicle crash, ending against a tree or another fixed object, or a rear-end collision with a stopped or slow-moving vehicle, while the driver had a clear view of the road ahead. Typical examples are a driver who misses a curve in a rural road and just continues to drive straight on (Davidse et al., 2011) and a driver who dozes off and runs into the back of a vehicle at the tail end of a traffic jam (Davidse et al., 2020). For both types of crashes, there are no signs that the driver had undertaken any action to prevent or mitigate the crash, for example, by applying harsh braking. The presence of other people in the car could possibly have prevented the driver from falling asleep in the first place but could also have helped to wake him up in time to undertake at least some action to prevent or mitigate the crash. The typical fatigue-related crash circumstances resemble those of a crash of an alcohol-intoxicated driver or a driver with a sudden indisposition. Hence, objectively assessable explanations for the crash have to be excluded before concluding that the crash was fatigue related.

2.1.6 WHICH DRIVERS ARE OVERREPRESENTED IN FATIGUE-RELATED ROAD CRASHES?

Certain groups of drivers are more often involved in fatigue-related road crashes than other groups. This overrepresentation in fatigue-related crashes relates to the type of traffic participation, physical aspects, lifestyle, and a combination of these factors. Groups that are relatively often involved in a fatigue-related crash are (SWOV, 2019):

- (long-distance) truck drivers;
- shift workers
- young men;
- people with untreated sleep disorders;
- taxi drivers.

2.1.6.1 (LONG-DISTANCE) TRUCK DRIVERS

Truck drivers, and in particular long-distance truck drivers, are particularly prone to fatigued driving for several reasons. Despite working and driving time regulations, they have lengthy hours of work, with relatively long periods behind the wheel, especially during the night (Vitols & Voss, 2021). (Co-)drivers often have to sleep in their truck under noisy, vibrating, and high-temperature conditions, resulting in short periods of poor-quality sleep (Baulk & Fletcher, 2012; Vitols & Voss, 2021). Additionally, drivers' lifestyle, which includes a lack of physical exercise and related obesity, increases the likelihood of obstructive sleep apnoea, which is known to decrease sleep quality and, hence, increase crash risk (Sieber et al., 2014; Wiegand, Hanowski & McDonald, 2009; see also Chapter 3.3 of this book).

2.1.6.2 SHIFT WORKERS

Shift workers are particularly prone to fatigue as shift work interferes with normal sleep patterns. Shift work prevents people from getting sufficient, and sufficiently good quality, sleep. Shift work also requires people to perform tasks at times when the physiological processes that regulate the sleep/wake cycle prepare the body for sleep and, consequently, when they are less attentive and functional. Both professional drivers (when driving during a night shift) and shift workers (when driving home after a night shift or a series of night shifts) have an increased risk of being involved in a road crash. For example, based on a driving simulator study with police officers, James and Vila (2015) found that driving after five consecutive night shifts resulted in more collisions and greater lane deviations than did driving after five consecutive daytime shifts. Lee et al. (2016), based on a study in real traffic, also showed that driving after one night shift was associated with increased objective and subjective drowsiness as well as degraded driving performance.

2.1.6.3 YOUNG MEN

Young male drivers are another group that have a high risk of falling asleep behind the wheel. Results of the large-scale ESRA survey showed that fatigued driving is most common among drivers between 18 and 24 years of age and generally also more common for men than for women (Goldenbeld & Nikolaou, 2019). The over-involvement of young male drivers in fatigue-related crashes is likely to be related to lifestyle, resulting in, on average, more night-time activities and more night-time driving as well as less sleep or less high-quality sleep at night (Radun, 2009; Shinar, 2017). Moreover, young men, or young adults in general, are more vulnerable to the effects of insufficient sleep than are older adults (Zitting et al., 2018).

2.1.6.4 PEOPLE WITH UNTREATED SLEEP DISORDERS

Sleep disorders notably include obstructive sleep apnoea (temporary respiratory arrest while sleeping) and narcolepsy (tendency to suddenly fall asleep, also by day). If these disorders are not treated, they will lead to excessive daytime sleepiness even after sufficient night-time sleep. As such they lead to an increased risk of a fatigue-related crash (Smolensky et al., 2011). A review by Talbot and Filtness (2016) showed that drivers with untreated sleep apnoea are two to three times more likely to be involved in a crash than drivers without sleep apnoea. The same review suggests that the crash risk of truck drivers with untreated sleep apnoea is potentially even higher than for other drivers. Sleep apnoea often goes hand in hand with being overweight. If sleep apnoea is treated successfully, crash risk can be reduced substantially (Tregear et al., 2010).

2.1.6.5 TAXI DRIVERS

Several studies have identified taxi drivers as another risk group for fatigue-related crashes (Fletcher & Mitchell, 2011; Meng et al., 2015). The over-representation is likely to be related to the nature of their work, which includes long shifts, also after midnight. Li et al. (2019), based on a questionnaire survey, compared taxi drivers with a high and a low fatigue-related crash risk and identified four main factors that distinguished these groups. The high-risk drivers generally had longer driving hours per working day, a lower rest ratio and less driving experience than low-risk drivers. These high-risk drivers were also more confident than low-risk drivers about their ability to resist fatigue, which may indicate that these drivers underestimate their fatigue and thus perceive less difficulty in fatigued driving. Like for truck drivers, obesity, and thus sleep apnoea, is relatively common among taxi drivers (Lim & Chia, 2015).

2.1.7 CONCLUSIONS

Fatigued driving is a common phenomenon, not only for long-distance commercial drivers, but also for ordinary passenger car drivers during everyday trips. Around 20 to 25% of passenger car drivers reported that they had been driving while seriously fatigued. For commercial drivers and, in particular, long-distance drivers, the prevalence of fatigued driving is much higher. Around two-thirds of commercial drivers reported that they regularly feel tired when driving and around one-third reported that they fell asleep at the wheel at least once in the previous year.

It is difficult to assess objectively whether fatigue played a role in a crash, and different studies have provided different estimates. On average, it can be assumed that driver fatigue plays a role in 15 to 20% of road crashes. Overall, the risk of getting involved in a crash increases considerably when a driver is fatigued. Again, it is difficult to quantify the risk increase and results of individual studies vary widely.

Road crashes in general are associated with considerable socio-economic costs, estimated to just over 3% of the GDP for high-income countries and between 1 and 3% for low- and middle-income countries. As 15 to 20% of road crashes can be assumed to be fatigue related, the economic impact of fatigue-related crashes amounts to up to one-fifth of these costs, that is, 0.66% of the GDP for high-income countries annually.

Most fatigue-related crashes occur between midnight and dawn, on a high-speed road without passengers, with the vehicle running off the road or colliding with a stopped or slow-moving vehicle, while the driver had a clear view of the road ahead. Specific groups of road users—notably (long-distance) truck drivers, shift workers, young men, people with untreated sleep disorders, and taxi drivers—are more prone to getting involved in a fatigue-related crash than others.

SUMMARY POINTS FOR PRACTITIONERS

- Fatigued driving is a common phenomenon, not only for long-distance commercial drivers, but also for ordinary passenger car drivers during everyday trips:
  - Around two-thirds of commercial drivers reported that they regularly feel tired when driving and around one-third reported that they fell asleep at the wheel at least once in the previous year.
  - Of the passenger car drivers surveyed, 20 to 25% indicated that, during the previous month, they had driven while they were seriously fatigued.
- It is impossible to assess objectively whether fatigue played a role in a crash. Different types of studies provide different estimates. Overall, it can be assumed that:
  - 15 to 20% of road crashes are fatigue related.
  - Fatigued driving results in a substantial increase of crash risk.
  - In high-income countries, the socio-economic cost of fatigue-related crashes amounts to 0.66% of its GDP annually.
- Most fatigue-related crashes:
  - occur during the night, on a quiet motorway or other high-speed road, without passengers; and
  - are single vehicle or rear-end crashes, without indications that the driver tried to prevent or mitigate the crash.
- Some groups are more prone to getting involved in a fatigue-related crash than are others. Notably, (long-distance) truck drivers, shift workers, young men, people with untreated sleep disorders, and taxi drivers.

NOTES

1   In this chapter, when using "driving", in principle this also refers to riding a (powered) two-wheeler, although research so far almost exclusively focuses on drivers of private cars, buses/coaches, and trucks.
2   ESRA: E-Survey of Road users' Attitudes—www.esranet.eu/en/

REFERENCES

Armstrong, K., Filtness, A. J., Watling, C. N., Barraclough, P., & Haworth, N. (2013). Efficacy of proxy definitions for identification of fatigue/sleep-related crashes: An Australian evaluation. *Transportation Research Part F: Traffic Psychology and Behaviour*, *21*, 242–252. https://doi.org/10.1016/j.trf.2013.10.002

Baulk, S.D., & Fletcher, A. (2012). At home and away: Measuring the sleep of Australian truck drivers. *Accident Analysis & Prevention, 45*, 36–40. https://doi.org/10.1016/j.aap.2011.09.023

Craft, R. (2007). The large truck crash causation study. Analysis brief Federal Motor Carrier Safety Administration Office of Research and Analysis. Publication No. FMCSA-RRA-07-017. Washington, NHTSA. www.fmcsa.dot.gov/research-and-analysis/research/large-truck-crash-causation-study

Davidse, R.J., Doumen, M.J.A., van Duijvenvoorde, K., & Louwerse, W.J.R. (2011). *Run-off-road crashes in the Province of Zeeland: Characteristics and possible solutions; Results of an in-depth study.* [in Dutch with extended English Summary] R-2011-20. SWOV, Leidschendam.

Davidse, R.J., van Duijvenvoorde, K., Boele-Vos, M.J., Louwerse, W.J.R., et al. (2019). Scenarios of crashes involving light mopeds on urban bicycle paths. *Accident Analysis & Prevention, 129*, 334–341. https://doi.org/10.1016/j.aap.2019.05.016

Davidse, R.J., van Duijvenvoorde, K., & Louwerse, W.J.R. (2020). *Fatal road crashes on national roads in 2019; Analysis of crash and injury factors and resulting potential countermeasures.* [in Dutch with extended English Summary] R-2020-29. SWOV, Den Haag.

Dawson, D., Reynolds, A.C., van Dongen, H.P.A., & Thomas, M.J.W. (2018). Determining the likelihood that fatigue was present in a road accident: A theoretical review and suggested accident taxonomy. *Sleep Medicine Reviews, 42*, 202–210. https://doi.org/10.1016/j.smrv.2018.08.006

Dingus, T.A., Guo, F., Lee, S., Antin, J. F., Perez, M., Buchanan-King, M., & Hankey, J. (2016). Driver crash risk factors and prevalence evaluation using naturalistic driving data. *PNAS: Proceedings of the National Academy of Sciences of the United States of America, 113*(10), 2636–2641. https://doi.org/10.1073/pnas.1513271113

ETSC (2001). *The role of driver fatigue in commercial road transport crashes.* Brussels, European Transport Safety Council.

ETSC (2011). *Tackling fatigue: EU social rules and heavy goods vehicle drivers.* Brussels, European Transport Safety Council.

European Commission (2021a). *Road safety thematic report–Fatigue.* European Road Safety Observatory. Brussels, European Commission, Directorate General for Transport.

European Commission (2021b). *Report from the Commission to the European Parliament and the Council on the implementation in 2017–2018 of Regulation (EC) No 561/2006 on the harmonisation of certain social legislation relating to road transport and of Directive 2002/15/EC on the organisation of the working time of persons performing mobile road transport activities.* Brussels, European Commission.

Filtness, A.J., Armstrong, K., Watson, A., & Smith, S. (2017). Sleep-related crash characteristics: Implications for applying a fatigue definition to crash reports. *Accident Analysis & Prevention, 99*, 440–444. https://doi.org/10.1016/j.aap.2015.11.024

Fletcher, A., & Mitchell, P. (2011). *Fatigue-related risks for Queensland taxi drivers.* Queensland Government, Australia.

Goldenbeld, C. (2017). Driving hours and rest time / hours of service regulations for commercial drivers. European Road Safety Decision Support System, developed by the H2020 project SafetyCube. Retrieved from www.roadsafety-dss.eu on 7 June 2022.

Goldenbeld, C., Davidse, R.J., Mesken, J., & Hoekstra, A.T.G. (2011). *Driver fatigue: Prevalence and state awareness of drivers of passenger cars and trucks. A questionnaire study among driving licence holders in the Netherlands.* R-2011-4 [In Dutch–summary in English]. SWOV, Leidschendam.

Goldenbeld, C., & Nikolaou, D. (2019). *Driver fatigue. ESRA2 Thematic report Nr. 4 (updated version). ESRA project (E-Survey of Road users' Attitudes)*. The Hague, Netherlands Institute for Road safety Research SWOV.

Horne, J., & Reyner, L. (2001). Sleep-related vehicle accidents: some guides for road safety policies. *Transportation Research Part F: Traffic Psychology and Behaviour*, *4*, 63–74. https://doi.org/10.1016/S1369-8478(01)00014-6

Jackson, P., Hilditch, C., Holmes, A., Reed, N., Merat, N., & Smith, L. (2011). Fatigue and road safety: A critical analysis of recent evidence. *Road Safety Web Publication*, No. 21. Great Britain, London, Department for Transport.

James, S., & Vila, B. (2015). Police drowsy driving: Predicting fatigue related performance decay. *Policing: An International Journal of Police Strategies & Management*, *38*(3), 517–538. http://dx.doi.org/10.1108/PIJPSM-03-2015-0033

Lee, M.L., Howard, M.E., Horrey, W.J., Liang, Y., Anderson, C., Shreeve, M.S., O'Brien, C.S., & Czeisler, C.A. (2016). High risk of near-crash driving events following night-shift work. *Proceedings of the National Academy of Sciences*, *113*(1), 176–181. https://doi.10.1073/pnas.1510383112

Léger, D., Pepin, E., & Caetano, G. (2019). The economic burden of sleepy driving. *Sleep Medicine Clinics*, 14(4), 423–429. https://doi.org/10.1016/j.jsmc.2019.07.004

Li, M.K., Yu, J.J., Ma, L., & Zhang. (2019). Modeling and mitigating fatigue-related accident risk of taxi drivers. *Accident Analysis & Prevention*, *123*, 79–87. https://doi.org/10.1016/j.aap.2018.11.001

Lim, S.M., & Chia, S.E. (2015). The prevalence of fatigue and associated health and safety risk factors among taxi drivers in Singapore. *Singapore Medical Journal*, *56*, 92–97. https://doi.org/10.11622/smedj.2014169

Matthews, G., Wohleber, R., Lin, J., Funke, G., et al. (2019). monitoring task fatigue in contemporary and future vehicles: A review. In: Cassenti, D.N. (red.), *Advances in Human Factors in Simulation and Modeling*. Cham, Switzerland: Springer International Publishing, , pp. 101–112. https://doi.org/10.1007/978-3-319-94223-0_10

McKernon, S. (2009). A literature review on driver fatigue among drivers in the general public. Research Report 342. Land Transport New Zealand, Wellington.

Meng, F., Li, S., Cao, L., Li, M., Peng, Q., Wang, C., & Zhang, W. (2015). Driving fatigue in professional drivers: A survey of truck and taxi drivers. *Traffic Injury Prevention*, *16*(5), 474–483. https://doi.org/10.1080/15389588.2014.973945

Moradi, A., Nazari, S.S.H., & Rahmani, K. (2019). Sleepiness and the risk of road traffic accidents: A systematic review and meta-analysis of previous studies, *Transportation Research Part F: Traffic Psychology and Behaviour*, *65*, 620–629. https://doi.org/10.1016/j.trf.2018.09.013

NETS (2021). *The cost of motor vehicle crashes to employers–2019*. Vienna, USA, the Network of Employers for Traffic Safety.

Otte, D., Pund, B., & Jänsch, M. (2009). A new approach of accident causation analysis by seven steps ACAS. In: *Proceedings of the 21st International Technical Conference on the Enhanced Safety of Vehicles (ESV)*, Stuttgart, Germany, 15–18 June 2009.

Radun, I. (2009). *Fatigued driving: Prevalence, risk factors and groups, and the law*. Doctoral dissertation. University of Helsinki.

Radun, I, Ohisalo, J., Radun, J., Wahde, M., & Kecklund, G. (2013). Driver fatigue and the law from the perspective of police officers and prosecutors. *Transportation Research Part F: Traffic Psychology and Behaviour*, *18*, 159–167. https://doi.org/10.1016/j.trf.2013.01.001

Salo, I., Parkkari, K., Sulander, P., & Keskinen, E. (2006). In-depth on-the-spot road accident investigation in Finland. Paper presented at the 2nd International conference on ESAR

"Expert Symposium on Accident Research", 1–2 September 2006, Hannover Medical School. Berichte der Bundesanstalt für Straßenwesen. Heft F61. BASt, Bergisch Gladbach.

Shinar, D. (2017). Fatigue and driving. In: D. Shinar (Ed.), *Traffic Safety and Human Behavior*. Bingley: Emerald Publishing Limited, pp. 797–857. www.emerald.com/insight/publicat ion/doi/10.1108/9781786352217

Sieber, W.K., Robinson, C.F., Birdsey, J., Chen, G.X., et al. (2014). Obesity and other risk factors: The national survey of U.S. long-haul truck driver health and injury. *American Journal of Industrial Medicine*, 57, 615–626. https://doi.org/10.1002/ajim.22293

Smolensky, M.H., Di Milia, L., Ohayon, M.M., & Philip, P. (2011). Sleep disorders, medical conditions, and road accident risk. *Accident Analysis & Prevention*, 43, 533–548. https://doi.org/10.1016/j.aap.2009.12.004

SWOV (2019). Fatigue. SWOV Fact sheet, September 2019. SWOV, The Hague. www.swov.nl/en/facts-figures/factsheet/fatigue

Talbot, R., & Filtness, A. (2016). Fatigue–sleep disorders–obstructive sleep apnea. European Road Safety Decision Support System, developed by the H2020 project SafetyCube. Retrieved from www.roadsafety-dss.eu on 13 June 2022.

Talbot, R., & Filtness, A. (2017). Fatigue–Not enough sleep/driving while tired. European Road Safety Decision Support System, developed by the H2020 project SafetyCube. www.roadsafety-dss.eu 24 Jan 2022.

Thiffault, P. (2011). *Addressing human factors in the motor carriers industry in Canada*. Report prepared for the, Canadian Council of Motor Transport Administrators (CCMTA). www.bv.transports.gouv.qc.ca/mono/1081534.pdf.

Tregear, S., Reston, J., Schoelles, K., & Phillips, B. (2010). Continuous positive airway pressure reduces risk of motor vehicle crash among drivers with obstructive sleep apnea: Systematic review and meta-analysis. *Sleep*, 33, 1373–1380. https://dx.doi.org/10.1093%2Fsleep%2F33.10.1373

Van Schagen, I., & Sagberg, F. (2012). The potential benefits of naturalistic driving for road safety research: Theoretical and empirical considerations and challenges for the future. *Procedia–Social and Behavioral Sciences*, 48, 692–701 https://doi.org/10.1016/j.sbs pro.2012.06.1047

Vitols, K., & Voss, E. (2021). *Driver fatigue in European road transport*. Brussels, European Transport Workers' Federation (ETF).

Wiegand, D.M., Hanowski, R.J., & McDonald, S.E. (2009). Commercial drivers' health: A naturalistic study of body mass index, fatigue, and involvement in safety-critical events. *Traffic Injury Prevention*, 10, 573–579. https://doi.org/10.1080/1538958090 3295277

Wijnen, W. & Stipdonk, H. (2016) Social costs of road crashes: An international analysis. *Accident Analysis & Prevention*, 94, 97–106. https://doi.org/10.1016/j.aap.2016.05.005

Wise, J.M., Heaton, K., & Patrician, P. (2019). Fatigue in long-haul truck drivers: A concept analysis. *Workplace Health & Safety*, 67(2), 68–77. https://doi.org/10.1177/216507991 8800509

Wundersitz, L.N., & Baldock, M.R.J. (2011). *The relative contribution of system failures and extreme behaviour in South Australia crashes*. Centre for Automotive Safety Research, Adelaide.

Zitting, K.M., Münch, M.Y., Cain, S.W., Wang, W., Wong, A., Ronda, J.M., Aeschbach, D., Czeisler, C.A., & Duffy, J.F. (2018). Young adults are more vulnerable to chronic sleep deficiency and recurrent circadian disruption than older adults. *Science Reports*, 23;8(1), 11052. https://doi.10.1038/s41598-018-29358-x

2.2 Fatigue Risk in Great Britain's Railway Industry

Dan Basacik[1], Ann Mills[1], Mark Young[2], Ishbel Macgregor-Curtin[3], and Nora Balfe[3]

[1]Rail Safety and Standards Board, London, UK
[2]University of Southampton, Southampton, Hampshire, UK
[3]Iarnród Eireann Irish Rail, Dublin, Ireland

CONTENTS

2.2.1 CONTEXT

Thirty-five people died and almost 500 were injured in the 1988 Clapham Junction train collision where a signalling technician had performed safety-critical work for 13 consecutive weeks without a single day off. Thirty years later, a trackworker was killed at Stoats Nest Junction when he walked out of the protected area and onto a line that was open to rail traffic. He had only had about 3.5 hours sleep in the previous 24 hours, and 12 hours sleep in the 48 hours before the incident.

Rail transport is a complex safety-critical system, with interfaces between trains, tracks, structures, stations, signalling and level crossings, and involving passenger, freight, and maintenance operations. One of the key elements in the system is the people—the drivers, signallers, and maintenance workers who operate and maintain the railway 24 hours a day, seven days a week, contributing to its status as one of the safest modes of transport (RSSB, 2021a). This safety-critical work can occur at any time, day or night, in difficult circumstances and against demanding work schedules. Consequently, fatigue is an operational concern in the rail industry that needs to be

DOI: 10.1201/9781003213154-10

effectively managed, just like any other risk. The challenge for fatigue risk management in rail is the wide variety of tasks and working environments, from signal control rooms to train cabs, to out on the infrastructure itself, exposed to the elements.

Consider the roles of train drivers and signallers[1], which require individuals to maintain high levels of concentration, retain information, identify and anticipate risk, and have good attention to detail. This is often in the context of quite monotonous tasks with lengthy periods of limited activity, other than observing information on a control desk or monitoring the track ahead. Meanwhile, other roles can be quite physically strenuous, such as maintaining the track or operating Victorian era lever-frame signal boxes.

Despite the large differences in the type of work, the pattern of work, and the working environment between these safety-critical roles, research (McGuffog et al., 2005; Robertson et al., 2010) in Great Britain (GB) has identified that many of the factors contributing to an increased likelihood of fatigue are similar: long periods of duty, time of day (night duties and early starts), the timing and duration of breaks (e.g., too early or too late in the shift, or a single long break rather than shorter, more frequent breaks), consecutive duties, and inadequate recovery time.

A recent rail industry survey in GB (RSSB, 2019) also identified fatigue risks in areas previously not explored. For example, 14% of the respondents in that study said that they have on-call duties and, of those, 59% reported that they sometimes or always exceed their company's working time limits when on-call, while a further 40% of those said that nobody checks whether they are fit to continue to work.

Surprisingly to some, the rail industry in Britain has a significant presence on the road network, to support maintenance and operational activities. Thus, as an industry we are concerned not only with the impact of fatigue on railway operations, but also with its impact on road risk, especially when railway workers undertake journeys at night, following long shifts, night shifts, and potentially covering long distances.

Failure to manage rail staff fatigue properly can have disastrous consequences. For example, fatigue caused by excessive overtime was identified as a contributory factor in the 1988 Clapham Junction collision which killed 35 people and injured nearly 500 (Hidden, 1989). More recently, the Office of Rail and Road (ORR), GB's rail regulator, successfully prosecuted an infrastructure contracting firm for fatigue risk management failures that resulted in the deaths of two of its workers in a road crash (ORR, 2020), emphasising an ongoing cultural change in attitude to fatigue within the industry.

Similar to other places, in GB, all employers have a legal responsibility to control the risk from fatigue. As is the case in many high-risk industries, legislation has formally shifted the focus away from prescriptive working time limits which specified, for example, minimum rest intervals between shifts and maximum shift lengths, to a more systematic approach to managing fatigue risk, integrated within an organisation's wider safety management system (SMS). This is in recognition of the fact that, in order to reduce the likelihood of incidents in which fatigue is a contributing factor, effective controls are needed at individual, job, and organisational levels. At the heart of fatigue risk management systems (FRMS) is an acknowledgement that fatigue risk cannot be controlled by management or company systems alone;

individual employees also have various duties in relation to fatigue. In the industry fatigue survey (RSSB, 2019), railway staff members were asked to indicate who they thought has responsibilities for managing fatigue: the individual, the employer, or both. The majority of respondents (83%) said they thought that both the individual and the employer were responsible for fatigue risk management.

In GB, this shift towards the holistic management of fatigue risk within rail has been supported by collaboration between organisations, including companies that build, operate, and maintain the railway, ORR (the safety and economic regulator for GB rail), and other industry bodies. This collaboration is facilitated by the Rail Safety and Standards Board (RSSB), which develops and maintains standards and provides clear and honest advice based on assessment of the data, analysis, research, and findings that it produces. RSSB publishes research and guidance on fatigue risk management, with industry input. The Rail Accident Investigation Branch (RAIB) independently investigates rail accidents to improve safety. It has helped the industry understand how fatigue has contributed to accidents on the railway, and what the industry needs to do to manage this risk better. In this chapter we present some of the incident investigation and research work that has shaped our understanding of fatigue risk in the GB rail context. We then discuss some of the challenges that the industry faces in managing this complex risk and where we think there are opportunities for future work, both within the industry and with the scientific community.

2.2.2   EXTENT OF THE PROBLEM

The nature of the work carried out in the rail industry highlights a potential vulnerability to fatigue. Research has attempted to quantify the scale of the issue and understand the link between fatigue and railway safety outcomes.

The recent survey of almost 8,000 railway staff in GB found that 22% were experiencing excessive daytime sleepiness (RSSB, 2019) as measured using the Epworth Sleepiness Scale, which indicates a propensity to doze off during normal daytime activities (Johns & Hocking, 1997; see Chapter 1.2 for more on measuring fatigue). Figure 2.2.1 shows that a higher proportion (24%) of railway shiftworkers were experiencing excessive daytime sleepiness, compared to non-shiftworkers (17%) (RSSB, 2019), highlighting a link between shiftwork (i.e., work schedules that do not conform to standard daytime hours) and fatigue.

In the same survey, over one-third (34%) of respondents said that they had had to make an effort to stay awake while at work once a week or more, including 3% who said "every day" (RSSB, 2019), indicating that fatigue is not just an issue outside of work, but at work as well (see Figure 2.2.2).

A third piece of data from the survey showed that of the 73% of staff who often drive for work or to and from work, 68% said that they had driven while fatigued in the last 12 months (RSSB, 2019). To put that into context, fatigue is thought to cause 20% of all road crashes and 25% of all serious or fatal crashes (RSSB, 2013).

This research clarifies that railway staff do experience fatigue at work, and that this is not necessarily an infrequent occurrence. The links between fatigue and reduced

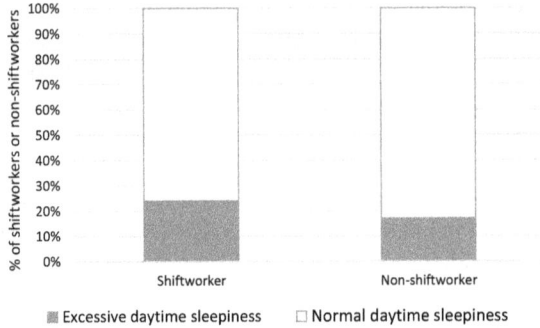

FIGURE 2.2.1 Shiftworkers' and non-shiftworkers' daytime sleepiness on the Epworth Sleepiness Scale (N=7208) (RSSB, 2019)—differences are statistically significant ($X^2(1, N=7208) = 47.22, p<0.001$).

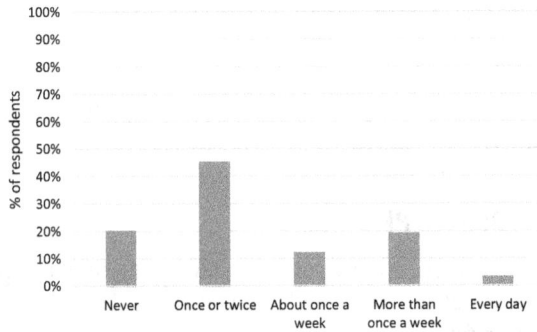

FIGURE 2.2.2 How often respondents have had to make an effort to stay awake at work during the last month (N=7222) (RSSB, 2019).

human performance have been explored in detail in the scientific literature and are summarised in Chapter 1.4 of this book. The implications are that fatigue is likely to cause deterioration in people's performance which, in turn, has the potential to impact safety on the rail and road networks, as well as worker health (Moreno et al., 2019; see also Chapter 3.5 of this book).

To explore the link between staff fatigue and railway incidents, Bowler and Gibson (2015) carried out an analysis of investigation reports into high-risk rail incidents, and found that fatigue was a factor in 21% of these events. This analysis demonstrates a clear link between fatigue and railway incidents. Interestingly, analysis of UK road crash data (DfT, 2011) and data looking at incidents across transport modes in the USA (Marcus & Rosekind, 2017) have found very similar figures in relation to the contribution of fatigue, suggesting that the issue is broader than any single industry and highlighting an opportunity to learn from each other's attempts and successes in managing this risk.

Bowler and Gibson (2015) also found that, according to the investigation reports, there was an almost equal contribution of home- and work-related factors contributing to fatigue in these incidents, while ill health was a third contributor to employee fatigue. This has significant implications for how to control fatigue risk. While work-related factors such as shift pattern and task design are key to managing a significant proportion of fatigue risk in the rail industry, focussing on working patterns alone would likely fail to control fatigue risk that is related to the person's sleeping environment, domestic and social activities, as well as ill health and medication.

The analyses described above do have limitations; for example, some of the investigation reports that Bowler and Gibson (2015) studied may, for various reasons, have failed to identify that fatigue did contribute to the incident. As railway companies develop more mature fatigue risk management systems, the accuracy of the fatigue risk data that they collect from their everyday operations (including incident investigations) will improve, and this will help the industry to better understand and monitor this risk. Nevertheless, the research taken as a whole has significantly improved the industry's understanding of the extent of the issue. It has shown that fatigue is not just a problem in theory, but a frequent experience for many staff, and one which leads to safety incidents. This type of analysis can be useful in persuading stakeholders to support the changes, or allocate resources, that are needed to manage fatigue risk. For example, in the GB rail industry, facts and figures from the research described above are displayed on the first page of a guidance document, *9 things you should consider for your fatigue risk management plan* (RSSB, 2020b). This document has helped safety managers in railway companies to get buy-in from their senior leadership teams, to focus on nine areas to improve how fatigue risk is managed.

2.2.3   FATIGUE AS A FACTOR IN INCIDENTS

Among the wider database of fatigue-related events described above, several have led to more serious incidents that have been the subject of detailed independent investigations. The body that carries out such investigations in GB, the RAIB, has so far identified fatigue to be a factor in 29 out of 496 of its reports (at the time of writing). Here, we present a selection of these to highlight some of the main impacts of fatigue in the rail industry.

The 24/7 nature of the rail industry means that shiftwork is a key contributor to fatigue. More specifically, this may relate to certain aspects of shiftwork, including long working hours or disruptions in circadian rhythm, which can lead to insufficient and poor-quality sleep. On 17 August 2010, all of these factors conspired against a freight train driver at Shap in Cumbria (north-west England), whose train slowed to a stop and then rolled back down a hill in an uncontrolled manner for more than two miles. The investigation report (RAIB, 2011) identified the immediate cause to be that the driver did not apply enough power to climb the gradient, nor the brakes to stop it from running back. In turn, the key causal factor was that the driver was not alert enough to notice the train slowing to a stop and rolling back because he was probably fatigued at the time. The incident occurred just after 02:00 hours, at a time when the driver was entering the window of circadian low (WOCL; see, e.g., Williamson &

Friswell, 2011 and Chapter 3.1 of this book). The driver was on his first night shift after a series of day shifts followed by only one rest day; he was therefore still in a diurnal pattern of sleep and had not yet adjusted to working at night. Because of this desynchronisation, he had woken up at around 08:00 hours on the day of his night shift, which began at 18:34 hours and was due to finish at 05:43 hours. By the time of the incident, then, the driver had been awake for over 18 hours, which is a known risk factor for fatigue affecting performance (Dawson & Reid, 1997).

That fatigue is "all about sleep" (cf. Dawson & McCulloch, 2005) was tragically demonstrated by a fatal tram derailment in Croydon, south London. On the morning of Wednesday 9 November 2016, a tram heading towards Croydon town centre derailed and overturned on a tight curve as it approached Sandilands Junction. The speed limit for the curve was 20 km/h, and the tram was travelling at about 73 km/h when it entered the curve. Seven people died in the incident, while a further 51 were taken to hospital, 16 of whom suffered serious injuries.

As with most major incidents involving complex sociotechnical systems (see, e.g., Hulme et al., 2021), there were several underlying and organisational factors identified in the RAIB report for this investigation (RAIB, 2017/2020), which resulted in 15 recommendations targeted at levels from design, through safety management, to regulation. However, among the more immediate causal factors, RAIB found it was likely that the driver, who survived, lost awareness of the driving task during a period of low workload, which possibly caused him to microsleep.

During the investigation, RAIB (2017/2020) considered the role of home–life and work–life-related fatigue. The tram driver worked a roster of permanent early shifts, which are a risk factor for fatigue due to the reduced opportunity for sleep. That said, there was nothing exceptional about the driver's shift on the morning of 9 November 2016 compared to his usual schedule. So, the investigation turned to consider the driver's sleep habits. The driver reported normally sleeping for around five and a half to six hours before an early start. This is less than the 7 to 8 hours of sleep that most people need each night, and may have resulted in a sleep debt (cf. Axelsson et al., 2008). Moreover, it is possible that the driver's sleep was further curtailed on the night before the incident, as there was evidence of activity on his mobile phone around four and a half hours before he woke up. The RAIB report also emphasised the role of task factors, since the incident occurred on a low workload stretch of track, which could have exacerbated the effect of any fatigue and acted as a catalyst for a microsleep (cf. Buckley et al., 2016; Desmond et al., 1998).

Nevertheless, the driver's stated belief was that his sleep pattern did not result in sleep deprivation. This raises other aspects of fatigue risk management at an organisational level, such as the culture around fatigue reporting and guidance on managing one's own fatigue. In the case of the incident at Sandilands, RAIB did not find sufficient evidence that these aspects were causally linked to the driver's possible fatigue on the day. (RAIB did, however, identify areas of potential improvement for fatigue risk management in a recommendation to the tram company which has since been implemented; see Chapter 5.1 of this book). Other RAIB investigations have revealed similar factors to be involved in fatigue-related incidents.

Two signal passed at danger (SPAD) incidents near Reading, Berkshire, in 2015 exhibited similar characteristics to each other in that they both involved freight trains whose drivers were nearing the end of a long night shift, and momentarily fell asleep on the approach to the signals concerned. Owing to the similarity of these incidents, RAIB investigated both of them together (RAIB, 2016), identifying factors associated with shift patterns as well as noting that neither driver reported as unfit for duty.

There are two parts to the challenge of fatigue reporting. The first is how to determine whether a member of staff is fit for duty, not just when they book on for duty, but also if they will remain so for the duration of their shift. The second, related challenge is how to accommodate staff who find that they become fatigued while on duty. There can be huge operational implications across the railway if a driver decides that they can no longer continue their journey; these pressures, along with a perception of consequent disciplinary action (whether or not that perception is justified), can act as strong barriers against drivers' willingness to report as fatigued. A "just" organisational culture (cf. Dekker, 2016) is crucial here in encouraging open and honest reporting, supported by suitable flexibility in dealing with the operational consequences. Moreover, engagement and education of staff about fatigue can facilitate the development of such a culture as well as go some way to raise awareness of fatigue. In many cases, staff are just unaware that they may be (or may become) fatigued, so it is essential that the causes, consequences, and countermeasures for fatigue are well known among the workforce.

The organisational implications reach even wider than this. In its investigation of a night-time fatality in November 2018 involving a track worker near Purley, south London, RAIB (2019) found that the rail industry's use of staff on so-called "zero-hours" contracts[2] made it difficult to manage fatigue effectively. Some of the staff involved in that incident had taken on additional daytime employment, which is not uncommon for zero-hours workers, but which increases the risk of fatigue. As well as the employer's responsibilities, then, there is an onus on the employee to manage their lifestyle outside of work such that they are suitably prepared and fit for duty.

Taken as a whole, valuable lessons have been learnt from these investigations about fatigue risk management in areas such as roster design, fitness for duty, fatigue reporting, education, training, and culture.

2.2.4 CHALLENGES AND FUTURE WORK

The GB rail industry's health and safety strategy (RSSB, 2020a) recognises fatigue risk management as one of 12 key risk areas to focus on in the coming years. Having a clear strategy has created momentum and provided a focus for action on fatigue risk management. In line with findings from the proactive survey and research studies, and the incident investigations and analysis described above, the strategy sets out five key challenges for the industry to overcome in order to improve how it manages this key risk.

2.2.4.1 PLANNED WORKING PATTERNS

The first of these challenges relates to the design of working patterns, including planned overtime and on-call status, to take into account employees' physiological processes such as sleep and circadian effects (Borbély, 1982; Darwent et al., 2015; Borbély et al., 2016). This was a key factor considered in the freight train rollback incident at Shap (RAIB, 2011) described above. It is also related to other important issues including railway finances, societal requirements for the timing and frequency of services, staff headcount, information technology, and staff working conditions.

In the decade since Shap, the industry has commissioned projects on developing numerical guidelines to avoid building fatiguing features into working patterns, and the appropriate use of biomathematical models to evaluate fatigue risk in sequences of shifts (Somvang et al., 2016; see also Chapter 4.3 of this book).

To truly manage fatigue risk related to working patterns, it is important to consider the bigger question of why companies evaluate rosters. Macgregor-Curtin et al.'s (2021) survey of railway companies revealed that all seven of the GB railway companies that took part used biomathematical models to bring rosters below an arbitrary[3] threshold or limit, but only four of these also reported that they would aim to reduce the scores to as low as reasonably practicable. The implication is that in some companies, simple changes that would further reduce fatigue risk would not be considered, because the focus is on compliance with a predefined threshold. Indeed, the UK's Health and Safety Executive has recently removed its biomathematical model, the Fatigue and Risk Index, from its website, citing that it was "being misused in order to justify work patterns that clearly require further action to reduce fatigue-related risk" (HSE, 2021). While this criticism is not necessarily directed at the rail industry, it shows the importance of culture and training in applying fatigue science to the rostering task.

A key focus for the rail industry in the coming years will be on broadening its application of existing tools and guidelines, and using them with a view to minimising fatigue risk as far as is reasonably practicable. The industry is also eager to see the scientific community refine and improve existing tools and guidelines to better account for a range of fatiguing factors such as cumulative fatigue and insufficient recovery from the effects of shiftwork (St Hilaire et al., 2017; Somvang et al., 2016; Van Dongen et al., 2004), and to develop tools which produce outputs that clearly express the safety risk from fatigue.

2.2.4.2 UNPLANNED CHANGES TO WORKING PATTERNS

The rail industry must deal with unplanned events such as staff absence, equipment failures, and engineering works, as part of its day-to-day operations. Responding to these types of challenges on the day is especially difficult for companies that work with low staff levels and limited contingency. Unplanned changes can result in working patterns that are very different from the planned roster, and this can have an impact on fatigue risk. Indeed, Balfe and Doyle's (2021) analysis of train depot incidents found that actual hours worked by staff carried a higher fatigue risk when compared with the planned (base) roster. However, the impacts of unplanned changes to the roster on fatigue risk are not always evaluated in detail, especially if this process is carried out manually.

A related challenge is about accurately recording actual hours worked by railway staff, to enable a retrospective analysis of the impact of changes "on the day" and to proactively consider the fatigue-related effects of those changes on the remainder of a roster. While some GB rail companies do this already (Macgregor-Curtin et al., 2021), for companies that do not have information technology systems that automate at least part of this process, this task presents an effortful administrative burden. Furthermore, and as discussed above in relation to the Purley incident (RAIB, 2019), casual work and zero-hours contracts have made it difficult for railway companies to maintain an awareness of the totality of their workers' schedules, which is a prerequisite for proactively or reactively assessing fatigue risk related to working patterns. As of autumn 2021, Network Rail's new contingent labour contracts aim to reduce the organisation's and its contractors' reliance on zero-hours contracts (RSSB, 2021a), and it is hoped that this will have a positive impact on the management of fatigue risk.

2.2.4.3 Fitness for Duty and Fatigue Reporting

As the incidents at Sandilands (RAIB, 2017/2020) and Reading (RAIB, 2016) highlighted, even with shift patterns that are aligned with good fatigue risk management practices, people might not get the sleep they need or may suffer from fatigue for other reasons. Therefore, a third challenge relates to making decisions about fitness for duty and reporting fatigue when needed.

The investigation into the SPADs near Reading (RAIB, 2016), in which one of the drivers was suffering from an undiagnosed sleep disorder, highlighted the importance of screening for such and providing treatment for sufferers, for which a number of options are now available (see Chapters 3.3, 4.9 and 5.3 for further discussion). Data from Macgregor-Curtin et al. (2021) suggest that of the seven GB rail companies that took part in the survey, three routinely assessed their staff for sleep disorders during regular medicals, and the remaining four only carried out assessments by exception. Considering fatigue more broadly, only two GB companies reported that fatigue was included explicitly in their company's fitness for duty rules (Macgregor-Curtin et al., 2021).

In recent years there have been scientific and technological developments towards more objective quantitative assessments of fatigue as a component of fitness for duty, ranging from self-reported sleep or actigraphy (e.g., Roach et al., 2010) coupled with a biomathematical model (Dorrian et al., 2019), to physiological tests (Martindale, 2012). A recent study by RSSB (2021b) evaluated two tools (one based on self-reported sleep and another based on actigraphy) that gave a fatigue-related prediction based on the user's recent sleep. The study concluded that more work is needed on these tools before they can be used on the railway to make decisions about fatigue at an individual level. In the meantime, the RSSB study recommended that the industry should integrate fatigue considerations into fitness for duty checking regimes through the use of rating scales (Åkerstedt & Gilberg, 1990) and rules of thumb about recent time asleep and time awake (Dawson & McCulloch, 2005; Wong et al., 2019). It is nevertheless important to judge each tool on its own merits and this is another area where the industry will benefit from scientific developments.

Alongside tools and processes, RSSB (2021b) also highlighted the importance of a mature, just organisational culture which we have discussed above in relation to RAIB's (2016) report on the Reading incidents.

2.2.4.4 EDUCATION AND TRAINING

A key enabler for a mature approach to managing fatigue risk is education and training (RSSB, 2012). For some years the focus of fatigue-related training in the GB rail industry has been on front-line staff. Further analysis of data from Macgregor-Curtin et al. (2021) showed that all seven of the GB rail companies that took part in the survey offer information to their staff on sleep, signs of fatigue, and managing fatigue on duty. Training on sleep and sleep hygiene, coupled with training in fatigue reporting procedures, is key to managing the significant risk of fatigue from home-life-related factors. However, the industry's health and safety strategy (RSSB, 2020a) recognises that, for a fatigue risk management system to work well, all staff who are allocated responsibilities under this system need to understand the risk and what they need to do to manage it. As discussed above, this is part of the solution to the current challenges around roster development, fitness for duty decisions, and fatigue reporting. This is also why the industry is looking at incorporating fatigue considerations into education and training for those involved in rostering, line managers, senior managers, and incident investigators.

2.2.4.5 USING DATA TO SUPPORT FATIGUE RISK MANAGEMENT

The types of research studies and analysis we have described above are effort-intensive and expensive, and are therefore not repeated frequently. Thus, the focus in the coming years must be on gathering and reporting the required data as part of day-to-day operations, to measure the "health" of companies' fatigue risk management systems.

The evaluation of fatigue risk controls is an integral part of fatigue risk management systems (RSSB, 2012). The Macgregor-Curtin et al. (2021) study showed that out of seven GB railway companies that responded to the survey, most set rostering rules around shift pattern design, but very few measured any key performance indicators (KPIs) to do with these rules. An ongoing cross-industry workstream aims to define a suite of KPIs, which companies can use to measure the "health" of their fatigue risk management system, and there are aspirations to anonymously report a subset to a relevant industry safety committee. These KPIs could be on, for example, rostering, fatigue training, and fatigue reports and incidents.

The contribution of fatigue to operational and safety incidents can be difficult to investigate, and even extreme cases of fatigue may not come to light if they do not lead to an incident or a fatigue report. The industry is also closely watching the developments in technology to monitor drowsiness and microsleeps (Dawson et al., 2014; Caldwell et al., 2009), which could provide more granular and reliable data on fatigue occurrences than what is currently available. The industry is keen to see data on the evaluation of such technologies, including their sensitivity and specificity in identifying fatigue.

2.2.5 CONCLUSIONS

Fatigue is a complex issue which requires organisations to adopt a multi-layered approach to address the risks specific to their operation (RSSB, 2012). Since the introduction of GB legislation requiring a risk-based approach, there has been a shift in focus in terms of the management of fatigue. In GB, sector-based fatigue working groups have been formed within the rail industry to develop and share good practices in fatigue risk management, and these groups have produced guidance on specific aspects of fatigue risk management (e.g., RSSB, 2020b).

SUMMARY POINTS FOR PRACTITIONERS

In this chapter we have presented some insights into the GB rail industry's fatigue risk management journey to date, and discussed the challenges that the industry faces as it seeks to mature its approach to managing this risk. In summary:

- Fatigue is a factor in 21% of high-risk rail incidents in GB, according to an analysis of incident investigation reports. Research and thorough incident investigation are key to quantifying the risk from fatigue and creating an initial evidential base to persuade stakeholders to act. Over time, this evidence should be generated and reported within the operation in order to drive continuous improvement.
- It is very difficult to detect and predict fatigue. There is a strong need for industry and academia to work together on the development and evaluation of tools, such as fatigue detection or assessment methods and biomathematical models to support rostering.
- Companies in the rail industry are benefiting from collaboration on fatigue risk management, which allows them to share good practice and to resolve challenges such as tracking the working patterns of railway workers, who sometimes work across multiple companies.
- To transition from a compliance-driven approach to a risk management approach to fatigue risk management, all staff need education on fatigue risk, and all those with responsibilities under an FRMS need training on their role in managing the risk.
- Fatigue is experienced by the individual, so staff members are a vital source of intelligence on fatigue risk. Processes that are designed to be fair and supported by a just culture will increase the likelihood that staff members raise fatigue issues so that the risk can be managed and documented. Education and training, coupled with strong leadership from senior management, are critical to the development of a just culture.

NOTES

1   Signallers operate signals and points on rail infrastructure to facilitate the safe and timely movement of trains. In some other countries they are known as train dispatchers, traffic controllers, train controllers or train service controllers.

2   This is a type of contract in which employers do not have to provide a minimum amount of work to workers, and workers do not have to accept the work that is offered.
3   At the time of writing there were no scientifically validated thresholds for the biomathematical model used in the GB rail industry.

REFERENCES

Åkerstedt, T., & Gillberg, M. (1990). Subjective and objective sleepiness in the active individual. *The International Journal of Neuroscience*, 52(1–2), 29–37. https://doi.org/10.3109/00207459008994241

Axelsson, J., Kecklund, G., Akerstedt, T., Donofrio, P., Lekander, M., & Ingre, M. (2008). Sleepiness and performance in response to repeated sleep restriction and subsequent recovery during semi-laboratory conditions. *Chronobiology International*, 25(2), 297–308. https://doi.org/10.1080/07420520802107031

Balfe, N., & Doyle, K. (2021). Delving deeper: Applying human factors analysis to identify factors contributing to railway incidents. In *Proceedings of the 7th International Human Factors Virtual Rail Conference*. www.sparkrail.org/Lists/Records/DispForm.aspx?ID=27293

Borbély, A. A. (1982). A two process model of sleep regulation. *Human Neurobiology*, 1(3), 195–204.

Borbély, A. A., Daan, S., Wirz-Justice, A., & Deboer, T. (2016). The two-process model of sleep regulation: A reappraisal. *Journal of Sleep Research*, 25(2), 131–143. https://doi.org/10.1111/jsr.12371

Bowler, N., & Gibson, H. (2015). *Fatigue and Its Contribution to Railway Incidents*. RSSB. www.sparkrail.org/Lists/Records/DispForm. aspx?ID=22066

Buckley, R. J., Helton, W. S., Innes, C., Dalrymple-Alford, J. C., & Jones, R. D. (2016). Attention lapses and behavioural microsleeps during tracking, psychomotor vigilance, and dual tasks. *Consciousness and Cognition*, 45, 174–183. https://doi.org/10.1016/j.concog.2016.09.002

Caldwell, J. A., Mallis, M. M., Caldwell, J. L., Paul, M. A., Miller, J. C., & Neri, D. F. (2009). Fatigue countermeasures in aviation. *Aviation, Space, and Environmental Medicine*, 80(1), 29–59. https://doi.org/10.3357/asem.2435.2009

Darwent, D., Dawson, D., Paterson, J. L., Roach, G. D., & Ferguson, S. A. (2015). Managing fatigue: It really is about sleep. *Accident Analysis and Prevention*, 82, 20–26. https://doi.org/10.1016/j.aap.2015.05.009

Dawson, D., & McCulloch, K. (2005). Managing fatigue: It's about sleep. *Sleep Medicine Reviews*, 9(5), 365–380. https://doi.org/10.1016/j.smrv.2005.03.002

Dawson, D., & Reid, K. (1997). Fatigue, alcohol and performance impairment. *Nature*, 388(6639), 235. https://doi.org/10.1038/40775

Dawson, D., Searle, A. K., & Paterson, J. L. (2014). Look before you (s)leep: Evaluating the use of fatigue detection technologies within a fatigue risk management system for the road transport industry. *Sleep Medicine Reviews*, 18(2), 141–152. https://doi.org/10.1016/j.smrv.2013.03.003

Dekker, S. (2016). *Just Culture: Restoring Trust and Accountability in Your Organization* (3rd ed.). CRC Press. https://doi.org/10.1201/9781315590813

Desmond, P. A., Hancock, P. A., & Monette, J. L. (1998). Fatigue and automation-induced impairments in simulated driving performance. *Transportation Research Record*, 1628(1), 8–14. https://doi.org/10.3141/1628-02

DfT. (2011). *Fatigue and Road Safety: A Critical Analysis of Recent Evidence*, Road Safety Web Publication No. 21. Department for Transport. https://webarchive.nationalarchives.gov.uk/ukgwa/20121107103953/http://www.dft.gov.uk/pgr/roadsafety/research/rsrr/theme3/fatigueroadsafetyanalysis/pdf/rswp21report.pdf

Dorrian, J., Hursh, S., Waggoner, L., Grant, C., Pajcin, M., Gupta, C., Coates, A., Kennaway, D., Wittert, G., Heilbronn, L., Vedova, C. D., & Banks, S. (2019). How much is left in your "sleep tank"? Proof of concept for a simple model for sleep history feedback. *Accident Analysis and Prevention*, 126, 177–183. https://doi.org/10.1016/j.aap.2018.01.007

Hidden, A. (1989). *Investigation into the Clapham Junction Railway Accident*. Department for Transport. www.railwaysarchive.co.uk/documents/DoT_Hidden001.pdf

HSE. (2021, June). *RR446–The Development of a Fatigue / Risk Index for Shiftworkers*. Health and Safety Executive. www.hse.gov.uk/research/rrhtm/rr446.htm

Hulme, A., Stanton, N. A., Walker, G. H., Waterson, P., & Salmon, P. M. (2021). Complexity theory in accident causation: Using AcciMap to identify the systems thinking tenets in 11 catastrophes. *Ergonomics*, 64(7), 821–838. https://doi.org/10.1080/00140139.2020.1869321

Johns, M., & Hocking, B. (1997). Daytime sleepiness and sleep habits of Australian workers. *Sleep*, 20(10), 844–849. https://doi.org/10.1093/sleep/20.10.844

Macgregor Curtin, I., Balfe, N., & Leva, M.C. (2021). Managing and measuring fatigue: A survey of rail industry practices. In *Proceedings of the 7th International Human Factors Virtual Rail Conference*. www.sparkrail.org/Lists/Records/DispForm.aspx?ID=27293

Marcus, J. H., & Rosekind, M. R. (2017). Fatigue in transportation: NTSB investigations and safety recommendations. *Injury Prevention: Journal of the International Society for Child and Adolescent Injury Prevention*, 23(4), 232–238. https://doi.org/10.1136/injuryprev-2015-041791

Martindale V. E. (2012). Breathalyzer for fatigue: The "fatigualyzer". *Aviation, Space, and Environmental Medicine*, 83(1), 70–71. https://doi.org/10.3357/asem.3210.2012

McGuffog, A., Spencer, M.B., Stone, B.M., & Turner, C. (2005) *Guidelines for the Management and Reduction of Fatigue in Train Drivers, T059*. RSSB. www.sparkrail.org/Lists/Records/DispForm.aspx?ID=9342

Moreno, C., Marqueze, E. C., Sargent, C., Wright Jr, K. P., Ferguson, S. A., & Tucker, P. (2019). Working Time Society consensus statements: Evidence-based effects of shift work on physical and mental health. *Industrial Health*, 57(2), 139–157. https://doi.org/10.2486/indhealth.SW-1

ORR. (2020, May 13). *Contractor Renown Consultants Fined £450k*. Office of Rail and Road. www.orr.gov.uk/search-news/contractor-renown-consultants-fined-ps450k

RAIB. (2011). *Uncontrolled Freight Train Run-Back between Shap and Tebay, Cumbria 17 August 2010* (Report 15/2011). Rail Accident Investigation Branch, Department for Transport. https://assets.digital.cabinet-office.gov.uk/media/547c8fe9e5274a4290000018d/R152011_110815_Shap_Summit.pdf

RAIB. (2016). *Two Signal Passed at Danger Incidents, at Reading Westbury Line Junction, 28 March 2015, and Ruscombe Junction, 3 November 2015* (Report 18/2016). Rail Accident Investigation Branch, Department for Transport. https://assets.publishing.service.gov.uk/media/5ad9b47de5274a76c13dff84/R182016_160930_Reading_Ruscombe.pdf

RAIB. (2017/2020). *Overturning of a Tram at Sandilands Junction, Croydon 9 November 2016* (report 18/2017 version 2.2). Rail Accident Investigation Branch, Department for Transport. https://assets.publishing.service.gov.uk/media/5de79643e5274a06dee23a10/R182017_201022_Sandilands_v2.2.pdf

RAIB. (2019). *Track Worker Struck by a Train at Stoats Nest Junction, near Purley 6 November 2018 (Report 07/2019)*. Rail Accident Investigation Branch, Department for Transport. https://assets.publishing.service.gov.uk/government/uploads/system/uploads/attachme nt_data/file/920525/R072019_190711_Stoats_Nest_Junction.pdf

Roach, G. D., Darwent, D., & Dawson, D. (2010). How well do pilots sleep during long-haul flights?. *Ergonomics*, 53(9), 1072–1075. https://doi.org/10.1080/00140139.2010.506246

Robertson, K., Spencer, M., McGuffog, A., & Stone, B. (2010). *Fatigue and Shiftwork for Freight Locomotive Drivers and Contract Trackworkers: Implications for Fatigue and Safety (T699)*. RSSB. www.sparkrail.org/Lists/Records_StaffMembers/DispForm. aspx?ID=369

RSSB. (2012). *Managing Fatigue Risk: A Good Practice Guide* (RS/504 Issue 1). RSSB. www. rssb.co.uk/en/standards-catalogue/CatalogueItem/RS504-Iss-1

RSSB. (2013). *Managing Occupational Road Risk Associated with Driver Fatigue: A Good Practice Guide*. RSSB. www.rssb.co.uk/-/media/Project/RSSB/RssbWebsite/Docume nts/Registered/Research-Projects/2020/07/06/17/55/T997_Managing_occupational_ro ad_risk-GPG.pdf

RSSB. (2019). *The Rail Industry Fatigue Survey*. RSSB. www.rssb.co.uk/en/what-we-do/key-industry-topics/fatigue-and-alertness/the-rail-industry-fatigue-survey

RSSB. (2020a). *Leading Health and Safety on Britain's Railway*. RSSB. www.rssb.co.uk/en/ safety-and-health/leading-health-and-safety-on-britains-railway

RSSB. (2020b). *9 Things You Should Consider for Your Fatigue Risk Management Plan*. RSSB. www.rssb.co.uk/-/media/Project/RSSB/RssbWebsite/Documents/Registered/Registe red-content/Insight-and-News/Health-and-Wellbeing/9-things-to-consider-for-your-fati gue-risk-mngmt-plan.pdf

RSSB. (2021a). *Annual Health and Safety Report 2020/21*. RSSB. www.rssb.co.uk/-/media/ Project/RSSB/RssbWebsite/Documents/Public/Public-content/Improving-Safety-and-Health/ashr/ahsr-2021-summary.pdf?la=en&hash=16EFA9841103729DBA5A367E4 F7E2637

RSSB. (2021b). *Fitness for Duty Decision Aids (T1130)*. RSSB. www.sparkrail.org/Lists/Reco rds/DispForm.aspx?ID=27314

Somvang, V., Hayward, B., & Cabon, P. (2016). *Guidance Document on Biomathematical Fatigue Models (T1083)*. RSSB. www.sparkrail.org/Lists/Records/DispForm. aspx?ID=24303

St Hilaire, M. A., Rüger, M., Fratelli, F., Hull, J. T., Phillips, A. J., & Lockley, S. W. (2017). Modeling neurocognitive decline and recovery during repeated cycles of extended sleep and chronic sleep deficiency. *Sleep*, 40(1), zsw009. https://doi.org/10.1093/sleep/ zsw009

Van Dongen, H. P.A., Maislin, G., & Dinges, D. F. (2004). Dealing with inter-individual differences in the temporal dynamics of fatigue and performance: Importance and techniques. *Aviation, Space, and Environmental Medicine*, 75(3 Suppl), A147–A154.

Williamson, A., & Friswell, R. (2011). Investigating the relative effects of sleep deprivation and time of day on fatigue and performance. *Accident Analysis and Prevention*, 43(3), 690–697. https://doi.org/10.1016/j.aap.2010.10.013

Wong, I. S., Popkin, S., & Folkard, S. (2019). Working Time Society consensus statements: A multi-level approach to managing occupational sleep-related fatigue. *Industrial Health*, 57(2), 228–244. https://doi.org/10.2486/indhealth.SW-6

2.3 Awakening to the Challenge of Fatigue Management in Maritime Transportation

Nita Lewis Shattuck, Darian Lawrence-Sidebottom, Panagiotis Matsangas, and Matthew Nicholson

Operations Research Department, Naval Postgraduate School, Monterey, CA, USA

CONTENTS

2.3.1 INTRODUCTION

Startled into wakefulness by his morning alarm, US Navy Lieutenant (LT) Johnson looks at his phone. It reads "0400". "Just another day living the dream", he thinks to himself as he stumbles out of his rack and clumsily puts his uniform on. After getting ready, LT Johnson grabs a quick breakfast and heads to his stateroom to prepare for the ship getting underway. He reviews the Plan of the Day: A mid-morning underway, followed by ammunition loadout, flight operations, and small boat operations, all before transiting to a new area of operations overnight to conduct engineering drills the next morning.

DOI: 10.1201/9781003213154-11

After making it through a busy but uneventful day, LT Johnson seizes an opportunity for a quick nap. The hour of sleep seems to pass all too quickly. Exhausted, and with little time to waste, he fills up his coffee mug and heads to the bridge to start turnover for the 22:00 to 02:00 watch. As the rest of the bridge team conducts their respective turnovers, LT Johnson assumes his duties as Officer of the Deck (OOD)— the direct representative of the Commanding Officer, responsible for ensuring the general safety, navigation, and operation of the ship. It should be a nice night with moderate temperatures, good visibility, light seas, and some moonlight due to show up around halfway through watch. Letting out a sigh and taking another sip of much-needed coffee, he says to himself, "It's only four hours".

At roughly half-past midnight, LT Johnson inspects the radar and notices several contacts off the starboard bow not far off in the distance. "We need to identify those contacts and figure out their closest point of approach", he tells the Junior Officer of the Deck (JOOD). The JOOD looks through her binoculars and senses that they may be facing an impending collision if they don't take action. "We should slow down", she says. "No, that will only make it worse!" blurts Johnson, without properly communicating his thought process. Confused, the JOOD thinks "Fine, but we should at least be making a turn to starboard since we're the give-way vessel. There are three contacts and there is plenty of space to manoeuvre behind them… Why aren't we doing anything?" With the invisible weight of exhaustion bearing down on him, LT Johnson's mind struggles to decide on the appropriate course of action. A few minutes later, and a little unsure of himself, he gives the order to come right ten degrees. However, this course change inadvertently puts the ship on a more direct collision course than before. The bridge goes quiet as the crew scrambles to make sense of the unfolding situation. Following a position update of the contacts, the bridge team is shocked to hear that one of the vessels is dangerously close. Short on time and trying to maintain the safety of the crew, LT Johnson orders the ship to come hard right, but then second guesses himself and orders the ship to come hard left. It's too late. There isn't enough time or space to avoid the impending collision.

2.3.1.1 BACKGROUND

The story above is a fictional recreation of the events that may have transpired onboard the USS Fitzgerald, a US Navy Arleigh Burke-class destroyer, the day it collided with the ACX Crystal, a container ship bound for Japan. Seven crew members died on the USS Fitzgerald and three more were injured in the incident. Thankfully, the crew onboard the ACX Crystal were unharmed. Beyond the tragic loss of life, the Fitzgerald sustained damage costing "in excess of $300 million". In the post-incident investigation, a lack of fatigue mitigation, particularly on the side of the US Navy, was identified as a major contributing factor to the incident. Indeed, long work hours and shift work exacerbated the fatigue level and cognitive impairment of the Fitzgerald OOD, as is evident in the story above. In addition, several other parties—including the JOOD, the surface warfare coordinator, and the optical sight system operator— were identified as having excessive fatigue. In the ship's combat information centre (which is responsible for identifying nearby contacts and relaying information to the bridge), six bridge watch-standers and seven crew members did not provide sufficient communication, judgement, and decision-making support to avoid the collision. Despite having ample time and resources to make a straightforward decision and handle a temporary mission deviation, fatigue challenged the Fitzgerald's crew to perform some of the most basic functions of seamanship.

In the last 30 to 40 years, several other high-profile incidents involving ships have clearly highlighted the potentially catastrophic consequences of fatigue in the maritime environment. In 1989, two separate tankships ran aground: the Exxon Valdez and Royal Majesty. The passenger vessel, Star Princess, ran aground in 1995, and in 2003 the cargo ship, Jambo, ran aground. In 2011, another major collision involved the tankship, Eagle Otome. In 2017, two major ship collisions occurred within the US Navy, less than two months apart: the collision of the USS Fitzgerald with the ACX Crystal (described above), and the collision of the USS John S. McCain with the Alnic MC.

In the post-incident investigations of each of these groundings and collisions, fatigue was called out as a major factor for the human error that contributed to those incidents. Sleep loss and fatigue are ubiquitous in the maritime industry, with round-the-clock operations and limited crew common on many ships. Excessively long working hours, inadequate sleep opportunities, and shift work have been cited as sources of sleepiness and fatigue in crew and officers. Additionally, post-incident investigations have reported undiagnosed, or untreated, sleep disorders in individuals partially responsible for some of the maritime incidents. For example, the pilots of the Star Princess and Jambo were both found to have obstructive sleep apnoea (OSA; see also Chapters 3.3 and 5.3 of this book). Operating at night is also problematic for safety in the maritime industry, as most of the incidents discussed above occurred during the night or early morning when alertness is at its lowest and human errors are more likely to occur.

In this chapter, we will further delve into shipboard stressors that contribute to or amplify fatigue, including sailor job demands and unique conditions associated with the shipboard environment. We will also briefly discuss other factors that can exacerbate fatigue and fatigue-related risks in the maritime environment (e.g., time of day and biological factors).

2.3.2   THE SHIPBOARD STRESSOR COMPLEX

The maritime work environment is characterised by several different types of stressors that affect ship crews, ultimately taking a toll on crew members' psychological and physiological state. Based on earlier research and a series of studies conducted by the Crew Endurance Team at the Naval Postgraduate School (NPS), we have classified these fatigue-inducing stressors into six groups that are considered in this chapter (Figure 2.3.1).

2.3.3   MISSION REQUIREMENTS

The maritime sector features a wide range of operations, including cargo transport, fishing, and military operations, with diverse mission goals and requirements.

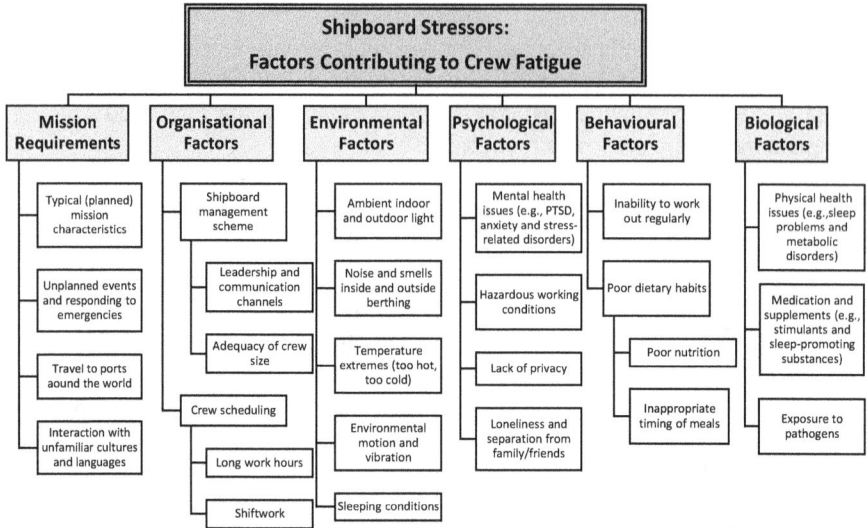

FIGURE 2.3.1   Shipboard stressors: factors contributing to maritime crew fatigue. (PTSD = post-traumatic stress disorder.)

Together, these maritime industries make for a busy global water-space with tremendous economic impact, with shipping accounting for an estimated 90% of global trade (International Maritime Organisation, 2009). Life at sea is largely determined by the operational requirements of a ship, as work conditions affect the seafarer's environment, responsibilities, and physical and mental workload. Scheduled tasks and unplanned events often contribute to exceptionally high workload, also called high operational tempo (OPTEMPO). The nature of international missions (e.g., for trade or military) requires ships to transit multiple time zones, which challenges circadian processes. Additionally, year-round navigation through congested ports and waterways to safely deliver goods on time can involve travel to countries with different cultures and languages.

2.3.4   ORGANISATIONAL FACTORS

2.3.4.1   SOCIAL FACTORS

The social structure aboard a ship is traditionally hierarchical but will vary according to leadership culture. The ship captain or "master" is responsible for overseeing all aspects of ship operations, including navigation, safety, and maintenance (Lützhöft, Grech, & Porathe, 2011; Oldenburg, Baur, & Schlaich, 2010). From there, the ship hierarchy is broken into departments and types of personnel. Personnel include officers, who primarily serve in leadership and managerial roles, and non-officers (e.g., enlisted personnel on naval ships), who perform more specialised work.

The organisational structure onboard ships often emphasises the "chain of command". Ship operations are governed by orders from the ship's captain and carried out through the respective departments. The chain-of-command provides clear translation and traceability of information flow. While this chain facilitates information flow from top to bottom of the organisation, it also necessitates that individuals higher up the chain be regularly informed of evolving situations. As a result, the captain is subjected to regular sleep disturbances when awakened by crew to make critical decisions or oversee dangerous shipboard evolutions.

Experience, age, and rank are closely aligned in the maritime industry, with more experienced and higher-ranking crew members tending to be older. The accepted sleep requirement for adults is 7 to 8 hours of sleep per night. However, younger adults and adolescents require more sleep and at later times (i.e., their circadian system is phase delayed). These factors appear to be related to sleep and fatigue on ships, where enlisted personnel (who tend to be younger) are more likely to report excessive daytime sleepiness, insomnia symptoms, and to be classified as poor sleepers than officers (Shattuck & Matsangas, 2022).

2.3.4.2 SCHEDULING CONSIDERATIONS

While at sea, the daily schedule or watch bill determines when crew members work, and defines the time available to eat, sleep, socialise, and tend to other personal activities. Shipboard culture often overlooks the importance of sleep for operational safety and effectiveness, as evidenced by the watch bills that limit opportunities for crew to obtain good sleep. Maritime operations generally run 24/7 and crew must be qualified (i.e., with appropriate training) to perform their duties. However, qualified crew members are limited, and regularly work long hours, often including nightshift work (Belenky, Lamp, Hemp, & Zaslona, 2014).

Longer shift durations are associated with greater levels of fatigue and poorer sleep (Gurubhagavatula et al., 2021). On the other hand, extremely short shift durations may interfere with crew situational awareness due to frequent hand-offs. Thus, the balance between shift duration and situational awareness is important when designing and implementing schedules. While a schedule may appear to involve reasonable working hours and provide adequate time for rest, crew members typically work more hours than prescribed by a schedule. In a study of crews working the 4/8 schedule (4 hours on watch and 8 hours off watch), sailors worked an average of 11.5 hours per day, with some individuals working more than 14 hours per day (Sanquist, Raby, Forsythe, & Carvalhais, 1997). This issue of extra, undocumented work duties is especially prevalent for crew members with more responsibilities, typically those who are more senior and those in command.

Nightshift work comes with increased risk because crew members are operating when alertness is at its lowest, and judgement and situational awareness are often impaired (Lützhöft et al., 2011). Not surprisingly, grounding mishaps occur more commonly during the late night and early morning hours when individuals are normally sleeping (Marine Accident Investigation Branch, 2004). In an assessment of US Navy sailors, nightshift workers exhibited greater impairment in sleep, sleepiness, and vigour compared to dayshift workers (Shattuck & Matsangas, 2020). Notably, dayshift workers also exhibited evidence of poor sleep and mood disturbance, demonstrating that, while working at night may exacerbate sleep and mood problems, fatigue is omnipresent in the maritime environment regardless of schedule timing.

To share the burden of nightshift work among crew members, rotating watch standing schedules are often used so that each person works all shifts at some point during the mission. While using a rotating schedule may seem like an equitable management decision, the imposition of a rotation—that is, forcing crew to regularly change their work and rest schedules—is another source of fatigue and risk, especially while the crew adapts to a new schedule. Following a schedule rotation, crew members may be working and sleeping at times that do not align with their natural circadian rhythms, ultimately contributing to performance impairment and disrupted sleep.

Unfortunately, schedules that do not align with the 24-hour day (also called "non-circadian watch bills") have been historically favoured in maritime operations. One of these rotating schedules is the "5/10" schedule, which involves a repeating cycle of 5 hours on-duty followed by 10 hours off-duty (Shattuck & Matsangas, 2015). In contrast, the 4/8, 6/6, and 3/9 schedules are commonly used fixed schedules that align with the 24-hour day (meaning that they are "circadian-based watch bills") (Comperatore, Rivera, & Kingsley, 2005; Lützhöft et al., 2011; Shattuck & Matsangas, 2016). Studies comparing circadian with non-circadian watch bills found that circadian watch bills were associated with better sleep and reduced fatigue (Shattuck & Matsangas, 2019). In 2015, the US Navy's submarine force abandoned their 6/12 non-circadian schedules that had been used for decades in favour of circadian-based 8/16 watch bills. All US Navy surface ships were directed in 2017 to adopt circadian-based watch bills, a clear attempt to mitigate the risks associated with fatigue and poor sleep in the maritime environment. However, this policy is not applied across maritime industries and does not address other sources of fatigue (e.g., long work hours).

Crew size is an important consideration for the selection of a watch bill because the number of qualified crew available directly affects possible shift durations. Larger crew sizes can accommodate watch bills with more sections (i.e., groups of crew members who work at different times), which allows each person to work shorter shifts, thereby reducing the workload for each person. Conversely, smaller crew sizes may be restricted to watch bills with few sections (e.g., two- or three-section watch bills), which are associated with longer shifts and fewer opportunities for rest.

2.3.5 ENVIRONMENTAL FACTORS

Crew members experience a host of environmental factors that are unique to the maritime domain, where ships may be exposed to severe weather conditions including rough seas, poor visibility, near-zero illumination nights, and extreme high and low temperatures (Comperatore et al., 2005; Lützhöft et al., 2011). Each of these environmental conditions may contribute to fatigue by interfering with sleep (directly or indirectly), altering OPTEMPO, and/or exacerbating physiological wear-and-tear and psychological stress (Comperatore et al., 2005; Lützhöft et al., 2011; Matsangas & Shattuck, 2017, 2021).

Light is the primary means by which our body entrains its circadian rhythm (see also Chapters 3.1 and 4.8 of this book). High energy visible (HEV) light suppresses melatonin secretion in the brain, thereby reducing the intensity of the biological "sleep" signal. Thus, exposure to light may pose a challenge for crew exposed to light at times that do not align with their circadian rhythm and sleep/wake schedule (e.g., during nightshift work). In a field study of US Navy sailors exclusively working night shifts, the sleep patterns of crew members working topside were contrasted with the sleep patterns of sailors working belowdecks (Matsangas & Shattuck, 2017; Miller & Nguyen, 2003). Sleep was significantly worse for the nightshift crew members who were exposed to natural light before bedtime (i.e., "topsiders") versus those who experienced only artificial light (i.e., their work was primarily belowdecks). Crew members working belowdecks even reported foregoing cigarettes in order to avoid the alerting effects of sunlight exposure before bedtime (Matsangas & Shattuck, 2017; Miller & Nguyen, 2003). Notably, because maritime operations are executed globally and at all times of the year, crew members may experience challenges from both natural and artificial lighting conditions. For example, in polar regions at extreme latitudes, light conditions vary throughout the year, with winter months characterised by periods of near-constant darkness and near-constant light in the summer months. Extremes in natural light conditions disrupt normal circadian rhythmicity, presenting challenges for maintaining healthy sleep habits.

The internal ship environment is largely determined by the external environment. Despite improvements in environmental control, shipboard temperatures are often at the mercy of regional climatic zones (Oldenburg, Jensen, Latza, & Baur, 2009). Cooler water temperatures typically result in cooler internal temperatures, whereas warmer water temperatures result in warmer internal temperatures. Further, certain compartments onboard a ship, such as the engine room or the catapult room onboard an aircraft carrier, can create excessive working temperatures—e.g., work in the engine room is often executed in temperatures exceeding 90°F/32 °C (Comperatore et al., 2005). Temperature is an important safety consideration; exposure to extreme ambient temperatures can contribute to fatigue and temperature in the sleeping space is known to affect sleep quality.

Ship motion can affect crew in a complex manner. Working in a moving environment can lead to motion-induced fatigue (Wertheim, 1998). Also, some individuals may experience motion sickness, which can be accompanied by sopite syndrome, a response to motion that is associated with significant drowsiness (Matsangas & McCauley, 2014). In a field study conducted aboard a high-speed US Navy ship, the HSV-2 *SWIFT,* crew members experienced extreme ship motion. Poor sleep outcomes (quality and duration) were most evident when the vessel was in particularly rough seas (Matsangas & Miller, 2006). Rough seas, however, can also be associated with increased sleep duration if crew members are motion sick and/or have symptoms of sopite syndrome (Matsangas, Shattuck, & McCauley, 2015).

While maritime platforms share many commonalities, environmental conditions may differ dramatically both within a ship and between different vessels which vary in terms of size, capabilities in rough seas, and habitability (Matsangas & Shattuck, 2017). Additionally, operational factors may affect environmental conditions such as location, OPTEMPO, and manning requirements.

2.3.6 PSYCHOLOGICAL FACTORS

Mariners are faced with several psychological stressors that are unique to working and living aboard sea-bound vessels. Their work is highly demanding and dangerous, as physical labour is often paired with personal risk. Further, maritime operations are often performed under significant time pressures. The wear and tear of this high OPTEMPO is exacerbated by inadequate opportunities for rest and recuperation. Additionally, most maritime missions require personnel to spend weeks or months at sea. These long underway periods result in extended separations from family, friends, and support networks (Comperatore et al., 2005; Lützhöft et al., 2011). In one study, sailors reported that the greatest source of stress was time away from home, followed by the demands of their work (Oldenburg et al., 2010). Unlike most other occupations, ship crews live and work in a confined environment for long periods of time. Loneliness on board, fatigue, multi-nationality (for mariners), inability to disengage from work, and limited recreation activities are some of the other factors that can be sources of psychosocial stress at sea (Bridger, Brasher, Dew, & Kilminster, 2011).

2.3.7 BEHAVIOURAL FACTORS

The relationship between physical activity and fatigue is bidirectional and often mediated by sleep. Acute and regular exercise has been shown to contribute to good sleep (Kredlow, Capozzoli, Hearon, Calkins, & Otto, 2015), and there is evidence that sleep also affects physical activity (Chennaoui, Arnal, Sauvet, & Léger, 2015). A study comparing fatigue and sleepiness in US Navy sailors found that those who reported low levels of fatigue tended to exercise more regularly than did those sailors with high levels of fatigue (Matsangas & Shattuck, 2016). Similarly, more frequent exercise while at sea may protect against the accumulation of sleepiness and negative mood states caused by extended underway periods (Dahlman, Matsangas, & Shattuck, 2017). Unfortunately, access to physical activity (e.g., exercise equipment and sports activities) is limited on ships. Unpublished data collected by the NPS Crew Endurance Team from 2009 to 2020 shows that only two-thirds of sailors on underway US Navy ships have a regular exercise routine. Inadequate physical activity while at sea may contribute to poor physical and mental health in sailors, exacerbating existing fatigue issues.

Limited timing for meals and reduced dietary options are characteristics of much of the maritime industry. Meals are offered at highly structured times during operations, so crew may have difficulty eating at times that best align with sleep/wake patterns and digestion. For example, eating at night, especially close to bedtime, is associated with negative physiological outcomes, such as higher percentage of body fat and higher prevalence of gastroesophageal reflux disease (Fujiwara et al., 2005; McHill et al., 2017). The timing of food availability may result in eating close to bedtime or skipping meals altogether. In an assessment of meal timing in relation to sleep onset, Shattuck and Matsangas (2021) found that approximately 20% of US Navy sailors had an average meal-to-sleep interval of less than 3 hours, with 10% of the measured meal-to-sleep intervals indicating that sailors ate within 15 minutes of bedtime. Individuals on a two-section watch bill ate closer to bedtime than those on three- or four-section watch bills. Meal timing also affects cognitive performance. Gupta and colleagues demonstrated an association between eating at night and impairments in vigilant attention and driving performance (Gupta et al., 2018). This reduction in performance is an important consideration for crew members who must perform duties at night.

Insufficient sleep produces changes in the regulation of the hormones responsible for signalling hunger and satiety (ghrelin and leptin), such that the body's hunger signal is generally stronger and the satiety signal is dampened (Taheri, Lin, Austin, Young, & Mignot, 2004). This effect is accompanied by increased intake of carbohydrates and weight gain (Markwald et al., 2013). While aboard a ship, crew have little control over food options, although most maritime industries are required to provide crews with meals of adequate nutritional quality to support health and well-being (Oldenburg, Harth, & Jensen, 2013). Nonetheless, sleep-restricted or shift working sailors may be more likely to select unhealthy foods, thereby contributing to obesity, poor metabolic health, and poor overall well-being.

2.3.8 BIOLOGICAL FACTORS

Physical issues and pathologies, including poor metabolic health, mental health issues, and sleep disorders, can contribute to fatigue in sailors. It is difficult to generalise health status to all seafarers, however, because the overall health and well-being of seafarers depends on many factors, including industry and working conditions. For example, military seafarers may be held to more stringent health requirements than those in other industries, where health problems may be more prevalent. A study of sailors working on Danish ships (e.g., container vessels and tankers) found that Nordic seafarers had a higher prevalence of being overweight or obese compared to the general Nordic population (Hoeyer & Hansen, 2005). Further, a recent meta-analysis identified metabolic syndrome, obesity, and cardiovascular/coronary heart disease as the main health issues that affect seafarers (Drylli et al., 2019). In a study conducted on a US Navy aircraft carrier, approximately 60% of sailors reported having experienced musculoskeletal symptoms over the course of a year. Symptomatic sailors reported greater levels of fatigue compared to sailors without musculoskeletal symptoms (Shattuck, Matsangas, Moore, & Wegemann, 2016).

Sleep disorders are characterised by degraded sleep quality and/or quantity. Insomnia and OSA are the most commonly diagnosed sleep disorders, with some studies estimating that up to one-third of the general population has insomnia (Bhaskar, Hemavathy, & Prasad, 2016). A recent study reported a drastic increase in the incidence of OSA and insomnia in the US military services, including the Navy and Marine Corps, from 2005 to 2019 (Moore, Tison, Palacios, Peterson, & Mysliwiec, 2021). However, the prevalence of diagnoses of both disorders was still far lower than in the general population (<5%), which suggests either that sleep disorders are underdiagnosed or truly less prevalent in US military sailors. We did not identify any published assessments of sleep disorders in other maritime sectors, highlighting that further research is needed to quantify the rates of sleep disorders in different maritime populations.

The use of pharmacological interventions can diminish or intensify fatigue. Caffeine may transiently promote alertness, thereby sustaining performance (Kamimori, Johnson, Thorne, & Belenky, 2005). However, excessive use of caffeine may result in greater tolerance and diminished effectiveness of its alerting properties. Synthetic melatonin can be used to promote better sleep when taken before bedtime (Krueger et al., 2011; Paul et al., 2001), and can also be used to shift circadian timing (Dawson & Armstrong, 1996). Further, melatonin may be more suitable for use in operational environments than other sleep-promoting substances because it does not degrade performance or result in grogginess upon awakening (Paul, Gray, Kenny, & Pigeau, 2003). Notably, using caffeine and melatonin to promote alertness and sleepiness, respectively, is most effective when circadian (i.e., biological time of day) and operational (e.g., performance requirements) factors are taken into account.

2.3.9 CONCLUSIONS

Considering the potentially catastrophic consequences of human error in maritime operations, increased fatigue and risk contribute to dangerous and potentially deadly conditions. In this chapter, we have detailed various factors present in the maritime environment that may produce fatigue. Each of these factors must be addressed to increase safety, optimise performance, and improve the health and well-being of crew members. The remedies listed will require changes to the status quo, involving a drastic shift in the maritime culture that has historically turned a blind eye to the consequences of a fatigued crew. It is crucial that fatigue mitigation efforts are prioritised by policymakers, ship commands, and individual seafarers, and that these groups work together to develop and implement fatigue mitigation plans. Importantly, these fatigue mitigation plans should address multiple sources of fatigue and should be based on best practices and recommendations from sleep and circadian experts.

SUMMARY POINTS FOR PRACTITIONERS

- Fatigue is highly prevalent in the maritime sector and has been identified as a major contributor to several catastrophic incidents involving ships.
- Mission requirements (e.g., job demands, unplanned events, and high operational tempo) and organisational factors, such as challenging work schedules or watch bills (e.g., long work hours and/or shift work), may cause or exacerbate fatigue levels in crew members.
- The shipboard environment often includes factors (e.g., light, noise, motion, and uncomfortable berthing spaces) that produce stress and interfere with good-quality sleep.
- The physiological and health status of sailors plays an important role in determining fatigue levels. It can be difficult to maintain healthy habits aboard ships and sailors may have poor mental and/or physical health, which further magnifies the fatigue produced by other factors present in the maritime environment.
- To optimise performance and well-being in crew members, thereby mitigating risk, it is crucial for policymakers, leaders, and individual sailors to reduce the effects of the shipboard stressor complex by implementing fatigue management techniques.

REFERENCES

Belenky, G., Lamp, A., Hemp, A., & Zaslona, J. L. (2014). Fatigue in the workplace. In M. Bianchi (Ed.), *Sleep Deprivation and Disease: Effects on the Body, Brain and Behavior* (pp. 243–268). New York: Springer Science.

Bhaskar, S., Hemavathy, D., & Prasad, S. (2016). Prevalence of chronic insomnia in adult patients and its correlation with medical comorbidities. *Journal of Family Medicine and Primary Care, 5*(4), 780–784. doi: 10.4103/2249-4863.201153

Bridger, R. S., Brasher, K., Dew, A., & Kilminster, S. (2011). Job stressors in naval personnel serving on ships and in personnel serving ashore over a twelve month period. *Applied Ergonomics, 42*(5), 710–718. doi: 10.1016/j.apergo.2010.11.005

Chennaoui, M., Arnal, P. J., Sauvet, F., & Léger, D. (2015). Sleep and exercise: A reciprocal issue? *Sleep Medicine Reviews, 20*, 59–72. doi: 10.1016/j.smrv.2014.06.008

Comperatore, C. A., Rivera, P. K., & Kingsley, L. (2005). Enduring the shipboard stressor complex: A systems approach. *Aviaton Space Environmental Medicine, 76*(6 Suppl.), B108–B118.

Dahlman, A. S., Matsangas, P., & Shattuck, N. L. (2017). The effect of habitual exercise on daytime sleepiness and mood of US Navy sailors. *Proceedings of the Human Factors and Ergonomics Society Annual Meeting, 61*(1), 522–526. doi: 10.1177/1541931213601615

Dawson, D., & Armstrong, S. M. (1996). Chronobiotics–drugs that shift rhythms. *Pharmacology and Therapeutics, 69*(1), 15–36. doi: 10.1016/0163-7258(95)02020-9

Drylli, A., Papanikolaou, V., Chrysovergis, A., Kanella, Z., Kikidis, D., & Kyrodimos, E. (2019). Seafarers' health problems, emergencies, diseases and risk factors: A systematic review of the literature. *International Journal of Medical and Health Research, 5*(2), 43–48.

Fujiwara, Y., Machida, A., Watanabe, Y., Shiba, M., Tominaga, K., Watanabe, T.,… . Arakawa, T. (2005). Association between dinner-to-bed time and gastro-esophageal reflux disease. *The American Journal of Gastroenterology, 100*(12), 2633–2636.

Gupta, C. C., Dorrian, J., Centofanti, S., Coates, A., Kennaway, D., Wittert, G.,… . Banks, S. (2018). Meal inertia: The impact of eating different sized meals on vigilant attention throughout the night. *Sleep, 41*(Abstract supplement 1), A67–A68.

Gurubhagavatula, I., Barger, L. K., Barnes, C. M., Basner, M., Boivin, D. B., Dawson, D.,… . Van Dongen, H. P. A. (2021). Guiding principles for determining work shift duration and addressing the effects of work shift duration on performance, safety, and health: Guidance from the American Academy of Sleep Medicine and the Sleep Research Society. *Sleep, 44*(11). doi: 10.1093/sleep/zsab161

Hoeyer, J. L., & Hansen, H. L. (2005). Obesity among Danish seafarers. *International Maritime Health, 56*(1–4), 48–55.

International Maritime Organization. (2009). *International Shipping and World Trade: Facts and Figures*. London, UK.

Kamimori, G. H., Johnson, D. E., Thorne, D., & Belenky, G. L. (2005). Multiple caffeine doses maintain vigilance during early morning operations. *Aviation Space and Environental Medicine, 76*(11), 1046–1050.

Kredlow, M. A., Capozzoli, M. C., Hearon, B. A., Calkins, A. W., & Otto, M. W. (2015). The effects of physical activity on sleep: A meta-analytic review. *Journal of Behavioral Medicine, 38*(3), 427–449. doi:10.1007/s10865-015-9617-6

Krueger, G. P., Bergoffen, G., Pickettt, R., Leaman, H. M., Murray, D., & Transportation Research Board. (2011). *Effects of Psychoactive Chemicals on Commercial Driver Health and Performance: Stimulants, Hypnotics, Nutritional, and Other Supplements.* Washington, DC: Transportation Research Board.

Lützhöft, M., Grech, M. R., & Porathe, T. (2011). Information environment, fatigue, and culture in the maritime domain. *Reviews of Human Factors and Ergonomics*, *7*(1), 280–322. doi: 10.1177/1557234X11410391

Marine Accident Investigation Branch. (2004). *Bridge Watchkeeping Safety Study*. Southampton, UK.

Markwald, R. R., Melanson, E. L., Smith, M. R., Higgins, J., Perreault, L., Eckel, H., & Wright Jr., K. P. (2013). Impact of insufficient sleep on total daily energy expenditure, food intake, and weight gain. *Proceedings of the National Academy of Science of the United States of America*, *110*, 5695–5700.

Matsangas, P., & McCauley, M. E. (2014). Sopite syndrome: A revised definition. *Aviation Space and Environmental Medicine*, *85*, 672–673.

Matsangas, P., & Miller, N. L. (2006). The effects of ship motion on the sleeping patterns of crewmembers aboard a high speed Naval vessel. *Sleep*, *29*(Suppl. S), A126–A126.

Matsangas, P., & Shattuck, N. L. (2016). Discriminating between fatigue and sleepiness in the naval operational environment. *Behavioral Sleep Medicine*, *16*(5), 427–436. doi: 10.1080/15402002.2016.1228645

Matsangas, P., & Shattuck, N. L. (2017). Exploring sleep-related habitability issues in berthing spaces on U.S. Navy ships. *Proceedings of the Human Factors and Ergonomics Society Annual Meeting*, *61*(1), 450–454.

Matsangas, P., & Shattuck, N. L. (2021). Habitability in berthing compartments and well-being of sailors working on United States Navy surface ships. *Human Factors*, *63*(3), 462–473. doi: 10.1177/0018720820906050

Matsangas, P., Shattuck, N. L., & McCauley, M. E. (2015). Sleep duration in rough sea conditions. *Aerospace Medicine and Human Performance*, *86*(10), 901–906. doi: 10.3357/AMHP.4250.2015

McHill, A. W., Phillips, A. J. K., Czeisler, C. A., Keating, L., Yee, K. E., Barger, L. K.,…. Klerman, E. B. (2017). Later circadian timing of food intake is associated with increased body fat. *The American Journal of Clinical Nutrition*, *106*, 1213–1219. doi: 10.3945/ajcn.117.161588

Miller, N. L., & Nguyen, J. L. (2003). *Working the nightshift on the USS John C. Stennis: Implications for enhancing warfighter effectiveness*. Paper presented at the Human Systems Integration Symposium (HSIS) 2003: Enhancing Human Performance in Naval & Joint Environments, Vienna, VA.

Moore, B. A., Tison, L. M., Palacios, J. G., Peterson, A. L., & Mysliwiec, V. (2021). Incidence of insomnia and obstructive sleep apnea in active duty United States military service members. *Sleep*, *44*(7). doi:10.1093/sleep/zsab024

Oldenburg, M., Baur, X., & Schlaich, C. (2010). Occupational risks and challenges in seafaring. *Journal of Occupational Health*, *52*(5), 249–256.

Oldenburg, M., Harth, V., & Jensen, H.-J. (2013). Overview and prospect: Food and nutrition of seafarers on merchant ships. *International Maritime Health*, *64*(4), 191–194. doi: 10.5603/imh.2013.0003

Oldenburg, M., Jensen, H. J., Latza, U., & Baur, X. (2009). Seafaring stressors aboard merchant and passenger ships. *International Journal of Public Health*, *54*, 96–105.

Paul, M. A., Brown, G., Buguet, A., Gray, G., Pigeau, R. A., Weinberg, H., & Radomski, M. (2001). Melatonin and zopiclone as pharmacologic aids to facilitate crew rest. *Aviation, Space, and Environmental Medicine*, *72*(11), 974–984.

Paul, M. A., Gray, G., Kenny, G., & Pigeau, R. A. (2003). Impact of melatonin, zaleplon, zopiclone, and temazepam on psychomotor performance. *Aviation, Space, and Environmental Medicine*, *74*(12), 1263–1270.

Sanquist, T. F., Raby, M., Forsythe, A., & Carvalhais, A. B. (1997). Work hours, sleep patterns and fatigue among merchant marine personnel. *Journal of Sleep Research*, *6*, 245–251.

Shattuck, N. L., & Matsangas, P. (2015). Operational assessment of the 5-h on/10-h off watchstanding schedule on a US Navy ship: Sleep patterns, mood, and psychomotor vigilance performance of crew members in the nuclear reactor department. *Ergonomics, 59*(5), 657–664. doi:10.1080/00140139.2015.1073794

Shattuck, N. L., & Matsangas, P. (2016). Comparison of the 3/9 and 6/6 watchstanding schedules for crewmembers of a U.S. Navy destroyer. *Proceedings of the Human Factors and Ergonomics Society 37th Annual Meeting, 60*(1), 881–885.

Shattuck, N. L., & Matsangas, P. (2019). *Assessment of the utility of circadian-based watchstanding schedules for sailors working on U.S. Navy surface vessels* (Technical Report No. NPS-OR-19-001R). Monterey, CA: Naval Postgraduate School.

Shattuck, N. L., & Matsangas, P. (2020). Does the quality of life differ for shift workers compared to day workers? *Chronobiology International, 37*(9–10), 1299–1303. doi:10.1080/07420528.2020.1810062

Shattuck, N. L., & Matsangas, P. (2021). Eating behaviors in sailors of the United States Navy: Meal-to-sleep intervals. *Nutrition and Health, 27*(1), 3–8. doi:10.1177/0260106020960878

Shattuck, N. L., & Matsangas, P. (2022). Who sleeps more and who works longer in the US Navy: Officers or enlisted personnel? *Sleep Health.* doi:10.1016/j.sleh.2022.03.007

Shattuck, N. L., Matsangas, P., Moore, J., & Wegemann, L. (2016). Prevalence of musculoskeletal symptoms, excessive daytime sleepiness and fatigue in the crewmembers of a U.S. Navy ship. *Military Medicine, 181*(7), 655–662.

Taheri, S., Lin, L., Austin, D., Young, T., & Mignot, E. (2004). Short sleep duration is associated with reduced leptin, elevated ghrelin, and increased body mass index. *PloS Med, 1*(3). doi:10.371/journal.pmed.0010062

Wertheim, A. H. (1998). Working in a moving environment. *Ergonomics, 41,* 1845–1858.

2.4 Fatigue-Related Consequences in Aviation

Katherine Wilson and Jana Price

National Transportation Safety Board,
Washington DC, USA

CONTENTS

The views expressed in this chapter do not necessarily represent the views of the NTSB or the United States.

2.4.1 INTRODUCTION

Charles Lindbergh (1953) recalled the fatigue that ensued during his 33-hour solo transatlantic flight in 1927, stating,

> My mind clicks on and off, as though attached to an electric switch with which some outside force is tampering. I try letting one eyelid close at a time when I prop the other open with my will. But the effort's too much. Sleep is winning. My whole body argues dully that nothing, nothing life can attain is quite so desirable as sleep.

Lindbergh's insightful observations are of interest to researchers and perhaps familiar to many pilots. In this chapter, we examine how fatigue manifests in aviation, both for pilots and others in the aviation system. We also discuss lessons from investigations that uncovered fatigue issues and how such investigations can inform the development of countermeasures to reduce the incidence of fatigue-related events.

The International Civil Aviation Organization (ICAO, 2011) defines fatigue as "a physiological state of reduced mental or physical performance capability resulting from sleep loss or extended wakefulness, circadian phase, or workload (mental and/ or physical activity) that can impair a crew member's alertness and ability to perform safety related operational duties". For this chapter, we focus on fatigue induced by circadian factors, sleep loss, and extended wakefulness (Cabon, 2011; Tassi & Muzet, 2000), rather than fatigue caused by physical exertion or workload.

The National Transportation Safety Board (NTSB) is tasked with investigating all civil aviation accidents[1] in the United States, as well as major accidents in other modes of transportation including highway, rail, marine, and pipeline. The goal of NTSB investigations is to determine the probable cause of the accident and to issue safety recommendations to prevent recurrences of similar events. Safety recommendations are issued to those organisations that are best able to take corrective action, such as regulatory agencies, vehicle manufacturers, operators, and industry associations. The NTSB advocates for implementation of its safety recommendations and tracks progress of their adoption.

The Civil Aeronautics Board (as the NTSB was previously called) was citing fatigue as causal or contributing to aviation accidents in the 1960s (Mohler, 1965). In the 1980s, the NTSB published several major reports in which truck, bus, boat, or train operator fatigue was determined to be a causal factor. In the investigation report for the 1993 American International Airways flight 808 collision with terrain on approach to Guantanamo Bay, Cuba, impaired judgement, decision-making, and flying abilities of the captain and flight crew due to the effects of fatigue were identified as causal factors (NTSB, 1994), and the agency included an analysis of crew fatigue factors conducted by the US National Aeronautics and Space Administration (NASA) Fatigue Countermeasures group as an appendix to that report. The NASA analysis, led by Dr Mark Rosekind, who would 17 years later become an NTSB Board Member, helped to shape the NTSB's current approach to investigating fatigue factors. Between 2001 and 2014, 27% of major aviation accidents in the US (the primary focus of this chapter) were attributed to fatigue (Marcus, 2021).

To determine if fatigue was a factor in an event, investigators seek to determine (1) if fatigue was present at the time of the event and, if so, (2) whether the actions that led to the event are consistent with the known effects of fatigue. Like other investigative agencies worldwide, the NTSB focuses on five factors to determine if fatigue was present:

1. quantity of sleep—hours of sleep obtained in previous 24 to 72 hours;
2. quality of sleep—how well an individual slept with consideration of any interruptions to sleep;
3. time since awakening—how long an individual has been awake since their last sleep period;

4. circadian factors—time of day or circadian desynchronisation from crossing time zones;
5. medical factors—medical conditions that directly or indirectly induce fatigue.

Any of these factors either alone or in combination can cause an operator to be fatigued. If fatigue was present at the time of the event, the investigator must then determine if the actions that led to the event were consistent with the known effects of fatigue.

As discussed in previous chapters of this book, fatigue can result in degradation of decision accuracy and timing, difficulty focusing, increased risk taking, attitude and mood changes, and even involuntary lapses into sleep, among other effects. Fatigue can also make individuals more susceptible to cognitive biases, such as expectation and confirmation biases. And while these effects have been identified in numerous aviation investigations, the ability to definitively establish cause and effect is not always black and white as it is in a laboratory setting.

In 1994, the NTSB reviewed 37 flight crew-related major aircraft accidents and evaluated how time since awakening, circadian factors (time of day and time zone crossings), and work schedules contributed to errors (NTSB, 1994). The study found an increase in flight crew vulnerability based on time since awakening. Specifically, the study found that first officers who had been awake for more than 11 hours and captains who had been awake for more than 12 hours made significantly more procedural and tactical decision errors than those who had been awake for less time. The study also noted that, when time since awakening was a factor, it was "somewhat confounded" with time of day. Additionally, tactical decision errors were more common in afternoon-evening events than those that occurred during morning-midday.

In some investigations, the link between fatigue and actions that led to an event is clear. Consider, for example, a crash that occurred on September 22, 2012, at 1:50 AM (NTSB, 2013b). The pilot was flying his newly purchased Cessna 172 from Pensacola, Florida, to Tampa, Florida. About 15 minutes after being cleared by air traffic control (ATC) for landing, the airplane descended below 1000' despite being 15 nautical miles from the airport. ATC contact went unanswered, and the airplane continued a gradual descent until impacting a pasture about 17 miles from the airport. There was no evidence of hypoxia or drugs or alcohol in the pilot's system. A review of the pilot's schedule showed evidence of long days and circadian shifts over the previous 9 days. Fatigue, which resulted in the pilot falling asleep during the initial descent, was cited as the probable cause.

In a more recent event near Hazelhurst, Wisconsin, that took place just before 11:00 PM on April 26, 2018, in-cockpit video showed a helicopter pilot slump to his left as the aircraft rolled to the right until impacting the ground (NTSB, 2020a). The pilot appeared incapacitated, but the investigation found no evidence of medical conditions or of alcohol or other drugs in his system. Ultimately, the investigation determined that the pilot likely fell asleep as a result of working at night at a time when he had been sleeping during the previous week, and the soporific effect of the cruise environment.

2.4.2   MORE THAN JUST FALLING ASLEEP AT THE YOKE

There is no blood test for fatigue, nor does every cockpit have a video feed to identify when a pilot falls asleep, making the role of fatigue at times difficult to pinpoint. And in many cases, the pilot does not fall asleep, but rather may experience cognitive lapses or make a series of missteps or errors. The effects of fatigue in transportation can vary widely; in some modes, it can have an immediate effect. Consider the consequences of a driver who nods off at the wheel and drifts into oncoming traffic or runs a red light; even a brief microsleep at the wrong time could result in a crash. In other modes, like aviation, fatigue could have an immediate effect (such as misjudging the altitude on final approach) or its effect may not be actualised until much later—for example, programming an onboard computer incorrectly, or forgetting a maintenance task.

In some cases, fatigue degraded a pilot's ability to respond to an unexpected event. For example, an agricultural pilot was unable to recover the airplane after encountering wake turbulence near Butte City, California, on May 15, 2013 (NTSB, 2013a). The pilot had been awake for 15 hours, had worked for 12 of those hours and was experiencing high workload at the time of the event. In another event, the pilot did not follow emergency procedures after experiencing fuel exhaustion and crashed into powerlines while performing a forced landing near Goodland, Kansas, on January 21, 2015 (NTSB, 2016). Although the crash occurred at 7:54 AM, the pilot had been awake for over 15 hours and had worked an overnight shift.

In other cases, fatigue-related lapses led to errors that resulted in crashes downstream. For example, on October 21, 2017, at 5:30 AM, in Anchorage, Alaska, an air ambulance pilot did not confirm that the landing gear was extended before landing, resulting in substantial damage to the airplane (NTSB, 2020b). After the crash, the pilot told investigators that he had worked a long duty day and had experienced fragmented sleep in the preceding days. These factors, in conjunction with operating during the window of circadian low—that is, the time of day when the drive for sleep is greatest—contributed to the pilot's fatigue, which led to his error and ultimately the crash.

A more severe example that involved a fatigue-related lapse that escalated occurred when UPS 1354 crashed on approach to Birmingham, Alabama, on August 14, 2013, fatally injuring both crew members (NTSB, 2014). Evidence showed that the first officer had mis-programmed the flight management computer about 5 minutes prior; as a result, the crew was provided meaningless vertical guidance to the runway. This error went undetected by both crewmembers and the captain erroneously believed the airplane was high on the approach. The crash occurred during the window of circadian low, which likely adversely impacted both the captain's and first officer's performance. Additionally, the first officer was experiencing acute sleep loss due to inadequate management of her off-duty time, which she had recognised but decided to remain on duty rather than report as unfit or request time off.

The effects of fatigue on operational safety have not only been documented in pilots. For example, in the December 7, 2011, fatal helicopter crash near Las Vegas, Nevada (NTSB, 2013c), the NTSB determined that inadequate maintenance caused the crash. The mechanic's work schedule shifted the day before the maintenance work was performed, which—combined with a lack of clearly delineated task steps to follow—resulted in improper maintenance. The investigation also found that the maintenance inspector was fatigued resulting in an inadequate inspection.

The US has also seen investigations in which fatigue was not deemed causal or contributing but was recognised as a safety issue. Colgan Air crashed on February 12, 2009, killing 49 passengers and crew, as well as one person on the ground (NTSB, 2010b). The investigation revealed that both flight crew members were likely experiencing fatigue at the time of the crash due to poor sleep quality from sleeping in an airport crew room and while commuting on another flight. The extent to which the crew's fatigue contributed could not be determined, but the NTSB highlighted its concerns with fatigue management in its investigative report and issued a recommendation to the FAA. Following the investigation, a major campaign by the families of the passengers led to the establishment of better duty and rest requirements for flight crews. On January 4, 2014, 14 CFR Part 117 became effective. This rule prescribed new flight- and duty-time regulations for all flight crew members and certificate holders conducting certain passenger operations; unfortunately, the rules do not cover all passenger and cargo operations.

2.4.3 LEARNING FROM NEAR MISSES

In an ideal world, fatigue would be detected and addressed before safety is compromised. Although the NTSB is not required to investigate events that do not result in "accidents" as defined by its authorising legislation, the agency has investigated a number of near-miss events in which fatigue was causal or contributing. Most notably, on July 7, 2017, Air Canada flight 759 erroneously lined up for landing on a taxiway at San Francisco International Airport where four other air carrier airplanes were awaiting clearance for take-off (NTSB, 2018). ATC issued a go around (i.e., to discontinue the landing) to the crew and the Air Canada flight reached a minimum altitude of 60 feet as it overflew the waiting aircraft on the taxiway.

The incident occurred at 11:56 PM, PDT; however, the crew was based on the eastern time zone where the time would have been 2:56 AM, approaching the window of circadian low and higher susceptibility to fatigue. The crew was also unable to take advantage of controlled rest (defined by ICAO as a "short sleep opportunity" to mitigate unexpected fatigue during flight) during the flight due to challenging/poor weather encountered along the route. As such, the captain had been awake for 19 hours at the time of the event. Research has shown that performance decrements from time awake occur 17 hours after awakening (Dawson & Reid, 1997).

Being fatigued left the Air Canada crew susceptible to expectation bias, or the manipulation of perceived elements to be consistent with an individual's expectation (Bhattacherjee, 2001) and increased their difficulty in overcoming expectation bias once it occurred (Harrison & Horne, 1999). The crew was unaware that runway 28L was closed, and so they misaligned the aircraft with the taxiway, mistaking light cues from the waiting aircraft as runway lighting. For example, wingtip navigation lights on the departing aircraft appeared to be runway edge lights and red flashing beacon lights were consistent with approach lighting. Even though the crew stated in post-incident interviews that they saw green taxiway centreline lights near the beginning of what appeared to be the runway threshold, they continued the approach despite conflicting cues.

The crew's fatigue provided an additional challenge to the identification and investigation of the incident. The captain delayed reporting the incident until the next morning, stating that he was "very tired", and it was "very late" after they landed. Air Canada dispatch was notified about 4:08 PM the next day and, as a result, the portion of the cockpit voice recording that captured the event flight had been overwritten before it could be preserved. While the crew provided useful insights, the recording could have supplied additional details into the crew's observations and decisions during the approach to better understand the event. In a similar incident, a Boeing 767 landed on taxiway M at Atlanta Hartsfield International Airport after being cleared to land on runway 27R on October 19, 2009 (NTSB, 2010a). A more serious incident was avoided as there were no aircraft on the taxiway at the time of the landing. During the overnight flight, one flight crew member became ill which prevented the two remaining crew members from taking their anticipated crew rest during the flight. At the time of the incident, the flight crew had been on duty for about 12 hours; additionally, the captain had been awake for over 22 hours and the first officer had been awake for at least 14 hours.

Fatigue has also contributed to events involving ATC. For example, on March 24, 2011, a controller working alone during the midnight shift at Reagan National Airport fell asleep for at least 24 minutes (NTSB, 2011). During that time, two air carrier aircraft landed at the airport without contact with the tower. A post-incident investigation revealed that the controller on duty was experiencing fatigue due to acute sleep loss in the 24 hours before the event and circadian disruption due to working his fourth midnight shift in a row. The controller recalled thinking, "I need to throw some water on my face" and he knew he "was dragging" prior to falling asleep. He thought he had only been out for a couple of minutes and after he "came out of the haze" he had a fogginess that lasted at least 3 or 4 minutes. He recalled that "the adrenaline was pumping" after he woke up and he was able to get through the shift although he recalled feeling tired, but not exhausted, after about 5 minutes of making transmissions.

2.4.4   FATIGUE MITIGATION STRATEGIES

An international group of fatigue experts concluded that fatigue is "the largest identifiable and preventable cause of accidents in transport operations," and its impact is often underestimated, leading "to the underutilisation of important countermeasures" (Åkertstedt, 2000). In some investigations, the NTSB has documented precursors of fatigue risk, such as an undiagnosed sleep disorder, that—if they had been recognised and addressed—may have prevented the crashes from occurring. In other investigations, the risk of fatigue is systemic and not as easily remedied due to the nature of operations, such as overnight cargo flying. Between 1972 and 2017, the NTSB issued 235 recommendations related to fatigue across all modes of transportation. In aviation, almost half of the 59 recommendations focused on scheduling policies and practices; other focus areas included education and raising awareness, organisational strategies, healthy sleep, research and evaluation, and fatigue management plans. These recommendations and lessons learnt from investigations can be used to minimise the risk of fatigue and further enhance a highly reliable aviation system. Sleep is a complex issue and there is no one strategy that can address all factors contributing to fatigue; rather, a combination of strategies or interventions, including safety programmes, self-reporting fatigue, scheduling, health screenings, biomathematical modelling, education, and technologies, is critical to mitigating the effects of fatigue to ensure aviation safety.

2.4.4.1 SAFETY PROGRAMMES

It is not enough for near misses to occur for safety to be improved. Rather, the near misses must be captured, precursors must be understood, lessons learnt must be communicated, and mitigations must be put into place if necessary. Safety programmes are critical to identifying not only specific events but also trends in data that if allowed to continue could impact safety. Safety reporting systems are one such programme of capturing near misses. For example, the Aviation Safety Reporting System was developed from a partnership between NASA, FAA, air carriers, and labour organisations to allow for voluntary, confidential reporting of events in which safety has been compromised. It receives about 265 reports each day and has received close to 2 million reports since 1981.

Since 2015, large air carriers in the US have been required to implement a safety management system (SMS) in the organisation, and specifically a fatigue risk management system (FRMS). FRMS is defined by ICAO (2011) as "a data-driven means of continuously monitoring and managing fatigue related safety risks, based upon scientific principles and knowledge as well as operational experience that aims to ensure relevant personnel are performing at adequate levels of alertness." Additionally, Advisory Circular (AC) 120-103A "Fatigue Risk Management Systems for Aviation Safety" provides guidance to operators (FAA, 2013). The AC states that by combining "schedule assessment, operational data collection, continuous and systematic analysis, and both proactive and reactive fatigue mitigations, guided by information provided by scientific studies of fatigue", flexibility is offered within the regulatory limitations to operators while still adhering to flight time, duty time, and rest period requirements. One critical component of an FRMS is a non-punitive reporting policy in which a pilot (or other safety critical personnel) can report being fatigued and immediately be removed from duty so as to not jeopardise safety. Unfortunately, even with these programmes in place, fatigue is not always managed as not all pilots (or safety critical personnel) utilise these programmes.

In the aforementioned UPS 1354 crash near Birmingham, Alabama, the first officer did not take advantage of available sleep opportunities during her off-duty time and had acquired a sleep debt of over 13 hours on the night of the event. Text messages from her cell phone and a conversation between the crew captured on the CVR just prior to the flight indicated that the first officer was aware of her fatigued state; however, she did not report her fatigue to the company and according to a friend she wanted to "fly under the radar". Had she reported her fatigue, company policy would have required her immediate removal from the schedule. The investigation concluded that the first officer's fatigue due to acute sleep loss and circadian factors, combined with the time compression and the change in approach modes, likely resulted in the multiple errors she made during the flight.

Although not specific to only fatigue-related events, certain operators also use flight data monitoring programmes, in which flight data is regularly downloaded from the aircraft flight data recorder and analysed, to improve operational safety and efficiency. These operators also utilise a programme known as the Aviation Safety Action Program to encourage voluntary reporting of safety-related issues and events, including alleged violations of regulations.

2.4.4.2 SELF-REPORTING FATIGUE

The importance of self-reporting fatigue cannot be underestimated. In a survey of regional airline pilots, about one in three reported that they had fallen asleep while in the cockpit and about one in five reported that their company's attendance policies did not apply to calling in fatigued (Freiwald & O'Toole, 2015). Fatigue attendance policies were addressed in US commercial aviation passenger operations with the institution of 14 CFR Part 117. Unfortunately, individuals are not very good at rating their fatigue and fail to appreciate how tired they actually are until they are experiencing extreme levels of fatigue (Van Dongen et al., 2003). But even when individuals recognise their fatigue, they may fail to self-report, believing they can "push through" the fatigue or they may fear the consequences of calling in fatigued. In other cases, pilots may not recognise they are fatigued until they are in flight. Self-reporting fatigue to another crew member (if available) can facilitate discussions of options to minimise the impact of fatigue until the aircraft can be safely landed, or even reporting to ATC to receive priority landing if available. While some countries allow controlled rest in the cockpit to minimise fatigue, in-cockpit napping was excluded from US rest and duty regulations revised in 2010. Operating during the window of circadian low increases a pilot's risk of fatigue (see Chapter 4.10). As a result of the UPS 1354 investigation, the NTSB (2014) concluded that

> given the increased likelihood of fatigue during overnight operations, briefing the threat of fatigue before every flight would give pilots the opportunity to identify the risks associated with fatigue and mitigate those risks before taking off and throughout the flight.

The NTSB issued an accompanying recommendation to the FAA requiring "principal operations inspectors (POIs) to ensure that operators with flight crews performing... overnight operations brief the threat of fatigue before each departure, particularly those occurring during the window of circadian low". As of the time of this writing, the FAA did not act on this recommendation and the NTSB has designated it "Closed-Unacceptable Action." Controlled rest has been implemented in several places around the world (e.g., Canada, New Zealand, and Europe), and has been shown to be beneficial in laboratory studies (Rosekind et al., 1995). It must be implemented in such a way that it accounts for factors such as phase of flight/time until landing and sleep inertia.

2.4.4.3   HEALTH SCREENINGS

On February 13, 2008, both pilots of Go! Airlines flight 1002 unintentionally fell asleep in the cockpit on a flight from Honolulu to Hilo, Hawaii (NTSB, 2009). The flight travelled about 26 nautical miles past the destination airport before the crew awoke, reversed course, and landed safely in Hilo. A post-incident medical evaluation diagnosed the captain with severe obstructive sleep apnoea (OSA) for which symptoms (such as snoring) and risk factors (such as obesity) were present before the incident. The evaluating physician wrote that the captain's condition provided "an etiology for significant fatigue". Severe OSA has been associated with reduced sleep quality, daytime fatigue, and cognitive dysfunction. The captain's undiagnosed OSA in combination with multiple days of an early duty start time likely contributed to his falling asleep during the incident flight. The NTSB made three safety recommendations about OSA screening and detection because of this event. Since this incident, much has been learnt about the effects of OSA and its short-term and long-term effects on individual performance and chronic health issues. The FAA now requires aviation medical examiners (AMEs) to evaluate all pilots for OSA when performing medical examinations (or assessments). Early screening of OSA (and other sleep disorders) can lead to treatment that can improve safety as well as avoiding or mitigating chronic illnesses (for more on sleep disorders, see Chapter 3.3).

2.4.4.4   BIOMATHEMATICAL MODELLING

With the understanding that both sleep/wake periods and circadian factors affect fatigue, performance, and crash risk, researchers have endeavoured to design models that use sleep/wake data or work schedule data to predict fatigue levels and their likely effects on performance during trips. Such models can then be used proactively to design schedules or to make crew assignments (Van Dongen, Balkin, & Hursh, 2017; see also Chapters 4.3 and 4.4). A number of models exist today, including the McCauley Model, Harvard Model, and SAFTE-FAST Model (Martinez, Quintero, & Flynn-Evans, 2015). These models are not exclusive to aviation and have been used in rail and commercial trucking as well. Additionally, FAA uses modelling data as part of its evaluation of alternative means of compliance for duty hours rules.

2.4.4.5   FATIGUE EDUCATION

Another mitigation that can help aviation personnel to understand not only fatigue and its impact on performance, but also strategies for how to recognise fatigue in oneself and others, is fatigue education. Following the NTSB recommendations resulting from the Go! Airlines event in 2008, the FAA has focused its efforts on fatigue education for AMEs and pilots. Specifically, the FAA has implemented an AME education programme on OSA. Additionally, the FAA published a safety brochure about OSA (FAA, 2016) and included information regarding sleep hygiene and sleep apnoea in the Aeronautical Information Manual. Additionally, FAA requires all operators operating under 14 CFR Part 117 to implement a fatigue education and awareness programme and offers guidance to operators in Advisory Circular 117-2 (FAA, 2012).

2.4.4.6 Technology-Based In-vehicle Solutions

While fatigue education is relatively easy and cost-effective to implement, it cannot overcome a pilot's impairment due to fatigue (e.g., Caldwell, 2001; Watson et al., 2015). Further, a fatigued individual often experiences multiple lapses or performance errors before a fatigue-related event occurs. In-vehicle technologies have the potential to detect and alert vehicle operators before or when a fatigue-related event occurs. For example, researchers have identified patterns of automobile steering wheel movements that were used to predict the onset of a drowsiness-related lane departure 6 seconds before it occurred (McDonald et al., 2014). Additionally, analyses of crashes from a large-scale naturalistic driving study found that in 9.5% of all crashes the driver was showing eye lid closure behaviours characteristic of fatigue in the 3 minutes that preceded the crash (Owens et al., 2018). Observing driver behaviour that happens prior to a crash offers insights into how fatigue may be detected before a crash occurs. In the aviation context, a recent study by Naeeri and colleagues (2021) used eye tracking to predict fatigue in a simulated cockpit environment. The data showed that as pilot fatigue increased, so did eye fixation duration and eye movement. Conversely, as fatigue increased, there was a decrease in eye fixation number and pupil size. These findings are encouraging as non-invasive eye tracking could be used to predict fatigue in flight crews.

Not commonly used in aviation, technology-based fatigue countermeasures have been employed in other transportation modes such as highway and rail. Some systems track an operator (e.g., an operator's physiology or eye movements) whereas other systems track vehicle performance (e.g., lane departure). Such systems could potentially prevent events in aviation caused by a wide range of human performance impairments, including fatigue, distraction, drug/alcohol use, or medical impairment. However, to ensure such systems are employed effectively, their validity and reliability should be considered.

2.4.5 CONCLUSIONS

Investigations are an important component in improving aviation safety. Ideally, fatigue mitigations, such as those discussed in this chapter, would prevent *all* fatigue-related events, but history has taught us that it will repeat itself. The aviation system is inherently safe; redundant systems abound. But more work can be done to prevent future, albeit rare, fatigue-related events from occurring. The desire for around-the-clock aviation operations pushes the limits of pilots (and other safety-critical personnel) and it is important that we do not forget these limitations. By discussing lessons learnt from investigations, we can recognise fatigue risk and its impact. Further, ongoing research and consideration of those mitigation strategies discussed will provoke critical and creative thinking into how we can mitigate fatigue risks moving forward.

SUMMARY POINTS FOR PRACTITIONERS

- Fatigue is a hazard in the aviation industry and manifests in crashes and near misses.
- Lessons learnt from investigations can inform the development of counter-measures to reduce the incidence of fatigue-related events.
- Near misses provide an invaluable opportunity to understand systemic issues related to fatigue that could result in a crash.
- Fatigue is a by-product of a 24-hour global system and requires a multipronged approach to manage it effectively.

NOTES

1   The US Code of Federal Regulations (49 CFR Part 830), which describes the NTSB's authority, defines an aircraft accident as,

> An occurrence associated with the operation of an aircraft which takes place between the time any person boards the aircraft with the intention of flight and all such persons have disembarked, and in which any person suffers death or serious injury, or in which the aircraft receives substantial damage.

Note that this chapter generally does not use the term "accident" except when referring to this authorisation language.

REFERENCES

Åkertstedt, T. (2000). Consensus statement: Fatigue and accidents in transport operations. *Journal of Sleep Research, 9,* 395–395. doi:10.1046/j.1365-2869.2000.00228.x

Bhattacherjee, A. (2001). Understanding information systems continuance: An expectation-confirmation model. *MIS Quarterly, 25*(3), 351–370. doi:10.2307/3250921

Cabon, P. (2011). Fatigue in air traffic control. *Hindsight, 13,* 55–59.

Caldwell, J. A. (2001). Efficacy of stimulants for fatigue management: The effects of Provigil® and Dexedrine® on sleep-deprived aviators. *Transportation Research Part F: Traffic Psychology and Behaviour, 4,* 19–37. https://doi.org/10.1016/S1369-8478(01)00011-0

Dawson, D., & Reid, K. (1997). Fatigue, alcohol and performance impairment. *Nature, 388,* 235–237. doi:10.1038/40775

Federal Aviation Administration (FAA). (2012). *AC 117-2–Fatigue Education and Awareness Training Program.* www.faa.gov/documentLibrary/media/Advisory_Circular/AC%20 117-2.pdf

FAA. (2013). *AC 120-103A–Fatigue Risk Management Systems for Aviation Safety.* www.faa. gov/documentLibrary/media/Advisory_Circular/AC_120-103A.pdf

FAA. (2016). *Obstructive Sleep Apnea: Overview for the Aerospace Community.* Accessed January 5, 2022, from www.faa.gov/pilots/safety/pilotsafetybrochures/media/Sleep_Apnea.pdf

Freiwald, D. R., & O'Toole, M. F. (2015). The effect of regional airline attendance policies on pilot self-removal from duty for illness or fatigue. *International Journal of Aviation, Aeronautics, and Aerospace, 2*(2), 1–16.

Harrison, Y., & Horne, J. A. (1999). One night of sleep loss impairs innovative thinking and flexible decision making. *Organizational Behavior and Human Decision Processes, 8*(2), 128–145.

International Civil Aviation Organisation (ICAO). (2011). *Fatigue Risk Management Systems: Implementation Guide for Operators.* www.icao.int/safety/fatiguemanagement/frms%20 tools/frms%20implementation%20guide%20for%20operators%20july%202011.pdf

Lindbergh, C. A. (1953). *The Spirit of St. Louis.* New York: Scribner's.

Marcus, J. (2021). *NTSB Fatigue Recommendations.* Human Fatigue Factors, July 16, 2021, NTSB Training Academy, Ashburn, VA. PowerPoint presentation.

Martinez, S.B., Quintero, L. O., & Flynn-Evans, E. (2015). *Validating and Verifying Biomathematical Models of Human Fatigue.* https://ntrs.nasa.gov/citations/2015 0015943

McDonald, A. D., Lee, J. D., Schwarz, C., & Brown, T. L. (2014). Steering in a random forest: Ensemble learning for detecting drowsiness-related lane departures. *Human Factors, 56*(5), 986–998.

Mohler, S.R. (1965). *Fatigue in Aviation Activities* (AM 65-13). Oklahoma City, Oklahoma: Federal Aviation Agency.

Naeeri, S., Kang, Z., Saptarshi, M. & Kwangtaek, K. (2021). Multimodal analysis of eye movements and fatigue in a simulated glass cockpit environment. *Aerospace, 8*(283), 1–19. doi:10.3390/aerospace8100283

National Transportation Safety Board (NTSB). (1994). *Safety Study: A Review of Flightcrew-Involved Major Accidents of U.S. Air Carriers, 1978 through 1990.* (NTSB/SS-94/01) Washington DC: NTSB.

NTSB. (2009). Hilo, Hawaii. https://data.ntsb.gov/carol-repgen/api/Aviation/ReportMain/ GenerateNewestReport/67542/pdf

NTSB. (2010a). Atlanta, Georgia. https://data.ntsb.gov/carol-repgen/api/Aviation/ReportMain/ GenerateNewestReport/74928/pdf

NTSB. (2010b). *Loss of Control on Approach, Colgan Air, Inc., Operating as Continental Connection Flight 3407, Bombardier DHC-8-400, N200WQ, Clarence Center, New York, February 12, 2009* (NTSB/AAR-10/01). Washington, DC.

NTSB. (2011). Arlington, Virginia. https://data.ntsb.gov/carol-repgen/api/Aviation/ReportM ain/GenerateNewestReport/78655/pdf

NTSB. (2013a). Butte City, California. https://data.ntsb.gov/carol-repgen/api/Aviation/Rep ortMain/GenerateNewestReport/86913/pdf

NTSB. (2013b). Land O'Lakes, Florida. http://saftiwfe01.ntsb.int/safti-repgen/api/Aviation/ ReportMain/GenerateNewestReport/85115/pdf

NTSB. (2013c). *Loss of Control, Sundance Helicopters, Inc., Eurocopter AS350-B2, N37SH, Near Las Vegas, Nevada, December 7, 2011* (NTSB/AAR-13/01). Washington, DC.

NTSB. (2014). *Crash During a Nighttime Nonprecision Instrument Approach to Landing, UPS Flight 1354, Airbus A300-600, N155UP, Birmingham, Alabama, August 14, 2013* (NTSB/AAR-14/02). Washington, DC.

NTSB. (2016). Goodland, Kansas. https://data.ntsb.gov/carol-repgen/api/Aviation/ReportM ain/GenerateNewestReport/90639/pdf

NTSB. (2018). *Taxiway Overflight, Air Canada Flight 759, Airbus A320-211, C-FKCK, San Francisco, California, July 7, 2017* (NTSB/AIR-18/01). Washington, DC.

NTSB. (2020a). Hazelhurst, Wisconsin. http://saftiwfe01.ntsb.int/safti-repgen/api/Aviation/ ReportMain/GenerateNewestReport/97118/pdf

NTSB. (2020b). Anchorage, Alaska. http://saftiwfe01.ntsb.int/safti-repgen/api/Aviation/Rep ortMain/GenerateNewestReport/96246/pdf

Owens, J. M., Dingus, T. A., Guo, F., Fang, Y., Perez, M., McClafferty, J. & Tefft, B. C. (2018). *Prevalence of Drowsy Driving Crashes: Estimates from a Large-Scale Naturalistic Driving Study* (Research Brief). Washington, D.C.: AAA Foundation for Traffic Safety.

Rosekind, M. R., Smith, R. M., Miller, D. L., Co, E. L., Gregory, K. B., Webbon, L. L., Gander, P. H., & Lebacqz, J. V. (1995). Alertness management: Strategic naps in operational settings. *Journal of Sleep Research, 4*(Suppl. 2), 62–66.

Tassi, P., & Muzet, A. (2000, August). Sleep inertia. *Sleep Medical Review, 4*(4), 341–353. https://doi.org/10.1053/smrv.2000.0098

Van Dongen, H. P. A., Balkin, T. J., & Hursh, S. R. (2017). Sleep and performance prediction modeling. In M. Kryger, T. Roth, & W. C. Dement (Eds.), *Principles and Practice of Sleep Medicine* (pp. 689–696). Elsevier. doi: 10.1016/B978-0-323-24288-2.00072-6

Van Dongen, H. P. A., Maislin, G., Mullington, J. M., & Dinges, D. F. (2003). The cumulative cost of additional wakefulness: Dose-response effects on neurobehavioral functions and sleep physiology from chronic sleep restriction and total sleep deprivation. *Sleep, 26,* 117–126. doi:10.1093/sleep/26.2.117

Watson, N. F., Badr, M. S., Belenky, G., Bliwise, D. L., Buxton, O. M., Buysse, D., Dinges, D. F., Gangwisch, J., Grandner, M. A., Kushida, C., Malhotra, R. K., Martin, J. L., Patel, S. R., Quan, S. F., & Tasali, E. (2015). Recommended amount of sleep for a healthy adult: A joint consensus statement of the American Academy of Sleep Medicine and Sleep Research Society. *Sleep, 38*(6), 843–844. doi:10.5665/sleep.4716

2.5 Telling the Story

How and Why Investigating for Fatigue Can Improve Safety in Transportation Operations

Christina M. Rudin-Brown, Geneviève Dubé, Michelle S. Gauthier, David Mohan, and Ari Rosberg

Transportation Safety Board of Canada, Gatineau, QC, Canada

CONTENTS

DOI: 10.1201/9781003213154-13

2.5.1   INTRODUCTION

The Transportation Safety Board of Canada (TSB) is an independent government agency that advances transportation safety by investigating occurrences[1] in the air, marine, pipeline, and rail modes of transportation. When warranted, the TSB makes formal recommendations to eliminate or reduce safety deficiencies that pose significant risks to the transportation system and warrant the attention of regulators and industry. From the early 1990s until mid-2022, the TSB made findings or issued safety messages about sleep-related fatigue in 99 occurrences: 38 in the air transportation sector, 29 in marine, and 32 in rail. It has also issued six Board recommendations—all in the marine mode—relating to fatigue management.

Since 2010, the TSB has published its "Watchlist" of key safety issues that need to be addressed to make Canada's transportation system safer. The issue of fatigue management in freight train operations was added to the Watchlist in 2016 and was expanded in 2018, 2020, and again in 2022 to include air and marine operations (TSB, 2022b).

Transportation industries operate in a challenging 24/7 environment, especially in Canada where, across six time zones, organisations need to accommodate extreme fluctuations in temperature, precipitation, and available daylight hours that characterise the landscape. Notwithstanding, the modern economics of essential services require transportation systems to incorporate crew scheduling into the 24/7 environment while at the same time ensuring the safety of employees and of the public. Compared to previous times that allowed for common day(s) of rest and generally consistent work schedules, the modernisation and globalisation seen today mean that consumers expect goods and services to be available every hour of every day regardless of holiday, religious observance, and social needs, and that transportation operations feeding the supply chain must be similarly active.

Social and familial needs and expectations have also evolved. Travel by air is no longer exclusive to the wealthy or elite, nor are flights confined to certain days and times. There is an expectation among the travelling, fare-paying public that (barring some unforeseen global event, such as a pandemic outbreak), wherever and whenever they want to travel, there will be a means to accomplish that travel. Unintended pressures by family and friends for workers to conform to a "normal" social and sleep schedule despite working at night, or at unpredictable shift times, can also exacerbate the risk of fatigue.

Compared to other industries, fatigue in transportation is made more likely because of challenges to the human body's circadian (daily) rhythm caused by shiftwork and travel across multiple time zones (see also Chapter 3.1 of this book). Crews often work long and irregular schedules—sometimes in challenging conditions—that are not always conducive to getting sufficient restorative sleep. Efforts have been made, in recent years and in the past, to improve safety and efficiency in operations by designing and implementing organisational and shift scheduling practices to min-imise the risk of employee fatigue. However, some of these practices can inadvert-ently introduce new fatigue safety risks. Investigation of transportation occurrences is one way to identify these unforeseen risks.

Investigating for fatigue using a systems approach, like the one used by the TSB (Rudin-Brown & Rosberg, 2021), can identify the factors that contribute to fatigue in transportation operations, document when fatigue does (and does not) contribute to an occurrence, and communicate the findings publicly. Investigating leads to safety improvements in the future by providing the opportunity for operators to learn from the experience of others. This chapter reviews the TSB's fatigue investigation meth-odology, including some of the challenges that may be encountered during the inves-tigation process. Special consideration is made of the methodology's applicability in the industrial and commercial transportation operations environments (as opposed to transportation that is undertaken by private citizens), using descriptions of some recent TSB investigations to illustrate the importance of the investigative process in identifying where organisational and/or shift scheduling practices contribute to fatigue risk.

2.5.2   TSB APPROACH TO INVESTIGATING FOR FATIGUE

Canada's TSB employs more than 100 specialised investigators who are experienced in air, marine, pipeline, or rail operations, various engineering disciplines, or human factors. Regardless of their background, the TSB trains all investigators to identify and collect reliable fatigue-related data to determine whether (1) people involved in an occurrence were experiencing fatigue (i.e., the test of *existence*), (2) the actions of those individuals were consistent with known fatigue-related perform-ance decrement(s) and that fatigue played a role in the occurrence (i.e., the test of *influence*), and (3) the operator had company and organisational practices in place to effectively manage the risks of fatigue (i.e., assess the company's or operation's fatigue management). For more detail on the TSB's fatigue investigation method-ology, see Rudin-Brown and Rosberg (2021).

Each year, between 3,000 and 4,000 transportation occurrences are reported to the TSB in accordance with the mandatory reporting requirements in the *Transportation Safety Board Regulations*. Practical considerations dictate that only a small proportion of these occurrences can be fully investigated. The TSB is not obligated to investigate all reported occurrences, and as such classifies occurrences according to their relative importance, complexity, and potential for yielding safety lessons. Nevertheless, as part of every investigation the TSB looks at the possibility that fatigue played a role. To do so, the TSB considers six risk factors, any one of which can indicate the exist-ence of fatigue: acute and chronic sleep disruption, continuous wakefulness, circa-dian rhythm effects, sleep disorders, and other medical and psychological conditions (and/or medicine or drugs) that affect sleep or sleepiness. The presence of more than one risk factor will increase the risk of fatigue. The TSB's Human Factors group has produced, since 1997, an internal Guide to Investigating for Sleep-Related Fatigue (TSB, 2022a).

The goal of data collection for any TSB fatigue investigation is to determine the involved individuals' optimal sleep-wake pattern when not working (to establish normal sleep requirements and sleep habits) and compare it to the comprehensive sleep-wake history for as far back as possible (at least 48 hours, and preferably up to 2 weeks) prior to the occurrence. Medical and psychological history is also important, and is determined mainly through interviews and, if necessary, by reviewing past medical records.

2.5.3 CHALLENGES IN INVESTIGATING FATIGUE IN TRANSPORTATION OPERATIONS

2.5.3.1 COLLECTING PERISHABLE DATA

Because some aspects of fatigue data can be "perishable" (i.e., that degrade significantly over time), they need to be collected carefully and deliberately, and in a timely manner. The sleep-wake history of crew in the day(s) leading up to an occurrence will be subject to memory fade if the information is not documented as soon as possible. The longer one waits, the more difficult it will be for a person to recall the necessary data as the information will likely be forgotten or modified through numerous recountings of the event. This possibility is made more likely if there are unforeseen delays before independent interviews can be conducted. It is not uncommon for crew members to be questioned by their company management, possibly multiple times and by multiple people, before they are formally interviewed. Sometimes advice may be given to workers, often unintentionally, by managers or others who may or may not have been involved in the occurrence. This can affect memory accuracy, and underscores the need for independent accident investigators to deploy quickly and begin interviews as soon as possible after an occurrence. It also illustrates the importance of collecting surrogate sources of sleep-wake information, for example, cellular device records, recordings, and time-stamped records like employee access or hotel key card use.

Humans remember habitual patterns of behaviour more easily than details about specific episodes (Freeman & Romney, 1987), making "optimal" sleep-wake information (sleep-wake patterns when one is not working) less perishable, or less likely to be forgotten over time. Other less-perishable fatigue data include the medical and psychological history of crew members—for example, if a crew member was being treated for a sleep disorder (see Chapter 3.3 of this book), or if there were medical or psychological conditions (or medications) that could disrupt sleep and increase fatigue. These data can be collected later in an investigation, and are often more appropriately explored during a follow-up interview.

2.5.3.2 LIMITED AVAILABILITY OF DATA

Collecting reliable fatigue data can be challenging when a crew member is deceased or seriously injured or otherwise not able to remember or describe the period preceding an occurrence. Sometimes, a deceased or injured crew's next of kin (NOK) may be reluctant or unable to provide potentially sensitive information regarding the individual's sleep history because of memory limitations or feelings of allegiance. An accident investigator should therefore gather information from other parties (e.g., colleagues or roommates) who were aware of a crew member's schedule and actions before the occurrence to corroborate sleep and wake times.

Sources of information to explore when investigating a company's fatigue management practices can also be challenging to access, depending on company characteristics such as size, maturity, and safety culture. Some potentially rich sources include inspection of crew rest facilities to estimate conduciveness for restorative sleep, documented fatigue management policies, training records, work scheduling practices, and opportunities for employees to take breaks and/or naps. As with personal information, companies may be reluctant to disclose information about their fatigue management practices (or lack thereof). Reminding them of the mandate of the TSB to advance transportation safety often improves cooperation.

2.5.3.3   CROSS-MODAL CHALLENGES

In addition to challenges collecting perishable and less-perishable data, difficulties can arise when investigating across multiple operational contexts or transportation modes. Accessing and understanding the different fatigue management regulations inherent to each context and/or mode of transportation can be difficult, especially when an investigator is deployed to a remote occurrence site with limited internet access. According to many industries' operating regulations, employees who occupy safety-sensitive positions have a responsibility to report for work rested and fit for duty. However, maximum and minimum permissible hours of work and rest can differ significantly among transportation modes. It is important to understand how the mode-specific regulations impact how fatigue is managed. Indeed, many TSB fatigue investigations have found that, while an operator's work schedule met regulatory requirements, a risk of fatigue nevertheless existed due to the company's not (properly) applying the principles of fatigue science when developing the work schedule, or not being required to do so (by regulation/oversight).

2.5.3.4   CHALLENGES WHEN ANALYSING DATA AND DRAWING CONCLUSIONS

Analysing data to conclusively identify fatigue as a causal or contributing factor can be tricky, as the effects of fatigue are often subtle. A good practice is to collect data from as many sources as possible, and use a multidisciplinary team approach to analysis. An evidence table can be very beneficial—this is a document that summarises all data sources and items, including those that support and those that oppose the fatigue findings, and the quality and strength of each item is evaluated and rated by a team of investigators. Biomathematical modelling software (e.g., see Chapter 4.3) that predicts the effects of shift scheduling practices and the quantity and quality of sleep on human performance can also be used retroactively to corroborate and support conclusions.

Drawing conclusions regarding fatigue and its role can similarly be challenging given the breadth of variables that can influence human performance. If an operator's actions are consistent with the known effects of fatigue, and they can be linked to unsafe action(s) or condition(s), then it can be concluded that fatigue likely caused or contributed to the occurrence. The investigator must always be aware, however, that multiple causes or contributing factors can be found in many occurrences. Investigators therefore need to conduct careful analysis, working in a multidisciplinary, team investigation approach and using proven investigation tools to build defensible conclusions.

2.5.4 THE "STORIES" BEHIND THE OCCURRENCES: HOW ORGANISATIONAL OR COMPANY SHIFT SCHEDULING PRACTICES CONTRIBUTED TO FATIGUE RISK

In any discussion about transportation accident investigation, it is important to consider the context that surrounds a vehicle operator and the larger operations. While there are typically between 3,000 and 4,000 aviation, marine, pipeline, and rail occurrences reported to the TSB each year under mandatory reporting requirements, practical considerations dictate that only about 2% are fully investigated by the TSB. Therefore, it is challenging to estimate statistically the prevalence of fatigue-related occurrences. Nevertheless, review of those investigations where fatigue was concluded to have played a role can increase our understanding of the issue. What follows are descriptions of some recent TSB investigations where one or more of the six TSB fatigue risk factors were identified as having contributed to, or increased the risk of, an occurrence and where organisational or company shift scheduling practices contributed to the fatigue risk.

2.5.4.1 "CRACK OF DAWN"—THE RISKS OF VERY EARLY MORNING SHIFTS AND BACKWARD-ROTATING SHIFT SCHEDULES

Early morning shifts are associated with shorter sleep periods and greater levels of stress than are shifts that begin later (Kecklund, Åkerstedt & Lowden, 1997). Employees working early morning shifts that curtail sleep are at an increased risk of sleepiness, fatigue-related impairment, and fatigue-related occurrences. Shift schedules that rotate forward (from morning to afternoon to night) facilitate circadian rhythm adjustment and lessen the risk of fatigue compared to backward shift rotation. Forward-rotating shift systems are associated with better sleep quality, increased sleep length, less fatigue, and fewer attention lapses than backward-rotating schedules (Driscoll, Grunstein & Rogers, 2007).

Early morning shifts and a backward-rotating shift schedule were found to increase the risk of fatigue for air crew in a runway incursion involving two commercial aircraft in August 2019 (TSB investigation A19O0117). In that occurrence, the crew of one aircraft misinterpreted an air traffic control communication as clearance for take-off. The captain had had only one day of rest following a 4-day evening shift schedule before beginning an early morning shift schedule that required him to wake up very early—before 5 AM. The captain suffered acute sleep disruption in the two days prior because the early morning shifts required much earlier start times than he was used to. He also experienced chronic sleep disruption, since the late evening shift end times on the days preceding the occurrence precluded him from getting full nights of restorative sleep on those nights. Despite the crew's schedule in the days leading to the occurrence having met Canadian aviation fatigue regulations, an increased risk of fatigue due to circadian rhythm desynchronisation was identified in any crew working a backward-rotating shift schedule similar to the occurrence crew. The report identified that, if crew members are not informed of the circadian rhythm desynchronisation that can happen with backward-rotating shift schedules, there is a risk that air crew will operate while fatigued.

2.5.4.2 "SUPERHERO"—EXTENDED WAKEFULNESS AND THE (MISTAKEN) BELIEF THAT THE EFFECTS OF FATIGUE CAN BE OVERCOME BY PERSONAL STRENGTH, MOTIVATION, AND WILL

In many transportation industries, fatigue is seen as something that can be overcome, if only one is strong and committed enough to overcome it. The marine industry, where a culture of working long hours is supported by current work and rest regulations, and where "rest" is often understood to be synonymous with relaxing (and not sleeping), is particularly prone to this type of belief and is often the context for fatigue-related occurrences. On 28 September 2012, at approximately 0430 local time, the Canadian fishing vessel *Viking Storm* collided with the American fishing vessel *Maverick* in thick fog (TSB investigation M12F0011). The crew of the *Maverick* had retired to bed around 19:45 the previous evening, leaving the wheelhouse unattended for the night. Meanwhile, a lone crew member was keeping watch on the *Viking Storm*. In the moments preceding the collision, the crew member on watch left the wheelhouse. Within seconds, the *Viking Storm*'s bow struck the *Maverick*'s port side, causing it to capsize and sink. Three of four crew members on board survived and were rescued by *Viking Storm*. The fourth crew member was never found and is presumed drowned.

The day before the occurrence, the mate of the *Viking Storm* woke at approximately 06:30 after approximately 4.5 hours of sleep. He remained awake and was involved in fishing operations until 23:00. The afternoon tow was long and afforded him only a 2-hour "rest" period during which time he ate, read, and watched TV. On the night of the occurrence, the mate had just 3 hours of sleep before being woken at 02:00 to take over the watch. Overall, the mate was awake for 19 out of 22 hours, with only a short rest period. The investigation concluded that his cognitive abilities were likely reduced due to the effects of fatigue at the time of the occurrence. Also, there was no specific fatigue management plan in place on the *Viking Storm*. As on other vessels, workers accepted fatigue, mostly related to physical exertion and long work days, as a normal part of doing business. There was limited understanding that consecutive hours of *sleep*, rather than "rest", are required to restore cognitive functions and remain safely on watch. The report warned that, if mariners equate resting with sleeping in terms of its restorative capacity, there is a risk that they will underestimate the continuous hours of sleep necessary to restore cognitive function.

2.5.4.3 "Surprise"—The Consequences of Unpredictable Shift Scheduling Practices on Workers' Health and Circadian Rhythm De-synchronisation

Although efforts have been made to improve fatigue management in some high-risk work groups by, for example, making it easier and more acceptable to report fatigue in oneself or colleagues, or to book time-off when fatigued, operational requirements that result in unpredictable and last-minute shift scheduling practices pose a risk to transportation safety by de-synchronising working time with times that employees would otherwise be awake (for more on circadian rhythm synchronisation, see Chapter 3.1). In 2012 and previously in 2004, the TSB investigated two occurrences, both involving the same marine pilot (TSB investigations M12L0147 and M04L0092) who, despite advances in marine pilot fatigue awareness training during that time, had fallen asleep in the same area in the St-Lawrence River and missed the same course change. As part of the later investigation, the pilot underwent a sleep study, and was diagnosed with mild obstructive sleep apnoea (OSA) and shift work sleep disorder. The physical environment of the bridge, which was dark and warm with monotonous engine noise, and the time of day (early morning in 2004, evening in 2012) would have also been conducive to sleep, especially for an individual with sleep disorders.

Both investigations noted that a marine pilot's work involves irregular and lengthy work hours, night shifts, unpredictable duty rosters, and commutes of various distances to and from their assignments, factors that contribute to fatigue by affecting how much restorative sleep they obtain. Both also stressed the importance of fatigue awareness training programmes, since individuals that have sleep disorders are often unaware and so may not recognise the symptoms in themselves or seek help to manage sleep-related issues. While there had been a fatigue awareness training programme for marine pilots introduced in Canada in the early 2000s, the training was not offered consistently or recurrently as of 2012, and the marine pilot had not taken it.

2.5.4.4 "Perfect Storm"—Interaction between Circadian Rhythm Timing and Unexpected Operational Delays

The time of day has a strong effect on an individual's alertness and performance because of changes in body physiology that are synchronised to the circadian rhythm. The human body is physiologically ready for sleep at night and for wakefulness during the day. Likewise, the overall performance and cognitive functioning are at their worst during the night-time circadian rhythm "trough", when fatigue increases significantly. Even if a person slept the previous night and is not feeling fatigued (Monk, Folkard & Wedderburn, 1996), overall performance may be degraded during the circadian rhythm trough.

Circadian rhythm timing can influence pilot performance. In November 2018, a Boeing 747-412F cargo aircraft (TSB investigation A18A0085) departed Chicago USA at 03:02 Atlantic time following a 13.5-hour flight delay. The aircraft touched down at Halifax, Canada at 05:06 during the hours of darkness, but failed to decelerate. It overran the runway's end, crossed a 3-m drop, and was damaged beyond repair. The three-person crew and one passenger survived with minor injuries.

The investigation considered the flight crew's work schedule, their sleep history, and circadian rhythm timing. Surrogate measures of sleep opportunity (hotel records and key cards, cell phone activity) were consulted. The analysis identified two fatigue risk factors that would have degraded the crew's performance during the flight and at the time of the occurrence by impairing working memory and problem-solving. First, the timing of the flight during the night corresponded to the crew's night-time circadian trough, when overall performance and cognitive functioning are at their worst. Second, because the 13.5-hour delay was not expected, and because they had been keeping a normal night-time sleep schedule in the week leading up to the flight that made it difficult to sleep during the afternoon and evening, the crew had been unable to obtain sufficient restorative sleep in the 24-hour period before the occurrence. The investigation found that the crew was experiencing sleep-related fatigue that degraded their performance and cognitive functioning during the approach and landing of the flight. An elevated level of stress and workload likely exacerbated the performance-impairing effects of fatigue to limit the crew's ability to determine the effect of a tailwind and influenced their decision to continue the approach despite conflicting information. This kind of limited flexibility to challenge the ongoing plan despite the existence of new and relevant information is consistent with some of the known performance impairment effects of fatigue (Harrison & Horne, 1999).

2.5.4.5 "Naptime"—Sleep Inertia and the Consequences of Mismanaged Controlled Rest

Sometimes, even efforts introduced to manage or relieve workers' fatigue can lead to unintentional negative consequences for safety. "Controlled rest" is a fatigue countermeasure that uses strategic napping to improve crew alertness during critical phases of operations. Rest periods are typically limited and, for flight operations, must be completed prior to top of descent. When the rest period is finished, the awakened pilot (or other vehicle operator) is provided a period of time without any duties before resuming normal duties.

The drive for sleep is increased during the night-time and, to a lesser extent, mid-afternoon circadian rhythm troughs, which are experienced by people who normally sleep at night and work or are active during the day. For example, because of the night-time trough, North American-based pilots flying night flights to Europe have an inherent risk of fatigue that can magnify performance decrements and increase sleep need. Investigation of transportation occurrences, such as a pitch excursion that happened over the Atlantic Ocean in January 2011 (TSB investigation A11F0012), illustrates why investigating for fatigue is important—especially after the introduction of fatigue countermeasures intended to improve safety. In that occurrence, the first officer (FO) of a commercial flight from Toronto, Canada to Zurich, Switzerland was provided an opportunity for controlled rest because of feeling fatigued from acute sleep disruptions in the 24 hours leading up to the flight. However, contrary to company directions, the FO was permitted to sleep more than the 40-minute maximum that was set as a defence against entering slow–wave (deep) sleep, which increases the likelihood of sleep inertia upon awakening (see Chapter 3.2). Shortly after awakening, the captain engaged the FO to visually search for an oncoming aircraft identified on the cockpit navigational display. The FO initially mistook the planet Venus for an aircraft, but the captain advised that the target aircraft was at the 12 o'clock position and 1,000 feet below. The FO continued to scan visually and, when he eventually saw the aircraft, he interpreted its position as being above and descending towards them. The FO reacted to the perceived imminent collision by pushing forward on the control column. The aircraft consequently experienced a 46-second pitch excursion and an altitude deviation of minus 120 m (400 feet) to plus 120 m (400 feet). Fourteen passengers and two flight attendants were injured. The investigation concluded that, at the time of the occurrence, the FO was experiencing a period of circadian low due to the time of day and fatigue due to acute sleep disruptions that increased the propensity for sleep. Napping for 75 minutes rather than the recommended 40-minute maximum meant that the FO was woken during slow-wave sleep and thus experienced sleep inertia upon awakening. By identifying the oncoming aircraft, the captain engaged the FO before the effects of sleep inertia had worn off.

2.5.4.6   "ALL OR NOTHING"—CHRONIC SLEEP DISRUPTION, SLEEP DISORDERS, AND THE POTENTIAL NEGATIVE INTERACTION WITH CONVENIENCE-BASED SHIFT SCHEDULING SYSTEMS

The vast size of Canada and its railway system means that many rail employees work in remote locations. A compressed shift scheduling system is sometimes used that is based on "drive-in/drive-out" (DIDO) or "fly-in/fly-out" (FIFO) models, where employees work for a number of days-on followed by days-off, with travel to and from the remote location considered non-work time, and employees being housed while working at a local company bunkhouse. This scheduling system offers benefits for employees such as predictability, the requirement to work mostly during daytime hours, and having multiple consecutive days-off in between work periods.

Despite their benefits, a TSB investigation found that these shift scheduling systems can be associated with an increased risk of fatigue. A collision between a freight train and hi-rail vehicle in March 2016 (TSB investigation R16H0024) occurred when the foreman responsible for managing track protection of the hi-rail vehicle and its crew forgot to protect the movement of the vehicle into another sector of track. Daytime scheduled shifts for these maintenance of way (MOW) workers, who were working a 7-days-on/7-days-off rotation, typically started at 07:00 and ended at 18:15. With minimal overtime, the number of work hours for each on-duty week was about 78.75, plus travel time. The investigation found that the foreman and the other worker involved had been working the 6th of 7 scheduled shifts on the day of the occurrence, and the foreman had worked an additional overtime shift the day prior to his normal work week. The occurrence happened at approximately 15:30, during the afternoon circadian trough. Because he complained of poor sleep in the months preceding the collision, the foreman underwent an overnight sleep study, which found that he had mild OSA and mild periodic limb movement disorder—a sleep disorder characterised by periodic episodes of repetitive, involuntary limb movements during sleep that can result in arousals and awakenings without the person's awareness. The investigation concluded that, at the time the foreman made the decision to depart where the MOW crew had been working, the foreman was experiencing a level of fatigue from several interacting factors, including the combined effects of two sleep disorders, the time of day during a circadian trough, and a demanding work schedule.

2.5.4.7 "SPLIT SHIFT"—SCHEDULES FOR "CAPTIVE" EMPLOYEES AND THE POTENTIAL FOR NEGATIVE INTERACTION WITH INDIVIDUAL FACTORS

Split work shifts comprise at least two distinct work periods in one 24-hour day, with a rest period in between. They offer an alternative to longer shift durations and make it so that employees who are otherwise confined to their work environment do not work too many consecutive hours in a row. Research on split duty shifts indicates that, compared to other singular shift types, they are associated with a greater risk of sleep inertia that is worse when awakenings occur during the morning hours, as compared to afternoons or evenings (Hilditch et al., 2016). The "6-hours-on, 6-hours-off" schedule that is particularly popular in marine operations can be especially risky in terms of the potential for performance impairment from fatigue (Härmä et al., 2008). This schedule presents a number of challenges that have been well documented by various studies and experts internationally, notably the difficulty in obtaining sufficient restorative rest during the off-duty periods. This is particularly the case for those workers who find it difficult to nap, or where the sleep environment is not conducive to daytime napping.

In October 2016, articulated tug-barge *Nathan E. Stewart* went aground near Athlone Island, British Columbia (TSB investigation M16P0378). The tug's hull was eventually breached and approximately 110,000 litres of diesel fuel released into the environment. The TSB investigation found that the second mate (who, contrary to Canadian regulations, was keeping watch alone on the bridge at the time leading up to the grounding) had fallen asleep and missed a planned course change. For more than two days prior, he had been working a "6-hours-on, 6-hours-off shift" schedule, alternating six hours of duty and six hours of rest. Opportunities to sleep had been provided, but his inability to nap, combined with the sleep-inducing conditions on the bridge at the time leading up to the grounding, led to increased fatigue. The investigation found that, despite the challenging conditions, there was no discussion between the master and the second mate prior to the shift regarding the second mate's preparedness for the watch, and the watchkeeper was not aware of the sleep-conducive conditions he was facing on the bridge that night.

2.5.5 CONCLUSIONS

Today's transportation operations—across all modes—need to negotiate deftly the challenges of 24/7 operations, while at the same time manage the safety of workers and of the travelling public. The importance of investigating for fatigue in every transportation occurrence, particularly those that occur in industrial or commercial operational contexts, is demonstrated through the review of several TSB investigations where fatigue was found to play a role. By documenting that role, the investigation reports serve to disseminate knowledge about fatigue-related safety hazards and how to mitigate them in future.

Organisations are encouraged to be forward-thinking in adopting more modern shift scheduling systems, fatigue management, and countermeasures that are based on the tenets of modern fatigue science and that consider operational context as well as employees' family and social constraints without relying solely on regulations and biomathematical fatigue modelling. Investigation is a flexible and effective way to identify risks and safety significant conditions and actions, especially in operational work environments.

Some challenges to investigating for fatigue in operations include the need to collect perishable data in a timely and effective way to minimise the effects of memory fade and unintended contamination, the importance of managing interviews with family, friends, and colleagues of those involved, difficulties in accessing sufficient and reliable information in interviews, and when analysing data and drawing conclusions when the effects of fatigue can be subtle or unclear. Regardless of whether it is used in the context of an organisation's safety and/ or fatigue management system, or by an independent national investigation board, fatigue investigation that leads to clearly articulated findings and related safety messaging is a proven, albeit reactive, method to learn from actual, real-world operations. The TSB ensures its ability to effectively investigate fatigue by training its investigators in the science behind, and need for, fatigue investigation to improve safety, and by providing and updating its Guide to Investigating for Sleep-Related Fatigue (TSB, 2022a) in both official languages (English and French).

Disclaimer: The views expressed in this chapter are those of the authors and not necessarily those of the Transportation Safety Board of Canada.

SUMMARY POINTS FOR PRACTITIONERS

- Investigating for fatigue in transportation occurrences can improve safety by documenting when fatigue does (and does not) play a role.
- Some challenges include the need to collect perishable data in a timely and effective way, the importance of managing interviews with family, friends, and colleagues, difficulties in accessing sufficient and reliable information, and drawing conclusions when the effects of fatigue are subtle or unclear.
- The importance of investigating for fatigue in every transportation occurrence, particularly those that occur in industrial or commercial operational contexts, is demonstrated through "stories" of several TSB investigations where fatigue was found to play a role.
- Regardless of whether it is used in the context of an organisation's safety and/or fatigue management system, or by an independent national investigation board, fatigue investigation that leads to clearly articulated findings and related safety messaging is a proven, albeit reactive, method to learn from actual, real-world operations.

NOTE

1   In this chapter, "occurrence" means a transportation event as defined in the Canadian Transportation Accident Investigation and Safety Board Act (2019). Generally speaking, an occurrence is any accident or incident associated with the operation of an aircraft, a marine vessel, a pipeline, or rolling stock on a railway. It may also extend to any situation or condition that the Board has reasonable grounds to believe could, if left unattended, induce an accident or incident.

REFERENCES

Canadian Transportation Accident Investigation and Safety Board Act (S.C. 1989, c. 3) (2019). https://laws-lois.justice.gc.ca/eng/acts/C-23.4/page-1.html#h-75348.

Chua, E. C. P., Fang, E., & Gooley, J. J. (2017). Effects of total sleep deprivation on divided attention performance. *PLoS One*, *12*(11), e0187098.

Driscoll, T. R., Grunstein, R. R., & Rogers, N. L. (2007). A systematic review of the neurobehavioral and physiological effects of shiftwork systems. *Sleep Medicine Reviews*, *11*(3) 179–194.

Freeman, L. C., & Romney, A. K. (1987). Words, deeds and social structure: A preliminary study of the reliability of informants. *Human Organization*, *46*, 330–334.

Härmä, M., Partinen, M., Repo, R., Sorsa, M., & Siivonen, P. (2008). Effects of 6/6 and 4/8 watch systems on sleepiness among bridge officers. *Chronobiology International*, *25*(2), 413–423.

Harrison, Y., & Horne, J. A. (1999). One night of sleep loss impairs innovative thinking and flexible decision making. *Organizational Behavior and Human Decision Processes*, *78*, 128–145.

Hilditch, C. J., Short, M., Van Dongen, H. P. A., Centofanti, S. A., Dorrian, J., Kohler, M., & Banks, S. (2016). Sleep inertia during a simulated 6-h on/6-h off fixed split duty schedule. *Chronobiology International*, *33*(6), 685–696.

Kecklund, G., Åkerstedt, T., & Lowden, A. (1997). Morning work effects of early rising on sleep and alertness. *Sleep*, *20*(3), 215–233.

Monk, T., Folkard, S., & Wedderburn, A. A. I. (1996). Maintaining safety and high performance on shiftwork. *Applied Ergonomics*, *27*(1), 17–23.

Rudin-Brown, C. M., & Rosberg, A. (2021). Applying principles of fatigue science to accident investigation: Transportation Safety Board of Canada (TSB) fatigue investigation methodology. *Chronobiology International*, *38*(2), 296–300.

[TSB] Transportation Safety Board. (2022a). Guide to investigating sleep-related fatigue. Human Factors and Macro Analysis division. (Internal report).

[TSB] Transportation Safety Board. (2022b). Watchlist 2022: Fatigue management. www.tsb.gc.ca/eng/surveillance-watchlist/multi-modal/2022/multimodal-03.html

2.6 Fatigue's Effects on Occurrence Survivability

Sarah Harris

Transportation Safety Board of Canada, Gatineau, QC, Canada

CONTENTS

2.6.1 INTRODUCTION

Fatigue can be a risk factor in the cause of, or contributor to, many incidents and accidents. As such, there is a focus on trying to ensure that operators are fit to effectively perform their duties. However, there is typically much less understanding, and therefore less focus, on the need to ensure that these operators will also be fit to *survive* should an emergency occur. Furthermore, there is even less focus on *passenger* fatigue and the effect this may have on *their* ability to survive.

As fatigue can affect vigilance, processing, memory, and decision-making, as discussed in detail in other chapters in this book, it may therefore affect an individual's ability to perceive and process any available survival information and to ultimately "be ready" to perform the required survival actions. This chapter focuses on how fatigue can affect individuals during actual emergency scenarios. In particular, it addresses the *readiness to detect and prepare for an imminent emergency, emergency performance,* and *surviving until rescue* phases of the occurrence sequence (see Figure 2.6.1). It also covers how drugs, alcohol, and medications can exacerbate fatigue and affect the likelihood of survival. To conclude, the chapter addresses how fatigue could be mitigated to optimise an individual's chance of survival.

DOI: 10.1201/9781003213154-14

2.6.2 READINESS TO DETECT AND PREPARE FOR AN IMMINENT EMERGENCY

There are four main phases to an emergency scenario: the *pre-hazard phase*, the *hazard onset phase*, the *survival phase*, and the *rescue* phase (see Figure 2.6.1, a modified version of the accident timeline taken from Harris, 2011 and Harris, 2015). Although these phases may overlap to some degree, there will be important survival information available to individuals within each of these phases. During the first phase of an emergency scenario, the *pre-hazard phase*, there is often important information available to individuals to prepare them for an emergency, even though there is not yet a fully developed emergency scenario. This is likely to be in the form of *early warning cues*, such as unusual visual or audible cues, physical sensations, or possibly smells. These cues may be perceived directly, for example, by observing increasingly rough sea conditions, or via a person's "sixth sense", that is, they are not aware of identifying any specific cue but they just "feel" something isn't right. Perception of such information in this *pre-hazard phase* can provide individuals with the opportunity to perform some early preparatory actions, such as putting on or tightening their seat belt or life jacket, bracing themselves or moving nearer to an exit, "just in case". It can also increase their vigilance and cross-checking of their environment, which improves their survival readiness for further emergency cues.

During the subsequent *hazard on-set phase*, when the emergency actually occurs, there will be further information available. In this phase, the cues may now be more pronounced, such as alarms in the flight deck or locomotive, aggressive vessel movements, or the presence of smoke or fire. For operators, the detection of

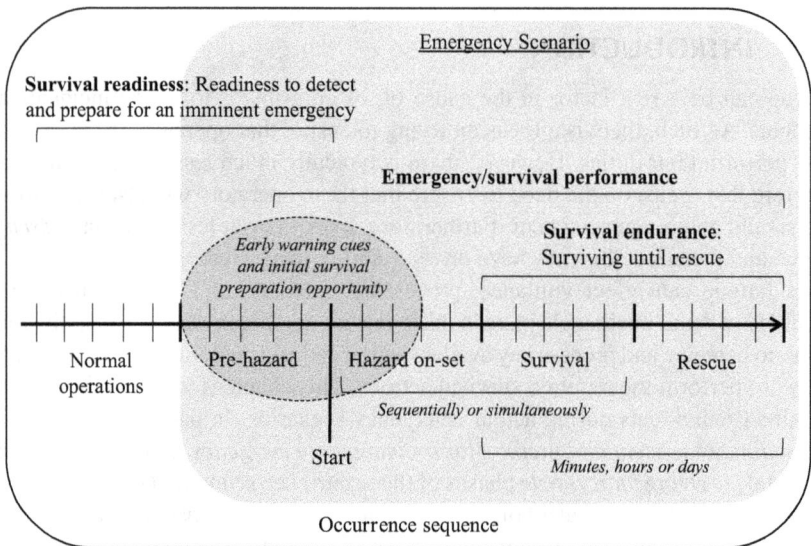

FIGURE 2.6.1 Phases and survival requirements during an emergency—a modified version of the accident timeline taken from Harris (2011) and Harris (2015).

these hazardous cues is imperative. Unless the hazard can be successfully resolved, operators will need to start planning and performing as soon as practicable, the actions required for survival. This may include sounding alarms, issuing mayday calls, providing emergency commands, donning survival equipment, or preparing to egress or abandon ship. Only at this point will any passengers formally receive *their* survival instructions, if the situation requires operators to provide such instructions. If the individual missed the *early warning cues* in the *pre-hazard phase* (or if there were no cues), then the emergency in the *hazard on-set phase* can appear "suddenly", which can startle and confuse people. Particularly, if the emergency is abruptly catastrophic, such as a sudden impact or capsize, there may not be any further opportunity to acknowledge, prepare, or respond to the emergency. It is for this reason that an individual's *survival readiness* should be optimised in order to maximise their *survival preparation opportunity*.

Although there is always variability in what information people attend to, being fatigued can reduce any levels of attention and vigilance (Lim et al., 2010). This will be particularly and obviously the case, if individuals are actually asleep. As a result, fatigue can impair an individual's *survival readiness*. In several marine investigations, vessel crews have not responded to increasing risk in the environment. Although in some instances this could be partly attributed to other factors such as a possible risk-taking culture on a vessel, many scenarios were exacerbated by the presence of fatigue. Some crews, who had been taking ad hoc opportunities to rest in non-sleep conducive environments for several days, which likely resulted in acute fatigue and circadian rhythm disruptions, became less vigilant in looking out for and detecting environmental deteriorations, such as changes to weather, sea conditions, and vessel movements. In some instances, despite environmental deteriorations and increasing risk, crew members elected to nap or rest inside the vessel, which meant they missed the *early warning cues*. As a result, when the emergency was abruptly catastrophic and the vessel "suddenly" and "unexpectedly" capsized, they were unprepared as they had missed their *survival preparation opportunity*. Conversely, in some air accidents, passengers *have* detected early warning cues in the *pre-hazard phase*, typically resulting in them sitting upright, tightening their seat belt, and bracing themselves. These individuals had less initial impact injuries compared to those that were napping during the critical take-off or landing phase of flight, who had missed their *survival preparation opportunity*.

2.6.3 EFFECTS OF DRUGS AND ALCOHOL ON SURVIVAL READINESS

Taking certain prescription and non-prescribed over-the-counter (OTC) medications, or using drugs and alcohol, may cause or exacerbate any fatigue and therefore also have the potential to impair an individual's *survival readiness*. Some prescription and OTC medications have side effect(s) that directly cause "drowsiness". These are usually marked with warning labels such as "may cause drowsiness, do not drive or operate machinery". In fact, some medications may be prescribed and taken purposefully to induce sleep before a shift, such as temazepam for aircrew or military personnel (Hancock et al., 2008a). However, these medications are tightly controlled in that they must be taken a certain number of hours before reporting for duty, so that there are no residual fatiguing effects. Some prescribed and OTC medications do not directly cause drowsiness but can still affect the individual's sleep pattern. For example, medications that contain stimulants such as amphetamines affect the quality and quantity of sleep, which can lead to acute or chronic fatigue in the following days. These medications are not necessarily labelled with a warning, and so people may take them without anticipating any such sleep effects. Similarly, alcohol can increase the risk of fatigue if taken before the day in question, as it disrupts the individual's sleep architecture, or how sleep phases are structured. If alcohol and cannabis are taken whilst on duty or whilst travelling, they may exacerbate any on-the-day fatigue. However, the degree to which it affects existing fatigue depends on a multitude of factors, such as the amount taken, the individual's tolerance and health, and the exact type of the substance. For example, one person may take one type of cannabis and feel euphoric and energised, whereas another person may take a different type and dosage and feel relaxed and fall asleep. Either way, cannabis can cause impairments to cognitive functioning, particularly with respect to attention, vigilance, processing new information, and dealing with unexpected events (Newman, 2004), as well as mood changes, such as panic reactions (NHTSA, 2014).

Although operators are typically aware of the restrictions on drinking alcohol whilst on duty, some operators and most passengers typically do not understand how alcohol, cannabis, or their medications may affect their levels of fatigue or their *survival readiness*. In one recent air occurrence, for example, those passengers that had consumed cannabis prior to the flight, which did exacerbate their fatigue, did not perceive the *early warning cues* during take-off, despite many of the other passengers doing so. They remained unaware, or not clearly aware, that there was a developing emergency and that there was likely to be an imminent impact. As a result, they did not make any survival preparations, whereas other passengers braced themselves. Further, on impact, they remained confused for a longer period of time, unable to process the unexpected events, which had a significant impact on their subsequent emergency performance. With the recent (2018) legalisation of cannabis in Canada, the number of passengers boarding transport whilst affected by the drug is becoming increasingly more common.

Some passengers will *intentionally* take alcohol, cannabis, and/or a prescription or OTC medication, such as Benadryl, to *induce* sleep for part or all of their journey. These individuals are unlikely to perceive any *early warning cues* and will also be less efficient and less effective at any kind of emergency response.

2.6.4   EMERGENCY PERFORMANCE

As an emergency develops into the *survival phase* and individuals realise that survival actions are required, assuming that there is still some *survival preparation opportunity* remaining, the efficiency and effectiveness of their *emergency performance* will often determine their probability of survival.

The associated workload and stress of an emergency will often reduce an individual's cognitive capacity and possibly narrow their visual and auditory attention (Wickens et al., 1999a), reducing their ability to understand, and respond effectively to, unusual information and events. It is for this reason that crew members *practise* emergency actions during training, so that they develop skills until they can perform survival actions *automatically* (Wickens et al., 1999b) and without much mental effort, despite the probable onset of some level of emergency stress. However, such training may not be enough to overcome the presence of both stress *and* fatigue, as both can impair general cognitive functioning, slow reaction time, and reduce the ability to solve complex problems. With the addition of fatigue in a stressful emergency, even skilled crew members may be slower at understanding *what* just happened and *what* survival actions are actually required. They may be slower at performing time-sensitive actions, such as mustering passengers, and may forget critical actions, such as remembering to take survival kits and manifests when evacuating an aircraft. For ineffectively trained crew members and passengers, the onset of emergency stress may be debilitating, as they do not have *any* skills or experience to rely on. In particular, these individuals may not have enough mental resources remaining in a new scenario to "figure things out", such as how to find and don their own life jacket, deploy a life raft, evacuate an aircraft or open an emergency window. The additional presence of fatigue in these instances would significantly exacerbate such impaired emergency performance.

Although there are many scenarios where crew members and passengers have overcome their emergency stress, with an adrenalin-fuelled focus that enables them to perform survival actions that they would not normally be able to do, the additional presence of fatigue usually hinders such performance in one way or another. Waking *during* an emergency is a particular issue. If awoken, an individual may experience *sleep inertia,* which is a period of confusion and decreased alertness (for more on the effects of sleep inertia, see Chapter 3.2 of this book). Although individual differences may vary, typically, when being suddenly awoken, sleep inertia can affect performance for several minutes, especially with respect to complex tasks. In some recent marine accidents, the crew members were already fatigued prior to sleep as a result of several days of sleep disruptions and this fatigue was exacerbated, when they were abruptly awoken during a capsize. The combined effect of these fatigue factors impaired their alertness during the subsequent emergency sequences. In particular, it affected their ability to "figure things out", for example, how to perform *unpractised* survival tasks whilst under stress, such as retrieving and donning their immersion suits and manually deploying the life raft.

2.6.5   SURVIVING UNTIL RESCUE

Even if an individual can perform some survival actions throughout the *hazard onset phase* and the *survival phase*, they will still need to survive until the *rescue phase* is complete. Although some emergencies are short lived, others can continue for hours, or days. In these instances, the required survival actions may be extensive and *survival performance* turns into *survival endurance*.

In certain survival scenarios, there are many *physical* factors that actually *cause* fatigue. In the water, for example, a person uses a lot of physical energy trying to tread water or swim, whilst also trying to keep their mouth above the water line. This could be for several minutes or even hours. If the water is cold, they also have to cope with the effects of cold-water shock, cold incapacitation, and, possibly, hypothermia. In rougher water conditions, even more energy is required to sustain survival. If the individual is shivering, this will sap energy, making survival actions harder to achieve. Even if the person is on land, they may need to sustain long hikes or climbs and, if also cold, they will use energy as a result of shivering and hypothermia. There may also be other factors, such as the effects of altitude, extreme weather or terrain, disabilities, injuries, hunger, or thirst.

In one recent air accident, crew and passengers had to survive an impact with terrain, perform a physically challenging evacuation from damaged wreckage, hike in freezing temperatures at night whilst also significantly injured and, then, keep themselves alive until they reached medical attention (see Transportation Safety Board [TSB] investigation A17C0146 [TSB, 2017]). In one recent marine accident (see TSB investigation M21P0030 [TSB, 2021]), a crew member had to survive sudden immersion in cold water at night, whilst out at sea and with no flotation aid. They then had to deploy a life raft from within the cold water, physically board the raft and stay alive for hours until rescue. Even upon rescue, they had to use energy to keep alive for several more hours until they finally reached a medical facility. In other instances, such as in 2015 when a whale watching vessel capsized off the coast of Tofino, British Columbia (see TSB investigation M15P0347 [TSB, 2015]), passengers have had to use physical energy to escape from inside a capsized vessel, then swim through cold rough sea conditions to a flotation object, then tread water for hours whilst trying to keep hold of the flotation object, then get in a rescue boat and keep themselves alive until they finally reached an ambulance.

Regardless of the *physical* demands of an emergency scenario, the individual nearly always has to contend with the *psychological* effects of the emergency, such as stress, anxiety, confusion, and disorientation, as well as the associated *physiological* effects, such as an increased heart rate, trembling, weakness, nausea, and erratic breathing patterns. If a person has to survive for many hours or days, or the survival period is at a time when the person would normally be sleeping, they may also become sleepy, just as anyone would who had their sleep pattern disturbed. These psychological and physiological effects alone can rapidly become fatiguing.

Overall, the combined physical, psychological, and physiological demands of an emergency are fatiguing, which is likely to impair an individual's *survival endurance*. In some rescue scenarios, people have succumbed to exhaustion as soon as they thought the immediate threat to life had subsided (for further reading, see Leach 1994). This may be as soon as they exited the aircraft, as soon as they boarded the life raft, or as soon as they reached land. However, this is not necessarily when they have reached safety. After the initial peak of the emergency response, they may still need to remain vigilant for a possible rescue opportunity. They may also need to perform periodic survival actions, such as deploying a flare, making sure their rescue light is still on, keeping their life jacket inflated and blowing their whistle. If on land, they may need to light and maintain a fire, or build a shelter. These actions, especially attempts at continued vigilance, can exacerbate ongoing stress and fatigue (Hancock et al., 2008b).

Due to the natural limitations of humans in extreme environments, it is reasonable to understand how someone may rapidly become fatigued (for further reading, see Ashcroft, 2001). Although it is not possible to predict and prepare for every type of emergency scenario demand or to estimate how quickly someone will become fatigued, it is possible to maximise their probability of survival by ensuring they are suitably rested, as much as practicable, at the start of the emergency. Entering into a survival scenario *already* fatigued will almost certainly escalate the survival-induced fatigue, impairing the individual's *survival endurance* from the outset.

2.6.6 OPTIMISING SURVIVAL WITH AN INTEGRATED APPROACH TO EMERGENCY FATIGUE MANAGEMENT

Although there are a multitude of factors that contribute to whether or not someone survives an accident, some of the factors relating to fatigue and survivability can be mitigated. Mitigations could include suitable emergency-related training, equipment and services, and for passengers, suitable safe travel information and safety briefings. These mitigations are often considered as part of an overall safety management system (SMS), usually as some kind of *emergency safety plan*. The SMS may also document general fatigue mitigations, usually through a *fatigue management plan*. However, fatigue management is not often integrated with emergency management; in particular, fatigue management is not often integrated as part of any *passenger safety management plan*. Integrating *fatigue management* with *emergency management* could optimise the way both are addressed. For example, **emergency duties training** courses for crew members and their managers could increase awareness of how important *survival readiness* is and how demanding *survival performance* and *survival endurance* can be. Such training could then go on to explain the detrimental effects of fatigue and sleep inertia on survival probability and how drugs, alcohol, and certain medications can cause or exacerbate fatigue. **Crew scheduling** may sometimes focus on ensuring that crew members are fit for duty at the *start* of their shift. However, this does not necessarily mean that they will remain alert long enough to manage an emergency *throughout* their shift, or particularly towards the end of a shift, especially if it is long and/or spread over several days with sporadic, poor-quality rest periods that have disrupted their normal sleep pattern. Instead, where possible, **operational risk assessments** and crew scheduling could optimise the probability of survival by factoring in the potential demands of an emergency. In particular, they could ensure that crew members are able to work an entire shift with enough reserve levels of alertness and effectiveness (as practicable), to detect and respond to an emergency *and* (within reason) survive until rescue.

For those that experience shift patterns that are unavoidably long, **operating procedures** could ensure that crew members take sufficient, effective rest periods only at a time when other crew members are able to retain effective *survival readiness*. Further, to avoid the effects of sleep inertia during a critical period of *survival performance*, procedures could require that all crew members remain awake and prepared when there is, or about to be, an increased risk in the operating scenario.

For passengers, some of these mitigations are not necessarily as applicable. However, there are other approaches, which mainly centre around improving **passenger awareness** of fatigue's effects on survivability. Most passengers are not aware of what is actually required to detect, respond to, and survive an emergency and most passengers are not aware of how fatigue, whether a result of natural tiredness or a fatigue that is exacerbated by drugs, alcohol, or certain medications, can affect their probability of survival. Further, most passengers depend on the crew members, assuming that *they* will be the ones responsible for *survival readiness*. For example, in a 2008 air investigation (see TSB investigation A08O0233 [TSB 2008]), the TSB concluded that, as a result of fatigue, both passengers fell asleep during the flight, leaving the pilot to fly the aeroplane and to safely monitor the flight. However, as the pilot was also fatigued, the pilot also fell asleep and the aeroplane continued in its trimmed condition until it struck the ground. The investigation concluded that as the passengers were asleep, they were unable to identify, and therefore respond to, the unsafe flight scenario. In this air example, passengers unwittingly relinquished any control over or involvement in their own *readiness to detect and prepare for an imminent emergency*.

Similarly, passengers in road vehicles often fall asleep and rely on the driver to drive the vehicle and to safely monitor the road scenario. However, a driver may not necessarily remain alert, for example, as a result of fatigue from staying up all night or getting up early for the journey, which may reduce *their* ability to identify and respond to the scenario. As with the air scenario, sleeping car passengers will not have any *readiness to detect and prepare for an imminent emergency* or at best, a substantially reduced window of time to realise what is happening and to prepare for appropriate action.

Improving passenger awareness of fatigue's effects on survivability, therefore, can at least in part contribute to some kind of passenger fatigue management. To start, a general government-wide awareness-raising initiative could promote the import-ance of passengers always maintaining a general level of *fitness to travel*, to optimise their health and safety throughout their journey. This could include addressing how taking drugs, alcohol, or certain medications could affect their fitness levels, par-ticularly with respect to responding to any unusual or unexpected events. Ideally, such an initiative would aim at promoting **passenger responsibility**, so passengers would take a more active, rather than passive, role in their well-being whilst travel-ling. This approach is similar to what was taken with respect to counter-terrorism, when governments promoted a *"remain alert"* and *"if you see something, say some-thing"* passenger campaign.

Once aboard the mode of transport, *passenger responsibility* could be reinforced. For example, with air passengers, the probability of having to detect and respond to a survival situation is most likely to happen during take-off or landing. In par-ticular, therefore, passengers could be encouraged to maintain their levels of alertness and safety awareness by staying awake and abstaining from drinking alcohol during these phases of flight. For other modes of transport, such as marine and rail, the risks of an emergency are more evenly spread throughout the different phases of travel. However, *passenger responsibility* and *fitness to travel* can still be reinforced once onboard. For times when there is an increased risk in the scenario, for example, when the weather deteriorates during a passenger ferry crossing, then crew members could periodically reinforce the requirement for passengers to remain awake and aware of the location of the vessel's safety equipment.

A step further than this would be to create more restrictive *passenger regulations*, as there are with crew regulations. For example, most crew members are ideally fit for duty at the start of a shift and are not allowed to drink alcohol or take drugs whilst on duty. Transport Canada and other transport organisations and regulators also require medical monitoring for certain crew members, which includes monitoring for prescribed or non-prescribed medications. However, there are currently minimal (if any) such regulations for passengers. Although the Canadian Aviation Regulations (CARS 602.04) (CARS, 2022) require that *no operator of an aircraft shall allow a person to board the aircraft, where there are reasonable grounds to believe that the person's faculties are impaired by alcohol or a drug to an extent that may present a hazard to the aircraft or to persons on board the aircraft,* this is aimed more at passengers who are significantly impaired. There are no such restrictions for those passengers that have smoked cannabis or drunk moderate levels of alcohol in the departure lounge, or who have arrived for their flight fatigued, for example. Although most operators cannot control passenger behaviour and condition prior to boarding, and although it is reasonable that most operators do not want to appear too restrictive for commercial reasons, a balance is still required. This brings us back to the more feasible approach of increasing *passenger awareness* and promoting *passenger responsibility*, an approach that relies more on motivating voluntary passenger-driven behavioural changes, as opposed to applying travel enforcements.

On a final note, *fatigue in emergencies* should also be part of any SMS requirement for occurrence reporting and investigation. This includes documenting and investigating the *presence* of any pre-emergency fatigue for both crew members and passengers, the *influence* of this fatigue on the detection and management of the emergency and the overall influence fatigue had on occurrence survivability.

2.6.7   CONCLUSIONS

Vehicle operator and crew fatigue can occur prior to a shift and/or whilst on duty. Passenger fatigue can also occur prior to travel and/or whilst travelling. Taking certain medications, or using drugs and alcohol, can cause or exacerbate any such fatigue. Regardless of the cause, these actions would result in fatigue being present prior to any emergency. If present, fatigue could influence the *pre-hazard, hazard onset, survival,* and *rescue phases* of an emergency. In particular, it can impair an individual's *survival readiness* and their ability to perceive any *early warning cues,* reducing their *survival preparation opportunity.* Once ready to respond to an emergency, fatigue can also impair *survival performance* and the degree of *survival endurance.* However, integrating *fatigue management* with *emergency management* in an SMS can mitigate the risk of pre-emergency fatigue, for example, through *emergency duties training, operational risk assessments, crew scheduling,* and *operating procedures.* For passengers, the risk of pre-emergency fatigue can be at least partially mitigated through *passenger awareness* and the promotion of *passenger responsibility.* To complete such an approach, a company's SMS should also make *emergency fatigue* part of any incident reporting and occurrence investigation, particularly with respect to any survivability aspects.

DISCLAIMER

The views expressed in this chapter are those of the author and not necessarily those of the Transportation Safety Board of Canada.

SUMMARY POINTS FOR PRACTITIONERS

- Fatigue can develop prior to, or on the day of an emergency, usually as a result of some kind of sleep or rest disturbance. Certain medications, drugs, and alcohol can cause or exacerbate any such fatigue.
- The presence of fatigue *prior* to an emergency can significantly decrease the probability of detecting, understanding, responding to, and surviving an emergency.
- Integrating fatigue management with emergency management in a company's SMS can mitigate the risk of pre-emergency fatigue, optimising the probability that crew members at least enter an emergency scenario as fit and as ready as practicable.
- Improving passenger awareness and promoting passenger responsibility can partially mitigate the risk of pre-emergency fatigue, optimising the probability that passengers at least enter an emergency scenario as fit and as ready as practicable.
- An SMS should facilitate the reporting, and investigation, of the presence and influence of any pre-emergency fatigue on survival activities.

REFERENCES

Ashcroft, A. (2001). *Life at the extremes: The science of survival*. Flamingo.

[CARS] Canadian Aviation Regulations (2022). *Part VI General Operating and Flight Rules. Subpart 2 Operating and Flight* Rules. Section 602.04 Alcohol or drugs–passengers.

Hancock, P.A., & Szalma, J. L. (2008a). *Performance under stress. Human factors in Defence*. Ashgate. Ch. 12 Fatigue and its effect on performance in military environments.

Hancock, P.A. & Szalma, J. L. (2008b). *Performance under stress. Human factors in Defence*. Ashgate. Ch. 7 Vigilance, workload and stress.

Harris, S. (2011). Human factors investigation methodology. *Proceedings International Symposium on Aviation Psychology*, Dayton, US, 2–5 May.

Harris, S. (2015). Errors and accidents. In D. P. Gradwell and D. J. Rainford (Eds.), *Ernsting's aviation and space medicine* (5th ed., pp. 707–722). CRC Press.

Leach, J. (1994). *Survival psychology*. McMillan Press Ltd. Page 60.

Lim, J., & Dinges, D. (2010). A meta-analysis of the impact of short-term sleep deprivation on cognitive variables. *Psychological Bulletin*, 136(3), 375–389.

[NHTSA] National Highway Traffic Safety Administration. (2014). Drugs and human performance fact sheets. U.S. Department of Transportation Report No. DOT HS 809 725. Available at: www.nhtsa.gov/sites/nhtsa.gov/files/809725-drugshumanperformfs.pdf

Newman, D. G. (2004). Alcohol and human performance from an aviation perspective: A review. Australian Transport Safety Bureau (ATSB) research report discussion paper. Available at: www.atsb.com.au/media/36525/Alcohol_and_human_performance.pdf

[TSB] Transportation Safety Board of Canada. (2008). Investigation Report A08O0233. Available at: www.tsb.gc.ca/eng/rapports-reports/aviation/2008/a08o0233/a08o0233. html?wbdisable=true

[TSB] Transportation Safety Board of Canada. (2015). Investigation Report M15P0347. Available at: www.bst-tsb.gc.ca/eng/enquetes-investigations/marine/2015/m15p0347/ m15p0347.html.

[TSB] Transportation Safety Board of Canada. (2017). Investigation Report A17C0146. Available at: www.tsb.gc.ca/eng/rapports-reports/aviation/2017/a17c0146/a17c0146.html

[TSB] Transportation Safety Board of Canada. (2021). Investigation Report M21P0030. Available at: www.tsb.gc.ca/eng/rapports-reports/marine/2021/m21p0030/m21p0030.html

Wickens, C. D., & Hollands, J. G. (1999a). *Engineering psychology and human performance* (3rd ed.). Ch. 12: Stress.

Wickens, C. D., & Hollands, J. G. (1999b). *Engineering psychology and human performance* (3rd ed.). Ch. 10: Manual Control.

2.7 Regulatory and Legal Frameworks for Managing Fatigue in Transportation

Drew Dawson, Madeline Sprajcer, and Matthew J.W. Thomas

Appleton Institute, Central Queensland University, Wayville, SA, Australia

CONTENTS

2.7.1 INTRODUCTION AND CONTEXT

This chapter sets out some broad principles of legal and regulatory accountability with respect to fatigue-related risk in transportation. The chapter is comprised of two parts. The first part sets out a brief history of regulatory frameworks and some factors that have shaped their evolution over time. Current regulatory frameworks are then explored as a series of stages, that is, a work-in-progress, and an attempt made to situate different jurisdictional approaches within broader historical trends in the field of work health and safety (WHS)—specifically, as part of the broader shift from prescription towards performance-based approaches, from compliance-based systems to risk- and safety-management systems' approaches. Furthermore, the potential applicability of performance-based approaches to the transport sector is considered.

There has always been a complex intersection between fatigue management and the legal and regulatory frameworks that exist to ensure safety in transport industries.

DOI: 10.1201/9781003213154-15

In the context of fatigue-related transport safety incidents worldwide, there are comparatively few clear examples where individual operators have been convicted for fatigue-related offences, especially outside the context of road traffic crashes. Of these, the UK Selby rail disaster provides an exemplar. In this case, a driver who was experiencing fatigue due to severe sleep restriction was found to have fallen asleep at the wheel, subsequently running off the road, leading to a collision between two trains and the deaths of 10 people. The car driver was found to have caused death by dangerous driving, with the driver's culpability being established in terms of the driver suffering sleepiness prior to falling asleep at the wheel, thus demonstrating knowledge of the risks of driving while in a state of fatigue (Rajaratnam & Jones, 2004).

The purpose of this chapter is not to exhaustively document current regulatory approaches and case law around fatigue. Rather, this chapter aims to identify key trends, challenges, and principles that underlie the evolution of fatigue management internationally and help the reader understand why traditional approaches are no longer the preferred way of managing fatigue-related risk. The strengths and weaknesses of the varying approaches and the likely future direction of fatigue management over the next decade or two are also explored.

With respect to legal frameworks, this chapter identifies key current and emerging areas of litigation, the underlying legislation and principles, and the way courts are interpreting the laws to determine guilt, liability, consequence, and compensation. When discussing legislation and regulation, this chapter addresses not only fatigue management practices within organisations, but also fitness for work, and fatigue regulation in the non-work transportation context. This chapter presents an overview of the legal principles from criminal, civil, and WHS law most likely to (1) influence their own attempts at policy formulation at the local level and (2) determine individual, executive, and directorial liability accountability in the event of an accident.

2.7.2   THE EVOLUTION OF LEGAL AND REGULATORY FRAMEWORKS RELATING TO FATIGUE

The way in which fatigue is regulated has undergone a profound transformation in recent decades. Historically, fatigue was typically managed as part of the labour contract between employees and employers. Starting in the late 19th century, working hours were increasingly restricted to:

(a) reduce the injuries due to the muscular fatigue associated with long hours of work in physically demanding occupations and, to a lesser extent;

(b) ensure an adequate opportunity to discharge family, social, and community responsibilities;

(c) increase employment by reducing the hours an individual could work; and

(d) increase financial compensations via overtime payments where long working hours were required.

Brooks, 1956; Huberman & Minns, 2007

Because the accumulation of physical fatigue can be quite accurately characterised as a simple linear function of the amount of time-on and time-off a task, the regulatory frameworks were understandably based around simple rules prescribing maximum shift durations, minimum break durations, and limits on aggregate total hours worked over nominal periods (e.g., a week, fortnight, month or year, etc.). By and large this was a simple and effective way to regulate physical fatigue and was the basis of regulatory frameworks for the best part of the century between 1850 and 1950.

Over the 20th century, and particularly after the Second World War, the physical demands of work diminished significantly as a direct consequence of mechanisation and automation. At the same time, the nature of work became more cognitively and less physically demanding, requiring a greater reliance on knowledge-based skills, symbolic manipulation, and complex decision-making/judgement. These cognitive demands, in addition to time of day and prior sleep wake behaviour, have an equal and sometimes greater influence on mental fatigue or sleepiness than mere time-on/ off task.

Despite evidence to the contrary, a hundred and fifty years of union and management negotiations had established a long-held, but arguably erroneous, belief that fatigue was best managed via the working time arrangement as part of the labour contract rather than as a hazard under WHS legislation. From this perspective, a safe-system-of-work (vis-à-vis fatigue) could be easily defined on simple (or more correctly simplistic) rules around scheduling work and rest. Compliance with this negotiated contractual rule set provided an unambiguous definition of what was safe (or not) and work outside these limits was proscribed, overlooked, or compensated with higher pay or time-off in lieu.

There is no doubt that simplistic rules relating to the scheduling of work and rest can be attractive to key stakeholders. Compliance can be easily determined albeit substituted as merely a proxy for safety. Additional work can be compensated with overtime and penalty rates ("danger" or "dirt" money in common parlance) to compensate workers for the social inconvenience and WHS risks associated with elevated fatigue. In an economy with high levels of unionisation and centralised wage fixing, such approaches are not without merit. In the period 1870 to 1970, fatigue due to extended hours of work was not a common practice in developed countries, and prescriptive approaches limited most working time arrangements. However, ironically, these restrictions were often realised due to arguments predicated on the financial penalties to employers and the social penalties to employees of working longer hours, rather than on arguments based on health and safety.

With the advent of significant neoliberal "reforms" starting in the 1980s and the decline of union influence on working time arrangements, there has been a significant "deregulation" of working time arrangements in many developed economies. Shift durations and weekly limits on working time arrangements have been relaxed considerably in many occupations and real income growth has been maintained primarily via work intensification until the early years of this century. For full-time employees, average working hours and workload have broadly increased and staffing levels have significantly declined over the last 40 years. The transport sector appears to have not been immune to such pressures, and in sectors such as commercial light vehicle and passenger transport, long working hours across a week have become a normalised mechanism to ensure earning capacity for individual operators in some parts of the world.

There is little doubt that these changes have resulted in significant increases in labour productivity and corporate profitability. There is also strong evidence that real income growth for employees over this period was also similar (although much less so in the last decade). However, these changes in the ideological landscape have reduced the capacity of labour contracts to control the health and safety risks associated with extended working hours. Many corporate and union leaders, as well as employees, have been willing to overlook the additional risks associated with work intensification in order to realise short-term productivity and income gains associated with extended working time arrangements.

In effect, the neoliberal drive for productivity and flexibility was a success, but many of the costs were externalised or delayed in the new economic landscape. Nowhere was this more evident than in the area of fatigue management. In parallel with the de facto deregulation of the workplace (i.e., the relaxation of strict hours of work limitations) there was an increasing focus on the role of fatigue in mediating workplace safety. From the early 1990s there has been an increasing focus on the relationship between extended working hours, fatigue, and workplace safety.

On the left of the political divide (i.e., for those involved in labour movements and/or those aligned with left-leaning policies or parties) was an increasing awareness that deregulation, often acceded to by unions and employees to buttress income, had resulted in an increased likelihood of employee fatigue while working and/or commuting. In some cases, there was clear evidence of increased risk of accident and injury (Folkard & Åkerstedt, 2004). Unfortunately, however, decentralisation of working time arrangements and the political challenges of accessing large-scale corporate and regulatory accident and injury data made it difficult to produce incontrovertible evidence of a significant reduction in workplace safety directly attributable to fatigue.

On the right, there was an increasing frustration with the very poor link between compliance and safety and the disproportionate costs associated with black and white interpretations of prescriptive rules relating to scheduling of work and rest. Exceeding prescribed limits on shift durations by small amounts to enable greater flexibility (and income) was (a) demonstrably safe in many cases but not permitted by the regulations and (b) was safer than many other permitted practices (often in similar industries with different labour agreements) that were demonstrably unsafe. The lack of concordance between working hours compliance and safety, along with the decentralisation of the industrial/labour relations process, placed increasing pressure on politicians and regulators to find new ways to regulate fatigue.

In some jurisdictions, the initial response to the need for novel strategies for regulating fatigue was to "tighten" regulatory frameworks. Shift maxima, break minima, and total aggregate hours were restricted below the currently permitted values. The idea was that this would reduce excessive hours and fatigue-related risk. The difficulty with this approach is that it is politically fraught since many operators have established workplace practices and infrastructure based on maximum limits, and small changes can carry expensive adjustment costs that can often outweigh the safety benefits. In many jurisdictions this results in significant political interference via lobbying, and changes can be stalled for years if not decades as the actors argue about the net economic benefit.

Starting in the early 2000s, there was considerable academic and industry pressure to reduce the reliance on industrial/labour relations contracts as the primary mechanism through which to regulate fatigue. Drawing on the broader changes in Occupational Health and Safety (OHS) legislation/regulation across much of the developed world, key actors in the academy and industry argued for a shift to performance-based regulation as is commonly applied to all safety hazards (for a more detailed discussion of this topic, the reader is referred to the Robens Report commissioned by the UK Parliament (Robens, 1972) and the subsequent UK Health and Safety Act (Health and Safety at Work etc. Act, 1974)).

According to the principles of a performance-based regulatory framework, employers are required to ensure "a safe system of work" but the means to do that are not prescribed in detail by the regulator. It is up to the employer to identify relevant hazards, and to document and manage the risk to as low as is reasonably practicable. It is up to the employer to determine how best to do this based on current best practice and relative risk. Depending on the jurisdiction, this system may be "approved" by a regulator, or in other jurisdictions, the regulator may not be required to approve but merely prosecute an employer for failing to provide a safe-system-of-work after an event has occurred. Indeed, in some jurisdictions, an accident is considered prima facie evidence of the failure to provide a safe system of work.

While there has been a shift towards deregulation of hours of work in many industries, the transport sector—in most jurisdictions—remains a last bastion of prescriptive working time arrangements. Strict limitations on, for example, driving hours (in road transport or rail) are used to both manage the contractual component (i.e., enterprise bargaining) and as a proxy for fatigue management. Given the potential consequences of a fatigue-related error for transport operators, it has been considered reasonable to impose strict regulations on the amount of time one can spend "on task" (i.e., at work). However, employing a strict prescriptive hours of work system by design conflates safety with compliance. By solely limiting hours of work to nominally "manage fatigue", the need for actual monitoring and control of the hazard is removed. As such, it is possible, and indeed likely, that undetected and unmanaged fatigue is present within industries that are bound by even strict hours of work guidelines.

2.7.3   AN INTERNATIONAL SNAPSHOT ACROSS TRANSPORT INDUSTRIES

Given the complex evolution of legal and regulatory approaches to fatigue in the transport industries, the early 21st century has seen the emergence of an approach in most transport industries that attempts to mix prescriptive rule sets with risk-based approaches to fatigue management.

2.7.3.1   REGULATORY FRAMEWORKS IN ROAD TRANSPORT

The international regulatory approach to fatigue in road transport is perhaps the most complex of the transportation industries, with various layers of law and regulation influencing the overall management of fatigue. Three critical layers are relevant for road transport in many jurisdictions worldwide, including: (1) criminal and civil law; (2) work health and safety law and regulation; and (3) specific law and regulation relating to commercial road transport (Thomas et al., 2021).

Criminal and civil law play an important role in road safety, and in most jurisdictions act as a *general deterrent* to driving while fatigued. In most jurisdictions worldwide, the act of driving while fatigued is not in and of itself an offence, even though there is long-standing evidence that fatigue is associated with significant risk from a road safety perspective (Horne & Reyner, 1999). Rather, it is only when a crash occurs due to fatigue-related impairment that fatigue is seen as a factor contributing to culpable driving. Further, it is also usually necessary to establish that the driver is aware of their levels of fatigue, or sleepiness, and therefore knowing the risks to safety, in achieving prosecution of drivers involved in crashes for culpable driving offences (Rajaratnam & Jones, 2004). In general, this can be seen as a *reactive* regulatory approach to managing the risks of fatigue in transportation, where drivers are deterred from driving while fatigued in case that fatigue causes an accident for which they will be held culpable and punished.

In only a few jurisdictions worldwide, driving while fatigued is seen as an actual criminal offence. For instance, in the Nordic countries of Denmark, Norway, Sweden, and Finland, driving while impaired by fatigue is an offence in and of itself, among other factors that can impair driving performance (Radun et al., 2012). Similarly, in the US state of New Jersey, the so-called "Maggie's Law" sets out that causing a road crash that results in death while driving fatigued (defined as having been without sleep for more than 24 hours) can result in prosecution for vehicular homicide (Dawson et al., 2021).

The impacts of fatigue on driving performance cannot be used as a defence in criminal law, and for many years it has also been established that fatigue cannot be used as a factor in civil law to reduce liability (Jones et al., 2003). Indeed, civil liability is another legal mechanism by which driving while fatigued may be associated with penalty. Civil law is built around the concept of causing loss to another individual, and rests on standards of acceptable behaviour and duties of care. To this end, if a driver causes loss to an individual due to fatigue-related impairment causing an accident, the driver may be held responsible and be required to pay compensation for that loss (Barker et al., 2012).

In most English-speaking jurisdictions, to establish liability it is incumbent on the state/claimant to establish that the driver was (1) aware of their level of impairment and (2) was aware of the risk to self and others. Needless to say, the burden of proof in these cases is high, especially in criminal proceedings, and juries often appear reluctant to find defendants guilty given the (perceived) difficulty in quantifying a driver's level of fatigue and the lack of clear community standards on how tired is too tired to drive.

It has been suggested that the legal implications of driving while impaired due to fatigue could be aligned with the legal implications of driving while under the influence of drugs or alcohol. Driving while intoxicated was not a "crime" until community attitudes changed in the middle of the 20th century. First alcohol and later drug driving were proscribed irrespective of whether an accident had occurred or not.

Risky behaviour itself became the offence. It is likely that the same process may possibly influence fatigued driving regulation. Where a community accepts that fatigued driving is a significant risk factor that is reasonably foreseeable based on prior sleep-wake behaviour and time-of-day, it would not be unreasonable to see fatigued driving as the equivalent of driving while intoxicated. It is likely that this reflects a longer-term trend in community attitudes towards all impaired driving (e.g., also distracted driving). However, most legal and regulatory frameworks in transportation industries do not provide clear guidance on what constitutes operating while fatigued and, unlike drink or drug driving, investigations must rely on expert evidence to deem an operator impaired. A recent review paper from the authors of this chapter indicates that, based on the available evidence, it may be appropriate to deem an individual impaired due to fatigue if they have had less than 5 hours of sleep in the preceding 24 hours (Dawson et al., 2021). However, this is an emerging area of research, and any regulation or legislation deeming drivers to be impaired due to fatigue would require significant consultation with community members and relevant stakeholders, in addition to scientific evidence regarding impairment.

Specific laws and regulations relating to commercial road transport have been in place in jurisdictions worldwide for many decades. With respect to fatigue, many of these laws and regulations include provisions for prescriptive hours of work limitations to manage fatigue-related risk. Limiting driving time, mandating the frequency and duration of rest periods, and capping cumulative hours of work across consecutive days are all common features of prescriptive rule sets in the road transport industries in many countries. In some jurisdictions, such as Australia, these traditional prescriptive hours of work limitations have been more recently augmented by risk-based approaches to fatigue management, whereby organisations can develop their own tailored hours of work limitations if they are able to demonstrate enhanced risk management through factors such as improved design of working time arrangements, training in fatigue management strategies for drivers and schedulers, and the use of advanced fatigue detection technologies.

WHS laws and regulations in many jurisdictions worldwide are relevant to fatigue and driving that occur as part of employment. Since the latter part of the 20th century, WHS laws and regulations in many jurisdictions have moved away from simple prescriptive (rule-based) approaches to safety management, and now pivot around a basic duty for employers to provide for a safe system of work. Most jurisdictions adopt an approach that requires organisations to create the outcome of a safe system of work through the process of identifying hazards, assessing their risk, and putting in place appropriate forms of risk mitigation. To this end, several international standards have been developed to assist organisations in this process. Specifically, the standards ISO 45001:2018 Occupational Health and Safety Management Systems and ISO 31000:2018 Risk Management set out the frameworks adopted in many jurisdictions worldwide to meet the duties and obligations set out in WHS legislation (International Organisation for Standardisation [ISO], 2018). While prescriptive hours of work rules may form a component of risk management, they are increasingly seen as insufficient to manage the risks of fatigue from a WHS perspective.

2.7.3.2 REGULATORY FRAMEWORKS IN RAIL TRANSPORT

For many years, prescriptive rules governing working time arrangements have been the dominant form of fatigue risk management in the rail industry worldwide, as has been the case with other transport industries. Over the years, these prescriptive rules have become more limiting in many jurisdictions, as illustrated by recent (2020) changes to duty time limits in the Canadian rail industry (Table 2.7.1).

In Australia, national regulations stipulate that rail operators must have a safety management system that includes a Fatigue Risk Management Programme (FRMP). The FRMP must meet the requirements set out in Regulation 29 of the National Regulations which identifies the key fatigue-related risk factors that must be taken into account within the FRMP (Office of the National Rail Safety Regulator, 2020). These fatigue-related risk factors are provided in Table 2.7.2.

2.7.3.3 REGULATORY FRAMEWORKS IN MARITIME TRANSPORT

Unlike road transport or rail, fatigue management in the maritime domain is guided by overarching international regulation through the International Maritime Organisation

TABLE 2.7.1
Example Changes in Duty Time Limits–Canadian Rail Industry

Factor	2011 Work/Rest Rules	2020 Updated Duty/Rest Rules
Length of duty period	Up to 16 hours per duty period No fatigue mitigation measures	12-hour limit Fatigue assessment and intervention measures for shifts ending during overnight hours
Total work hours	No weekly, monthly, or annual limits	60 hours in a 7-day period; 192 hours in a 28-day period; 2500 hours per year
Rest periods	6 hours at home 8 hours away	12 hours at home 10 hours away
Deadheading (the authorised transportation of operating employees from one location to another)	Lack of clarity between time spent commuting versus deadheading	Commuting time versus deadheading defined. Adjustment to hours of rest based on time spent deadheading
Time away from work	No allowance	32 hours every 7 days with two 8-hour rest periods for freight railway operations
Fatigue management plans	Minimal requirements	Set of extensive, prescriptive requirements related to specific elements of the new rules and grounded in fatigue science.

Source: www.canada.ca/en/transport-canada/news/2020/11/updated-workrest-rules-for-railway-operating-employees.html

TABLE 2.7.2
Example of Fatigue Risk Factors from Australian Rail Regulation

Fatigue Risk Factor

Scheduling of work and non-work periods, including time-on-task and rest opportunities in shifts and the total period of time in which work is being carried out;

Call-in, on-call, and lift-up and lay-back arrangements, and extended hours of work, including overtime;

The impact of work scheduling and relief practices generally on social and psychological factors that may impact performance and safety, including the effect of scheduling practices, schedule predictability and irregularity, and control over work hours on sleep loss, performance, and safety;

Physiological factors arising out of work practices affecting rail safety workers, such as the effect on worker alertness and recovery of the time when work is undertaken, the length and frequency of breaks, commuting time, circadian effects, extended wakefulness, chronic sleep loss effects, and sleep inertia;

The kinds of rail safety work being carried out, including—

(i) work that requires significant physical exertion or high cognitive task demand; and

(ii) the degree of monotony or boredom or low cognitive task demand of the work;

The variations in shifts and rest periods that may be required by different rail safety work requirements, including different routes, crew-call practices and predictability of working hours;

The suitability of rest environments, including barracks, rest houses, and relay vans provided for rail safety workers by the operator;

The physical environment in which rail safety work is to be carried out, including climatic conditions, noise, vibration, and fumes;

Fatigue risks arising from any one-off or occasional circumstances in which rail safety work may be required to be carried out, including in emergencies or under degraded or abnormal conditions, subject to the working hours being dependent on the rail safety workers' indication of their fitness to continue;

Relevant developments in research related to fatigue and any technology that may be applied to manage work-related fatigue.

(IMO). For vessels operating outside and across individual domestic jurisdictions, a set of governing principles and prescriptive limits can be found in IMO conventions.

International Convention on Standards of Training Certification and Watchkeeping for Seafarers (STCW), 1978 (as amended) makes clear provisions with respect to fatigue management that include a requirement to "establish and enforce rest periods for watchkeeping personnel and those whose duties involve designated safety, security and prevention of pollution duties". Rest periods are specified in the STCW Code as a minimum of 10 hours in any 24-hour period, broken into no more than two periods, of which one rest period must be 6 hours or longer, and a minimum of 70 hours rest must be provided in every 7 days. Of course, for domestic shipping and other maritime activities, individual jurisdictions are able to set more limiting requirements for their crew.

In recent years, guidance material for the international maritime industry has followed the lead of other transport industries and highlighted the need to move towards a less singularly prescriptive and more risk-based approach to the management of fatigue.

2.7.3.4 REGULATORY FRAMEWORKS IN AVIATION

Like the case of the international maritime industry, a single international regulatory body, the International Civil Aviation Organisation (ICAO), has been established through international convention, and through the Standards and Recommended Practices (SARPs), provides guidance to member states with respect to minimum requirements for fatigue management in commercial air transportation.

As has traditionally been the case in transportation industries worldwide, prescriptive rules around working time arrangements have for many years formed the basis of fatigue management in civil aviation (International Civil Aviation Organisation, 2011). While ICAO does not set out specific prescriptive limits for member states, individual regulatory bodies have developed broadly similar approaches to flight and duty time limitations worldwide.

In more recent years, the aviation industry has been a leader in the establishment of risk-based approaches to fatigue management, and now a structured framework for Fatigue Risk Management Systems (FRMS) is set out in ICAO SARPs and guidance materials (IATA et al., 2015).

2.7.4 FUTURE CHALLENGES

Within some transportation industries, such as commercial aviation, the shift from prescriptive to a performance-based regulatory approach has been slow but steady. Progress has been fastest in those modes organised within large international bodies, such as aviation, who are often self-insured, can afford the cost of subject matter experts and advanced fatigue detection technologies, and have the safety culture and infrastructure necessary to support such a transition. On the other hand, road transport has been probably one of the slower transport sectors in evolving towards performance-based oversight, since the industry is typically national, dominated by small to medium enterprises who lack the culture and infrastructure at the firm level.

The slow (or non-existent) transition from prescriptive to performance- or risk-based fatigue management in part reflects ongoing tensions between industrial agreements and safety or regulatory requirements. In many cases, this difficulty stems from the fact that both sides aim to cover similar components of a work arrangement. From the industrial side, there is a need to manage working time arrangements to ensure that appropriate compensation and similar worker protections are in place. It is generally from this perspective that unions may be involved in supporting (or rejecting) certain working time arrangements and/or associated limitations. However, it must be noted that industrial agreements designed to limit workload, hours, or to manage compensation are typically created without serious consideration for safety (though they may note that limiting hours of work is expected to have positive implications for safety). Furthermore, many organisations, having established working hour limitations based on industrial agreements, believe that their fatigue management responsibilities have been met—and their workers are therefore "safe". It is not uncommon to see an organisation that, when asked to provide their fatigue management documentation, simply points to an enterprise agreement. Despite this, work hour limitations and other fatigue risk management strategies would ideally be within the purview of safety management and/or regulation systems due to the direct link to accident and injury risk.

In practice, individual regulators and jurisdictions have often moved towards performance-based approaches and then stalled or even moved back towards prescription or settled for hybrid models. An example of this was the prolonged regulatory reform process relating to flight and duty limits and implementation of FRMS in the civil aviation sector in Australia, which saw some sectors of the industry return in recent years to more prescriptive flight and duty limits than had previously existed under a regime of "standard industry exemptions" to previous flight and duty limits. Regardless, many academics have suggested, and a significant proportion of regulators have now accepted, in principle, that (1) prescriptive frameworks for managing fatigue have significant limitations and (2) performance-based approaches hold considerable promise to improve the management of fatigue-related risk (Sprajcer et al., 2021). Specifically, it is now well accepted that prescriptive rules are not well suited to effectively manage fatigue as a hazard because they do not provide a good match between compliance and safety. One only needs to consider the fact that a very significant percentage of workplace fatigue is directly attributable to non-work causes, and compliance with prescriptive hours of work rule set can never address these. (For a detailed discussion of the potential benefits and drawbacks of prescriptive and risk-based systems of fatigue management, see Chapter 4.1).

When considering the future of fatigue management and regulation, we must also consider the legal implications of fatigue outside of the workplace context. In particular, the degree of liability faced by driving while fatigued, and the potential consequences for the driver in the event of a fatigue-related vehicle crash, is the subject of current debate (Dawson et al., 2021). To date, most prosecutions for fatigue-related offences have been at the egregious end of the spectrum where fatigue-related impairment was incontrovertible (e.g., 24 hours of wakefulness), since few, if any, governments have provided clear community guidance on the amount of sleep required in order to drive or work safely. This is in stark contrast to the laws around drink and drug-impaired driving where blood alcohol concentrations are used as a well-accepted (but equally debatable) proxy measure of impairment. While there is no doubt that it may be more difficult to prove how many hours of sleep a driver has (or has not) obtained, where it is possible to demonstrate definitively that the minimum amount of sleep has not been obtained, prosecution should be straightforward in the presence of clear community expectations and guidance on the amount of sleep needed to drive or work safely. Arguably such guidance already exists (Dawson et al., 2021).

SUMMARY POINTS FOR PRACTITIONERS

- In most transport industries, fatigue has been managed through prescriptive limits on working time arrangements, such as maximum shift length and minimum rest break.

- The very act of operating while fatigued is rarely made explicit as an offence in legislation and regulation worldwide.
- Difficulties remain in determining an individual's level of fatigue-related impairment, and in the absence of specific bio-markers of fatigue-related impairment, surrogate measures such as the amount of sleep or wakefulness experienced by an individual must be used to determine fatigue likelihood.
- Increasingly risk-based approaches that adopt many elements of performance-based safety management systems are being utilised to manage fatigue, mirroring the changes to the management of Work Health and Safety risks seen in jurisdictions worldwide.

REFERENCES

Barker, K., Cane, P., Lunney, M., & Trindade, F. (2012). *The Law of Torts in Australia*. Oxford University Press.

Brooks, G. (1956). History of union efforts to reduce working hours. *Monthly Labor Review*, 1271–1273.

Dawson, D., Sprajcer, M., & Thomas, M. (2021). How much sleep do you need? A comprehensive review of fatigue related impairment and the capacity to work or drive safely. *Accident Analysis & Prevention, 151*, 105955.

Folkard, S., & Åkerstedt, T. (2004). Trends in the risk of accidents and injuries and their implications for models of fatigue and performance. *Aviation, Space, and Environmental Medicine, 75*(3), A161–A167.

Health and Safety at Work etc. Act (1974).

Horne, J. A., & Reyner, L. A. (1999). Vehicle accidents related to sleep: A review. *Occupational and Environmental Medicine, 56*(5), 289–294.

Huberman, M., & Minns, C. (2007, 2007/10/01/). The times they are not changin': Days and hours of work in Old and New Worlds, 1870–2000. *Explorations in Economic History, 44*(4), 538–567. https://doi.org/https://doi.org/10.1016/j.eeh.2007.03.002

IATA, ICAO, & IFAPLA. (2015). *Fatigue Management Guide for Airline Operators* (2nd ed.). IATA.

International Civil Aviation Organisation (ICAO). (2011). *Guidance Material for the Development of Prescriptive Fatigue Management Regulations (Annex 6, Part I, Ammendment 37)*. ICAO.

International Organisation for Standardisation (ISO). (2018). *Risk Management: ISO 31000*. International Organisation for Standardisation. www.iso.org/files/live/sites/isoorg/files/store/en/PUB100426.pdf

Jones, C., Dorrian, J., & Dawson, D. (2003). Legal implications of fatigue in the Australian transportation industries. *Journal of Industrial Relations, 45*(3), 344–359.

Office of the National Rail Safety Regulator. (2020). *Fatigue Risk Management–ONRSR Guideline*. ONRSR.

Radun, I., Ohisalo, J., Radun, J., & Rajalin, S. (2012). Law defining the critical level of driver fatigue in terms of hours without sleep: Criminal justice professionals' opinions and fatal accident data. *International Journal of Law, Crime and Justice, 40*(3), 172–178.

Rajaratnam, S. M., & Jones, C. B. (2004). Lessons about sleepiness and driving from the Selby rail disaster case: R v Gary Neil Hart. *Chronobiology International, 21*(6), 1073–1077.

Robens, A. (1972). *Safety and Health at Work. Report of the Committee 1970–1972.* www. mineaccidents.com.au/uploads/robens-report-original.pdf

Sprajcer, M., Thomas, M. J., Sargent, C., Crowther, M. E., Boivin, D. B., Wong, I. S., Smiley, A., & Dawson, D. (2021). How effective are fatigue risk management systems (FRMS)? A review. *Accident Analysis & Prevention*, 106398.

Thomas, M. J. W., Gupta, C. C., Sprajcer, M., Demasi, D., Sach, E., Roach, G., Sargent, C., Dawson, D., & Ferguson, S.A. (2021). *Fatigue and Driving: An International Review.* Appleton Institute–Central Queensland University, Adelaide, Australia.

Section 3

---

*Factors that Contribute
to Fatigue and Sleepiness
in Transportation*

3.1 Sleep Pressure and Circadian Rhythms

Anastasi Kosmadopoulos

Central Queensland University, Wayville, SA, Australia

CONTENTS

3.1.1 SLEEP AND CIRCADIAN PHYSIOLOGY

3.1.1.1 WHAT IS SLEEP?

Sleep has been described behaviourally as "a natural and reversible state of reduced responsiveness to external stimuli and relative inactivity, accompanied by a loss of consciousness" (p. 681; Rasch & Born, 2013). The ability to monitor brain activity in the early 20th century altered the prevailing view of sleep as a passive brain state to an active one composed of neuronal activity substantially different from that observed during wakefulness (Berger, 1929). Sleep or sleep-like states are believed to occur in all animals and considered to be essential for optimal healthy functioning. (Campbell & Tobler, 1984; Siegel, 2008). However, the required amount, frequency, and timing vary from species to species. The timing and duration of episodes of sleep are influenced by interacting homeostatic and circadian physiological processes (Borbély, 1982). While there is substantial variation in the sleep requirements of individuals influenced by genetic, behavioural, medical, and environmental factors, it is recommended that people sleep at least 7 hours per night on a regular basis to promote health and well-being (Watson et al., 2015).

DOI: 10.1201/9781003213154-17

3.1.1.2 SLEEP STAGES AND SLEEP ARCHITECTURE

Sleep is comprised of multiple stages that differ in terms of their recuperative value and ease of arousal (Carskadon & Dement, 2017; Dement & Kleitman, 1957). These stages can be identified by distinct patterns in the frequency and amplitude of neuronal activity (electroencephalography), as well as changes in eye movement (electrooculography, EOG), and muscle tone (electromyography, EMG) (Aserinsky & Kleitman, 1953; Dement & Kleitman, 1957). Sleep stages may be categorised as one of two main types: rapid eye movement (REM) sleep or non-rapid eye movement (non-REM) sleep (Aserinsky & Kleitman, 1953; Berry et al., 2017). REM and non-REM sleep rotate throughout a sleep episode in approximately 80 to 120 min cycles (Dement & Kleitman, 1957; Dijk, 2009).

REM sleep comprises a single distinct stage renowned for its association with dreaming and characterised by random movement of the eyes, loss of muscle tone, and high-frequency low-amplitude neuronal activity resembling that found during wakefulness (Aserinsky & Kleitman, 1953; Dement & Kleitman, 1957). This stage is believed to be important for memory, learning, and creativity (Cai et al., 2009; Walker et al., 2002; Walker & Stickgold, 2004). In contrast, non-REM sleep is conventionally subdivided into three stages (N1, N2, and N3) that span a continuum of increasing sleep depth (Aserinsky & Kleitman, 1953; Berry et al., 2017). Stage N3 sleep, the deepest stage of sleep, is commonly referred to as slow-wave sleep (SWS) after its distinctive high proportion of low-frequency slow-wave activity (Berry et al., 2017; Blake & Gerard, 1937; Carskadon & Dement, 2017; Williams et al., 1964). This stage is believed to be important for recuperation, restoration, growth, immune function, and memory consolidation (Cairney et al., 2014; Hardin, 2009; Opp & Krueger, 2015).

3.1.1.3 SLEEP-WAKE REGULATION

The human sleep-wake cycle is usually composed of a single period of wake and a major sleep episode every 24 hours. This alternation of sleep and wake normally coincides with the daily light-dark cycle, such that sleep occurs at night and wake occurs during the day. Over the last century, this rhythmicity has come to be understood as a product of internally generated biological mechanisms rather than culturally engendered habit.

The Two-Process Model

Sleep and wake are primarily regulated by two separate but interacting physiological processes that affect the timing, intensity, and duration of sleep (Achermann & Borbély, 2003; Dijk & von Schantz, 2005). These processes comprise a sleep homeostatic component and a circadian component, representing amalgams of complex physiological systems (Borbély, 1982). According to this conceptualisation, the homeostatic process functions to maintain sleep homeostasis by reducing differences between an individual's sleep requirements and their behaviour (Borbély, 1982). Stated differently, a sleep homeostat helps individuals meet their biological sleep needs by (i) progressively increasing the physiological drive for sleep, that

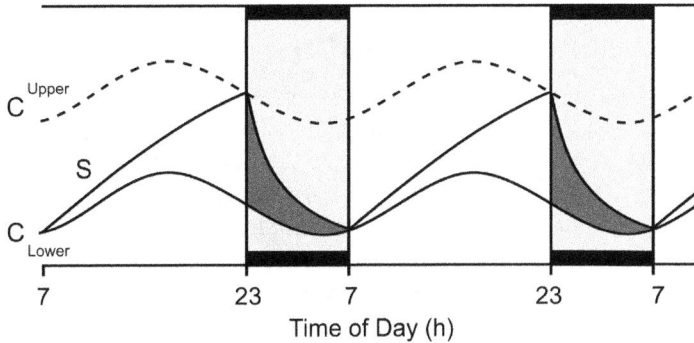

FIGURE 3.1.1 Schematic of the homeostatic and circadian components involved in the regulation of sleep. The homeostatic component is a sleep-dependent process (S) that increases the drive for sleep during periods of wakefulness and dissipates during sleep. The circadian component (C) produces an alerting signal during the day which peaks and then declines in the evening. These processes interact to facilitate and maintain the timing and consolidation of sleep at night and wake during the day. Homeostatic upper (sleep) and lower (wake) thresholds fluctuate with circadian phase. (Figure inspired by Borbély [1982]).

is, sleepiness, during periods of wakefulness and (ii) exponentially reducing this drive during sleep as requirements are satiated (Figure 3.1.1). The circadian process, which operates on near 24-hour cycles, provides regular "windows of opportunity" for sleep consolidation by influencing the propensity for sleep and wakefulness across the day (Borbély, 1982; Daan et al., 1984). According to the model, sleep is initiated when the homeostat reaches an upper threshold of sleep pressure and ends when it reaches a lower threshold. The circadian process interacts with the sleep homeostat to adjust these upper and lower bounds, making it easier to meet the sleep threshold at night and the wake threshold during the day (Figure 3.1.1). Combined, individuals are likely to be most ready for sleep at night after a prolonged period of wakefulness (Borbély, 1982; Dijk & Czeisler, 1994).

Physiological Basis of the Circadian and Homeostatic Regulatory Processes

The homeostatic drive for sleep is proposed to reflect the accumulation and dissipation of sleep-promoting substances in the brain, such as adenosine, which increases with prolonged wakefulness and decreases during sleep (Basheer et al., 2000; Huang et al., 2011). These substances are proposed to have this soporific effect by inhibiting the expression of wake-promoting neurons (Basheer et al., 2000; Huang et al., 2011). The circadian component of sleep regulation has a physiological basis in the suprachiasmatic nucleus (SCN) of the hypothalamus in the brain, the body's central pacemaker (i.e., "master clock" or "body clock"). The SCN is synchronised to the light-dark cycle and is responsible for maintaining the rhythmicity of physiological and behavioural rhythms. This central pacemaker generates wake-promoting rhythms that oppose the sleep-promoting homeostat during the day and subside during the night (Dijk & Lockley, 2002).

3.1.2 CONTRIBUTORS TO SLEEP- AND CIRCADIAN-RELATED FATIGUE IN TRANSPORTATION

Transportation employees in aviation, railway, road, and maritime sectors are often required to sleep away from home in suboptimal conditions and work long hours in various shift work systems designed to extend operations around the clock (Dorrian et al., 2011; Onninen et al., 2021; Petrilli et al., 2006). Despite sharing similar functions, these work schedules may differ from each other in multiple ways, including the timing of the start, end, and duration of shifts; the frequency and duration of breaks; the length of the work cycle; whether rostered shifts are permanent, rotating, or irregular; and, if rotating, the speed and direction of rotation. These characteristics are important to consider for fatigue management because they not only restrict the opportunities available for recuperative sleep but also affect the times at which employees must maintain alertness.

3.1.2.1 EXTENDED WAKEFULNESS AND TOTAL SLEEP DEPRIVATION

The greatest sleep-related risks to safety are those involving total sleep deprivation (TSD) and extended wakefulness as these often combine the extremes of accumulated homeostatic sleep pressure with the circadian trough in alertness (Borbély, 1982; Doran et al., 2001) (Figure 3.1.2). In an occupational context, extended wakefulness (usually ≥ 16 hours awake) is often a result of long work hours that encroach upon habitual bedtimes. TSD is an extreme form of extended wakefulness (≥24 hours) that

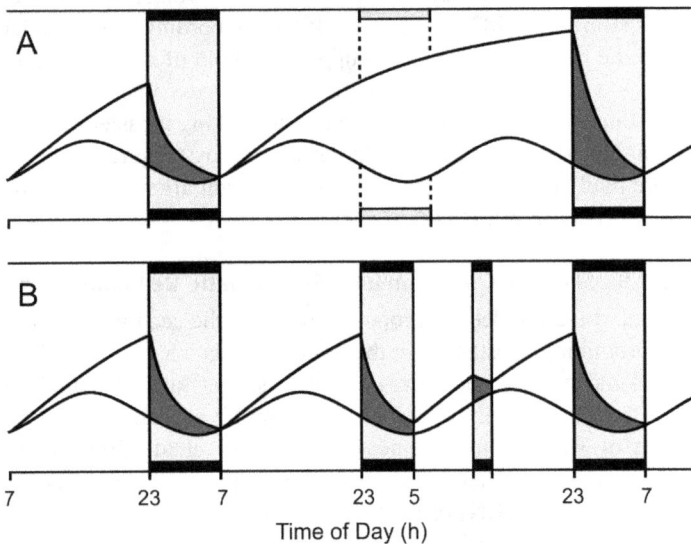

FIGURE 3.1.2 Schematic of the time course of the interaction between the homeostatic sleep-wake and circadian components of sleep regulation during a night of sleep deprivation (panel A) and after supplementing short sleep with a nap (panel B). The x-axis depicts time of day. (Figure inspired by Borbély [1982] and Achermann and Borbély [2003]).

can occur in the context of night work, particularly during the transition to the first night shift (Santhi et al., 2007).

During periods of uninterrupted wakefulness, sleepiness increases and the ability to maintain alertness becomes increasingly more variable (Doran et al., 2001). Dawson and Reid (1997) were able to equate cognitive psychomotor performance on a tracking task after 17 hours of wakefulness with that of performance at a blood alcohol concentration (BAC) of 0.05%. Subsequent studies with other measures of neurobehavioural function, including a simulated driving task, have documented impairment equivalent to BAC of 0.08% to 0.10% at approximately 20 to 25 hours of wakefulness (Arendt et al., 2001; Lamond & Dawson, 1999).

3.1.2.2 PARTIAL SLEEP DEPRIVATION

Partial sleep deprivation occurs when individuals obtain less sleep than is needed to satiate their physiological homeostatic requirements. This often happens in the context of late bedtimes or early waketimes when there is little or no opportunity to accommodate corresponding adjustments to waketimes and bedtimes, respectively. Indeed, Roach et al. (2012) found that short-haul aeroplane pilots obtained less sleep prior to duty periods commencing between 04:00 h and 05:00 h (i.e., 5.4 hours) than prior to duty periods commencing between 09:00 h and 10:00 h (i.e., 6.6 hours). Similar observations regarding earlier and later work start times have also been made for train drivers and truck drivers (Ingre et al., 2008; Philip et al., 2002). In these afore-mentioned studies, sleep was curtailed by the "Wake Maintenance Zone" (Folkard & Barton, 1993; Lavie, 1986), a period of time in the biological evening when it is difficult to initiate and maintain sleep, that prevents the appropriate advancement of bedtimes.

While few experience TSD on a regular basis, it is common for shift workers to obtain less sleep than desired or required to function optimally (Anderson & Horne, 2008). It has long been demonstrated that a single night of restriction to 4 hours or less of time in bed can cause fatigue and substantial impairment to both alertness and cognitive function (Tilley & Wilkinson, 1984). In other studies, comparatively mod-erate restriction to between 4 and 7 hours in bed has also produced deficits, though less pronounced (Dinges et al., 1997; Herscovitch & Broughton, 1981). Anderson and Horne (2013) demonstrated that restricting sleep to 5 hours increases the propen-sity of drivers to become distracted and thus more likely to have distraction-related incidents. An investigation by the US Department of Transportation found that drivers who reported sleeping 5 to 6 hours in the 24 hours before a crash had almost double the odds of being deemed culpable as those reporting 7 to 10 hours of sleep (Tefft, 2018). Further, another study found that drivers who slept 5 hours or less had almost triple the odds of being involved in a serious or fatal crash compared with drivers who reported sleeping more (Connor et al., 2002).

3.1.2.3 CHRONIC SLEEP LOSS

Chronic sleep loss refers to the experience of regularly obtaining insufficient sleep for an extended or ongoing period over several weeks or months. In transportation, the cause of chronic sleep loss is often attributable to work schedules that restrict sleep opportunities to inadequate durations or to times of day when sleep is difficult to maintain (Lemke et al., 2016; Roach et al., 2003). Indeed, in a study of train drivers, the amount of sleep obtained during 12-hour breaks between consecutive shifts averaged as much as 8 hours when the breaks occurred at night but as little as 3 hours when they happened during the day (Roach et al., 2003). Sallinen et al. (2003) also observed effects of different shift sequences for train drivers and railway traffic controllers, particularly in relation to night work. Sleep periods between consecutive night shifts were reduced by an average of 3 to 3.5 hours (Sallinen et al., 2003). Long work hours can also contribute to sleep loss: Lemke et al. (2016) found that 70% of long-haul truck drivers reported working for more than 11 hours per day and 44% reported violating the 14-hour regulated daily maximum. In turn, more than one-third (37.5%) of the drivers obtained less than 6.5 hours on workdays, compared to 17% on days off (Lemke et al., 2016).

The systematic restrictions imposed by these schedules mean that frequently working overtime or working evening/night, early morning, or irregular shifts can result in an accumulation of sleep debt and excessive daytime sleepiness (Garbarino et al., 2016; Onninen et al., 2021). Indeed, as one example, Onninen et al. (2021) observed that 45% of long-haul truck drivers working irregular shifts for 2 weeks accumulated more than 6 hours of sleep loss at least once in the 72-hour window before the end of a shift (Onninen et al., 2021).

Two important investigations into the cumulative effects of sleep loss on neurobehavioural function were published by Van Dongen et al. (2003) and Belenky et al. (2003). Participants were restricted to one of several daily sleep "doses" across consecutive nights. Van Dongen et al. (2003) limited time in bed to 8, 6, or 4 hours per day for 14 days or TSD (0 hours) for 3 days, while Belenky et al. (2003) limited time in bed to 9, 7, 5, or 3 hours per day over a period of 7 days. They demonstrated that restriction to 7 hours or less in bed per night can impair cognitive performance. The extent of impairment was dose dependent, such that nightly restriction to 6 hours for 2 weeks produced deficits equivalent to 1 night of TSD, while restriction to 4 hours produced deficits equivalent to 2 nights of TSD (Van Dongen et al., 2003).

The long-term effects of chronic partial sleep restriction on fatigue appear to be longer lasting than that of TSD and extended wakefulness (Banks et al., 2010; Belenky et al., 2003). While a full return to normal baseline neurobehavioural function following TSD is possible with a single night of long-duration recovery sleep (Yamazaki et al., 2020), complete recovery from chronic sleep restriction may not be observed in all areas of functioning after even three or four nights (Belenky et al., 2003; Yamazaki et al., 2020). Given the findings that self-reported "catch-up sleep" on weekends is often insufficient to compensate for sleep debt accumulated across a work week (Leger et al., 2020), transportation workers may need to consider strategies to maximise sleep across the work cycle.

3.1.2.4 Circadian Disruption and Misalignment

Work times are important to consider in fatigue management because they can coincide with phases of the circadian master clock during which the brain and body are prepared for sleep (Figure 3.1.2). Many studies have described a reliable peak in crash risk between midnight and early hours of the morning, consistent with increased fatigue due to circadian physiology (Folkard et al., 2006; Horne & Reyner, 1995). Constraints caused by schedules also mean that when night-working transportation workers do sleep during the daytime, it is frequently shorter and of poorer quality than the sleep achieved by day workers during the night time (Jeong et al., 2018; Lemke et al., 2016). This has been observed in many transportation sectors, including aviation, railway, and maritime (Gander et al., 2008; Philip & Åkerstedt, 2006; Roach et al., 2003; Roach et al., 2012). Chronic sleep loss has been demonstrated to exacerbate fatigue-related decline in performance associated with being awake at night (Kosmadopoulos et al., 2017; Matthews et al., 2012). This highlights the need for proactive implementation of both preventative and protective strategies for transportation workers engaging in night work (e.g., napping and caffeine).

3.1.3 SLEEP STRATEGIES FOR MITIGATING SLEEP-RELATED FATIGUE

The sum of research into the homeostatic-circadian regulation of alertness indicates that sleep duration, prior wakefulness, and circadian time are dependent on each other. Where one factor is not ideal for sustaining alertness, fatigue may be mitigated by the others. For example, fatigue attributed to being awake at night may be alleviated by obtaining sufficient sleep during the day and wakefulness not exceeding the habitual duration (Bonnet, 1991). Conversely, fatigue attributed to insufficient sleep may be moderated by ensuring wakefulness is not prolonged and occurs during the daytime (Belenky et al., 2003). A growing body of research suggests that obtaining multiple short sleep episodes per day can satisfactorily sustain alertness provided the total duration is sufficient (Cousins et al., 2021; Jackson et al., 2014; Kosmadopoulos et al., 2014; Roach et al., 2017; Sargent et al., 2022). As such, supplementing inadequate sleep with naps may be one of the most effective ways to minimise overall daily sleep loss (Rosekind et al., 1995).

In workplaces that permit on-shift napping (e.g., for "on-call" work), opportunities could be strategically utilised to serve the dual purposes of satiating sleep need and mitigating fatigue (Bonnet, 1991; Lovato et al., 2009). Compensatory naps obtained during the night have been shown to alleviate accumulated fatigue and improve night-time performance (Ficca et al., 2010; Ruggiero & Redeker, 2014). Conversely, prophylactic naps could be obtained in preparation for scheduled sleep loss, especially when nocturnal functioning is required (e.g., before extended night-time shifts or commutes) (Figure 3.1.2) (Bonnet, 1991; Kosmadopoulos et al., 2016; Lovato et al., 2009; Macchi et al., 2002; Sargent et al., 2022).

3.1.4 CONCLUSIONS

Sleep loss and circadian rhythm disruption are significant contributors to fatigue in transportation and represent the most important factors to target mitigations. This chapter explored the sleep-wake and circadian regulatory processes that drive the physiological pressure for sleep during the day and night, as well as their roles in alertness and cognitive function. Disruption of these processes caused by work schedules that limit sleep, extend periods of wakefulness, and desynchronise the circadian system can exacerbate the accumulation of fatigue and impair the quality of subsequent sleep.

SUMMARY POINTS FOR PRACTITIONERS

- Sleepiness and alertness are influenced by two separate but interacting physiological processes that regulate the timing and duration of sleep and wake—i.e., a sleep homeostat and a circadian pacemaker. Thus, people are biologically predisposed to be sleepiest at night and after long durations of wakefulness.
- Total sleep time is critical for optimal function and reducing sleepiness. Individuals should aim to regularly obtain a total of 7 to 9 hours of sleep per day, whether in a single consolidated period at night or distributed across the day in multiple shorter periods.
- Sustained wakefulness of 17 hours following a regular night of sleep produces levels of fatigue and impairment of cognitive function equivalent to that observed with a blood alcohol concentration of 0.05%.
- Individuals who are required to sustain operations during the night can take strategically-timed naps to dissipate the homeostatic drive for sleep.
- Sleep quality is important for maximising its recuperative and prophylactic benefits. Good sleep is best facilitated by a dark, quiet, and comfortable environment free from distraction.

REFERENCES

Achermann, P., & Borbély, A. A. (2003). Mathematical models of sleep regulation. *Frontiers in Bioscience*, *8*, s683–s693.

Anderson, C., & Horne, J. A. (2008). Do we really want more sleep? A population-based study evaluating the strength. *Sleep Medicine*, *9*(2), 184–187. https://doi.org/10.1016/j.sleep.2007.02.006

Anderson, C., & Horne, J. A. (2013). Driving drowsy also worsens driver distraction. *Sleep Medicine*, *14*(5), 466–468. https://doi.org/10.1016/j.sleep.2012.11.014

Arendt, J. T., Wilde, G. J. S., Munt, P. W., & MacLean, A. W. (2001). How do prolonged wakefulness and alcohol compare in the decrements they produce on a simulated driving task? *Accident Analysis and Prevention*, *33*(3), 337–344. https://doi.org/10.1016/S0001-4575(00)00047-6

Aserinsky, E., & Kleitman, N. (1953). Regularly occurring periods of eye motility, and concomitant phenomena, during sleep. *Science*, *118*, 273–274.

Banks, S., Van Dongen, H. P. A., Maislin, G., & Dinges, D. F. (2010). Neurobehavioral dynamics following chronic sleep restriction: Dose-response effects of one night for recovery. *Sleep*, *33*(8), 1013–1026. https://doi.org/10.1093/sleep/33.8.1013

Basheer, R., Porkka-Heiskanen, T., Strecker, R. E., Thakkar, M. M., & McCarley, R. W. (2000). Adenosine as a biological signal mediating sleepiness following prolonged wakefulness. *Neuro-Signals*, *9*(6), 319–327. www.karger.com/DOI/10.1159/000014655

Belenky, G., Wesensten, N. J., Thorne, D. R., Thomas, M. L., Sing, H. C., Redmond, D. P., Russo, M. B., & Balkin, T. J. (2003). Patterns of performance degradation and restoration during sleep restriction and subsequent recovery: A sleep dose-response study. *Journal of Sleep Research, 12*(1), 1–12. https://doi.org/10.1046/j.1365-2869.2003.00337.x

Berger, H. (1929). Uber das Elektrenkephalogramm des Menschen. *Archiv Psychiatrie und Nervenkrankheiten, 87,* 527–570.

Berry, R. B., Brooks, R., Garnaldo, C. E., Harding, S. M., Lloyd, R. M., Quan, S. F., Troester, M. M., & Vaughn, B. V. (2017). *The AASM Manual for the Scoring of Sleep and Associated Events: Rules, Terminology and Technical Specifications* (2nd ed.). American Academy of Sleep Medicine.

Blake, H., & Gerard, R. W. (1937). Brain potentials during sleep. *American Journal of Physiology, 119,* 692–703.

Bonnet, M. H. (1991). The effect of varying prophylactic naps on performance, alertness and mood throughout a 52-hour continuous operation. *Sleep, 14*(4), 307–315.

Borbély, A. A. (1982). A two process model of sleep regulation. *Human Neurobiology, 1*(3), 195–204.

Cai, D. J., Mednick, S. A., Harrison, E. M., Kanady, J. C., & Mednick, S. C. (2009). REM, not incubation, improves creativity by priming associative networks. *Proceedings of the National Academy of Sciences, 106*(25), 10130–10134. https://doi.org/doi:10.1073/pnas.0900271106

Cairney, S. A., Durrant, S. J., Power, R., & Lewis, P. A. (2014). Complementary roles of slow-wave sleep and rapid eye movement sleep in emotional memory consolidation. *Cerebral Cortex, 25*(6), 1565–1575. https://doi.org/10.1093/cercor/bht349

Campbell, S. S., & Tobler, I. (1984). Animal sleep: A review of sleep duration across phylogeny. *Neuroscience & Biobehavioral Reviews, 8*(3), 269–300. https://doi.org/10.1016/0149-7634(84)90054-X

Carskadon, M. A., & Dement, W. C. (2017). Normal human sleep: An overview. In M. H. Kryger, T. Roth, & W. C. Dement (Eds.), *Principles and Practice of Sleep Medicine* (6th ed., pp. 15–24). Elsevier, Inc. https://doi.org/10.1016/B978-0-323-24288-2.00002-7

Connor, J., Norton, R., Ameratunga, S., Robinson, E., Civil, I., Dunn, R., Bailey, J., & Jackson, R. (2002). Driver sleepiness and risk of serious injury to car occupants: Population based case control study. *British Medical Journal, 324*(7346), 1125. https://doi.org/10.1136/bmj.324.7346.1125

Cousins, J. N., Leong, R. L. F., Jamaluddin, S. A., Ng, A. S. C., Ong, J. L., & Chee, M. W. L. (2021). Splitting sleep between the night and a daytime nap reduces homeostatic sleep pressure and enhances long-term memory. *Scientific Reports, 11*(1), 5275. https://doi.org/10.1038/s41598-021-84625-8

Daan, S., Beersma, D. G. M., & Borbély, A. A. (1984). Timing of human sleep: Recovery process gated by a circadian pacemaker. *American Journal of Physiology–Regulatory, Integrative and Comparative Physiology, 246,* R161–R183.

Dawson, D., & Reid, K. (1997). Fatigue, alcohol and performance impairment. *Nature, 388*(6639), 235–235. https://doi.org/10.1038/40775

Dement, W., & Kleitman, N. (1957). Cyclic variations in EEG during sleep and their relation to eye movements, body motility, and dreaming. *Electroencephalography and Clinical Neurophysiology, 9*(4), 673–690. https://doi.org/10.1016/0013-4694(57)90088-3

Dijk, D.-J. (2009). Regulation and functional correlates of slow wave sleep. *Journal of Clinical Sleep Medicine: JCSM: Official Publication of the American Academy of Sleep Medicine, 5*(2 Suppl), S6–S15. www.ncbi.nlm.nih.gov/pubmed/19998869; www.ncbi.nlm.nih.gov/pmc/articles/PMC2824213/

Dijk, D. J., & Czeisler, C. A. (1994). Paradoxical timing of the circadian rhythm of sleep propensity serves to consolidate sleep and wakefulness in humans. *Neuroscience Letters, 166*(1), 63–68.

Dijk, D.-J., & Lockley, S. W. (2002). Invited review: Integration of human sleep-wake regulation and circadian rhythmicity. *Journal of Applied Physiology*, *92*(2), 852–862. https://doi.org/10.1152/japplphysiol.00924.2001

Dijk, D.-J., & von Schantz, M. (2005). Timing and consolidation of human sleep, wakefulness, and performance by a symphony of oscillators. *Journal of Biological Rhythms*, *20*(4), 279–290. https://doi.org/10.1177/0748730405278292

Dinges, D. F., Pack, F., Williams, K., Gillen, K. A., Powell, J. W., Ott, G. E., Aptowicz, C., & Pack, A. I. (1997). Cumulative sleepiness, mood disturbance and psychomotor vigilance performance decrements during a week of sleep restricted to 4–5 hours per night. *Sleep*, *20*(4), 267–277.

Doran, S. M., Van Dongen, H. P. A., & Dinges, D. F. (2001). Sustained attention performance during sleep deprivation: Evidence of state instability. *Archives Italiennes de Biologie*, *139*(3), 253–267. https://doi.org/10.4449/aib.v139i3.503

Dorrian, J., Baulk, S. D., & Dawson, D. (2011). Work hours, workload, sleep and fatigue in Australian Rail Industry employees. *Applied Ergonomics*, *42*(2), 202–209. https://doi.org/10.1016/j.apergo.2010.06.009

Ficca, G., Axelsson, J., Mollicone, D. J., Muto, V., & Vitiello, M. V. (2010). Naps, cognition and performance. *Sleep Medicine Reviews*, *14*, 249–258.

Folkard, S., & Barton, J. (1993). Does the 'forbidden zone' for sleep onset influence morning shift sleep duration? *Ergonomics*, *36*(1–3), 85–91.

Folkard, S., Lombardi, D. A., & Spencer, M. B. (2006). Estimating the circadian rhythm in the risk of occupational injuries and accidents. *Chronobiology International*, *23*(6), 1181–1192. https://doi.org/10.1080/07420520601096443

Gander, P. H., van den Berg, M., & Signal, L. (2008). Sleep and sleepiness of fishermen on rotating schedules. *Chronobiology International*, *25*, 389–398. https://doi.org/10.1080/07420520802106728

Garbarino, S., Durando, P., Guglielmi, O., Dini, G., Bersi, F., Fornarino, S., Toletone, A., Chiorri, C., & Magnavita, N. (2016). Sleep apnea, sleep debt and daytime sleepiness are independently associated with road accidents. A cross-sectional study on truck drivers. *PloS One*, *11*(11), e0166262. https://doi.org/10.1371/journal.pone.0166262

Hardin, K. A. (2009). Sleep in the ICU: Potential mechanisms and clinical implications. *Chest*, *136*(1), 284–294.

Herscovitch, J., & Broughton, R. J. (1981). Performance deficits following short-term partial sleep deprivation and subsequent recovery oversleeping. *Canadian Journal of Psychology*, *35*(4), 309–322. https://doi.org/10.1037/h0081197

Horne, J. A., & Reyner, L. A. (1995). Sleep related vehicle accidents. *British Medical Journal*, *310*, 565–567.

Huang, Z.-L., Urade, Y., & Hayaishi, O. (2011). The role of adenosine in the regulation of sleep. *Current Topics in Medicinal Chemistry*, *11*(8), 1047–1057. https://doi.org/http://dx.doi.org/10.2174/156802611795347654

Ingre, M., Kecklund, G., Åkerstedt, T., Söderström, M., & Kecklund, L. (2008). Sleep length as a function of morning shift-start time in irregular shift schedules for train drivers: Self-rated health and individual differences. *Chronobiology International*, *25*(2–3), 349–358. https://doi.org/10.1080/07420520802110704

Jackson, M. L., Banks, S., & Belenky, G. (2014). Investigation of the effectiveness of a split sleep schedule in sustaining sleep and maintaining performance. *Chronobiol Int*, *31*(10), 1218–1230. https://doi.org/10.3109/07420528.2014.957305

Jeong, I., Park, J. B., Lee, K. J., Won, J. U., Roh, J., & Yoon, J. H. (2018). Irregular work schedule and sleep disturbance in occupational drivers-A nationwide cross-sectional study. *PloS One*, *13*(11), e0207154. https://doi.org/10.1371/journal.pone.0207154

Kosmadopoulos, A., Sargent, C., Darwent, D., Zhou, X., Dawson, D., & Roach, G. D. (2014). The effects of a split sleep-wake schedule on neurobehavioural performance and predictions of performance under conditions of forced desynchrony. *Chronobiology International*, *31*(10), 1209–1217. https://doi.org/10.3109/07420528.2014.957763

Kosmadopoulos, A., Sargent, C., Zhou, X., Darwent, D., Matthews, R. W., Dawson, D., & Roach, G. D. (2017). The efficacy of objective and subjective predictors of driving performance during sleep restriction and circadian misalignment. *Accident Analysis and Prevention*, *99*(Pt B), 445–451. https://doi.org/10.1016/j.aap.2015.10.014

Kosmadopoulos, A., Zhou, X., Roach, G. D., Darwent, D., & Sargent, C. (2016). No first night shift effect observed following a nocturnal main sleep and a prophylactic 1-h afternoon nap. *Chronobiology International*, *33*(6), 716–720. https://doi.org/10.3109/07420 528.2016.1167727

Lamond, N., & Dawson, D. (1999). Quantifying the performance impairment associated with fatigue. *Journal of Sleep Research*, *8*(4), 255–262. https://doi.org/10.1046/ j.1365-2869.1999.00167.x

Lavie, P. (1986). Ultrashort sleep-waking schedule: III. 'Gates' and 'forbidden zones' for sleep. *Electroencephalography and Clinical Neurophysiology*, *63*(5), 414–425.

Leger, D., Richard, J.-B., Collin, O., Sauvet, F., & Faraut, B. (2020). Napping and weekend catchup sleep do not fully compensate for high rates of sleep debt and short sleep at a population level (in a representative nationwide sample of 12,637 adults). *Sleep Medicine*, *74*, 278–288. https://doi.org/https://doi.org/10.1016/j.sleep.2020.05.030

Lemke, M. K., Apostolopoulos, Y., Hege, A., Sonmez, S., & Wideman, L. (2016). Understanding the role of sleep quality and sleep duration in commercial driving safety. *Accident Analysis and Prevention*, *97*, 79–86. https://doi.org/10.1016/ j.aap.2016.08.024

Lovato, N., Lack, L., Ferguson, S., & Tremaine, R. (2009). The effects of a 30-min nap during night shift following a prophylactic sleep in the afternoon. *Sleep and Biological Rhythms*, *7*(1), 34–42.

Macchi, M. M., Boulos, Z., Ranney, T., Simmons, L., & Campbell, S. S. (2002). Effects of an afternoon nap on nighttime alertness and performance in long-haul drivers. *Accident Analysis and Prevention*, *34*(6), 825–834. https://doi.org/10.1016/s0001-4575(01)00089-6

Matthews, R. W., Ferguson, S. A., Zhou, X., Sargent, C., Darwent, D., Kennaway, D. J., & Roach, G. D. (2012). Time-of-day mediates the influences of extended wake and sleep restriction on simulated driving. *Chronobiology International*, *29*(5), 572–579. https:// doi.org/10.3109/07420528.2012.675845

Onninen, J., Pylkkönen, M., Tolvanen, A., & Sallinen, M. (2021). Accumulation of sleep loss among shift-working truck drivers. *Chronobiology International*, *38*(9), 1344–1353. https://doi.org/10.1080/07420528.2021.1929280

Opp, M. R., & Krueger, J. M. (2015). Sleep and immunity: A growing field with clinical impact. *Brain, Behavior, and Immunity*, *47*, 1–3. https://doi.org/10.1016/j.bbi.2015.03.011

Petrilli, R. M., Roach, G. D., Dawson, D., & Lamond, N. (2006). The sleep, subjective fatigue, and sustained attention of commercial airline pilots during an international pattern. *Chronobiology International*, *23*(6), 1357–1362. https://doi.org/10.1080/07420520601085925

Philip, P., & Åkerstedt, T. (2006). Transport and industrial safety, how are they affected by sleepiness and sleep restriction? *Sleep Medicine Reviews*, *10*(5), 347–356. https://doi. org/10.1016/j.smrv.2006.04.002

Philip, P., Taillard, J., Léger, D., Diefenbach, K., Åkerstedt, T., Bioulac, B., & Guilleminault, C. (2002). Work and rest sleep schedules of 227 European truck drivers. *Sleep Medicine*, *3*(6), 507–511. https://doi.org/https://doi.org/10.1016/S1389-9457(02)00138-7

Rasch, B., & Born, J. (2013). About Sleep's Role in Memory. *Physiological Reviews*, *93*(2), 681–766. https://doi.org/10.1152/physrev.00032.2012

Roach, G. D., Reid, K. J., & Dawson, D. (2003). The amount of sleep obtained by locomotive engineers: Effects of break duration and time of break onset. *Occupational and Environmental Medicine*, *60*(12), e17. https://doi.org/10.1136/oem.60.12.e17

Roach, G. D., Sargent, C., Darwent, D., & Dawson, D. (2012). Duty periods with early start times restrict the amount of sleep obtained by short-haul airline pilots. *Accident Analysis and Prevention*, *45S*, 22–26. https://doi.org/10.1016/j.aap.2011.09.020

Roach, G. D., Zhou, X., Darwent, D., Kosmadopoulos, A., Dawson, D., & Sargent, C. (2017). Are two halves better than one whole? A comparison of the amount and quality of sleep obtained by healthy adult males living on split and consolidated sleep-wake schedules. *Accident Analysis and Prevention*, *99*, 428–433. https://doi.org/10.1016/j.aap.2015.10.012

Rosekind, M. R., Smith, R. M., Miller, D. L., Co, E. L., Gregory, K. B., Webbon, L. L., Gander, P. H., & Lebacqz, J. V. (1995). Alertness management: Strategic naps in operation settings. *Journal of Sleep Research*, *4*(Suppl. 2), 62–66. https://doi.org/10.1111/j.1365-2869.1995.tb00229.x

Ruggiero, J. S., & Redeker, N. S. (2014). Effects of napping on sleepiness and sleep-related performance deficits in night-shift workers: A systematic review. *Biological Research for Nursing*, *16*(2), 134–142. https://doi.org/10.1177/1099800413476571

Sallinen, M., Härmä, M., Mutanen, P., Ranta, R., Virkkala, J., & Müller, K. (2003). Sleep–wake rhythm in an irregular shift system. *Journal of Sleep Research*, *12*(2), 103–112. https://doi.org/https://doi.org/10.1046/j.1365-2869.2003.00346.x

Santhi, N., Horowitz, T. S., Duffy, J. F., & Czeisler, C. A. (2007). Acute sleep deprivation and circadian misalignment associated with transition onto the first night of work impairs visual selective attention. *PloS One*, *2*(11), e1233. https://doi.org/10.1371/journal.pone.0001233

Sargent, C., Kosmadopoulos, A., Zhou, X., & Roach, G. D. (2022). Timing of sleep in the breaks between consecutive night-shifts: The effect of different strategies on daytime sleep and night-time neurobehavioural function. *Nature and Science of Sleep*, *14*, 231–242. https://doi.org/10.2147/NSS.S336795

Siegel, J. M. (2008). Do all animals sleep? *Trends in Neurosciences*, *31*(4), 208–213. https://doi.org/10.1016/j.tins.2008.02.001

Tefft, B. C. (2018). Acute sleep deprivation and culpable motor vehicle crash involvement. *Sleep*, *41*(10), 1–11. https://doi.org/10.1093/sleep/zsy144

Tilley, A. J., & Wilkinson, R. T. (1984). The effects of a restricted sleep regime on the composition of sleep and on performance. *Psychophysiology*, *21*(4), 406–412. https://doi.org/10.1111/j.1469-8986.1984.tb00217.x

Van Dongen, H. P. A., Maislin, G., Mullington, J. M., & Dinges, D. F. (2003). The cumulative cost of additional wakefulness: Dose-response effects on neurobehavioral functions and sleep physiology from chronic sleep restriction and total sleep deprivation. *Sleep*, *26*(2), 117–126. https://doi.org/10.1093/sleep/26.2.117

Walker, M. P., Liston, C., Hobson, A., & Stickgold, R. (2002). Cognitive flexibility across the sleep-wake cycle: REM-sleep enhancement of anagram problem solving. *Cognitive Brain Research*, *14*, 317–324. https://doi.org/10.1016/S0926-6410(02)00134-9

Walker, M. P., & Stickgold, R. (2004). Sleep-dependent learning and memory consolidation. *Neuron, 44*(1), 121–133. https://doi.org/10.1016/j.neuron.2004.08.031

Watson, N. F., Badr, M. S., Belenky, G., Bliwise, D. L., Buxton, O. M., Buysse, D., Dinges, D. F., Gangwisch, J., Grandner, M. A., Kushida, C., Malhotra, R. K., Martin, J. L., Patel, S. R., Quan, S. F., & Tasali, E. (2015). Recommended amount of sleep for a healthy adult: A joint consensus statement of the American Academy of Sleep Medicine and Sleep Research Society. *Journal of Clinical Sleep Medicine, 11*(6), 591–592. https://doi.org/10.5664/jcsm.4758

Williams, H. L., Hammack, J. T., Daly, R. L., Dement, W. C., & Lubin, A. (1964). Responses to auditory stimulation, sleep loss and the EEG stages of sleep. *Electroencephalography and Clinical Neurophysiology, 16*, 269–279.

Yamazaki, E. M., Antler, C. A., Lasek, C. R., & Goel, N. (2020). Residual, differential neurobehavioral deficits linger after multiple recovery nights following chronic sleep restriction or acute total sleep deprivation. *Sleep, 44*(4). https://doi.org/10.1093/sleep/zsaa224

3.2 Jet Lag, Sleep Timing, and Sleep Inertia

Cassie J. Hilditch[1] and Dorothee Fischer[2]

Fatigue Countermeasures Laboratory, Department of
Psychology, San José State University, San José, CA, USA
[2]Institute for Aerospace Medicine, German Aerospace
Center, Cologne, Germany

CONTENTS

3.2.1 INTRODUCTION

This chapter explores the causes, consequences, and countermeasures related to jet lag, mistimed sleep, and sleep inertia. The core processes underpinning these topics are described in the three-process model of sleep regulation. How desynchrony within, and interactions between, these processes can lead to fatigue and ultimately reduced cognitive performance is outlined. For each topic, we highlight the relevance to the transportation industry and discuss how to mitigate or manage fatigue resulting from these factors.

DOI: 10.1201/9781003213154-18

3.2.2 JET LAG

3.2.2.1 WHAT IS JET LAG?

After flying across multiple time zones, most people experience a transient state of desynchrony, known as jet lag, between the new local clock time and the body's biological clock that governs rhythms in physiology and cognition (Herxheimer, 2014). Across the jet lag literature, the term has been used to refer to different aspects, describing the cause, mechanism, or symptoms of jet lag. Jet lag usually occurs after a flight across time zones resulting in a rapid shift of the local day-night cycle, for example, people arrive at their destination in bright daylight, while it is night-time at their location of departure (this is the cause). The rapid shift causes desynchrony between the timing of an individual's biological rhythms and the timing of day and night (in other words, light and darkness) at the new destination (this is the mechanism). The desynchrony manifests downstream as jet lag disorder, an official classification by the American Academy of Sleep Medicine, with symptoms ranging from indigestion to sleep disturbances, fatigue, and cognitive impairments (this is the symptomatology) (Sack et al., 2007). Severity and duration of jet lag symptoms are largely determined by travel-specific factors, particularly the direction of travel (eastward vs. westward) and the number of time zones crossed; in-flight factors, such as the opportunity and ability to sleep while travelling; and environmental factors at the destination that have the potential to realign the body clock with the new local clock time, including the timing of light, meals, and exercise. The scheduled exposure to (and avoidance of) these factors are used as non-pharmacological strategies to alleviate jet lag, often supplemented with the use of pharmacological substances (e.g., melatonin).

3.2.2.2 WHAT CAUSES JET LAG?

In millions of years of evolution, all living organisms have evolved a mechanism that enables them to measure time and predict cyclic environmental changes, for example, daily and seasonal changes in photoperiod and temperature that determine the availability of food and potential presence of predators. This mechanism is the circadian clock, regulating the timing of virtually all physiological functions, including gene expression (Brown et al., 2005), metabolism (Bass, 2012), immune system (Scheiermann et al., 2013), and cognitive functions (Schmidt et al., 2012). In humans, the circadian clock resides in the brain, in the suprachiasmatic nucleus (SCN). The SCN synchronises to the 24-hour day in an active process, called entrainment, using environmental signals of light and dark that reach the SCN via a direct pathway from the eyes to the brain. In situations of jet lag, the entrainment process is disrupted since light-dark signals have abruptly changed due to crossing multiple time zones. Accordingly, the circadian clock needs to re-entrain to the new local light-dark cycle, which happens naturally after a few days but can be accelerated by exposing oneself to bright light and avoiding it at the appropriate times (or slowed down if exposed at inappropriate times). "Appropriate" times are determined by the so-called *phase response curves* (PRC) that describe how light affects the circadian clock depending on the timing of the light exposure.

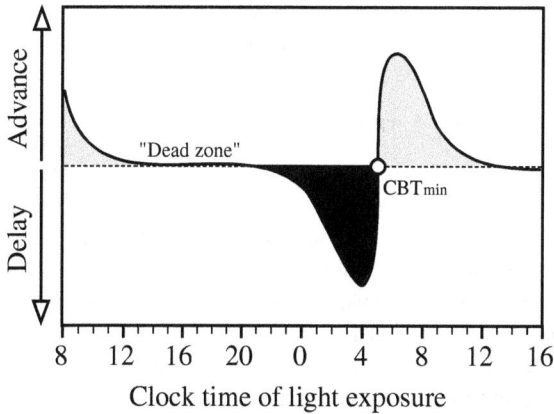

FIGURE 3.2.1 The phase response curve (PRC) to light in humans. CBTmin = core body temperature minimum.

Figure 3.2.1 shows the PRC to light in humans. Light delays the circadian clock when presented in the late afternoon/evening (i.e., sleep onset is later compared to a scenario with no such light exposure). In contrast, light advances the clock when presented in the early morning hours (i.e., sleep onset is earlier compared to a scenario with no such light exposure). The delaying and advancing areas of the PRC are separated by a "dead zone" (around noon), during which light has no effect on the circadian clock. It is essential to note that terms such as "late afternoon/evening" are not defined in reference to clock time but in reference to the individual's biological time (as determined, for instance, by the rhythm of core body temperature). The distinction is especially important in situations of jet lag: the exposure to light cannot be scheduled to local clock time, since clock time has changed due to crossing time zones (e.g., 18:00 at the destination is not 18:00 at the place of departure). Because biological time (i.e., phase of the circadian clock) changes non-linearly during re-entrainment, there is no straightforward estimation of it in jet lag situations. Mathematical models exist to dynamically estimate circadian phase in changing light-dark cycles (Jewett & Kronauer, 1998), but in most real-world applications, the best timing of light exposure to facilitate adaptation is crudely approximated by local time at the place of departure (see also sub-section 3.2.2.5). To make matters more complex, biological time also varies across individuals, which will be described in more detail in sub-section 3.2.3.1.

3.2.2.3 WHAT ARE THE CONSEQUENCES OF JET LAG?

Consequences of jet lag include disturbed sleep (e.g., shortened duration, poor quality, and irregular timing), fatigue, excessive daytime sleepiness, reduced cognitive performance, and somatic symptoms such as indigestion (Morgenthaler et al., 2007). Symptoms eventually disappear due to complete circadian adaptation after a few days, but they can occasionally have severe consequences, for example, in safety-critical occupations such as aviation, where the performance effects of jet lag-induced fatigue can have potentially fatal consequences.

3.2.2.4   EXAMPLES OF JET LAG IN AVIATION

Flight crew frequently experience travel jet lag, potentially resulting in increased fatigue, reduced capacity to perform cognitively, and an increased risk for safety incidents (e.g., a crash). A study investigating circadian adaptation and performance in pilots on flights from the United States (US) west coast to Asia (an 8-hour change in time zones) found that adaptation was complete after four days in Asia, with cognitive performance improving continuously across subsequent days post-arrival (Signal et al., 2013). Another study in pilots flying repeatedly between the US east coast and Japan (an 11-hour change in time zones) found that reaction times on the psychomotor vigilance test (a simple reaction time task) were more strongly correlated with predicted circadian phase than with the local clock time of the flights, with pilots reacting slower when tested at a detrimental circadian time (i.e., during their biological night) (Gander et al., 2016). A third study approximating circadian phase by local home base clock time reported a similar association between response speed and circadian timing when in a different time zone, with generally slower reaction times at circadian times that signal rest and sleep, instead of activity and wakefulness (Gander et al., 2015). Fatigue risk management systems have been implemented by airlines to help manage adverse consequences of jet lag for flight crew performance, recommending strategies that either increase the speed of circadian adaptation to a local layover time or try to keep flight crew on home base time, depending on the desired outcome. For example, if the timing of the return flight is a night flight based on the layover local time, it may be better to maintain home base circadian timing so that the return flight is not operated during the pilots' circadian low (Holmes et al., 2012). In practice, however, it can be very difficult to maintain home base time at the layover destination due to social pressures such as meal availability (Holmes et al., 2012). How and when flight crew choose to sleep on layover is currently an under-researched area.

3.2.2.5   HOW CAN JET LAG BE MANAGED?

There is no universal treatment for jet lag. Recommended mitigation strategies aim at maintaining the proper timing of (environmental) signals with the potential to reset the circadian clock. These signals are called *zeitgebers* (German for "signal-giver"). The best-studied zeitgebers to treat jet lag are light exposure and melatonin (Waterhouse & Reilly, 2009).

Bright Light

Properly timed exposure to and avoidance of bright light has been shown to facilitate adaptation to a new time zone (Simmons et al., 2015). Dark sunglasses can help block out light when isolation indoors is not possible or feasible. Exposure to light can be achieved using light-emitting devices mounted onto goggles, bright light boxes for home use, or by simply going outdoors during daytime. As described in sub-section 3.2.2.2, the effect of light on the circadian clock depends on the timing of its exposure, summarised in PRCs (Figure 3.2.1). In general, the circadian system adapts faster to westward travel (requiring a phase delay, i.e., going to bed later) than to eastward travel (requiring a phase advance, i.e., going to bed earlier). The schedule for timing of light exposure therefore differs for westward and eastward travel. Recommended times for light exposure to entrain faster have been summarised, based on the direction of travel and the numbers of time zones crossed (Simmons et al., 2015). Multiple mobile phone apps have been developed that help travellers schedule their sleep-wake cycle before, during, and after travel, to optimise re-synchronisation while considering their individual sleep-wake behaviour (Christensen et al., 2020). The importance of individual differences in sleep-wake behaviour will be further described in sub-section 3.2.3.

Melatonin

Melatonin is a circadian-controlled hormone, primarily secreted by the pineal gland in the brain. In humans, it is released during night-time darkness and suppressed by light, leading to its popular name "darkness hormone". Orally administered melatonin can induce circadian phase-shifts by signalling back to the circadian clock. As for the phase-shifting effects of light, a PRC for melatonin has been demonstrated in humans (Lewy et al., 1992). When administered before the endogenous dim-light onset of melatonin (DLMO; start of "normal" melatonin secretion in the early evening), oral melatonin induces a phase advance and promotes sleep; however, when administered after DLMO, it creates a phase delay, extending the biological night. Recommended times and doses of melatonin for travel purposes have been summarised (Simmons et al., 2015). The literature on the efficacy of melatonin for jet lag treatment is, however, mixed, likely due to the challenge of carefully timing oral melatonin administration and controlling light exposure while in the field (Arendt, 2018). A meta-analysis carefully selecting studies with appropriate criteria included nine randomised trials in airline passengers, airline staff, or military personnel (Herxheimer & Petrie, 2002). It found that melatonin taken close to the desired bedtime at the destination (between 22:00 and 00:00) significantly reduced subjective jet lag symptoms after crossing ≥ 5 time zones.

The most common symptom of jet lag is disturbed sleep, caused by a mismatch between the body's biological clock and the external day-night cycle. As such, *mistimed sleep* is an important part of jet lag, requiring travellers to sleep at times that are in conflict with circadian physiological functions. Mistimed sleep can also occur outside of air travel (e.g., in shift work), with no change in the solar light-dark cycle to help re-entrain the circadian clock.

3.2.3   SLEEP TIMING

The alternation between wakefulness and sleep is one of the most important biological rhythms in humans. Sleep is primarily regulated by two internal processes: a sleep homeostatic process and a circadian process (Borbély et al., 2016). The sleep homeostatic process is the increasing drive for sleep, the longer one is awake. The circadian process is the endogenous daily rhythm in the drive for sleep that originates from the master pacemaker in the brain, the circadian clock (the SCN). The homeostatic and the circadian processes interact in such a way that sleep is consolidated during the night, providing a biological sleep "window". Attempting to sleep outside of this window often results in reduced sleep duration and quality, as seen in jet lag and in shift workers required to sleep during the day (Åkerstedt & Wright, 2009). However, the specific timing of this sleep window (and with it the timing of physiological, behavioural, and cognitive rhythms) varies greatly among individuals. These inter-individual differences in sleep timing preferences are known as *chronotypes*.

3.2.3.1 WHAT ARE CHRONOTYPES?

An individual's chronotype results from the synchronisation process of the circadian clock to the 24-hour day, with rhythms in sleep, physiology, and cognition occurring accordingly earlier or later (Kerkhof & Van Dongen, 1996). Chronotypes range on a continuum from very early ("larks") to very late ("owls"). Late types exhibit later sleep onset times, the ability to extend their sleep into the day (e.g., after a night shift), as well as more variable day-to-day sleep times (Fischer et al., 2016). The difference in sleep timing between extremely early and extremely late chronotypes can be as much as 10 to 12 hours (Fischer, Lombardi, Marucci-Wellman, et al., 2017). Chronotype changes with age and sex: Both males and females become later types throughout adolescence, reaching a peak in "lateness" at around 20 years of age, and become earlier again with increasing age. On average, males tend to be later chronotypes than females before the age of 40 to 50 years, but this difference is reported to either disappear (Roenneberg et al., 2004) or be reversed (Fischer, Lombardi, Marucci-Wellman, et al., 2017) beyond that age.

Chronotype is a factor that potentially contributes to fatigue via individual differences in the daily timing of sleep, sleepiness, and cognitive performance. In shift work, early chronotypes adjust less well to night shifts than late types (Fischer et al., 2021), showing shorter sleep, reduced sleep quality, and more frequent napping (Kervezee et al., 2021), lower cognitive performance (Vetter et al., 2012), and increased sleepiness and fatigue (Reinke et al., 2015). Compared with early chronotypes, late types report higher daytime sleepiness (Hidalgo et al., 2003) and show worse driving performance (Del Rio-Bermudez et al., 2014), decreased vigilance (Correa et al., 2014), and impaired memory (Hidalgo et al., 2004) when tested during their non-optimal time of day, i.e., during morning hours. One underlying mechanism for the link between chronotype and fatigue/cognitive impairment is circadian disruption. That is, a misalignment between an individual's sleep-wake rhythm and external demands, such as work schedules that require people to be awake and active at the "wrong" time.

3.2.3.2 WHAT ARE THE CONSEQUENCES OF MISTIMED SLEEP?

Circadian Disruption

The term "circadian disruption" broadly refers to a mismatch between an external environmental rhythm and an internal circadian rhythm. Typical examples include the misalignment between work schedules and the sleep-wake cycle, such that the opportunity to sleep is restricted by work hours. Such a misalignment results in mistimed sleep as well as in mistimed wakefulness, both of which can contribute to fatigue.

There is a critical difference between the desynchrony experienced during jet lag and circadian disruption as described here; while for jet lag, the change in the solar light-dark cycle drives re-entrainment and eventually resolves the desynchrony, there is no such change in the solar light-dark cycle for circadian disruption. Thus, changes in circadian rhythms during jet lag are necessary to re-synchronise to the new clock time and reflect the natural adaptability of the circadian clock, whereas variations in circadian rhythms against the backdrop of an unchanged light-dark cycle are potentially detrimental.

There is a large body of research linking circadian disruption with adverse outcomes for safety and health, including incidents/injuries (Williamson et al., 2011), impaired cognitive performance (Taillard et al., 2021), and endocrine, metabolic, and cardiovascular diseases (Bedrosian et al., 2016; Maury, 2019; Portaluppi et al., 2012). While associated risks are well-documented, the assessment of circadian disruption is often challenging given that its magnitude depends on both the exposure (e.g., shift work) and the individual (e.g., chronotype). The same individual is likely to experience different levels of circadian disruption when exposed to different challenges (e.g., delaying a shift schedule by 2 vs. 6 hours). Yet, given the same exposure (e.g., working the same shift schedule), individuals can experience different levels of circadian disruption. For example, early chronotypes experience higher levels of circadian disruption on night shifts than late types do (Kervezee et al., 2021). Individuals with higher levels of circadian disruption, based on the combination of exposure and chronotype, are also likely to experience higher levels of fatigue, sleepiness, and impaired cognitive performance. These detrimental effects can be mitigated by aligning shifts and chronotype, thus reducing circadian disruption (Vetter et al., 2015).

Examples of Circadian Disruption

Shift work is one of the most common causes of circadian disruption. Adverse effects of shift work for health, safety, and general well-being are well documented, including cardiovascular diseases (Vyas et al., 2012), obesity and diabetes (Proper et al., 2016), and incidents and injuries (Fischer, Lombardi, Folkard, et al., 2017). Shift work can involve "permanent" night shifts and/or rapid alternations of work times that span the 24-hour day (e.g., rotation between morning, evening, and night shifts). There is ongoing debate as to whether permanent or rotational schedules are better in terms of health and safety. A review and meta-analysis concluded that although night shifts on rotating schedules reduced sleep duration (i.e., a risk factor for health and safety outcomes) more than permanent night shifts, slowly rotating schedules had, overall, the least detrimental impact on sleep (Pilcher et al., 2000). Complete circadian adaptation to permanent night work is achieved in less than 3% of workers (Folkard, 2008), suggesting that benefits of permanent night shift schedules are limited by the inability of the circadian system to adapt to a nocturnal lifestyle. Yet, permanent schedules can help maintain regular sleep-wake, dietary, and social behaviours. Sleep-wake patterns in rotational shift workers are often highly irregular, in response to highly irregular work schedules. **Irregular sleep** (variable sleep timing between days) is associated with a wide range of health and safety outcomes, often in cases where other dimensions of sleep behaviour, such as sleep duration, show no association with these outcomes (Lunsford-Avery et al., 2018). This is possibly because irregular sleep may be a proxy for variability in other rhythms, such as light exposure, meals, and exercise and, therefore, reflects certain aspects of circadian disruption that average sleep duration and timing do not capture. Accordingly, associations between irregular sleep and fatigue, performance, and health outcomes could be mediated not by sleep itself, but by irregularity in other co-occurring factors, including light exposure. While irregular sleep frequently occurs in response to irregular work schedules, it is also widespread, with 80% of the general population experiencing at least some degree of irregularity by shifting sleep times between weekdays and weekends (Roenneberg et al., 2012). This phenomenon has been coined "**Social Jetlag**" to describe a discrepancy between the circadian clock and the social clock (e.g., work/school times, social/family events) (Roenneberg et al., 2019). Social jetlag is a modern phenomenon that for most is characterised by earlier and shorter sleep on weekdays and later and longer catch-up sleep on weekends. This irregular but systematic sleep-wake pattern is due to rise times for school and work that are too early for most people's endogenous sleep-wake rhythms. Social jetlag is, therefore, most pronounced in late chronotypes and has been associated with a wide range of adverse outcomes, including lower academic performance (Zerbini et al., 2017) and increased risks for physical and mental health issues (Henderson et al., 2019; Parsons et al., 2015).

3.2.3.3 How Can Mistimed Sleep Be (re-)Aligned?

What the above-described causes of circadian disruption have in common is not only a misalignment between sleep and work times, but also their collective misalignment with the solar alternation of day (i.e., natural light) and night (i.e., natural darkness). Accordingly, the strategies previously described in sub-section 3.2.2.5 to manage jet lag also apply to managing mistimed sleep, using the timed exposure to, and avoidance of, light as an effective way to (re-)align sleep, reduce circadian disruption, and reduce fatigue and cognitive impairment.

3.2.4 SLEEP INERTIA

3.2.4.1 What Is Sleep Inertia?

The term "sleep inertia", coined by Lubin and colleagues in 1976 (Lubin et al., 1976), describes the transient period of reduced alertness and impaired cognitive performance experienced immediately after waking from sleep (Hilditch & McHill, 2019). Thus, to account for this rather unintuitive phenomenon of "waking up tired", a third process was added to the two-process model of sleep/wake regulation (Folkard & Åkerstedt, 1992). As shown in Figure 3.2.2, sleep inertia has a relatively brief influence on overall alertness. However, if sleep inertia coincides with safety-critical activities, this period of reduced performance can have catastrophic consequences. The symptoms of sleep inertia typically dissipate within 15 to 30 minutes of waking (Brooks & Lack, 2006), but recovery to full alertness may take as long as 2 hours in scenarios in which symptoms are particularly severe or persistent (Achermann et al.,

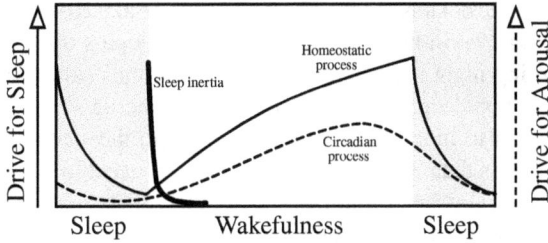

FIGURE 3.2.2 The three-process model of sleep/arousal regulation. Adapted from Hilditch and McHill (2019).

1995). Early studies of sleep inertia describe performance impairments on a range of tasks from simple reaction time tests (Langdon & Hartman, 1961) to putting on a space suit (Seminara & Shavelson, 1969), while others describe "hypnopompic intrusions" with participants speaking semi-coherently during the testing period immediately after waking (Dinges, 1990).

3.2.4.2 WHAT CAUSES SLEEP INERTIA?

Studies of the underlying neurophysiological profile of the brain during the transition from sleep to wakefulness suggest that several neurophysiological processes are slow to recover to wakeful levels after sleep. Importantly, the time course of restoration and regions of impairment appear to match the recovery from neurobehavioural symptoms under different conditions (Balkin et al., 2002; Hilditch, Bansal et al., 2022; Vallat et al., 2019). Therefore, the unique milieu of brain activity observed during the awakening period appears to underlie the symptoms experienced during sleep inertia and may, therefore, serve as novel targets for future interventions that manipulate these physiological processes.

There are several known factors that can exacerbate sleep inertia severity. These factors are often related to the interaction between sleep inertia and the two-process model of alertness regulation. For example, sleep inertia interacts with the circadian rhythm, such that waking during the biological night (i.e., when melatonin is high, core body temperature is low, and the body is primed for sleep) is related to greater sleep inertia than waking during the day (Scheer et al., 2008). Prior sleep loss, either acute (e.g., due to extended wakefulness, or one night of sleep restriction) (Dinges et al., 1985; Tassi et al., 2006) or chronic (e.g., losing a few hours of sleep across several nights) (McHill et al., 2019), increases homeostatic pressure and subsequently increases sleep inertia severity. There is also some evidence that waking from slow wave sleep (SWS, also known as *deep sleep*) or waking from sleep episodes with increased slow wave activity can exacerbate sleep inertia symptoms (Dinges et al., 1985; Tassi et al., 2006). SWS is homeostatically controlled, so the amount of SWS may be a proxy for underlying sleep debt and homeostatic pressure.

Interactions of sleep inertia with the body clock and prior sleep/wake patterns mean that waking from a nap at night following extended wakefulness is more likely to produce severe sleep inertia symptoms than, for example, waking from a short nap during the day (Brooks & Lack, 2006; Hilditch et al., 2016; Hilditch, Dorrian, Centofanti, et al., 2017). In an operational context, this puts transportation workers who may be working night shifts and long hours, and thus suffering from circadian misalignment and poor sleep, at a higher risk of sleep inertia symptoms. Under these conditions, SWS is also more likely to occur earlier in the sleep episode, such that restricting a nap to less than 30 minutes may not be sufficient to avoid SWS (Hilditch et al., 2016; Hilditch, Dorrian, Centofanti, et al., 2017). Therefore, while napping to mitigate fatigue is a well-supported countermeasure (Ruggiero & Redeker, 2014), recognition and management of sleep inertia symptoms in the period immediately after waking is critical to re-establish alertness before undertaking safety-critical tasks.

It is important to note that sleep inertia can occur even in the absence of exacerbating factors. For example, sleep inertia can occur following naps as short as 10 minutes (Hilditch, Dorrian, Centofanti, et al., 2017), when waking in the morning after an 8-hour sleep episode (Wertz et al., 2006), and following sleep episodes without any SWS (Hilditch, Dorrian, & Banks, 2017). Therefore, it is important to be aware of potential sleep inertia symptoms following *every* wake-up.

3.2.4.3 What Are the Consequences of Sleep Inertia?

Most literature on fatigue focuses on the effects of sleep loss and circadian misalignment. Indeed, disruptions to these two processes can have significant impacts on alertness and performance. However, perhaps due to its brief duration of effects, sleep inertia has received far less attention in fatigue research. It is worth considering the effects of sleep inertia relative to those caused by sleep loss or circadian misalignment, to fully understand the potential impact of the awakening process on performance and fatigue.

Sleep inertia, like sleep loss and circadian misalignment, impacts performance on a range of cognitive tasks from simple reaction time tests (Santhi et al., 2013) to higher-order tasks including decision-making (Bruck & Pisani, 1999; Horne & Moseley, 2011), memory (Achermann et al., 1995), mental arithmetic (Dinges et al., 1985; Wertz et al., 2006), and spatial configuration (Burke et al., 2015). Further, tasks emulating real-world scenarios such as military exercises (Horne & Moseley, 2011), firefighting strategies (Bruck & Pisani, 1999), or putting on protective equipment (Seminara & Shavelson, 1969) have shown increased errors during the sleep inertia period. It is difficult to determine whether some tasks are more or less susceptible to sleep inertia given the variation in methodologies used within a rather small subset of the literature on this topic (Burke et al., 2015; Santhi et al., 2013). Operationally, both vigilant attention and visual scanning are relevant to many transportation occupations in which monitoring dashboards and searching for threats in the environment are critical performance tasks.

Subjectively, sleep inertia can be very salient with reports of greater sleepiness post-sleep compared to pre-sleep (Brooks & Lack, 2006). Surveys of nurses (Fallis et al., 2011) and emergency medical pilots (Gregory et al., 2010) reveal that shift workers are aware of the impact of sleep inertia on alertness, such that workers may avoid napping in order to avoid the consequences of sleep inertia. However, self-reported alertness ratings do not always correlate with performance outcomes

(Achermann et al., 1995). Further, when asked to self-rate their performance during the sleep inertia period, people tend to not recognise their impairment and may even report *improved* performance despite a clear reduction on objective measures (Dinges, 1990; Hilditch et al., 2016). Therefore, self-assessment of alertness immediately after waking is not necessarily a reliable indicator of cognitive performance.

Despite the relatively brief nature of sleep inertia, the impact on cognitive performance can be as bad as, or even worse than, sleep loss and circadian misalignment combined. A study tracking performance on a mental arithmetic task from 2 minutes to 24 hours after waking observed that performance after 2 minutes of wakefulness was approximately three times worse than performance after 24 hours of wakefulness (Wertz et al., 2006). In studies of up to 64 hours of sleep deprivation, performance after recovery naps has been shown to be worse for up to an hour, compared to having no recovery sleep at all (Hilditch et al., 2016; Naitoh et al., 1993). For context, performance after 24 hours of continuous wakefulness following a morning wake time has been compared to performance impairment with a blood alcohol content of ~0.08% (Dawson & Reid, 1997). These studies highlight the potential severity of sleep inertia symptoms, however brief.

Naps relieve fatigue during extended wakefulness and following sleep loss, however, these benefits are often masked by sleep inertia for up to an hour after waking. When implementing napping as a countermeasure, consideration should be given to this potential delay in nap benefits and period of impaired performance. Countermeasures to help accelerate the dissipation of sleep inertia are discussed in sub-section 3.2.4.4.

Examples of Sleep Inertia in Transportation

Sleep inertia has been cited as a contributing factor in several incidents across multiple transportation sectors. In aviation, 158 people died in a 2010 plane crash in India after the captain, who had just woken from a long nap, overruled the first officer's requests for a "go-around" and continued with the landing. The aircraft subsequently overran the runway (Government of India Ministry of Civil Aviation, 2010). As described in Chapter 2.5, in another incident, a first officer woke from a nap on the flight deck and, in a disorientated state, mistook Venus for an oncoming plane (Transportation Safety Board of Canada, 2011). In military aviation, sleep inertia was identified as a contributing factor in a published case report detailing the near crash of a US military aircraft which stalled during the descent, dropping 4,000 feet before being recovered 773 feet above sea level (Armentrout et al., 2006). In this scenario, all three crew members were sleep deprived and two had woken from a nap shortly before the descent, leading to poor communication and low situational awareness. Further, a Israeli Air Force review of over 400 incidents showed that errors were most common during the first hour after waking, suggesting that sleep inertia may be at least partially responsible for the spike in incidents during this time (Ribak et al., 1983).

In a maritime incident, evidence suggested that the chief officer of the platform supply vessel, *Skandi Foula*, was suffering from sleep inertia when the vessel under his control made heavy contact with another vessel. The chief officer had missed his morning wake-up call and was subsequently woken only 4 minutes before arriving on the bridge to be briefed on the situation and make critical decisions (Marine Accident Investigation Branch, 2011). Napping is a recommended fatigue countermeasure for long-haul truck drivers, who often take naps in their truck cabin (Darwent et al., 2012). Sleeping in the truck cabin berth, instead of at home or a motel, may increase the chance of operating the vehicle very soon after waking. Observations of truck drivers waking from naps immediately prior to disembarking ferries support this possibility. While the strategy to take a nap is a good one, consideration should be given to the time required to fully awaken before undertaking a task requiring skill and concentration, such as manoeuvring a large vehicle at a ferry dock. It is important to educate truck drivers—and all transportation workers—of the importance of allowing time to fully wake up after sleep (Dawson et al., 2021).

In all of these incidents, while sleep inertia was not the only contributing factor, it was deemed to have had a significant influence. Given the potential for catastrophic events associated with sleep inertia, the need for a better understanding of its presence, cause, and effect in shift work scenarios is crucial. With greater knowledge, we can develop evidence-based guidance for transport workers who are required to perform safety-critical duties soon after waking.

3.2.4.4 How Can Sleep Inertia Be Managed?

There are two main approaches to sleep inertia management: proactive and reactive. Proactive management involves avoiding factors that are known to exacerbate sleep inertia—for example, waking during the day, limiting prior sleep loss and hours of wakefulness, and keeping naps short to reduce the probability of entering and waking from deep sleep. In reality, though, the need for sleep is driven by these factors, so napping often occurs under these conditions and the chances that one or more of these factors are present upon waking is almost unavoidable. This is especially true for shift workers, who are often exposed to sleep loss and circadian misalignment and make up approximately one-third of the transportation industry (Australian Bureau of Statistics, 2012).

Caffeine has been shown to effectively mitigate sleep inertia when administered before (orally) or during (via intravenous catheter) a sleep episode (Centofanti et al., 2020; Van Dongen et al., 2001). Caffeine takes approximately 20 minutes to take effect, so administering *before* a short nap aligns the stimulating effects with the most critical sleep inertia period. Other studies have investigated the use of light exposure before awakening to help aid the awakening process, with some success (Van De Werken et al., 2010). These proactive countermeasures may work in situations where sleep length and wake time are predetermined, but are of limited use in scenarios in which awakenings are unpredictable (e.g., on-call work). The realities of shiftwork and on-call work, coupled with the acknowledgement that sleep inertia can occur even in the absence of exacerbating factors, drive the need for reactive countermeasures. That is, strategies and interventions that can be applied *after* waking.

A literature review investigating reactive countermeasures to sleep inertia highlighted promising interventions, but also a critical need for more robust research in this area (Hilditch et al., 2016). Research teams around the world have since responded and have added valuable data to help evaluate the effectiveness of reactive countermeasures. Research into the use of bright, short wavelength-enriched light has been perhaps the most successful to date, with studies showing promising improvements in subjective alertness (Hilditch et al., 2022; Santhi et al., 2013) and vigilant attention (Hilditch et al., 2022). Further research investigated the potential for exercise as a countermeasure (Kovac et al., 2020), with one study showing improvement in subjective alertness, but not objective cognitive performance, following a short bout of high-intensity exercise (Kovac et al., 2021). A review of auditory countermeasures (McFarlane et al., 2020) highlighted important specifications for developing alarms to alert people upon awakening, and olfactory stimuli or temperature interventions (Kräuchi et al., 2004) are still yet to be investigated. A caffeine chewing gum with a faster absorption rate yielded some promising results for shortening the length of sleep inertia effects, but was not able to reduce symptoms in the first 12 minutes after waking (Kamimori et al., 2002). Together, these studies demonstrate that some countermeasures may be effective only subjectively, or only after a delay, or only in certain scenarios (e.g., dependent on time of day, prior sleep/wake history, or sleep stage prior to wake). Therefore, further research is needed in this area, investigating (i) novel countermeasures, (ii) established countermeasures in different scenarios, and (iii) countermeasures in combination, with the goal to provide evidence-based guidance to transportation workers on a suite of countermeasure options. When investigating these countermeasures, it is also important to consider the impact on subsequent sleep episodes for those workers who may need to return to sleep soon after a false alarm, or short activity (Gupta et al., 2021). For now, though, the best advice is to delay safety-critical activities for at least 15 to 30 minutes after waking, and to employ additional mitigations during the first hour after waking to manage any additional fatigue risk during the awakening period.

3.2.5 CONCLUSIONS

For those working in the transportation industry, careful consideration of jet lag, sleep timing, and sleep inertia is needed to mitigate and manage fatigue. The real-world consequences of mismanaged fatigue from these factors highlight the need for evidenced-based guidance to equip workers with the power to recognise and manage these—often unavoidable—consequences of shift work in the transportation industry.

SUMMARY POINTS FOR PRACTITIONERS

- Jet lag occurs due to the desynchrony between the internal body clock and external light/dark environment caused by trans-meridian air travel. The duration of jet lag symptoms can be minimised by strategic exposure to light and use of melatonin. The optimal timing of these exposures is often difficult to estimate but there are applications to guide these decisions (see Figure 3.2.1).
- Mistimed sleep—and thus mistimed wakefulness—can occur due to shiftwork, disrupting the circadian system. Circadian disruption is associated with adverse

effects for health and safety, including elevated fatigue and daytime sleepiness. Jet lag management strategies (e.g., light exposure and melatonin) can be adapted to help re-align sleep/wake patterns.

- Individual differences can play a large role in sleep timing and fatigue outcomes. Early chronotypes are less able to cope with night shifts, while late chronotypes perform poorly on early shifts.
- Sleep inertia should be recognised as a fatigue risk following any wake-up, especially when under conditions of prior sleep loss and waking at night. Where possible, safety-critical tasks should be avoided in the first 15 to 30 minutes after waking, and additional countermeasures put in place where this is not possible.

REFERENCES

Achermann, P., Werth, E., Dijk, D.-J., & Borbely, A. (1995). Time course of sleep inertia after nighttime and daytime sleep episodes. *Archives Italiennes de Biologie, 134*(1), 109–119.

Åkerstedt, T., & Wright, K. P., Jr. (2009). Sleep loss and fatigue in shift work and shift work disorder. *Sleep Medicine Clinics, 4*(2), 257–271. https://doi.org/10.1016/j.jsmc.2009.03.001

Arendt, J. (2018). Approaches to the pharmacological management of jet lag. *Drugs, 78*(14), 1419–1431. https://doi.org/10.1007/s40265-018-0973-8

Armentrout, J. J., Holland, D. A., O'Toole, K. J., & Ercoline, W. R. (2006). Fatigue and related human factors in the near crash of a large military aircraft [Case Reports]. *Aviation, Space, and Environmental Medicine, 77*(9), 963–970. www.ncbi.nlm.nih.gov/pubmed/16964748

Australian Bureau of Statistics. (2012). *Working time arrangements* (6342.0). Commonwealth of Australia.

Balkin, T. J., Braun, A. R., Wesensten, N. J., Jeffries, K., Varga, M., Baldwin, P.,.... Herscovitch, P. (2002). The process of awakening: A PET study of regional brain activity patterns mediating the re-establishment of alertness and consciousness. *Brain, 125*(10), 2308–2319. https://doi.org/10.1093/brain/awf228

Bass, J. (2012). Circadian topology of metabolism. *Nature, 491*(7424), 348–356. https://doi.org/10.1038/nature11704

Bedrosian, T. A., Fonken, L. K., & Nelson, R. J. (2016). Endocrine effects of circadian disruption. *Annual Reviews of Physiology, 78*, 109–131. https://doi.org/10.1146/annurev-physiol-021115-105102

Borbély, A. A., Daan, S., Wirz-Justice, A., & Deboer, T. (2016). The two-process model of sleep regulation: a reappraisal. *Journal of Sleep Research, 25*(2), 131–143. https://doi.org/10.1111/jsr.12371

Brooks, A., & Lack, L. (2006). A brief afternoon nap following nocturnal sleep restriction: Which nap duration is most recuperative? *Sleep, 29*(6), 831–840. www.ncbi.nlm.nih.gov/pubmed/16796222

Brown, S. A., Fleury-Olela, F., Nagoshi, E., Hauser, C., Juge, C., Meier, C. A.,.... Schibler, U. (2005). The period length of fibroblast circadian gene expression varies widely among human individuals. *PLoS Biol, 3*(10), e338. https://doi.org/10.1371/journal.pbio.0030338

Bruck, D., & Pisani, D. L. (1999). The effects of sleep inertia on decision-making performance. *Journal of Sleep Research, 8*(2), 95–103. www.ncbi.nlm.nih.gov/pubmed/10389091

Burke, T. M., Scheer, F. A., Ronda, J. M., Czeisler, C. A., & Wright Jr, K. P. (2015). Sleep inertia, sleep homeostatic and circadian influences on higher-order cognitive functions. *Journal of Sleep Research*, 24(4), 364–371.

Centofanti, S., Banks, S., Coussens, S., Gray, D., Munro, E., Nielsen, J., & Dorrian, J. (2020). A pilot study investigating the impact of a caffeine-nap on alertness during a simulated night shift. *Chronobiology International*, 37(9–10), 1469–1473.

Christensen, S., Huang, Y., Walch, O. J., & Forger, D. B. (2020). Optimal adjustment of the human circadian clock in the real world. *PLoS Comput Biol*, 16(12), e1008445. https://doi.org/10.1371/journal.pcbi.1008445

Correa, A., Molina, E., & Sanabria, D. (2014). Effects of chronotype and time of day on the vigilance decrement during simulated driving. *Accident Analysis and Prevention*, 67, 113–118. https://doi.org/10.1016/j.aap.2014.02.020

Darwent, D., Roach, G., & Dawson, D. (2012). How well do truck drivers sleep in cabin sleeper berths? *Applied Ergonomics*, 43(2), 442–446. https://doi.org/https://doi.org/10.1016/j.apergo.2011.06.019

Dawson, D., Ferguson, S. A., & Vincent, G. E. (2021). Safety implications of fatigue and sleep inertia for emergency services personnel. *Sleep Medicine Reviews*, 55, 101386.

Dawson, D., & Reid, K. (1997). Fatigue, alcohol and performance impairment. *Nature*, 388(6639), 235. https://doi.org/10.1038/40775

Del Rio-Bermudez, C., Diaz-Piedra, C., Catena, A., Buela-Casal, G., & Di Stasi, L. L. (2014). Chronotype-dependent circadian rhythmicity of driving safety. *Chronobiology International*, 31(4), 532–541. https://doi.org/10.3109/07420528.2013.876427

Dinges, D., Orne, M., & Orne, E. (1985). Assessing performance upon abrupt awakening from naps during quasi-continuous operations. *Behavior Research Methods*, 17(1), 37–45. https://doi.org/10.3758/bf03200895

Dinges, D. F. (1990). Are you awake? Cognitive performance and reverie during the hypnopompic state. In R. R. Bootzin, J. F. Kihlstrom, & D. L. Schacter (Eds.), *Sleep and Cognition* (pp. 159–175). American Psychological Association. https://doi.org/10.1037/10499-012

Fallis, W. M., McMillan, D. E., & Edwards, M. P. (2011). Napping during night shift: Practices, preferences, and perceptions of critical care and emergency department nurses. *Critical Care Nurse*, 31(2), e1–e11. https://doi.org/10.4037/ccn2011710

Fischer, D., Lombardi, D. A., Folkard, S., Willetts, J., & Christiani, D. C. (2017). Updating the "Risk Index": A systematic review and meta-analysis of occupational injuries and work schedule characteristics. *Chronobiology Int*, 34(10), 1423–1438. https://doi.org/10.1080/07420528.2017.1367305

Fischer, D., Lombardi, D. A., Marucci-Wellman, H., & Roenneberg, T. (2017). Chronotypes in the US–Influence of age and sex. *PLoS One*, 12(6), e0178782. https://doi.org/10.1371/journal.pone.0178782

Fischer, D., Roenneberg, T., & Vetter, C. (2021). Chronotype-specific sleep in two versus four consecutive shifts. *Journal of Biological Rhythms*, 36(4), 395–409. https://doi.org/10.1177/07487304211006073

Fischer, D., Vetter, C., & Roenneberg, T. (2016). A novel method to visualise and quantify circadian misalignment. *Scientific Reports*, 6, 38601. https://doi.org/10.1038/srep38601

Folkard, S. (2008). Do permanent night workers show circadian adjustment? A review based on the endogenous melatonin rhythm. *Chronobiology International*, 25(2), 215–224. https://doi.org/10.1080/07420520802106835

Folkard, S., & Åkerstedt, T. (1992). A three-process model of the regulation of alertness-sleepiness. In R. J. Broughton & R. D. Ogilvie (Eds.), *Sleep, Arousal, and Performance* (pp. 11–26). Birkhäuser.

Gander, P., Mulrine, H. M., van den Berg, M. J., Wu, L., Smith, A., Signal, L., & Mangie, J. (2016). Does the circadian clock drift when pilots fly multiple transpacific flights with 1–to 2-day layovers? *Chronobiology International, 33*(8), 982–994. https://doi.org/10.1080/07420 528.2016.1189430

Gander, P. H., Mulrine, H. M., van den Berg, M. J., Smith, A. A. T., Signal, T. L., Wu, L. J., & Belenky, G. (2015). Effects of sleep/wake history and circadian phase on proposed pilot fatigue safety performance indicators. *Journal of Sleep Research, 24*(1), 110–119.

Government of India Ministry of Civil Aviation. (2010). *Report on accident to Air India Express Boeing 737–800 aircraft VT-AXV on 22nd May 2010 at Mangalore.*

Gregory, K. B., Winn, W., Johnson, K., & Rosekind, M. R. (2010). Pilot fatigue survey: Exploring fatigue factors in air medical operations. *Air Medical Journal, 29*(6), 309–319. https://doi.org/10.1016/j.amj.2010.07.002

Gupta, C. C., Dominiak, M., Kovac, K., Reynolds, A. C., Ferguson, S. A., Hilditch, C. J.,... . Vincent, G. E. (2021). On-call work and sleep: The importance of switching on during a callout and switching off after a call. *Industrial Health, 60*(2), 91–96.

Henderson, S. E. M., Brady, E. M., & Robertson, N. (2019). Associations between social jetlag and mental health in young people: A systematic review. *Chronobiology International, 36*(10), 1316–1333. https://doi.org/10.1080/07420528.2019.1636813

Herxheimer, A. (2014). Jet lag. *BMJ Clinical Evidence*, 2014.

Herxheimer, A., & Petrie, K. J. (2002). Melatonin for the prevention and treatment of jet lag. *Cochrane Database Syst Rev* (2), Cd001520. https://doi.org/10.1002/14651858. Cd001520

Hidalgo, M. P., de Souza, C. M., Zanette, C. B., & Nunes, P. V. (2003). Association of daytime sleepiness and the morningness/eveningness dimension in young adult subjects in Brazil. *Psychological Reports, 93*(2), 427–434. https://doi.org/10.2466/pr0.2003.93.2.427

Hidalgo, M. P., Zanette, C. B., Pedrotti, M., Souza, C. M., Nunes, P. V., & Chaves, M. L. (2004). Performance of chronotypes on memory tests during the morning and the evening shifts. *Psychological Reports, 95*(1), 75–85. https://doi.org/10.2466/pr0.95.1.75-85

Hilditch, C. J., Bansal, K., Chachad, R., Wong, L. R., Bathurst, N. G., Feick, N. H.,... . Flynn-Evans, E. E. (2022). Reconfigurations in brain networks upon awakening from slow wave sleep: Interventions and implications in neural communication. *Network Neuroscience, 7*(1), 102–121. https://doi.org/10.1162/netn_a_00272

Hilditch, C. J., Centofanti, S. A., Dorrian, J., & Banks, S. (2016). A 30-minute, but not a 10-minute nighttime nap is associated with sleep inertia. *Sleep, 39*(3), 675–685.

Hilditch, C. J., Dorrian, J., & Banks, S. (2016). Time to wake up: Reactive countermeasures to sleep inertia. *Industrial Health, 54*, 1–14.

Hilditch, C. J., Dorrian, J., & Banks, S. (2017). A review of short naps and sleep inertia: Do naps of 30 min or less really avoid sleep inertia and slow-wave sleep? *Sleep Medicine, 32*, 176–190.

Hilditch, C. J., Dorrian, J., Centofanti, S. A., Van Dongen, H. P., & Banks, S. (2017). Sleep inertia associated with a 10-min nap before the commute home following a night shift: A laboratory simulation study. *Accident Analysis and Prevention, 99*, 411–415.

Hilditch, C. J., & McHill, A. W. (2019). Sleep inertia: Current insights. *Nature and Science of Sleep, 11*, 155–165.

Hilditch, C. J., Wong, L. R., Bathurst, N. G., Feick, N. H., Pradhan, S., Santamaria, A.,... . Flynn-Evans, E. E. (2022). Rise and shine: The use of polychromatic short-wavelength-enriched light to mitigate sleep inertia at night following awakening from slow-wave sleep. *Journal of Sleep Research*, e13558.

Holmes, A., Al-Bayat, S., Hilditch, C., & Bourgeois-Bougrine, S. (2012). Sleep and sleepiness during an ultra long-range flight operation between the Middle East and United States. *Accident Analysis and Prevention*, *45*, 27–31.

Horne, J., & Moseley, R. (2011). Sudden early-morning awakening impairs immediate tactical planning in a changing 'emergency' scenario *Journal of Sleep Research*, *20*(2), 275–278. https://doi.org/10.1111/j.1365-2869.2010.00904.x

Jewett, M. E., & Kronauer, R. E. (1998). Refinement of limit cycle oscillator model of the effects of light on the human circadian pacemaker. *J Theor Biol*, *192*(4), 455–465.

Kamimori, G. H., Karyekar, C. S., Otterstetter, R., Cox, D. S., Balkin, T. J., Belenky, G. L., & Eddington, N. D. (2002). The rate of absorption and relative bioavailability of caffeine administered in chewing gum versus capsules to normal healthy volunteers. *International Journal of Pharmaceutics*, *234*(1–2), 159–167. https://doi.org/http://dx.doi.org/10.1016/S0378-5173(01)00958-9

Kerkhof, G. A., & Van Dongen, H. P. (1996). Morning-type and evening-type individuals differ in the phase position of their endogenous circadian oscillator. *Neuroscience Letters*, *218*(3), 153–156. https://doi.org/10.1016/s0304-3940(96)13140-2

Kervezee, L., Gonzales-Aste, F., Boudreau, P., & Boivin, D. B. (2021). The relationship between chronotype and sleep behavior during rotating shift work: A field study. *Sleep*, *44*(4). https://doi.org/10.1093/sleep/zsaa225

Kovac, K., Ferguson, S. A., Paterson, J. L., Aisbett, B., Hilditch, C. J., Reynolds, A. C., & Vincent, G. E. (2020). Exercising caution upon waking–can exercise reduce sleep inertia? *Frontiers in Physiology*, *11*, 254.

Kovac, K., Vincent, G. E., Paterson, J. L., Reynolds, A., Aisbett, B., Hilditch, C. J., & Ferguson, S. A. (2021). The impact of a short burst of exercise on sleep inertia. *Physiology & Behavior*, *242*, e113617.

Kräuchi, K., Cajochen, C., & Wirz-Justice, A. (2004). Waking up properly: Is there a role of thermoregulation in sleep inertia? *Journal of Sleep Research*, *13*(2), 121–127. https://doi.org/10.1111/j.1365-2869.2004.00398.x

Langdon, D. E., & Hartman, B. (1961). *Performance Upon Sudden Awakening. Technical Report SAM-TDR*. Brooks AFB, TX: USAF School of Aerospace Medicine. www.ncbi.nlm.nih.gov/pubmed/14462063

Lewy, A. J., Ahmed, S., Jackson, J. M., & Sack, R. L. (1992). Melatonin shifts human circadian rhythms according to a phase-response curve. *Chronobiology International*, *9*(5), 380–392. https://doi.org/10.3109/07420529209064550

Lubin, A., Hord, D. J., Tracy, M. L., & Johnson, L. C. (1976). Effects of exercise, bedrest and napping on performance decrement during 40 hours. *Psychophysiology*, *13*(4), 334–339. https://doi.org/10.1111/j.1469-8986.1976.tb03086.x

Lunsford-Avery, J. R., Engelhard, M. M., Navar, A. M., & Kollins, S. H. (2018). Validation of the sleep regularity index in older adults and associations with cardiometabolic risk. *Scientific Reports*, *8*(1), 1–11.

Marine Accident Investigation Branch. (2011). *Heavy Contact by Skandi Foula with OMS Resolution, Aberdeen Harbour 29 May 2010. Accident Report No. 15/2011.*

Maury, E. (2019). Off the clock: From circadian disruption to metabolic disease. *International Journal of Molecular Sciences*, *20*(7). https://doi.org/10.3390/ijms20071597

McFarlane, S. J., Garcia, J. E., Verhagen, D. S., & Dyer, A. G. (2020). Alarm tones, voice warnings, and musical treatments: A systematic review of auditory countermeasures for sleep inertia in abrupt and casual awakenings. *Clocks & Sleep*, *2*(4), 416–433.

McHill, A. W., Hull, J. T., Cohen, D. A., Wang, W., Czeisler, C. A., & Klerman, E. B. (2019). Chronic sleep restriction greatly magnifies performance decrements immediately after awakening. *Sleep*, *42*(5), zsz032.

Morgenthaler, T. I., Lee-Chiong, T., Alessi, C., Friedman, L., Aurora, R. N., Boehlecke, B.,.... Zak, R. (2007). Practice parameters for the clinical evaluation and treatment of circadian rhythm sleep disorders. An American Academy of Sleep Medicine report. *Sleep*, *30*(11), 1445–1459. https://doi.org/10.1093/sleep/30.11.1445

Naitoh, P., Kelly, T., & Babkoff, H. (1993). Sleep inertia: best time not to wake up? *Chronobiology International*, *10*(2), 109–118. www.ncbi.nlm.nih.gov/pubmed/8500187

Parsons, M. J., Moffitt, T. E., Gregory, A. M., Goldman-Mellor, S., Nolan, P. M., Poulton, R., & Caspi, A. (2015). Social jetlag, obesity and metabolic disorder: Investigation in a cohort study. *International Journal of Obesity (London)*, *39*(5), 842–848. https://doi.org/10.1038/ijo.2014.201

Pilcher, J. J., Lambert, B. J., & Huffcutt, A. I. (2000). Differential effects of permanent and rotating shifts on self-report sleep length: A meta-analytic review. *Sleep*, *23*(2), 155–163.

Portaluppi, F., Tiseo, R., Smolensky, M. H., Hermida, R. C., Ayala, D. E., & Fabbian, F. (2012). Circadian rhythms and cardiovascular health. *Sleep Medicine Reviews*, *16*(2), 151–166. https://doi.org/10.1016/j.smrv.2011.04.003

Proper, K. I., van de Langenberg, D., Rodenburg, W., Vermeulen, R. C. H., van der Beek, A. J., van Steeg, H., & van Kerkhof, L. W. M. (2016). The relationship between shift work and metabolic risk factors: A Systematic Review of Longitudinal Studies. *American Journal of Preventative Medicine*, *50*(5), e147–e157. https://doi.org/10.1016/j.amepre.2015.11.013

Reinke, L., Özbay, Y., Dieperink, W., & Tulleken, J. E. (2015). The effect of chronotype on sleepiness, fatigue, and psychomotor vigilance of ICU nurses during the night shift. *Intensive Care Medicine*, *41*(4), 657–666. https://doi.org/10.1007/s00134-015-3667-7

Ribak, J., Ashkenazi, I. E., Klepfish, A., Avgar, D., Tall, J., Kallner, B., & Noyman, Y. (1983). Diurnal rhythmicity and air force flight accidents due to pilot error. *Aviation, Space, and Environmental Medicine*, *54*(12 Pt 1), 1096–1099.

Roenneberg, T., Allebrandt, K. V., Merrow, M., & Vetter, C. (2012). Social jetlag and obesity. *Current Biology*, *22*(10), 939–943.

Roenneberg, T., Kuehnle, T., Pramstaller, P. P., Ricken, J., Havel, M., Guth, A., & Merrow, M. (2004). A marker for the end of adolescence. *Current Biology*, *14*(24), R1038–R1039. https://doi.org/10.1016/j.cub.2004.11.039

Roenneberg, T., Pilz, L. K., Zerbini, G., & Winnebeck, E. C. (2019). Chronotype and social jetlag: A (self-)critical review. *Biology (Basel)*, *8*(3). https://doi.org/10.3390/biology8030054

Ruggiero, J. S., & Redeker, N. S. (2014). Effects of napping on sleepiness and sleep-related performance deficits in night-shift workers: A systematic review. *Biological Research for Nursing*, *16*(2), 134–142. https://doi.org/10.1177/1099800413476571

Sack, R. L., Auckley, D., Auger, R. R., Carskadon, M. A., Wright, K. P., Jr., Vitiello, M. V., & Zhdanova, I. V. (2007). Circadian rhythm sleep disorders: Part I, basic principles, shift work and jet lag disorders. An American Academy of Sleep Medicine review. *Sleep*, *30*(11), 1460–1483. https://doi.org/10.1093/sleep/30.11.1460

Santhi, N., Groeger, J. A., Archer, S. N., Gimenez, M., Schlangen, L. J., & Dijk, D.-J. (2013). Morning sleep inertia in alertness and performance: Effect of cognitive domain and white light conditions. *PLoS One*, *8*(11), e79688.

Scheiermann, C., Kunisaki, Y., & Frenette, P. S. (2013). Circadian control of the immune system. *Nature Reviews Immunology*, *13*(3), 190–198. https://doi.org/10.1038/nri3386

Schmidt, C., Peigneux, P., Leclercq, Y., Sterpenich, V., Vandewalle, G., Phillips, C.,.... Collette, F. (2012). Circadian preference modulates the neural substrate of conflict processing across the day. *PLoS One*, *7*(1), e29658. https://doi.org/10.1371/journal.pone.0029658

Seminara, J. L., & Shavelson, R. J. (1969). Effectiveness of space crew performance subsequent to sudden sleep arousal. *Aerospace Medicine, 40*(7), 723–727. www.ncbi.nlm.nih.gov/pubmed/4389321

Signal, T. L., Gander, P. H., van den Berg, M. J., & Graeber, R. C. (2013). In-flight sleep of flight crew during a 7-hour rest break: Implications for research and flight safety. *Sleep, 36*(1), 109–115. https://doi.org/10.5665/sleep.2312

Simmons, E., McGrane, O., & Wedmore, I. (2015). Jet lag modification. *Current Sports Medicine Reports, 14*(2), 123–128. https://doi.org/10.1249/jsr.0000000000000133

Taillard, J., Sagaspe, P., Philip, P., & Bioulac, S. (2021). Sleep timing, chronotype and social jetlag: Impact on cognitive abilities and psychiatric disorders. *Biochemical Pharmacology, 191*, 114438. https://doi.org/10.1016/j.bcp.2021.114438

Tassi, P., Bonnefond, A., Engasser, O., Hoeft, A., Eschenlauer, R., & Muzet, A. (2006). EEG spectral power and cognitive performance during sleep inertia: The effect of normal sleep duration and partial sleep deprivation *Physiology & Behavior, 87*(1), 177–184. https://doi.org/10.1016/j.physbeh.2005.09.017

Transportation Safety Board of Canada. (2011). *Pitch Excursion: Air Canada, Boeing 767–333, C-GHLQ, North Atlantic Ocean, 55°00'N 029°00'W, 14 January 2011. Aviation Investigation Report No. A11F0012.*

Vallat, R., Meunier, D., Nicolas, A., & Ruby, P. (2019). Hard to wake up? The cerebral correlates of sleep inertia assessed using combined behavioral, EEG and fMRI measures. *Neuroimage, 184*, 266–278.

Van De Werken, M., Giménez, M. C., De Vries, B., Beersma, D. G., Van Someren, E. J., & Gordijn, M. C. (2010). Effects of artificial dawn on sleep inertia, skin temperature, and the awakening cortisol response. *Journal of Sleep Research, 19*(3), 425–435. https://doi.org/10.1111/j.1365-2869.2010.00828.x

Van Dongen, H. P., Price, N. J., Mullington, J. M., Szuba, M. P., Kapoor, S. C., & Dinges, D. F. (2001). Caffeine eliminates psychomotor vigilance deficits from sleep inertia. *Sleep, 24*(7), 813–819.

Vetter, C., Fischer, D., Matera, J. L., & Roenneberg, T. (2015). Aligning work and circadian time in shift workers improves sleep and reduces circadian disruption. *Current Biology, 25*(7), 907–911. https://doi.org/10.1016/j.cub.2015.01.064

Vetter, C., Juda, M., & Roenneberg, T. (2012). The influence of internal time, time awake, and sleep duration on cognitive performance in shiftworkers. *Chronobiology International, 29*(8), 1127–1138. https://doi.org/10.3109/07420528.2012.707999

Vyas, M. V., Garg, A. X., Iansavichus, A. V., Costella, J., Donner, A., Laugsand, L. E.,.... Hackam, D. G. (2012). Shift work and vascular events: Systematic review and meta-analysis. *BMJ, 345*, e4800. https://doi.org/10.1136/bmj.e4800

Waterhouse, J., & Reilly, T. (2009). Managing jet lag. *Sleep Medicine Reviews, 13*(4), 247–248. https://doi.org/10.1016/j.smrv.2008.10.001

Wertz, A. T., Ronda, J. M., Czeisler, C. A., & Wright, K. P., Jr. (2006). Effects of sleep inertia on cognition. *JAMA, 295*(2), 163–164. https://doi.org/10.1001/jama.295.2.163

Williamson, A., Lombardi, D. A., Folkard, S., Stutts, J., Courtney, T. K., & Connor, J. L. (2011). The link between fatigue and safety. *Accident Analysis and Prevention, 43*(2), 498–515.

Zerbini, G., van der Vinne, V., Otto, L. K. M., Kantermann, T., Krijnen, W. P., Roenneberg, T., & Merrow, M. (2017). Lower school performance in late chronotypes: Underlying factors and mechanisms. *Scientific Reports, 7*(1), 4385. https://doi.org/10.1038/s41598-017-04076-y

3.3 Sleep Disorders and Driving

Walter T. McNicholas

University College Dublin, Department of Respiratory and Sleep Medicine, Dublin, Ireland

CONTENTS

3.3.1 INTRODUCTION

There are specific characteristics pertaining to the driver that increase the likelihood of having a motor vehicle collision (MVC), including excessive speed and alcohol consumption. Consequently, every developed country has specific regulations limiting highway speed and alcohol level while driving. Sleep disturbances and disorders also represent a major risk factor for MVC and recognition of this risk has grown progressively over recent decades (Bioulac et al., 2017). The scale of the problem is demonstrated by reports indicating that about 20% of serious MVCs have driver fatigue or sleepiness as a major contributing factor (Czeisler et al., 2016; Maia, Grandner, Findley, & Gurubhagavatula, 2013; Tefft, 2012). Furthermore, a recent European survey of 12,434 drivers reported that the average prevalence of drivers falling asleep at the wheel in the previous 2 years was 17%, and 7% of those falling asleep experienced a sleep-related collision (Gonçalves et al., 2015). The growing recognition of the risk of drowsy driving has led regulatory authorities in

DOI: 10.1201/9781003213154-19

some countries to implement restrictions on driver licencing for patients with specific sleep-related disorders such as obstructive sleep apnoea (OSA), most notably the regulations recently introduced by the European Union (EU) on driving in OSA (Bonsignore et al., 2016). This development is particularly important as the increased MVC risk associated with OSA exceeds the risk associated with many other medical disorders already specified in the driving licence regulations of many jurisdictions (Vaa, 2003). However, general restrictions targeting sleepy drivers are difficult to formulate as it is difficult to reliably quantify sleepiness in contrast to the highly specific criteria available for speed and alcohol level. Potential causes of driver fatigue and sleepiness include behavioural factors such as inadequate sleep, medical disorders associated with daytime sleepiness including OSA and narcolepsy, and insomnia. Since OSA is the most common medical disorder associated with daytime sleepiness and is the subject of specific driving regulations in many jurisdictions, the discussion will especially focus on this aspect.

3.3.2   OBSTRUCTIVE SLEEP APNOEA

OSA is the most prevalent medical disorder associated with excessive daytime sleepiness (EDS), affecting up to one billion people worldwide (Benjafield et al., 2019). The disorder is due to recurring obstruction of the upper airway (UA) during sleep, largely due to an inability of the UA dilating muscles to overcome the collapsing forces within the UA during inspiration (breathing in). EDS is a major feature of OSA and EDS while driving is an important factor in MVC or work-related collisions (McNicholas & Rodenstein, 2015) The medicolegal consequences of OSA principally relate to collision risk with its associated economic and legal consequences (Krieger et al., 2002). Several jurisdictions, notably the EU and United Kingdom (UK), have implemented regulations restricting the ability of patients with OSA to drive until effective treatment is demonstrated (McNicholas, 2019). Such regulations typically include objective severity of OSA demonstrated by the frequency of apnoeas and hypopnoeas per hour of sleep (the apnoea-hypopnoea index [AHI]) measured in a sleep study, in addition to self-reported sleepiness. The importance of including both measures is emphasised by the poor association between AHI and subjective sleepiness measured by the Epworth Sleepiness Scale (ESS) score (Deegan & McNicholas, 1996; Kingshott, Sime, Engleman, & Douglas, 1995) and the continuing uncertainty about the relative importance of AHI and sleepiness in predicting collision risk (McNicholas & Rodenstein, 2015)

3.3.2.1   EPIDEMIOLOGY OF MOTOR VEHICLE COLLISIONS IN PATIENTS WITH OSA

OSA has been reported for several decades to be associated with an increased risk of MVC (Findley, Unverzagt, & Suratt, 1988), and this risk has been quantified in various studies to range between two and seven times the risk of control populations (Tregear, Reston, Schoelles, & Phillips, 2009). The risk is mainly associated with occurrence of EDS, usually assessed as subjective sleepiness by an ESS score ≥11/24. The risk of MVC has long been recognised as having extra implications for long-haul truck drivers, where drowsiness while driving is common (Mitler, Miller, Lipsitz, Walsh,

& Wylie, 1997) and the MVC risk is enhanced by other factors such as alcohol consumption (Terán-Santos, Jimenez-Gomez, & Cordero-Guevara, 1999) and short sleep duration (Howard et al., 2004; Pack et al., 2006). It is also common for OSA patients who have had a crash to report a preceding history of near miss events, although the relationship with near miss MVC differs between reports (Catarino, Spratley, Catarino, Lunet, & Pais-Clemente, 2014; Ward et al., 2013). Thus, it is appropriate to consider the history of previous MVC as part of the process of issuing or renewing a driving license.

Most studies of MVC risk in OSA were cross-sectional association studies based on self-administered questionnaires such as Epworth (Johns, 1991) or Berlin (Netzer, Stoohs, Netzer, Clark, & Strohl, 1999) and a history of previous MVC, in addition to anthropometric measurements. In non-commercial drivers, sleepiness and OSA risk were associated with increased risk of MVC in some reports (Al-Abri et al., 2018; Gonçalves et al., 2015; Quera Salva et al., 2014), but not in others (Philip et al., 2010; Vaz Fragoso, Araujo, Van Ness, & Marottoli, 2008, 2010). In elderly subjects, the risk of OSA was not associated with MVC (Vaz Fragoso et al., 2010). In commercial drivers, the response rates were low but self-reported sleepiness was associated with increased risk of MVC (Catarino et al., 2014; Vennelle, Engleman, & Douglas, 2010; Zwahlen, Jackowski, & Pfaffli, 2016).

Systematic reviews and meta-analyses support an increased risk of MVC in both professional and non-professional drivers with untreated OSA (Garbarino, Guglielmi, Sanna, Mancardi, & Magnavita, 2016; Tregear et al., 2009). An increased risk of MVC was reported in untreated OSA (AHI>5), with a median odds ratio (OR) of 2.83 (95% confidence interval [CI]: 2.72 to 3.08) (Garbarino, Ottavia Guglielmi, et al., 2016). Dose–effect relationships were reported between OSA severity and risk of MVC in the general population (Masa, Rubio, & Findley, 2000), but short sleep duration and/or self-reported sleepiness also played a role (Howard et al., 2004). Sleepiness is a major factor in the increased risk of MVC in patients with OSA, with some reports indicating this to be more important than measures obtained by polysomnography (PSG), which records sleep stage, breathing, and oxygen saturation, among other variables (Kingshott et al., 2004). In professional drivers, the same trend was observed (Garbarino, Durando, et al., 2016; Karimi, Hedner, Häbel, Nerman, & Grote, 2015; Meuleners, Fraser, Govorko, & Stevenson, 2015; Wu et al., 2017), with some studies underlining a major role for sleep deprivation (Carter, Ulfberg, Nystrom, & Edling, 2003), or sleepiness (Karimi et al., 2013), or nocturnal hypoxaemia, typically measured by the oxygen saturation (Wu et al., 2017). Conversely, Stevenson et al. (2014) found no difference in MVC occurrence between heavy-vehicle drivers with and without moderate or severe OSA. Patients with severe OSA and young males with OSA are especially at risk (Arita et al., 2015; Horstmann, Hess, Bassetti, Gugger, & Mathis, 2000)

3.3.2.2 ROLE OF SLEEPINESS

EDS is reported as a contributing factor in 5 to 7% of MVC, and in up to 17% of collisions involving fatalities (Tefft, 2012). A recent meta-analysis reported that sleepiness at the wheel was associated with an increased risk for MVC with an OR of

2.51 (Bioulac et al., 2017). Sleepiness is a major factor contributing to the occurrence of MVCs and disorders associated with EDS are recognised risk factors (Carter et al., 2003). A role for nocturnal hypoxaemia in predicting EDS has been reported in several studies (Barbe et al., 1998; Karimi et al., 2013; Stevenson et al., 2014) and sleep fragmentation was associated with ESS scores in some reports (Bennett, Langford, Stradling, & Davies, 1998; Roure et al., 2008; Seneviratne & Puvanendran, 2004), but not in others (Chen et al., 2011; Gonçalves et al., 2015; Mediano et al., 2007). EDS may have many contributing factors and not only those relating to OSA.

A strong association between subjective EDS and depression in OSA has been reported (Lang et al., 2017). Depression and obesity predicted EDS better than AHI in a large cohort of OSA patients at diagnosis (Pamidi, Knutson, Ghods, & Mokhlesi, 2011) and a meta-analysis found that EDS decreased after weight loss without evident relationship with changes in AHI (Ng et al., 2017). In patients undergoing bariatric surgery, EDS was related more to metabolic variables and depression than to AHI (Dixon, Dixon, Anderson, Schachter, & O'Brien P, 2007; Dixon, Schachter, & O'Brien, 2005). A longitudinal study in the general population reported changes in EDS associated with weight gain or loss, and a significant influence of comorbidities and depression over a follow-up of 7.5 years (Fernandez-Mendoza et al., 2015).

3.3.2.3 EVALUATION OF SLEEPINESS

The evaluation of sleepiness, especially in large populations, is difficult, and simple objective tools are not available (see also Chapters 1.2 and 1.3). Thus, a detailed objective evaluation of EDS may be most appropriately performed in a specialist centre, especially for professional drivers, although subjective evaluation by the ESS score can be performed by General Practitioners (GPs). Furthermore, fitness to drive in this context should not be viewed as exclusively related to sleepiness; other factors such as vigilance may be equally important (Warm, Parasuraman, & Matthews, 2008). Several objective and subjective tests have been developed to assess the effects of sleep deprivation on vigilant attention, and the results have been extrapolated to driving ability (Gupta, Pandi-Perumal, Almeneessier, & BaHammam, 2017). These tests include the Psychomotor Vigilance Test (PVT), which is easy to perform and is reported to be impaired in untreated OSA (Cori et al., 2018). The Maintenance of Wakefulness Test (MWT) is a more complex test that has been demonstrated to correlate with the ability to perform on a driving simulator in patients with untreated OSA (Mazza et al., 2005; Pizza, Contardi, Mondini, Trentin, & Cirignotta, 2009; P. Sagaspe et al., 2007). The Oxford Sleep Resistance (OSLER) test is a simpler form of MWT (Bennett, Stradling, & Davies, 1997; Cori et al., 2018) and poor performance has been shown to be associated with previous episodes of MVC (Karimi, Hedner, Habel, Nerman, & Grote, 2015).

3.3.2.4 EFFECTIVENESS OF CPAP TREATMENT IN OSA ON COLLISION RISK

Effective treatment with nasal Continuous Positive Airway Pressure (CPAP) substantially reduces the increased collision risk associated with OSA, and several reports indicate that the risk may be reduced to a level similar to that of the general population (Antonopoulos, Sergentanis, Daskalopoulou, & Petridou, 2011; Tregear, Reston, Schoelles, & Phillips, 2010). In fact, the risk of near miss events in truck drivers decreased to normal after two years of CPAP treatment.(Garbarino et al., 2016). A meta-analysis also found a significant reduction in collisions after treatment (Antonopoulos et al., 2011), which has obvious benefits in financial and human costs (Sassani et al., 2004). In the trucking industry, CPAP-adherent patients had crash risks similar to controls, whereas non-adherent patients had a fivefold greater crash risk after 6 years of follow-up (Burks et al., 2016). Many studies indicate that CPAP improves sleepiness after as little as one night of treatment, although few of those studies used a randomised experimental design—making the results less robust (Engleman, Martin, Deary, & Douglas, 1994; Hack et al., 2000; Hoekema et al., 2007; Phillips et al., 2013). Improvements in vigilance were found after 1 year treatment (Cassel et al., 1996) and CPAP therapy was associated with objectively improved reaction times and sustained attention in OSA drivers (Alakuijala, Maasilta, & Bachour, 2014). However, continuing regular treatment is essential to maintain benefit, and CPAP cannot compensate for other factors such as inadequate sleep time.

3.3.2.5 European Union Regulations on Driving in Patients with OSA

An important milestone in the official regulation of driving ability in patients with sleep disorders was the implementation in 2014 by the EU of an official legal directive that introduced regulations on fitness to drive in patients with OSA. The directive is now mandatory throughout the EU and thus covers a population of about 450 million people. The directive specifies that patients with AHI $\geq$15 and associated sleepiness should not drive until effective treatment is demonstrated and physician certification is required to confirm suitability to continue driving (Bonsignore et al., 2016). While the regulations do not distinguish between professional and non-professional drivers in the OSA criteria that determine driving restriction, the requirements for monitoring of professional drivers are more stringent (Bonsignore et al., 2016), Also, some European countries, such as France and Spain, have introduced stricter regulations than those specified by the EU directive such as requiring an MWT test for professional drivers, resulting in a large variation in legislation between different countries.

3.3.2.6 Evaluation of Fitness to Drive in OSA

The problem of evaluating fitness to drive in OSA has been extensively investigated in the last 30 years, but the level of evidence regarding fitness remains insufficient. In addition, there is a lack of normative data regarding most tests of vigilance and results of driving simulators. We still lack simple instruments that are suitable to apply on a large scale, which could reliably indicate that a subject with OSA is fit to drive or not. Although several questionnaires have been used, their sensitivity and specificity vary according to the people being assessed (McNicholas, 2016). A fast sleep latency (time taken to fall asleep) during the MWT is used in some European countries to document increased sleepiness in OSA patients, but the resource requirements of the test make it unsuitable to evaluate large numbers, and may be more appropriate for selected groups such as commercial truck drivers and drivers where the subjective reports of sleepiness are questioned. Attention should be paid to potentially important risk factors, such as a history of previous MVCs, especially where sleepiness was a likely contributing factor, or the presence of obesity, where weight reduction measures may also be appropriate. Unfortunately, this is often not the case, as shown by recent surveys of physicians where considerable uncertainty regarding the necessary criteria to medically approve continued driving persists (Alkharboush et al., 2017; Dwarakanath et al., 2015; Mets, Alford, & Verster, 2012). Stricter criteria for the issuing or renewal of driving licenses for commercial drivers have been adopted in several countries. These drivers have a higher exposure to the risk of MVC compared to non-commercial drivers since long-haul journeys and driving on divided highways are associated with greater risk than short urban journeys. A fast-track approach for sleepy drivers with OSA to allow rapid initiation of CPAP therapy has recently been tested in the UK (West et al., 2017).

The allocation of responsibility for driver licensing is also an important consideration. While it should be the responsibility of the physician to suspect OSA and request diagnostic examination in the case of patients who are renewing their driving license, the primary responsibility for issuing the driving licence should remain with the relevant licensing authority.

In the case of CPAP-treated patients, the evaluation is more straightforward as daily CPAP compliance and efficacy can be quantified by data downloaded from their device, and there is good evidence that effective CPAP treatment greatly decreases MVC risk (Tregear et al., 2010). A recent statement from the European Respiratory Society indicated that documented use of CPAP for at least 4 hours for at least 70% of nights is considered enough evidence to regard a treated patient as fit to drive (Bonsignore et al., 2020).

3.3.3 NARCOLEPSY

The most important central disorder associated with excessive sleepiness is narcolepsy, although some cases of sleepiness cannot be clearly defined and are referred to as idiopathic hypersomnolence. Narcolepsy is a lifelong disorder of hypersomnolence characterised by multiple daily periods of irrepressible urge to sleep, or frequent daytime lapses into sleep. Type 1 narcolepsy is also associated with cataplexy, which is a phenomenon where strong emotions precipitate bilateral loss of muscle tone with retained consciousness, sometimes resulting in collapse. It is also associated with sleep paralysis.

Although far less common than OSA, sleepiness while driving is a major concern in patients with narcolepsy and is especially serious because sleepiness is difficult to resist, regardless of the circumstances. In this respect, sleepiness associated with narcolepsy may carry a higher risk of MVC than sleepiness associated with OSA. Indeed, narcolepsy has been reported to confer up to a fourfold greater risk for sleep-related collisions than other sleep disorders (McCall & Watson, 2020; Philip et al., 2010). Furthermore, patients with narcolepsy are more likely to enter rapid eye movement (REM) sleep during brief episodes of sleep, wherein muscle tone is lost, thus leading to higher risk of MVC. Also, cataplexy occurring in response to strong emotion can cause loss of skeletal muscle tone, which also increases the risk of an MVC.

The increased risk of MVC in subjects with narcolepsy has been estimated at 3.16 in a French population study (Philip et al., 2010), which is supported by data from the Second Strategic Highway Research Program Naturalistic Driving Study from the USA (Liu, Perez, & Lau, 2018), although the number of subjects with narcolepsy was small in this latter report. An early survey report involving 180 patients with narcolepsy indicated that driving was greatly affected, with 66% of patients reporting having fallen asleep at the wheel and 29% having experienced cataplexy while driving (Broughton et al., 1981).

3.3.3.1 Evaluation of Driving Ability in Narcolepsy

The MWT and PVT have poor ability to predict impaired driving in patients with narcolepsy or idiopathic hypersomnolence. This limits their use for clinical evaluation of fitness to drive, making real-time monitoring of sleepiness while driving a more reliable measure in these patients (Bijlenga et al., 2022). The relationship between real and simulated driving performance and the objective level of alertness as measured by the MWT was evaluated in a small cohort of patients with narcolepsy (Sagaspe et al., 2019). Untreated patients demonstrated shorter sleep latencies on the MWT and worse simulated driving performance ($P< 0.001$) than treated patients. Drug treatment for narcolepsy includes wake promoting agents such as modafinil and anti-cataleptic agents such as venlafaxine. While treated patients still exhibited shorter sleep latencies on the MWT than control subjects, driving performance was identical in both groups. Similar results were found in an earlier report from Germany, where driving simulator performance was reported as superior to neuropsychological testing in the evaluation of fitness to drive in patients with narcolepsy (Kotterba et al., 2004).

3.3.3.2 Impact of Treatment

Mitigating strategies to reduce the risk of drowsy driving crashes in patients with narcolepsy should optimally account for all the associated risks of sleepiness, cataplexy, and sleep paralysis. Treatments, such as the wake-promoting agent modafinil, may improve driving ability and has been demonstrated to result in improved real driving performance in patients with narcolepsy and idiopathic hypersomnolence. These performance effects also correlated with improvements in MWT (Philip et al., 2014). However, the impact of other treatments, such as stimulants and sodium oxybate, on driving ability has not been well studied.

Behavioural and lifestyle modifications may also reduce crash risk associated with narcolepsy, including scheduled naps, driving only short distances, and avoiding driving after meals, sedating medications, and alcohol intake. Even with effective treatment, alertness in patients with narcolepsy may never reach that of normal drivers, although studies have suggested that narcolepsy patients may be able to drive safely with appropriate limitations such as driving short distances only and avoiding late night driving (McCall & Watson, 2020). Patients with narcolepsy have impaired objective on-the-road driving ability, which persists despite conventional treatment (van der Sluiszen et al., 2021), although a recent report indicates that the newer wake-promoting agent, solriamfetol, improves driving performance in patients with narcolepsy (Vinckenbosch et al., 2021). Thus, overall, while medications typically used in the treatment of patients with narcolepsy improve driving ability and safety, they do not appear to result in the same level of improvement typically associated with successful CPAP therapy in patients with OSA. Some jurisdictions such as the United Kingdom specify narcolepsy as a disorder that restricts the ability to drive unless adequate control of symptoms is demonstrated.

3.3.4 INADEQUATE SLEEP, SLEEP DISTURBANCE, AND INSOMNIA

The most common deficit in sleep quality and quantity is inadequate time in bed because of lifestyle factors. Modern lifestyles often result in people going to bed late and getting up early, which results in less time spent in bed than the recommended 8 hours. Sleep restriction and poor sleep hygiene have been associated with increased collision risk (Philip, Taillard, & Micoulaud-Franchi, 2019). However, acute sleep loss was not associated with increased near miss collision risk in one questionnaire-based report (Quera Salva et al., 2014), although another study involving long-haul driving reported that sleep restriction combined with fatigue significantly affected reaction time behind the wheel (Philip et al., 2003).

A questionnaire-based study reported a threefold increase in the rate of serious driving collisions among workers with insomnia compared to control workers (Léger, Massuel, & Metlaine, 2006). Another multinational questionnaire-based study of subjects reporting sleep disturbance concluded that reduced total sleep time may be one factor explaining the high risk of collisions in individuals who complain of insomnia (Léger et al., 2014). However, more recent objective evidence indicates that patients with insomnia perform as well as control subjects in an urban test of driving with original risk scenarios and a car-following test performed during the middle afternoon (Perrier, Amato, Berthelon, & Bocca, 2019). Another report found that insomniacs treated with hypnotic medications showed no differences in driving performance and driving-related skills compared to non-insomniac control subjects (Leufkens, Ramaekers, de Weerd, Riedel, & Vermeeren, 2014). However, patients with primary insomnia have been reported to demonstrate performance decrements during a simulated monotonous driving task, but were able to drive safely for a short time (Perrier et al., 2014). Thus, sleep restriction and insomnia appear to have a complex relationship with driving ability and may be particularly associated with increased crash risk in long-haul monotonous driving situations such as on motorways.

3.3.5 CONCLUSIONS

Sleep disorders represent a highly prevalent cause of sleepiness and fatigue while driving. The most prevalent medical cause of sleepiness is OSA, which is highly relevant in that effective treatment of OSA is associated with major reductions in these complaints with consequent benefits to personal and public safety. However, other factors such as inadequate sleep should be considered in the overall context of patient management.

SUMMARY POINTS FOR PRACTITIONERS

- Sleepiness and fatigue while driving are as much a collision risk as excessive speed and alcohol consumption.
- The most common medical disorder associated with sleepiness is obstructive sleep apnoea, which affects up to one billion people worldwide.
- The collision risk associated with sleep apnoea is about three times that of the general driving population but is reversed by effective treatment.
- Narcolepsy, although relatively rare, is associated with a very high collision risk because of the associated manifestations of uncontrollable sleepiness and cataplexy.
- Sleep restriction and insomnia may also increase collision risk, especially in long-haul monotonous driving scenarios.

REFERENCES

Al-Abri, M. A., Al-Adawi, S., Al-Abri, I., Al-Abri, F., Dorvlo, A., Wesonga, R., & Jaju, S. (2018). Daytime sleepiness among young adult Omani car drivers. *Sultan Qaboos University Medical Journal, 18*(2), e143–e148. doi:10.18295/squmj.2018.18.02.004

Alakuijala, A., Maasilta, P., & Bachour, A. (2014). The Oxford Sleep Resistance test (OSLER) and the Multiple Unprepared Reaction Time Test (MURT) detect vigilance modifications in sleep apnoea patients. *J Clin Sleep Med, 10*(10), 1075–1082. doi:10.5664/jcsm.4104

Alkharboush, G. A., Al Rashed, F. A., Saleem, A. H., Alnajashi, I. S., Almeneessier, A. S., Olaish, A.H.,.... . AS, B. (2017). Assessment of patients' medical fitness to drive by primary care physicians: A cross-sectional study. *Traffic Inj Prev, 18*(5), 488–492.

Antonopoulos, C. N., Sergentanis, T. N., Daskalopoulou, S. S., & Petridou, E. T. (2011). Nasal continuous positive airway pressure (nCPAP) treatment for obstructive sleep apnoea, road traffic accidents and driving simulator performance: A meta-analysis. *Sleep Med Rev, 15*(5), 301–310. doi:10.1016/j.smrv.2010.10.002

Arita, A., Sasanabe, R., Hasegawa, R., Nomura, A., Hori, R., Mano, M.,.... . Shiomi, T. (2015). Risk factors for automobile accidents caused by falling asleep while driving in obstructive sleep apnoea syndrome. *Sleep Breath, 19*(4), 1229–1234. doi:10.1007/s11325-015-1145-7

Barbe, Pericas, J., Munoz, A., Findley, L., Anto, J. M., & Agusti, A. G. (1998). Automobile accidents in patients with sleep apnoea syndrome. An epidemiological and mechanistic study. *Am J Respir Crit Care Med, 158*(1), 18–22. doi:10.1164/ajrccm.158.1.9709135

Benjafield, A. V., Ayas, N. T., Eastwood, P. R., Heinzer, R., Ip, M. S. M., Morrell, M. J.,.... . Malhotra, A. (2019). Estimation of the global prevalence and burden of obstructive sleep apnoea: A literature-based analysis. *Lancet Respir Med, 7*(8), 687–698. doi:10.1016/s2213-2600(19)30198-5

Bennett, L. S., Langford, B. A., Stradling, J. R., & Davies, R. J. (1998). Sleep fragmentation indices as predictors of daytime sleepiness and nCPAP response in obstructive sleep apnoea. *Am J Respir Crit Care Med, 158*(3), 778–786. doi:10.1164/ajrccm.158.3.9711033

Bennett, L. S., Stradling, J. R., & Davies, R. J. (1997). A behavioural test to assess daytime sleepiness in obstructive sleep apnoea. *J Sleep Res, 6*(2), 142–145. doi:10.1046/j.1365-2869.1997.00039.x

Bijlenga, D., Urbanus, B., van der Sluiszen, N. N. J. J. M., Overeem, S., Ramaekers, J. G., Vermeeren, A., & Lammers, G. J. (2022). Comparing objective wakefulness and vigilance tests to on-the-road driving performance in narcolepsy and idiopathic hypersomnia. *J Sleep Res, n/a*(n/a), e13518. doi:https://doi.org/10.1111/jsr.13518

Bioulac, S., Franchi, J.-A. M., Arnaud, M., Sagaspe, P., Moore, N., Salvo, F., & Philip, P. (2017). Risk of motor vehicle accidents related to sleepiness at the wheel: A systematic review and meta-analysis. *Sleep, 40*(10), zsx134–zsx134. doi:10.1093/sleep/zsx134

Bonsignore, M. R., Randerath, W., Riha, R., Smyth, D., Gratziou, C., Gonçalves, M., & McNicholas, W. T. (2016). New rules on driver licensing for patients with obstructive sleep apnoea: European Union Directive 2014/85/EU. *J Sleep Res, 25*(1), 3–4. doi:10.1111/jsr.12379

Bonsignore, M. R., Randerath, W., Schiza, S., Verbraecken, J., Elliott, M. W., Riha, R.,.... . McNicholas, W. T. (2020). European Respiratory Society statement on sleep apnoea, sleepiness and driving risk. *Eur Respir J*, Oct 2:2001272. doi: 10.1183/13993003.01272–2020. Online ahead of print. doi:10.1183/13993003.01272-2020

Broughton, R., Ghanem, Q., Hishikawa, Y., Sugita, Y., Nevsimalova, S., & Roth, B. (1981). Life effects of narcolepsy in 180 patients from North America, Asia and Europe compared to matched controls. *Can J Neurol Sci, 8*(4), 299–304. doi:10.1017/s0317167100043419

Burks, S. V., Anderson, J. E., Bombyk, M., Haider, R., Ganzhorn, D., Jiao, X.,.... . Kales, S. N. (2016). Nonadherence with employer-mandated sleep apnoea treatment and increased risk of serious truck crashes. *Sleep, 39*(5), 967–975. doi:10.5665/sleep.5734

Carter, N., Ulfberg, J., Nystrom, B., & Edling, C. (2003). Sleep debt, sleepiness and accidents among males in the general population and male professional drivers. *Accid Anal Prev, 35*(4), 613–617. doi:10.1016/s0001-4575(02)00033-7

Cassel, W., Ploch, T., Becker, C., Dugnus, D., Peter, J. H., & von Wichert, P. (1996). Risk of traffic accidents in patients with sleep-disordered breathing: Reduction with nasal CPAP. *Eur Respir J, 9*(12), 2606–2611. doi:10.1183/09031936.96.09122606

Catarino, R., Spratley, J., Catarino, I., Lunet, N., & Pais-Clemente, M. (2014). Sleepiness and sleep-disordered breathing in truck drivers. *Sleep Breath, 18*(1), 59–68. doi:10.1007/s11325-013-0848-x

Chen, R., Xiong, K. P., Lian, Y. X., Huang, J. Y., Zhao, M. Y., Li, J. X., & Liu, C. F. (2011). Daytime sleepiness and its determining factors in Chinese obstructive sleep apnoea patients. *Sleep Breath, 15*(1), 129–135. doi:10.1007/s11325-010-0337-4

Cori, J. M., Jackson, M. L., Barnes, M., Westlake, J., Emerson, P., Lee, J.,.... . Howard, M. (2018). The differential effects of regular shift work and obstructive sleep apnoea on sleepiness, mood and neurocognitive function. *J Clin Sleep Med, 14*(6), 941–951. doi:10.5664/jcsm.7156

Czeisler, C. A., Wickwire, E. M., Barger, L. K., Dement, W. C., Gamble, K., Hartenbaum, N.,.... . Hirshkowitz, M. (2016). Sleep-deprived motor vehicle operators are unfit to drive: A multidisciplinary expert consensus statement on drowsy driving. *Sleep Health, 2*(2), 94–99. doi:https://doi.org/10.1016/j.sleh.2016.04.003

Deegan, P. C., & McNicholas, W. T. (1996). Predictive value of clinical features for the obstructive sleep apnoea syndrome. *Eur Respir J, 9*(1), 117–124.

Dixon, J. B., Dixon, M. E., Anderson, M. L., Schachter, L., & O'Brien P. E. (2007). Daytime sleepiness in the obese: Not as simple as obstructive sleep apnoea. *Obesity, 15*(10), 2504–2511. doi:10.1038/oby.2007.297

Dixon, J. B., Schachter, L. M., & O'Brien, P. E. (2005). Polysomnography before and after weight loss in obese patients with severe sleep apnoea. *Int J Obes (Lond), 29*(9), 1048–1054. doi:10.1038/sj.ijo.0802960

Dwarakanath, A., Twiddy, M., Ghosh, D., Jamson, S. L., Baxter, P. D., & Elliott, M. W. (2015). Variability in clinicians' opinions regarding fitness to drive in patients with obstructive sleep apnoea syndrome (OSAS). *Thorax, 70*(5), 495–497. doi:10.1136/thoraxjnl-2014-206180

Engleman, H. M., Martin, S. E., Deary, I. J., & Douglas, N. J. (1994). Effect of continuous positive airway pressure treatment on daytime function in sleep apnoea/hypopnoea syndrome. *Lancet, 343*(8897), 572–575. doi:10.1016/s0140-6736(94)91522-9

Fernandez-Mendoza, J., Vgontzas, A. N., Kritikou, I., Calhoun, S. L., Liao, D., & Bixler, E. O. (2015). Natural history of excessive daytime sleepiness: Role of obesity, weight loss, depression, and sleep propensity. *Sleep, 38*(3), 351–360. doi:10.5665/sleep.4488

Findley, L. J., Unverzagt, M. E., & Suratt, P. M. (1988). automobile accidents involving patients with obstructive sleep apnoea. *Am Rev Respir Dis, 138*(2), 337–340. doi:10.1164/ajrccm/138.2.337

Garbarino, S., Durando, P., Guglielmi, O., Dini, G., Bersi, F., Fornarino, S.,... . Magnavita, N. (2016). Sleep apnoea, sleep debt and daytime sleepiness are independently associated with road accidents. A cross-sectional study on truck drivers. *PLoS One, 11*(11), e0166262. doi:10.1371/journal.pone.0166262

Garbarino, S., Guglielmi, O., Campus, C., Mascialino, B., Pizzorni, D., Nobili, L.,.... Ferini-Strambi, L. (2016). Screening, diagnosis, and management of obstructive sleep apnoea in dangerous-goods truck drivers: to be aware or not? *Sleep Med, 25*, 98–104. doi:10.1016/j.sleep.2016.05.015

Garbarino, S., Guglielmi, O., Sanna, A., Mancardi, G. L., & Magnavita, N. (2016). Risk of occupational accidents in workers with obstructive sleep apnoea: Systematic review and meta-analysis. *Sleep, 39*(6), 1211–1218. doi:10.5665/sleep.5834

Gonçalves, M., Amici, R., Lucas, R., Åkerstedt, T., Cirignotta, F., Horne, J.,... . Grote, L. (2015). Sleepiness at the wheel across Europe: A survey of 19 countries. *J Sleep Res, 24*(3), 242–253.

Gupta, R., Pandi-Perumal, S. R., Almeneessier, A. S., & BaHammam, A. S. (2017). Hypersomnolence and traffic safety. *Sleep Med Clin, 12*(3), 489–499. doi:10.1016/j.jsmc.2017.03.018

Hack, M., Davies, R. J., Mullins, R., Choi, S. J., Ramdassingh-Dow, S., Jenkinson, C., & Stradling, J. R. (2000). Randomised prospective parallel trial of therapeutic versus subtherapeutic nasal continuous positive airway pressure on simulated steering performance in patients with obstructive sleep apnoea. *Thorax, 55*(3), 224–231.

Hoekema, A., Stegenga, B., Bakker, M., Brouwer, W. H., de Bont, L. G., Wijkstra, P. J., & van der Hoeven, J. H. (2007). Simulated driving in obstructive sleep apnoea-hypopnoea; effects of oral appliances and continuous positive airway pressure. *Sleep Breath, 11*(3), 129–138. doi:10.1007/s11325-006-0093-7

Horstmann, S., Hess, C. W., Bassetti, C., Gugger, M., & Mathis, J. (2000). Sleepiness-related accidents in sleep apnoea patients. *Sleep, 23*(3), 383–389.

Howard, M. E., Desai, A. V., Grunstein, R. R., Hukins, C., Armstrong, J. G., Joffe, D.,.... Pierce, R. J. (2004). Sleepiness, sleep-disordered breathing, and accident risk factors in commercial vehicle drivers. *Am J Respir Crit Care Med, 170*(9), 1014–1021. doi:10.1164/rccm.200312-1782OC

Johns, M. W. (1991). A new method for measuring daytime sleepiness: The Epworth sleepiness scale. *Sleep, 14*(6), 540–545.

Karimi, M., Eder, D. N., Eskandari, D., Zou, D., Hedner, J. A., & Grote, L. (2013). Impaired vigilance and increased accident rate in public transport operators is associated with sleep disorders. *Accid Anal Prev, 51*, 208–214. doi:10.1016/j.aap.2012.11.014

Karimi, M., Hedner, J., Habel, H., Nerman, O., & Grote, L. (2015). Sleep apnoea-related risk of motor vehicle accidents is reduced by continuous positive airway pressure: Swedish Traffic Accident Registry data. *Sleep, 38*(3), 341–349. doi:10.5665/sleep.4486

Kingshott, R. N., Cowan, J. O., Jones, D. R., Flannery, E. M., Smith, A. D., Herbison, G. P., & Taylor, D. R. (2004). The role of sleep-disordered breathing, daytime sleepiness, and impaired performance in motor vehicle crashes-a case control study. *Sleep Breath, 8*(2), 61–72. doi:10.1007/s11325-004-0061-z

Kingshott, R. N., Sime, P. J., Engleman, H. M., & Douglas, N. J. (1995). Self assessment of daytime sleepiness: patient versus partner. *Thorax, 50*(9), 994–995.

Kotterba, S., Mueller, N., Leidag, M., Widdig, W., Rasche, K., Malin, J.-P.,... . Orth, M. (2004). Comparison of driving simulator performance and neuropsychological testing in Narcolepsy. *Clin Neurol Neurosurg, 106*(4), 275–279. doi:https://doi.org/10.1016/j.clineuro.2003.12.003

Krieger, J., McNicholas, W. T., Levy, P., De Backer, W., Douglas, N., Marrone, O.,... . Rodenstein, D. (2002). Public health and medicolegal implications of sleep apnoea. *Eur Respir J, 20*(6), 1594–1609. doi:10.1183/09031936.02.00404502

Lang, C. J., Appleton, S. L., Vakulin, A., McEvoy, R. D., Vincent, A. D., Wittert, G. A.,... . Adams, R. J. (2017). Associations of undiagnosed obstructive sleep apnoea and excessive daytime sleepiness with depression: An Australian population study. *J Clin Sleep Med, 13*(4), 575–582. doi:10.5664/jcsm.6546

Léger, D., Bayon, V., Ohayon, M. M., Philip, P., Ement, P., Metlaine, A.,... . Faraut, B. (2014). Insomnia and accidents: Cross-sectional study (EQUINOX) on sleep-related home, work and car accidents in 5293 subjects with insomnia from 10 countries. *J Sleep Res, 23*(2), 143–152. doi:10.1111/jsr.12104

Léger, D., Massuel, M. A., & Metlaine, A. (2006). Professional correlates of insomnia. *Sleep, 29*(2), 171–178.

Leufkens, T. R., Ramaekers, J. G., de Weerd, A. W., Riedel, W. J., & Vermeeren, A. (2014). On-the-road driving performance and driving-related skills in older untreated insomnia patients and chronic users of hypnotics. *Psychopharmacology (Berl), 231*(14), 2851–2865. doi:10.1007/s00213-014-3455-z

Liu, S.-Y., Perez, M. A., & Lau, N. (2018). The impact of sleep disorders on driving safety—findings from the Second Strategic Highway Research Program naturalistic driving study. *Sleep, 41*(4). doi:10.1093/sleep/zsy023

Maia, Q., Grandner, M. A., Findley, J., & Gurubhagavatula, I. (2013). Short and long sleep duration and risk of drowsy driving and the role of subjective sleep insufficiency. *Accid Anal Prev, 59*, 618–622. doi:10.1016/j.aap.2013.07.028

Masa, J. F., Rubio, M., & Findley, L. J. (2000). Habitually sleepy drivers have a high frequency of automobile crashes associated with respiratory disorders during sleep. *Am J Respir Crit Care Med, 162*(4 Pt 1), 1407–1412. doi:10.1164/ajrccm.162.4.9907019

Mazza, S., Pepin, J. L., Naegele, B., Plante, J., Deschaux, C., & Levy, P. (2005). Most obstructive sleep apnoea patients exhibit vigilance and attention deficits on an extended battery of tests. *Eur Respir J, 25*(1), 75–80.

McCall, C. A., & Watson, N. F. (2020). Therapeutic strategies for mitigating driving risk in patients with narcolepsy. *Ther Clin Risk Manag, 16*, 1099–1108.

McNicholas, W. T. (2016). Screening for sleep-disordered breathing: The continuing search for a reliable predictive questionnaire. *Lancet Respir Med, 4*(9), 683–685. doi:10.1016/s2213-2600(16)30119-9

McNicholas, W. T. (2019). Sleepiness and driving: The role of official regulation. *Sleep Med Clin, 14*(4), 491–498. doi:https://doi.org/10.1016/j.jsmc.2019.08.006

McNicholas, W. T., & Rodenstein, D. (2015). Sleep apnoea and driving risk: The need for regulation. *Eur Respir Rev, 24*(138), 602–606. doi:10.1183/16000617.0049-2015

Mediano, O., Barcelo, A., de la Pena, M., Gozal, D., Agusti, A., & Barbe, F. (2007). Daytime sleepiness and polysomnographic variables in sleep apnoea patients. *Eur Respir J, 30*(1), 110–113. doi:10.1183/09031936.00009506

Mets, M. A. J., Alford, C., & Verster, J. C. (2012). Sleep Specialists' Opinion on Sleep Disorders and Fitness to Drive a Car: The Necessity of Continued Education. *Ind Health, 50*(6), 499–508. doi:10.2486/indhealth.2012-0001

Meuleners, L., Fraser, M. L., Govorko, M. H., & Stevenson, M. R. (2015). Obstructive sleep apnoea, health-related factors, and long distance heavy vehicle crashes in Western Australia: a case control study. *J Clin Sleep Med, 11*(4), 413–418. doi:10.5664/jcsm.4594

Mitler, M. M., Miller, J. C., Lipsitz, J. J., Walsh, J. K., & Wylie, C. D. (1997). The sleep of long-haul truck drivers. *N Engl J Med, 337*(11), 755–762. doi:10.1056/nejm199709113371106

Netzer, N. C., Stoohs, R. A., Netzer, C. M., Clark, K., & Strohl, K. P. (1999). Using the Berlin questionnaire to identify patients at risk for the sleep apnoea syndrome. *Ann Intern Med, 131*(7), 485–491.

Ng, W. L., Stevenson, C. E., Wong, E., Tanamas, S., Boelsen-Robinson, T., Shaw, J. E.,... . Peeters, A. (2017). Does intentional weight loss improve daytime sleepiness? A systematic review and meta-analysis. *Obes Rev, 18*(4), 460–475. doi:10.1111/obr.12498

Pack, A. I., Maislin, G., Staley, B., Pack, F. M., Rogers, W. C., George, C. F. P., & Dinges, D. F. (2006). Impaired performance in commercial drivers. *Am J Respir Crit Care Med, 174*(4), 446–454. doi:10.1164/rccm.200408-1146OC

Pamidi, S., Knutson, K. L., Ghods, F., & Mokhlesi, B. (2011). Depressive symptoms and obesity as predictors of sleepiness and quality of life in patients with REM-related obstructive sleep apnoea: Cross-sectional analysis of a large clinical population. *Sleep Med, 12*(9), 827–831. doi:10.1016/j.sleep.2011.08.003

Perrier, J., Amato, J.-N., Berthelon, C., & Bocca, M.-L. (2019). Primary insomnia patients' performances during simulated car following and urban driving in the afternoon. *J Sleep Res, 28*(4), e12847. doi:https://doi.org/10.1111/jsr.12847

Perrier, J., Bertran, F., Marie, S., Couque, C., Bulla, J., Denise, P., & Bocca, M. L. (2014). Impaired driving performance associated with effect of time duration in patients with primary insomnia. *Sleep, 37*(9), 1565–1573. doi:10.5665/sleep.4012

Philip, P., Chaufton, C., Taillard, J., Capelli, A., Coste, O., Léger, D.,... . Sagaspe, P. (2014). Modafinil improves real driving performance in patients with hypersomnia: A randomized double-blind placebo-controlled crossover clinical trial. *Sleep, 37*(3), 483–487. doi:10.5665/sleep.3480

Philip, P., Sagaspe, P., Lagarde, E., Leger, D., Ohayon, M. M., Bioulac, B.,... . Taillard, J. (2010). Sleep disorders and accidental risk in a large group of regular registered highway drivers. *Sleep Med, 11*(10), 973–979. doi:https://doi.org/10.1016/j.sleep.2010.07.010

Philip, P., Sagaspe, P., Taillard, J., Moore, N., Guilleminault, C., Sanchez-Ortuno, M.,... . Bioulac, B. (2003). Fatigue, sleep restriction, and performance in automobile drivers: A controlled study in a natural environment. *Sleep, 26*(3), 277–280. doi:10.1093/sleep/26.3.277

Philip, P., Taillard, J., & Micoulaud-Franchi, J. A. (2019). Sleep restriction, sleep hygiene, and driving safety the importance of situational sleepiness. *Sleep Med Clin, 14*(4), 407-+. doi:10.1016/j.jsmc.2019.07.002

Phillips, C. L., Grunstein, R. R., Darendeliler, M. A., Mihailidou, A. S., Srinivasan, V. K., Yee, B. J.,... . Cistulli, P. A. (2013). Health outcomes of continuous positive airway pressure versus oral appliance treatment for obstructive sleep apnoea: a randomized controlled trial. *Am J Respir Crit Care Med, 187*(8), 879–887. doi:10.1164/rccm.201212-2223OC

Pizza, F., Contardi, S., Mondini, S., Trentin, L., & Cirignotta, F. (2009). Daytime sleepiness and driving performance in patients with obstructive sleep apnoea: Comparison of the MSLT, the MWT, and a simulated driving task. *Sleep, 32*(3), 382–391.

Quera Salva, M. A., Barbot, F., Hartley, S., Sauvagnac, R., Vaugier, I., Lofaso, F., & Philip, P. (2014). Sleep disorders, sleepiness, and near-miss accidents among long-distance highway drivers in the summertime. *Sleep Med, 15*(1), 23–26. doi:10.1016/j.sleep.2013.06.018

Roure, N., Gomez, S., Mediano, O., Duran, J., Pena Mde, L., Capote, F.,... . Barbe, F. (2008). Daytime sleepiness and polysomnography in obstructive sleep apnoea patients. *Sleep Med, 9*(7), 727–731. doi:10.1016/j.sleep.2008.02.006

Sagaspe, P., Micoulaud-Franchi, J.-A., Coste, O., Léger, D., Espié, S., Davenne, D.,.... Philip, P. (2019). Maintenance of Wakefulness Test, real and simulated driving in patients with narcolepsy/hypersomnia. *Sleep Med, 55*, 1–5. doi:https://doi.org/10.1016/j.sleep.2018.02.009

Sagaspe, P., Taillard, J., Chaumet, G., Guilleminault, C., Coste, O., Moore, N.,... . Philip, P. (2007). Maintenance of wakefulness test as a predictor of driving performance in patients with untreated obstructive sleep apnoea. *Sleep, 30*(3), 327–330.

Sassani, A., Findley, L. J., Kryger, M., Goldlust, E., George, C., & Davidson, T. M. (2004). Reducing motor-vehicle collisions, costs, and fatalities by treating obstructive sleep apnoea syndrome. *Sleep, 27*(3), 453–458. doi:10.1093/sleep/27.3.453

Seneviratne, U., & Puvanendran, K. (2004). Excessive daytime sleepiness in obstructive sleep apnoea: Prevalence, severity, and predictors. *Sleep Med, 5*(4), 339–343. doi:10.1016/j.sleep.2004.01.021

Stevenson, M. R., Elkington, J., Sharwood, L., Meuleners, L., Ivers, R., Boufous, S.,... . Wong, K. (2014). The role of sleepiness, sleep disorders, and the work environment on heavy-vehicle crashes in 2 Australian states. *Am J Epidemiol, 179*(5), 594–601. doi:10.1093/aje/kwt305

Tefft, B. C. (2012). Prevalence of motor vehicle crashes involving drowsy drivers, United States, 1999–2008. *Accid Anal Prev, 45*, 180–186. doi:https://doi.org/10.1016/j.aap.2011.05.028

Terán-Santos, J., Jimenez-Gomez, A., & Cordero-Guevara, J. (1999). The association between sleep apnoea and the risk of traffic accidents. *N Engl J Med, 340*(11), 847–851. doi:10.1056/nejm199903183401104

Tregear, S., Reston, J., Schoelles, K., & Phillips, B. (2009). Obstructive sleep apnoea and risk of motor vehicle crash: Systematic review and meta-analysis. *J Clin Sleep Med, 5*(6), 573–581.

Tregear, S., Reston, J., Schoelles, K., & Phillips, B. (2010). Continuous positive airway pressure reduces risk of motor vehicle crash among drivers with obstructive sleep apnoea: Systematic review and meta-analysis. *Sleep, 33*(10), 1373–1380.

Vaa, T. (2003). Impairments, diseases, age and their relative risks of accident involvement: Results from a meta-analysis. *Institute of Transport Economics, Oslo, Norway*.

van der Sluiszen, N. N. J. J. M., Urbanus, B., Lammers, G. J., Overeem, S., Ramaekers, J. G., & Vermeeren, A. (2021). On-the-road driving performance of patients with central disorders of hypersomnolence. *Traffic Inj Prev, 22*(2), 120–126. doi:10.1080/15389588.2020.1862804

Vaz Fragoso, C. A., Araujo, K. L., Van Ness, P. H., & Marottoli, R. A. (2008). Prevalence of sleep disturbances in a cohort of older drivers. *J Gerontol A Biol Sci Med Sci, 63*(7), 715–723. doi:10.1093/gerona/63.7.715

Vaz Fragoso, C. A., Araujo, K. L., Van Ness, P. H., & Marottoli, R. A. (2010). Sleep disturbances and adverse driving events in a predominantly male cohort of active older drivers. *J Am Geriatr Soc, 58*(10), 1878–1884. doi:10.1111/j.1532-5415.2010.03083.x

Vennelle, M., Engleman, H. M., & Douglas, N. J. (2010). Sleepiness and sleep-related accidents in commercial bus drivers. *Sleep Breath, 14*(1), 39–42. doi:10.1007/s11325-009-0277-z

Vinckenbosch, F., Lammers, G. J., Overeem, S., Chen, D., Wang, G., Carter, L.,.... Vermeeren, A. (2021). Effects of solriamfetol on driving performance in participants with narcolepsy. *Neurology, 96*(15).

Ward, K. L., Hillman, D. R., James, A., Bremner, A. P., Simpson, L., Cooper, M. N.,.... Mukherjee, S. (2013). Excessive daytime sleepiness increases the risk of motor vehicle crash in obstructive sleep apnoea. *J Clin Sleep Med, 9*(10), 1013–1021. doi:10.5664/jcsm.3072

Warm, J. S., Parasuraman, R., & Matthews, G. (2008). Vigilance requires hard mental work and is stressful. *Hum Factors, 50*(3), 433–441. doi:10.1518/001872008x312152

West, S. D., Downie, B., Olds, G., Tomlinson, M., Wotton, C., Firth, E., & McMillan, A. (2017). A 4-week wait 'fast-track' sleep service is effective at establishing vocational drivers on continuous positive airway pressure. *J Clin Med, 17*(5), 401–402. doi:10.7861/clinmedicine.17-5-401

Wu, W. T., Tsai, S. S., Liao, H. Y., Lin, Y. J., Lin, M. H., Wu, T. N.,.... Liou, S. H. (2017). Usefulness of overnight pulse oximeter as the sleep assessment tool to assess the 6-year risk of road traffic collision: Evidence from the Taiwan Bus Driver Cohort Study. *Int J Epidemiol, 46*(1), 266–277. doi:10.1093/ije/dyw141

Zwahlen, D., Jackowski, C., & Pfaffli, M. (2016). Sleepiness, driving, and motor vehicle accidents: A questionnaire-based survey. *J Forensic Leg Med, 44*, 183–187. doi:10.1016/j.jflm.2016.10.014

3.4 Task-Related Causes or Contributors to Fatigue and Sleepiness

Ann Williamson

Transport and Road Safety (TARS) Research Group,
UNSW, Sydney, NSW, Australia

CONTENTS

3.4.1   INTRODUCTION

In many activities, the nature of task is a major cause of fatigue. These task-related factors alone can cause fatigue and compromise performance, especially in transportation. While many transport tasks involve characteristics that challenge people's sleep needs and affect safe performance, such as 24-hour/7-day operations, they also involve task characteristics unrelated to sleep, such as difficult, high pressure tasks, multitasking or requiring long periods of sustained attention, which also adversely affect fatigue and performance. This chapter covers evidence for the importance of task-related fatigue compared to other

DOI: 10.1201/9781003213154-20

causes, describes task-related factors most likely to cause fatigue and performance effects, and summarises current thinking on the mechanisms that underlie
those effects. It also looks at current knowledge of ways of mitigating task-related
fatigue effects in transportation settings.

It is commonly held that the main causes of fatigue and sleepiness and their effects
on performance relate to sleep factors, including sleep loss, circadian rhythms, and
time awake. In fact, widely cited models of fatigue and sleepiness only include sleep-
related factors. For example, the three-process model of alertness and performance
(Åkerstedt & Folkard, 1997) includes sleep need (Process S), circadian influences
(Process C), and post-sleep factors or sleep inertia (Process W) and does not acknowledge factors relating to the task.

Some researchers acknowledge task-related factors, like task difficulty and duration, as specific causes of fatigue and distinguish them from sleep-related factors
which cause sleepiness (Balkin & Wesensen, 2011). The difficulty is that fatigue and
sleepiness often co-occur and are highly correlated and we have little understanding
of whether they have the same underlying physiological causes or whether they are
different.

Other views acknowledge task-related factors but maintain that rather than playing
an independent role in causing fatigue and performance deficits, task-related factors
unmask underlying or latent sleepiness (Carskadon & Dement, 1982). This treats
sleep-related problems as the predominant causes of fatigue-related performance
effects with task-related characteristics playing an incidental role. Based on these
views, many argue that fatigue management is all about sleep and sleep management
(e.g., Dawson & McCulloch, 2005).

Little research has compared the independent and combined effects of task-related
and sleep-related factors. As pointed out by May and Baldwin (2009), most studies
confound the effects of sleep-related and task-related fatigue.

An exception is a recent study which compared the relative effects of sleep-related
(sleep deprivation) and task-related (time-on-task) factors separately and in combination on ratings of sleepiness and alertness and simulator driving performance over a
2-hour monotonous country drive (Zeller, Williamson & Friswell, 2020). The results
showed that both task-related and sleep-related factors had independent effects on
performance. In fact, task-related time-on-task effects on driving performance were
greater than the effects of moderate sleep need alone. The combination of these two
factors however was markedly worse than each factor alone. This study clarified the
relative contributions of sleep and task-related fatigue on performance. An earlier
laboratory experiment also supported these findings showing that characteristics of
the task in the form of monotonous work was as harmful as moderate sleep loss
(4 hours of night-time sleep) for sleepiness and performance (Sallinen, Härmä
et al., 2004).

Importantly, these studies provide good evidence that fatigue and adverse effects
on performance can occur in response to characteristics of the task itself even when
the person is rested. It is vital therefore that action to manage fatigue in transportation
must include the influence of task-related factors. It is not all about sleep.

3.4.2 INDICATORS OF TASK-RELATED FATIGUE EFFECTS ON PERFORMANCE IN TRANSPORTATION

Task-related factors increase fatigue and reduce performance in transportation. For example, Cummings et al. (2001) demonstrated time-on-task effects in a matched case-control study of crashes during highway driving in the USA showing that crash risk more than doubled with each 100 miles travelled. Long periods of driving result in deteriorating performance (Philip et al., 2005) and driving conditions can also adversely affect driving performance (Matthews & Desmond, 2002).

Research evidence suggests that fatigue due to both sleep and task-related causes has similar effects on performance. Lapses in attention and performance are very common during sleep-related fatigue and task-related fatigue states (Dinges & Powell, 1985), including during monitoring tasks in non-sleep deprived people during normal waking time (Peiris et al., 2006). A systematic review of simulator studies of fatigue effects on driving (Soares et al., 2020) showed increased variability of lateral position in lane and steering wheel movements were common effects of both sleep- and task-related fatigue factors.

3.4.3 WHAT TASK-RELATED FACTORS MAKE FATIGUE AND PERFORMANCE DEFICITS MORE LIKELY?

Fatigue in transportation is an issue because it affects vehicle control and the need for effortful attention to the control tasks, especially during 24-hour operations. Desmond and Hancock (2000) distinguished two forms of task-related fatigue state relevant to transportation. Active fatigue occurs due to high demand conditions like driving in high-density traffic, low visibility, or when using a navigation system while driving. High demand tasks in transportation include local drivers with high pressured delivery schedules (Friswell & Williamson, 2008) and short haul commercial pilots doing multiple sectors over a work period (Powell et al., 2007). Passive fatigue occurs in low demand conditions such as country or monotonous highway driving and during long or extended trips. Many transport tasks involve low demand from passive monitoring such as long-haul road, rail, and air transport. So the task can be a source of cognitive stress from overload due to high task demands for effortful attention or workload, or from underload because task demand is low requiring sustained attention. Transport tasks that achieve a zone of performance comfort between the two extremes should maximise performance and minimise fatigue (Hancock & Warm, 1989).

A study by Saxby et al. (2013) compared effects of active and passive fatigue in 10- and 30-minute simulator drives. Active fatigue was induced by frequent strong wind gusts while driving requiring the driver to correct steering, while passive fatigue was induced by automating the driving task so requiring drivers to simply monitor. During the passive fatigue drives steering and braking responses were slower and collisions were more frequent than in the active fatigue drives, especially for the longer 30-minute drive. These results support the findings of an earlier driving simulator study (Matthews & Desmond, 2002) where more passive driving (straight sections of road) induced fatigue and poorer vehicle control than more active driving (difficult curved sections). While active fatigue should be avoided, these studies highlight underload or passive task-related fatigue as of particular concern.

Time-on-task is one of the most recognised causes of passive fatigue. This refers to the progressive decline in performance for tasks requiring vigilance, defined as monitoring for long periods. Multiple studies have investigated the effects of monitoring-type tasks on fatigue and performance and show that performance on sustained attention tasks decreases with time-on-task (Warm & Parasuraman, 1987). Long hours on tasks like operating a transport vehicle almost always involve sustained attention and monitoring and produce fatigue and deterioration of performance. These types of tasks are increasingly common with the advent of technology in vehicles where tasks that were once entirely performed by humans are now performed at least partly by computers. Downgrading the active role of the human operator to only supervising and monitoring increases passive fatigue effects (Korber et al., 2015).

These time-on-task effects are amplified if the task is monotonous and undemanding. Thiffault and Bergeron (2003) examined performance on two 40-minute simulator drives, one with monotonous road conditions and the other with diverse road conditions. Time-on-task-related decrements in steering wheel movements occurred within 15 to 20 minutes of driving especially in the monotonous driving conditions. Similar effects have been found on road (Farahmand & Boroujerdian, 2018) and in rail (Dunn and Williamson, 2012). Adverse effects on fatigue and performance occur after even short periods of sustained attention and monitoring, and especially in conditions with high background event rate but rare critical signals, or where critical signals are difficult to discriminate, have uncertain timing or location (Parasuraman et al., 1987). These characteristics are found in transport-relevant situations like air traffic control, long distance driving, or train control, where a major component of the task involves monitoring for rare, safety-critical events.

3.4.4 MECHANISMS UNDERLYING THE EFFECTS OF TASK CHARACTERISTICS ON FATIGUE AND PERFORMANCE

The causes of task-related fatigue are debated, especially those relating to time-on-task. All explanations involve the role of attention and effort required to perform monitoring tasks. Transport tasks, such as driving a vehicle, plane, or train, are primarily visual and cognitive, requiring drivers/pilots to maintain attention and respond to the demands of the task, often very quickly. Driving, for example, does not necessarily require a driver's full attention, but the driver must monitor and stay engaged with the task. Skilled drivers can manage the driving task by applying a comparatively low, but continuous level of attention to the task to respond to the general needs of the task including lateral and longitudinal control. Drivers need also to monitor navigation, and to check for and respond to unexpected hazards. Maintaining driving performance over time requires sufficient control of attention to ensure continuous focus and engagement on the important elements of the task.

A recent state-of-the-art review (Wickens, 2021) provides an excellent overview of current theories of attention relating to complex multitasking or information processing overload conditions which are highly relevant to transport to understand and manage demanding task conditions. Unfortunately, this review did not address theories of underload/sustained attention which are inherent in daily activities in most transport tasks. Consequently, the next sections summarise four current theories describing the processes underlying fatigue and performance effects over time-on-task.

3.4.4.1 AROUSAL-BASED THEORIES

Traditionally, time-on-task effects were attributed to a decline in arousal due to the under-stimulating effects of doing the same task for a long time, with the greatest fatigue and performance effects occurring with more monotonous and boring tasks (Welford, 1962). The earliest explanation of time-on-task effects is related to energy or physiological arousal critical for attention, including the classic U-shaped function (Yerkes & Dodson, 1908) where very high and very low levels of arousal disrupt performance and optimum performance is obtained in mid-level arousal.

Recent arousal theories, such as the mindlessness hypothesis (Robertson et al., 1997), hold that performance decrements occur because the repetitive, undemanding, long-enduring nature of sustained attention tasks does not maintain sufficient arousal and sufficiently strong representation of the task ("what was I doing?") so disrupting supervisory attentional control. Where this theory does not specify what happens to attention withdrawn from the monitoring task, mind wandering theory does (Smallwood & Schooler, 2006). Mind wandering theory holds that when tasks fail to maintain attention over time, attention becomes task-unrelated and temporarily unavailable for the monitoring task so explaining increased lapses and slowed responding with longer time-on-task. Drivers disengage from the task and their performance becomes routine and thoughtless. There is some neurological support for the concept of mind wandering from evidence of activity changes in the brain's default mode network (Esterman & Rothlein, 2019). These theories predict that enhancing interest in the monitoring task by increasing complexity or difficulty and encouraging task engagement should reallocate attention to the task and decrease the time-on-task effect. This is consistent with research evidence.

3.4.4.2 RESOURCE THEORIES

An alternative view of the time-on-task or vigilance effect is based on resource theories (Warm et al., 2008). According to these theories, information processing resources, especially attentional capacity, are finite. Advocates (e.g., Warm et al., 2008) argue that despite the apparent simplicity of monitoring tasks, they are demanding of attention and that performance decrements in monitoring are due to cognitive overload which depletes attentional resources rather than to underload due to boredom and mindlessness.

Support for the resource theory account comes from findings of increases in cerebral blood flow velocity which mirrored vigilance decrements (Warm et al., 2008). Resource theories however do not account for all evidence on time-on-task effects, especially that the effects can be overcome if a person is engaged in the task (Pop et al., 2012), nor the finding that mind wandering becomes more likely with longer time-on-task (Smallwood & Schooler, 2006).

3.4.4.3 MOTIVATION CONTROL THEORY

Hockey's motivation control theory (Hockey, 2013) argues that the task-related fatigue effect occurs because sustained attention requires prolonged effort so is taxing and stressful and, over time, depletes one's capacity to perform at high levels. This theory shares features of resource theories but adds the concept of motivational control of fatigue to explain changes in performance. Tasks that require high levels of effort increase fatigue and interrupt attention to the ongoing task, leading to reassessment of motivational goals at that point in time. Goal reassessment can involve lowering performance levels, taking a temporary break if possible or even abandoning the task. The control model includes three supervisory or executive functions of goal maintenance, performance monitoring and regulation of effort. When task performance begins to require more effort and fatigue increases, it is evaluated on whether goals are being maintained and whether effort needs to be adjusted or compensated.

This theory acknowledges that maintaining performance goals on some tasks requires little effort. These tasks include automatic activities that require little attention, tasks that involve a high-priority personal goal and tasks that are highly controllable and can be started, continued, or stopped at will. Hockey (2013) argues that fatigue and effort are caused not only by the task itself, but by the need to perform on tasks that are unliked or unwanted and require effort to maintain performance. This theory predicts that reductions in task-related fatigue can be achieved by increasing the level of task interest and personal commitment to the task.

3.4.4.4 RESOURCE CONTROL THEORY

Resource control theory attempts to address the limitations of arousal and resource theory explanations of time-on-task effects on fatigue and performance (Thomson et al., 2015). The theory holds that attentional resources available for a task are finite and do not change over time, and that mind wandering, being the default state, will tend to highjack resources that would otherwise be used for the primary monitoring task. The theory contends that executive control of attention is needed to avoid the diversion of attention and to keep focus on the primary task, but the struggle to maintain fading executive control over time-on-task requires effort and produces fatigue. Lastly, this theory points out, as does Hockey, that many monitoring tasks require only limited attentional resources which allows mind wandering to occur, but this does not produce adverse effects on fatigue and performance.

3.4.4.5 SYNTHESIS OF THEORIES

Theories help to summarise what is known about a phenomenon and help direct ideas for further action. As research findings emerge, theories should evolve. Table 3.4.1 summarises theories of the mechanisms of time-on-task effects discussed in this chapter. The earlier physiology-based theories of arousal in which time-on-task effects are attributed to low demand have been challenged by resource theories that maintain that time-on-task requires effort and is demanding. More recently, the motivation

TABLE 3.4.1
Summary of Characteristics of Current Theories of Sustained Attention: How and Why Fatigue and Performance Changes over Time-on-Task

	Arousal Theories	Resource Theory	Motivation Control Theory	Resource-Control Theory
Characteristics of theory				
Influence of task demand	Low	High	Low	Low
Role of effort?	No	Yes	Yes	Yes
Role of attention	Diverted from main task Task-unrelated thought	Diminishes due to finite resource	Diverted from main task	Diverted from main task Task-unrelated thought
Supervisory control	Not considered	Not considered	High	High
Factors that influence time-on-task effects on performance				
Task difficulty	↑performance	↓performance	↓↑performance	↓performance
Task interest/ engagement	↑performance	↓performance	↑performance	↑performance
Secondary task	↑performance	↓↑performance	↓↑performance	↑performance
Rest breaks	↑performance	↑performance	↑performance	↑performance
Feedback	-	-	-	↑performance
Increase motivation	No change	No change	↑performance	↑performance

Up = increase performance, down = decrease performance.

control and resource control theories have added nuance and complexity by including the roles of motivation and executive control of attention and effort to explain time-on-task effects. These quite significant differences in focus of each theory also imply different approaches to mitigate and reduce time-on-task effects. These are discussed in next sections.

3.4.5 STRATEGIES FOR REDUCING TASK-RELATED FATIGUE EFFECTS

Research on strategies to overcome task-related effects on fatigue and performance exists but is somewhat disorganised. This section summarises the current evidence on strategies for reducing task-related fatigue effects.

3.4.5.1 THE EFFECTS OF REST BREAKS

Evidence from transport and elsewhere shows safety benefits of strategic breaks. Two case-control studies of truck crashes in Australia (Stevenson et al., 2014) and the US (Chen & Xie, 2014) showed, respectively, that crash risk significantly increased when rest breaks were not taken within four hours of driving and significantly decreased when two 30-minute rest breaks were taken over a 10-hour trip.

More fine-grained analysis from driving simulator studies suggests that the effects of rest breaks are not straightforward. A study of 8-hour night drives (Phipps-Nelson et al., 2011) confirmed that 1-hour breaks every 2 hours improved driving performance immediately following the break, but did not prevent an overall 2.5-fold deterioration in performance across the drive. Other studies of breaks during non-driving tasks also showed breaks improve performance over 60 to 90 minutes (Begum & Lehr 1962). Some studies indicate greater benefits of a break than introducing a secondary task (e.g., Ralph et al., 2017; Helton & Russell, 2015); however, these studies involved short study periods and short periods of rest.

It is not very surprising that breaks from driving help keep driving performance high as they interrupt the task and reduce time-on-task. The simulator studies suggest that breaks arrest the decline in performance over time but may not eliminate the time-on-task effect. More research is needed to clarify the best use of breaks, especially their timing and duration and whether their benefits are due to the change of activity or the opportunity for sleep.

3.4.5.2 CHANGE OF ACTIVITY APPROACHES

Based on most theories of sustained attention, a strategy involving change of activity would make the primary task more interesting and engaging. In a simulator study of monotonous 3-hour train driving, driving performance improved when speed limits were presented as a simple arithmetic task on 30 occasions over the trip compared to limits presented normally (Dunn & Williamson, 2012). Another study using the same strategy in a 2-hour monotonous car simulator drive failed to overcome the time-on-task effect (Zeller, et al., 2020), suggesting that this strategy was not sufficiently interesting in the context of a more challenging car driving task.

It is often not feasible to enhance the task itself in many transport operations, but it is possible to introduce a secondary task. Doing so, however, raises issues of distraction during tasks like driving and flying (e.g., Regan, Lee & Young, 2009). To avoid distraction secondary tasks cannot interfere visually or physically with the transport task and ideally should be able to be postponed if the primary task requires more attention.

Evaluation of different types of tasks for overcoming task-related fatigue effects in driving has mostly shown performance improvements. Verbal interactions or conversations during simulator drives improved performance when they occurred in the last 10-minutes of a 90-minute drive, but not when presented continuously throughout the drive which showed no advantage over passively listening to the radio or no secondary task (Atcherley et al., 2014). Other studies showed benefits for driving performance of having to converse (Kubose et al., 2006) or talk on a handsfree phone (Neubauer et al., 2014) while driving rather than simply listening although, again, these studies looked only at overall performance, not changes with time-on-task across the drive.

Trivia-type quizzes enhanced performance while on drives up to 2 hours long, but the benefit only lasted during the trivia quiz itself (e.g., Oran-Gilad et al., 2008; Song et al., 2017). Performance continued to deteriorate with time-on-task over the drive.

Many types of secondary task have been evaluated including number shadowing and recall tasks (He et al., 2014), driver selected gamebox activities (Verwey & Zaidel, 1999), song recognition (Trumbo et al., 2017), and listening to interesting and boring audio clips (Horrey et al., 2017). All studies found some performance improvements in the presence of a secondary task but most focussed only on effects on driving during the secondary task, not at effects over time on the drive. The exceptions were two studies where the driver had choice over aspects of the secondary task. The study by Verwey and Zaidel (1999) allowed drivers to choose the game and when they played it during a 135-minute simulator drive. Compared to the same drive without games, drivers were less drowsy and showed better performance. In the study by Trumbo et al. (2017), drivers chose the type of music for a song-naming game conducted halfway through a 60-minute simulator drive. Compared to the drive with no song-naming task, no time-on-task deterioration occurred on the drive with the song-recognition task. These two studies suggest that an appropriate secondary task can reduce time-on-task fatigue effects during a long drive, but more research is needed on what types of task will be most effective. These two studies suggest that driver preferences for the type and timing of the secondary task may be important.

3.4.5.3 TECHNOLOGY SOLUTIONS TO TASK-RELATED FATIGUE IN TRANSPORTATION

New technologies have been introduced to counteract fatigue in most transport modes. These typically warn drivers of signs of fatigue/drowsiness and some technologies tackle driver fatigue by partially or fully automating vehicle control, requiring drivers to passively monitor the technology for the need to resume control. This presents significant problems of making the driving task even more monotonous so increasing task-related fatigue and of getting the operator "back in the loop" when, or if, they are required to take back control. Multiple studies show that when resuming vehicle control, drivers need at least 2 to 5 seconds to regain awareness of the context (see Vogelpohl et al., 2018 for a review), with stable control only returning 35 to 40 seconds after technology disengages (Merat et al., 2014). Rather than solving the fatigue problem, current technology-based approaches may be producing more problems, for driving at least. Hancock (2021) argues that we must do better than the poorly designed human–technology interfaces that simply require more and longer sustained monitoring. He argues that interfaces should be more engaging and interesting even when the underlying task is repetitive and boring. Certainly, applying this approach would assist in reducing task-related fatigue in transportation.

3.4.6 SUMMARY AND CONCLUSIONS

Research shows that task-characteristics alone can cause fatigue and adverse effects on performance in transport operations. Furthermore, these task-related fatigue effects can be greater than those caused by sleep-related factors. The combination of task- and sleep-related factors produces the worst effects and therefore this should be avoided as a priority; however, task-related fatigue factors should not be overlooked as fatigue management cannot occur without addressing both sets of characteristics. Task- and sleep-related factors cause similar performance deficits in transport tasks, like more attentional lapses, poorer detection of critical information, and overall poorer performance.

In transport, apparently passive monitoring tasks that require sustained attention are common and of particular concern. The repetitive and monotonous nature of these tasks over time increases fatigue and performance deterioration as these characteristics make it hard and effortful to sustain attention and engagement. Effective strategies to overcome task-related fatigue effects include providing breaks from the task, and/or making the primary monitoring task more engaging and interesting. Introducing a secondary task may be effective if it is interesting and engaging and can be used as needed, but it must not distract or interfere with the driving task. Conversation tasks and trivia games show promise, although they may only be temporarily effective since when they are withdrawn, the time-on-task decline in fatigue and performance continues. More research is needed on effective countermeasures especially for passive task-related fatigue and time-on-task effects.

SUMMARY POINTS FOR PRACTITIONERS

- Fatigue due to task-related factors is a problem for transport at least as important as that due to sleep-related factors.
- Task-related characteristics like high time pressure, multitasking, and long periods of sustained monitoring can cause high levels of fatigue and significant deterioration of performance even in rested individuals.
- The combination of task- and sleep-related factors has strong negative effects on fatigue and performance, so management of fatigue in transport should address both sets of characteristics. It is not just about sleep.
- Effective strategies for managing task-related fatigue in general include timely rest breaks and, for passive monitoring tasks, enhancing interest and engagement in the task.

REFERENCES

Åkerstedt, T., & Folkard, S. (1997). The Three-process model of alertness and its extension to performance, sleep latency, and sleep length. *Chronobiology International, 14*(2), 115–123. doi:10.3109/07420529709001149

Atchley, P., Chan, M., & Gregersen, S. (2014). A strategically timed verbal task improves performance and neurophysiological alertness during fatiguing drives. *Human Factors, 56*(3), 453–462. doi:10.1177/0018720813500305

Balkin, T. J., & Wesensten, N. J. (2011). Differentiation of sleepiness and mental fatigue effects. In P. L. Ackerman (Ed.), *Cognitive fatigue: Multidisciplinary perspectives on current research and future* (pp. 47–66). Washington, D.C.: American Psychological Association.

Begum, B.O., & Lehr, D.J. (1962). Visual performance as a function of interpolated rest. *Journal of Applied Psychology, 46*,425–427. Doi:10.1037/h0043505

Carskadon, M. A., & Dement, W. C. (1982). The multiple sleep latency test: What does it measure? *Sleep, 5*(2), S67–S72.

Chen, C., & Xie, Y. (2014). Modeling the safety impacts of driving hours and rest breaks on truck drivers considering time-dependent covariates. *Journal of Safety Research, 51*, 57–63. doi:10.1016/j.jsr.2014.09.006

Cummings, P., Koepsell, T. D., Moffat, J. M., & Rivara, F. P. (2001). Drowsiness, counter-measures to drowsiness, and the risk of a motor vehicle crash. *Injury Prevention, 7*(3), 194–199.

Dawson, D., & McCulloch, K. (2005). Managing fatigue: It's about sleep. *Sleep Medicine Reviews, 9*(5), 365–380. doi:10.1016/j.smrv.2005.03.002

Desmond, P. A., & Hancock, P. A. (2000). Active and passive fatigue states. In A. Hancock & P. A. Desmond (Eds.), *Stress, workload, and fatigue* (pp. 455–465). Mahwah, NJ: Lawrence Erlbaum Associates Publishers; US.

Dinges, D.F., & Powell, J.W. (1985). Microcomputer analyses of performance on a portable, simple visual RT task during sustained operations. *Behavior Research Methods, Instruments, & Computers, 17*(6), 652–655.

Dunn, N., & Williamson, A. (2012). Driving monotonous routes in a train simulator: The effect of task demand on driving performance and subjective experience. *Ergonomics, 55*(9), 997–1008. doi:10.1080/00140139.2012.691994

Esterman, M., & Rothlein, D. (2019). Models of sustained attention. *Current Opinion in Psychology*, 29, 174–180. Doi:10.1016/j.copsyc.2019.03.006

Farahmand, B., & Bouroujerdian, A.M. (2018). Effect of road geometry on driver fatigue in monotonous environments: A simulator study. *Transportation Research Part F: Traffic Psychology and Behaviour*, 56, 640–651. doi10.1015/j.trf.2018.06.021

Friswell, R., &Williamson, A. (2008). Exploratory study of fatigue in light and short haul transport drivers in NSW, Australia. *Accident Analysis and Prevention*. 40(1), 410–417.

Hancock, P.A. (2021). Months of monotony-moments of mayhem: Planning for the human role in a transitioning world of work. *Theoretical Issues in Ergonomics Science, 22*(1), 63–82. doi:10.1080/1463922X.2020.1753260

Hancock, P. A., & Warm, J. S. (1989). A dynamic model of stress and sustained attention. *Human Factors, 31*(5), 519–537. doi:10.1177/001872088903100503

He, J., McCarley, J. S., & Kramer, A. F. (2014). Lane keeping under cognitive load: Performance changes and mechanisms. *Human Factors, 56*(2), 414–426. doi:10.1177/00187208 13485978

Helton, W. S., & Russell, P. N. (2015). Rest is best: The role of rest and task interruptions on vigilance. *Cognition, 134*, 165–173. doi:10.1016/j.cognition.2014.10.001

Hockey,G.R.(2013). *The psychology of fatigue: Work, effort and control.* Cambridge: Cambridge University Press.

Horrey, W. J., Lesch, M. F., Garabet, A., Simmons, L., & Maikala, R. (2017). Distraction and task engagement: How interesting and boring information impact driving performance and subjective and physiological responses. *Applied Ergonomics, 58*, 342–348. doi:10.1016/j.apergo.2016.07.011

Körber, M., Cingel, A., Zimmermann, M., & Bengler, K. (2015). Vigilance decrement and passive fatigue caused by monotony in automated driving. *Procedia Manufacturing, 3*, 2403–2409. doi:10.1016/j.promfg.2015.07.499

Kubose, T. T., Bock, K., Dell, G. S., Garnsey, S. M., Kramer, A. F., & Mayhugh, J. (2006). The effects of speech production and speech comprehension on simulated driving performance. *Applied Cognitive Psychology, 20*(1), 43–63. doi:10.1002/acp.1164

Matthews, G., & Desmond, P. A. (2002). Task-induced fatigue states and simulated driving performance. *Quarterly Journal of Experimental Psychology, 55A*(2), 659–686.

May, J. F., & Baldwin, C. L. (2009). Driver fatigue: The importance of identifying causal factors of fatigue when considering detection and countermeasure technologies. *Transportation Research Part F: Traffic Psychology and Behaviour, 12*(3), 218–224. doi:10.1016/j.trf.2008.11.005

Merat, N., Jamson, H. A., Lai, F., & Carsten, O. (2014). Human factors of highly automated driving: Results from the EASY and CityMobil projects. In G. Meyer and S. Beiker (Eds.), *Road Vehicle Automation, Lecture Notes in Mobility.* doi:10.1007/978-3-319-05990-7_11

Neubauer, C., Matthews, G., & Saxby, D. (2014). Fatigue in the automated vehicle: Do games and conversation distract or energize the driver? *Proceedings of the human factors and ergonomics society annual meeting, 58*(1), 2053–2057. doi:10.1177/1541931214581432

Oron-Gilad, T., Ronen, A., & Shinar, D. (2008). Alertness maintaining tasks (AMTs) while driving. *Accident Analysis and Prevention, 40*(3), 851–860. doi:10.1016/j.aap.2007.09.026

Parasuraman, R. Warm, J. S. & Dember, W. N. (1987). Vigilance taxonomy and utility. In L.S. Mark, J.S. Warm & R.S. Huston, (Eds.*), Ergonomics and human factors: Recent research.* New York: Springer-Verlag, pp. 11–32.

Peiris, M. T. R., Jones,R. D., Davidson, P. R., Carroll,G. J. & Bones, P. J. (2006). Frequent lapses of responsiveness duri ng an extended visuomotor tracking task in non-sleep-deprived subjects. *Journal of Sleep Research, 15*, 291–300.

Philip, P., Sagaspe, P., Moore, N., Taillard, J., Charles, A., Guilleminault, C., & Bioulac, B. (2005). Fatigue, sleep restriction and driving performance. *Accident Analysis and Prevention, 37*(3), 473–478. doi:10.1016/j.aap.2004.07.007

Phipps-Nelson, J., Redman, J. R., & Rajaratnam, S. M. (2011). Temporal profile of prolonged, night-time driving performance: Breaks from driving temporarily reduce time-on-task fatigue but not sleepiness. *Journal of Sleep Research, 20*(3), 404–415. doi:10.1111/j.1365-2869.2010.00900.x

Pop, V. L., Stearman, E. J., Kazi, S., & Durso, F. T. (2012). Using engagement to negate vigilance decrements in the NextGen environment. *International Journal of Human-Computer Interaction, 28*, 99–106.

Powell, D. M. C., Spencer, M. B., Holland, D., Broadbent, E., & Petrie, K. J. (2007). Pilot fatigue in short-haul operations: Effects of number of sectors, duty length, and time of day. *Aviation, Space, and Environmental Medicine, 78*(7), 698–701.

Ralph, B. C., Onderwater, K., Thomson, D. R., & Smilek, D. (2017). Disrupting monotony while increasing demand: benefits of rest and intervening tasks on vigilance. *Psychological Research, 81*(2), 432–444. doi:10.1007/s00426-016-0752-7

Regan, M. A., Lee, J. D., & Young, K. L. (Eds.). (2009). *Driver distraction: Theory, effects, and mitigation.* Boca Raton, FL: CRC Press.

Robertson, I. H., Manly, T., Andrade, J., Baddeley, B. T., & Yiend, J. (1997). 'Oops!': Performance correlates of everyday attentional failures in traumatic brain injured and normal subjects. *Neuropsychologia, 35*(6), 747–758. doi:10.1016/s0028-3932(97)00015-8

Sallinen, M., Harma, M., Akila, R., Holm, A., Luukkonen, R., Mikola, H., Muller, K., & Virkkala, J., (2004). The effects of sleep debt and monotonous work on sleepiness and performance during a 12-h dayshift. *Journal of Sleep Research,* 13 (4), 285–294.

Saxby, D., Matthews, G., Warm, J. S., Hitchcock, E. M., & Neubauer, C. (2013). Active and passive fatigue in simulated driving: Discriminating styles of workload regulation and their safety impacts. *Journal of Experimental Psychology Applied, 19*(4), 287–300. doi:10.1037/a0034386

Smallwood, J., & Schooler, J. W. (2006). The restless mind. *Psychological Bulletin, 132*(6), 946–958. doi:10.1037/0033-2909.132.6.946

Soares, S., Ferreira, S., & Couto, A. (2020). Driving simulator experiments to study drowsiness: A systematic review. *Traffic Injury Prevention, 21*(1), 29–37. doi: 10.1080/15389588.2019.1706088

Song, W., Woon, F. L., Doong, A., Persad, C., Tijerina, L., Pandit, P.,... . Giordani, B. (2017). Fatigue in younger and older drivers: Effectiveness of an alertness-maintaining task. *Human Factors, 59*(6), 995–1008. doi:10.1177/0018720817706811

Stevenson, M. R., Elkington, J., Sharwood, L., Meuleners, L., Ivers, R., Boufous, S.,... . Wong, K. (2014). The role of sleepiness, sleep disorders, and the work environment on heavy-vehicle crashes in 2 Australian states. *American Journal of Epidemiology, 179*(5), 594–601. doi:10.1093/aje/kwt305

Thiffault, P., & Bergeron, J. (2003). Monotony of road environment and driver fatigue: A simulator study. *Accident Analysis and Prevention, 35*(3), 381–391. doi:10.1016/s0001-4575(02)00014-3

Thomson, D. R., Besner, D., & Smilek, D. (2015). A resource-control account of sustained attention: Evidence from mind-wandering and vigilance paradigms. *Perspectives in Psychological Science, 10*(1), 82–96. doi:10.1177/1745691614556681

Trumbo, M. C., Jones, A. P., Robinson, C. S. H., Cole, K., & Morrow, J. D. (2017). Name that tune: Mitigation of driver fatigue via a song naming game. *Accident Analysis and Prevention, 108*, 275–284. doi:10.1016/j.aap.2017.09.002

Verwey, W. B., & Zaidel, D. M. (1999). Preventing drowsiness accidents by an alertness maintenance device. *Accident Analysis and Prevention, 31*(3), 199–211. Retrieved from www.ncbi.nlm.nih.gov/pubmed/10196596

Vogelpohl, T., Kühn, M., Hummel, T., Gehlert, T., & Vollrath, M., (2018). Transitioning to manual driving requires additional time after automation deactivation. *Transportation Research Part F: Traffic Psychology and Behaviour, 55*, 464–482. doi: 10.1016/j.trf.2018.03.019

Warm, J. S., & Parasuraman, R. (Eds.) (1987). Vigilance: Basic and applied research (Special Issue). *Human Factors, 29.*

Warm, J. S., Parasuraman, R., & Matthews, G. (2008). Vigilance requires hard mental work and is stressful. *Human Factors, 50*(3), 433–441. doi:10.1518/001872008X312152

Welford, A. T. (1962). Arousal, channel-capacity and decision. *Nature, 194*(4826), 365–366.

Wickens, C. (2021). Attention: Theory, principles, models and applications. *International Journal Of Human-Computer Interaction, 37*(5), 403–417. doi:0.1080/10447318.2021.1874741

Yerkes, R. M., & Dodson, J. D. (1908). The relation of strength of stimulus to rapidity of habit-formation. *Journal of Comparative Neurology and Psychology, 18*(5), 459–482. doi:10.1002/cne.920180503

Zeller, R., Williamson, A., & Friswell, R. (2020). The effect of sleep-need and time-on-task on driver fatigue. *Transportation Research Part F: Traffic Psychology and Behaviour, 74*, 15–29. doi:10.1016/j.trf.2020.08.001

3.5 Lifestyle as a Mediator of Fatigue and Sleepiness

Melissa A. Ulhôa,[1] Elaine C. Marqueze,[2] and Claudia R. C. Moreno[3,4]

[1]Faculty of Medicine, Educational Union of Vale do Aço, Ipatinga, MG, Brazil
[2]Department of Epidemiology, School of Public Health, Catholic University of Santos, SP, Brazil
[3]Department of Health, Life cycles, and Society, School of Public Health, University of São Paulo, SP, Brazil
[4]Stress Research Institute, Psychology Department, Stockholm University, Stockholm, Sweden

CONTENTS

3.5.1 INTRODUCTION

A long-haul truck driver who works for a transportation company has many goals to achieve in order to fulfil his/her task. In general, work timing varies according to the load demand. This means it is difficult to control the delivery time since it depends on several factors, such as road condition, type of vehicle, traffic, and distance. According to the type of load, delivery time is crucial to keep the load safe. However, regardless of the type of load, there is always time pressure on the driver that can contribute to a fatigue condition.

DOI: 10.1201/9781003213154-21

Although fatigue is a factor that has been comprehensively studied among workers, the mediation of lifestyle factors to develop or aggravate fatigue is not commonly presented. In other words, to mitigate fatigue in the transportation sector, it is important to consider that the driver who has to deliver the load on time has to sleep, eat, and drink. Moreover, the driver should not take medications or any substance that can disturb driving. These factors are part of the driver's lifestyle, that is, how a person or group lives. This means that the driver's habits may influence his/her performance behind the wheel. This scenario is also applicable for other types of workers involved in the transportation sector. This chapter brings to the reader a discussion about how lifestyle is relevant to reducing or avoiding fatigue and how society can influence lifestyle.

3.5.2   LIFESTYLE AND FATIGUE/SLEEPINESS

Sleepiness per se is a biological behaviour characterised by an increased probability of falling asleep. Alertness is the opposite. When sleepiness is chronic, it is called excessive sleepiness or hypersomnia, in which the person has difficulty staying awake and alert. Fatigue, on the other hand, refers to mental and physical conditions, including sleepiness. Although sleepiness and fatigue are interlinked and can coincide, there is a difference between sleepiness and fatigue (Åkerstedt & Wright, 2009; Schwartz et al., 2009).

According to the Canadian Centre for Occupational Health and Safety (2017), fatigue is "the state of feeling very tired, weary or sleepy resulting from insufficient sleep, prolonged mental or physical work, or extended periods of stress or anxiety". Regardless of its origin, fatigue can strongly affect the functional ability and quality of life (Smith et al., 2005). According to Åkerstedt and Wright (2009), fatigue can be reduced by resting. Conversely, rest (without sleep) or engaging in a sedentary activity will exacerbate sleepiness.

Excessive sleepiness may occur due to several factors like chronic sleep deprivation, sleep disturbances, and the effects of drugs use (Bittencourt et al., 2005). On the other hand, fatigue is mainly due to working conditions such as irregular hours, long hours, and working in different time zones. Excessive sleepiness and fatigue are associated with individual factors such as age, health status, sedentary lifestyle, and alcohol consumption (Sack, 2010; van Drongelen et al., 2017). Some occupations present high risks of fatigue, specifically those that include night work and long working hours, as is the case with occupations in the transport sector.

It is essential to highlight that a large part of the population currently has short sleep episodes, that is, they sleep less than what is necessary for health maintenance. According to Shockey and Wheaton (2017), 36.5% of workers reported sleeping less than 7 hours per night on average. It is worth mentioning that sleep disturbances, long work hours, shift work, the effects of certain medications, lack of exposure to natural light, and exposure to artificial light often at odd hours cause reduced sleep (Caldwell et al., 2019; Moreno et al., 2019). In addition, food intake also appears to affect sleepiness. In a study of truck drivers, Martins et al. (2019) verified that, compared to unhealthy patterns, healthy dietary patterns were associated with low sleepiness ratings during the day.

The relationship between work and fatigue is not always intuitive. Several studies have analysed the impact of sleepiness and fatigue on work performance, accident risks, and lifestyle, as well as the inverse relationship—the impact of work on fatigue. Although physical activity is recommended as a strategy for improving sleep, compared to low physical activity occupations, those with intense physical effort requirements and more significant musculoskeletal fatigue are more likely to be associated with sleep disturbances (Martins et al., 2016).

Another fatigue-related organisational factor is demanding work schedules, such as those that require many consecutive workdays. Jeklin et al. (2021) found that lower heart rate variability (HRV) was correlated with high level of fatigue. According to the authors, these results demonstrated that the gradual development of fatigue ultimately affected rest days, leading to poorer sleep quality. In a systematic review on HRV and sleepiness, fatigue, and stress, the authors concluded that HRV is an important monitoring marker of these variables among car drivers, which can prevent accidents (Burlacu et al., 2021).

Besides that, workers and employers use different behavioural and environmental strategies to combat the effects of fatigue. Sagah Zadeh et al. (2018) identified the following popular strategies: dietary interventions, physical, cognitive, sensory, and social stimuli, healthier lifestyles, naps at work, and exposure to natural light. Similarly, there is guidance on scientifically proven strategies to improve sleep and minimise fatigue (Caldwell et al., 2019). These authors recommend providing educational guidelines for workers, management, and family about the dangers of fatigue and the importance of adequate sleep (quality and quantity). In addition, they suggest providing opportunities for naps during working hours, facilitating regular sleep schedules, using fatigue monitoring tools, and proposing pharmacological interventions when necessary.

Some studies indicate a bidirectional influence between lifestyle and fatigue, with physical and behavioural consequences. According to Kuo et al. (2022), fatigue is a barrier to the practice of physical activity, as well as to the adoption of healthy eating habits, thus directly reducing their quality of life. Moreover, fatigue might be a risk of worsening a pre-existing disease and a factor of reduced survival. On the other hand, several diseases and treatments can be risk factors for the development of fatigue, like anxiety, depression, insomnia, type 2 diabetes mellitus, and obesity (Kuo et al., 2022). Some of these diseases have a high prevalence among truck drivers, such as metabolic diseases, sleep problems, and mental disorders (Moreno et al., 2006; Marqueze et al., 2012; Martins et al., 2019; Rocha et al., 2022). In this way, we can conclude that fatigue interferes with the balance between work and personal life and that a bidirectional relationship exists between lifestyle and fatigue and sleepiness.

3.5.3 LIFESTYLE, BEHAVIOUR, STRESS, AND THEIR RELATIONSHIP WITH FATIGUE AND SLEEPINESS

Lifestyle is a way of living, habits, attitudes, moral standards, and other factors that together constitute the mode of living of a person or a group. This section presents how some aspects of lifestyle can mediate fatigue, regardless of its cause (Johansson et al., 2021). Physical activity, diet, use of medicines, tobacco, and alcohol consumption are some critical aspects of lifestyle that contribute to fatigue. Yet, others—such as spirituality, therapeutic practices, meditation, and how one organises one's rest-activity cycle—can lessen one's risk of experiencing fatigue. Some of these factors are presented below.

3.5.3.1 PHYSICAL ACTIVITY AND EXERCISE

Physical activity, for instance, can cause or relieve physical fatigue, depending on the intensity, duration, and frequency. Specifically, studies have found beneficial effects of aerobic exercises on fatigue when it is regular and performed with moderate intensity (Mohandas et al., 2017). Aerobic training was associated with improved energy and decreased fatigue since it reduced the amount of effort to accomplish regular daily activities. Physical exercise can be a non-pharmacological treatment for fatigue (Mohandas et al., 2017). Taylor and Dorn (2006) affirm that physical activity may improve driving performance and reduce accident risk. Exercises have enhanced sleep and alertness, reduced fatigue, and improved cognitive functioning. Non-sedentary lifestyle can improve psychological and physical health status. There is evidence in the literature that professional drivers are less active than the population in general, which should be changed for better personal and social outcomes. On the other hand, despite this known beneficial effect of moderate exercise, high-intensity and long duration training can lead to fatigue and sleep problems.

In fact, physical exercise increases functional capacity and decreases efforts to realise daily activities. Compared to rest, regular exercise on most days of the week can reduce fatigue. The timing of practicing physical exercise appears to be critical; for example, exercise near bedtime should be avoided to allow for good, restorative sleep (van Rensburg et al., 2020). Similarly, a 15-month prospective study of nurses' aides showed that physical leisure activities reduce the risk of developing persistent fatigue (Eriksen & Bruusgaard, 2004). In summary, physical activity can help fatigue symptoms if it is of short duration and mild intensity (or moderate, at most).

3.5.3.2 FOOD AND DRINK

Equally important to exercise is food intake since it may lead to fatigue. Food intake can affect the body's master circadian clock, situated in the suprachiasmatic nucleus (SCN) and the peripheral clocks, present in most cells of all body tissues. Fewer symptoms of fatigue were observed in cabin crew that had eaten three regular meals a day and were synchronised with the light-dark cycle on arrival local time (Ruscitto et al., 2017). Measuring the phase of the circadian system and adequate timing of meal interventions can be challenging in real life (van Rensburg et al., 2020). Then, food should be taken during the activities period of the day.

Caffeine is the most consumed and socially accepted stimulant worldwide. Caffeine is a stimulant because it acts as an antagonist on adenosine receptors in the nervous system, thus stimulating the release of excitatory neurotransmitters. Because of this effect, caffeine produces greater mental alertness, wakefulness, cognitive performance, reaction time improvement, and general motor performance (Meeusen &

Decroix, 2018; Repantis et al., 2021). Caffeine may not be useful if used excessively early before a shift begins or too late during or after a shift. Concerning its stimulant effects, caffeine consumption must be avoided near bedtime to achieve good sleep quality and duration (Gurubhagavatula et al., 2021).

Natural and herbal supplements may also impact fatigue. Meeusen and Decroix (2018) reviewed the effects of water and supplements on performance and found that mild hypohydration significantly increased minor driving errors while performing the same task in a hydrated condition. This result should be a consequence of reductions in concentration and alertness secondary to hypohydration (Watson & Mears, 2015). There is evidence that herbal extracts such as polyphenols, ginseng, ginkgo biloba, and guarana (*Paullinia cupana*, a stimulant derived from an Amazonian plant) are marketed as supplements that can be taken to avoid sleepiness and fatigue. These plants may influence brain functioning, but there is a need for well-controlled randomised studies on fatigue effects. Not a plant but an amino acid, tyrosine is fully necessary for the synthesis of some neurotransmitter systems (5-HT and dopamine) associated with feelings of fatigue, and fatigue and lethargy are associated with neurotransmitter imbalance in the central nervous system. Thus, tyrosine has been accepted by nutritionists and physicians as a supplement against fatigue (Meeusen & Decroix, 2018).

Consuming exogenous melatonin is another strategy to recover from fatigue (van Rensburg et al., 2020). Shift workers who invert their rest-activity cycle present changes in concentrations of melatonin, cortisol, ghrelin, and leptin, for example. These physiological changes can negatively affect sleep and contribute to sedentarism, unhealthy eating habits, and stress. Regarding stress, most studies indicate that working shifts (as opposed to a regular schedule), per se, is a stressor, and this condition is intensified when work is associated with job strain (Ulhôa et al., 2015). Thus, melatonin reduces the time needed for resynchronisation of the circadian system and helps manage fatigue and sleep disturbances following ingestion by long-haul travel and shift workers.

3.5.3.3 Sleep Hygiene

People should sleep enough to rest and recover from activities done during wakefulness. Sleep "hygiene" includes the following strategies: a predictable sleep routine; avoiding exercise near bedtime; daytime exposure to bright light and avoiding light near bedtime; minimising light and noise exposure (e.g., using a cell phone or television) near bedtime; taking a warm bath before bedtime; avoiding caffeine, nicotine, alcohol, and excessive food or fluid intake in the evening; and emptying the bladder just before going to bed. Naps may also help but should be limited to less than 1 hour and should be scheduled earlier in the day rather than near bedtime (Ulhôa et al., 2022).

3.5.3.4 Medications

There are many drugs available to treat sleep problems by improving sleep quality and duration, and some substances can also be used to reduce fatigue or diurnal sleepiness. Methylphenidate has positive effects on self-reported fatigue because of its psychostimulant properties. This substance is a catecholamine reuptake inhibitor mainly used in the treatment of attention-deficit/hyperactivity disorder (Repantis et al., 2021). It acts fast and is generally well-tolerated and safe. However, it should be used with caution in patients with heart disease and other conditions. Modafinil has been largely used to treat some sleep disorders, such as insomnia, for instance. It is a non-amphetamine central nervous system stimulant. It is also used to treat drowsiness and fatigue with positive results (Murillo-Rodríguez et al., 2018, Repantis et al., 2021). Carnitine is an important intermediary in fat metabolism. It seems a reasonable approach to fatigue for its metabolic cell effect and plays a vital role in energy production (Flanagan et al., 2010).

In people with idiopathic fatigue, antidepressant therapy is suggested for depressive symptoms, even if they do not meet the diagnostic criteria for major depression. In these cases, a selective serotonin reuptake inhibitor is often recommended.

Alcohol and tobacco have negative impacts on fatigue. Heavy alcohol consumption impairs sleep quality, which is associated with increased next day hangover severity (Devenney et al., 2019). As explained in earlier section, poor sleep quality is correlated to fatigue. Moreover, alcohol hangover and increased lapses were statistically associated with impairing simulated highway driving performance (Verster et al., 2014). Undoubtedly, driving under the influence of alcohol and fatigue are the most important factors contributing to the severity of large truck crashes (Li et al., 2020a). Then, avoiding alcohol and mitigating fatigue can prevent severe large truck crashes. Additionally, alcohol consumption is associated with a high risk of sleep apnoea and more generally poorer health outcomes (Devenney et al., 2019).

The acute effects of tobacco are related to sympathetic nervous system stimuli, and there are observed associations between tobacco and fatigue's impact on physical and psychosocial functioning. This suggests that smoking cessation is a potential target in fatigue management (Johansson et al., 2021). Moreover, non-smoking was associated with a lower impact of fatigue (Kahraman et al., 2021).

3.5.3.5 Other Cognitive-Behavioural Interventions

In contrast to other well-known interventions, there are cognitive-behavioural strategies to be considered to diminish fatigue, such as yoga, group therapy, and stress management. For example, for fatigue related to cancer and its treatment, Tai Chi and acupuncture have been found in clinical trials to minimise the effects of fatigue (Mohandas et al., 2017; Li et al., 2020b). Possible biological mechanisms for these effects have been suggested, such as decreasing inflammatory response.

Cognitive-behavioural therapy (CBT) and psychosocial interventions (including mindfulness-based stress reduction) are effective strategies for reducing fatigue. It is a non-invasive therapy that can make fatigue awareness, reorient behaviours, and help the patient gain control over fatigue symptoms. This intervention, combined with other strategies, can achieve better results in fatigue management (Johns et al., 2016; Mohandas et al., 2017).

Despite some scepticism, the literature shows evidence of the effect of spirituality/religiosity (S/R) on fatigue and health. Spirituality is the personal development that draws people to forge meaning in life through spiritual transcendence. It is associated with better physical health and psychological well-being. Trusting in God, prayer, optimistic spiritual connections, forgiveness, and other coping activities and beliefs activate coping strategies for better health outcomes (Counted et al., 2018). On the other hand, it is important to expose possible adverse effects of S/R on health. For example, some situations may lead to religious distress. Excessively rigid or intolerant precepts can be a source of S/R suffering, such as when attitudes include a "passive deferral to God", "attributing all problems to the devil", or "intolerant precepts leading to inappropriate guilt" (Moreira-Almeida et al., 2014). The positive effect of S/R on health seems to be due to how the body copes with distress and neurotransmitters in the nervous system. Correlations have been reported between S/R and biological marks such as dopamine, serotonin, vesicular transporters, and oxytocin. However, more research is needed in this area (Anderson et al., 2017). Overall, studies suggest that focusing on the spiritual or religious dimension might be an effective approach to fatigue and general health management.

3.5.4 SOCIETY AS A DRIVE TO DETERMINE LIFESTYLE

Lifestyle (how a person lives) is not only about individual choices but also about political, social, economic, and environmental issues. Some political decisions lead to the determination of school time, for example. The government regime of a country grants or does not offer autonomy to schools to choose the times at which classes start and end. Private schools generally have more freedom than public schools to make these choices. It is the same for factories, companies, and services, which follow the local demands, regulations, and policies. Our mandatory activities and behaviours (school, work, eating, sleeping, etc.) are thus regulated by somebody else's decisions instead of our own. In other words, we have to eat during our lunch break at work (no matter whether it lasts 15 minutes or 2 hours) and sleep when we are not working. This means that the range for choosing how to live our lives is quite limited.

Philosophers, sociologists, and historians analyse in detail the effects of the organisation of society on the lives of people in different population groups. Han and Butler (2015) provide an interesting analysis of contemporary society. According to them, society has gone through important transitions over the years. More recently, there was an incentive and, more than that, demand for production based on workers' motivation in what has been called a performance society. Marked by an excess of positivity, contemporary society imposes the idea that anything is possible if people try hard enough. Failing to achieve self-imposed goals leads individuals to depression, burnout, and complete exhaustion. These aspects are at the heart of Han and Butler's argument in which they conceptualise today's society as the burnout society (Han & Butler, 2015). This idea supports the observation that today's lifestyle is imposed by obligations we force ourselves to fulfil at any cost.

Another concept regarding the effects of the process of modernisation on our society has been proposed by Harmut Rosa, who refers to changes taking place in the temporal patterns and structures of society, what he called "social acceleration" (Rosa, 2013). The general feeling of time pressure, which Rosa acknowledges as a feature of modern societies, results from the fact that the time required to fulfil our tasks exceeds the available time. Modern societies organise life in a way that does not consider the limits of 24 hours a day or 365 days a year.

Work fills a large part of life. If we think about an 8-hour workday, there are only 16 hours left for personal and family care, food intake, sleep, and leisure. For many people, a 24-hour day is insufficient for everything we need (and want) to do. It is possible to speculate that this is why many people consider sleep a waste of time; however, sleep is essential to feel well-being and avoid accidents (Chaput, 2010).

Moreover, as mentioned previously, there is a common tendency in today's society that thinking positively makes anything possible. Why should I sleep if I have so little time left in the day for leisure, for example? The answer lies in thousands of studies on the adverse effects of sleep restriction, including the aggravation or development of numerous diseases. Furthermore, it is believed that sleep can happen at any time of day without causing any harm to health (Robbins et al., 2019).

What seems to be behind the concepts proposed by the mentioned authors is how a society deals with the demands of its economic system. We reach a situation of chronic fatigue in a fast-paced society that seeks the best performance, always confident, thinking positively that the time spent on work is the most important. The current lifestyle does not leave time for adequate sleep and rest. Next, we present the main consequences of reduced sleep and rest—fatigue and sleepiness, which in turn have been found to contribute to the development of several diseases.

3.5.5 CONCLUSIONS

Lifestyle can be a mediator of fatigue (Figure 3.5.1). Some habits can increase the symptoms of fatigue, such as excessive alcohol consumption, tobacco use, poor

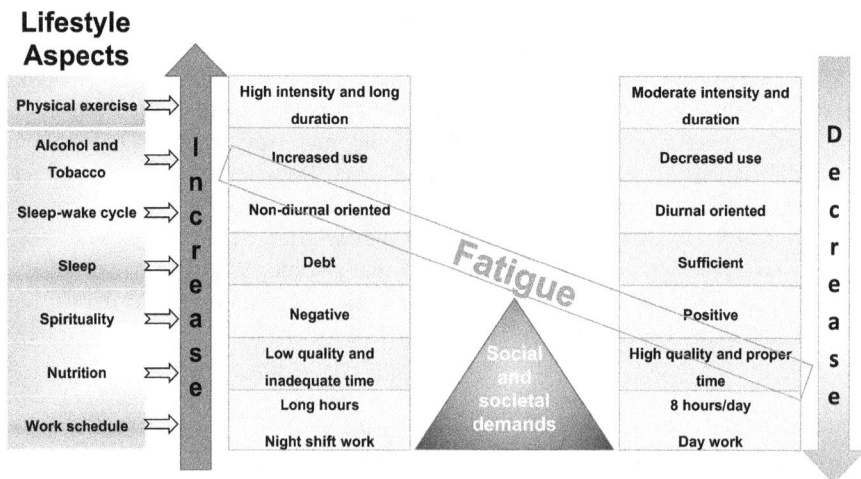

FIGURE 3.5.1　Lifestyle factors as a mediator for fatigue.

nutrition, and sleep debts. On the other hand, moderate physical activity, good nutrition, and sufficient sleep can minimise fatigue. It is essential to manage one's level of stress while at the same time keeping a balance between time dedicated to work and time for adequate sleep and social life (leisure).

Lifestyle varies according to location, work hours, socio-economic status, and many other aspects the individual does not necessarily choose. Political, social, economic, and environmental issues are directly linked to our lifestyle. Today's Western society imposes a rhythm of life that often makes a healthy lifestyle difficult or impossible to achieve. Some occupations are organised without considering adequate time for resting and leisure, which can increase the risk of fatigue and lead to accidents at work. Thus, work-related fatigue could be reduced with adequate work organisation and fatigue management.

Lastly, fatigue is interlinked to sleepiness, and both may occur simultaneously or not. Although sleepiness is a normal biological condition, it can occur at undesirable times and/or become chronic. In conclusion, fatigue has an interrelationship with lifestyle factors. Some of them can decrease (i.e., mild physical activity/good nutrition), and others can exacerbate fatigue (tobacco/alcohol/sleep problems). It is important to know about them to manage fatigue symptoms.

SUMMARY POINTS FOR PRACTITIONERS

- Political, social, economic, and environmental issues are directly linked to our lifestyle.
- From the individual point of view, the practice of physical activity and adequate nutrition avoid or minimise the development of fatigue.
- From the viewpoint of work organisation in the transport sector, it is necessary that working hours allow for adequate sleep duration and quality (according to individual needs).
- Spirituality and relaxation methods can help reduce fatigue.
- Tobacco, alcohol, and use of drugs can exacerbate fatigue.

REFERENCES

Åkerstedt, T., & Wright, K. P., Jr (2009). Sleep loss and fatigue in shift work and shift work disorder. *Sleep Medicine Clinics, 4*(2), 257–271. https://doi.org/10.1016/j.jsmc.2009.03.001

Anderson, M. R., Miller, L., Wickramaratne, P., Svob, C., Odgerel, Z., Zhao, R., & Weissman, M. M. (2017). Genetic correlates of spirituality/religion and depression: A study in offspring and grandchildren at high and low familial risk for depression. *Spirituality in Clinical Practice (Washington, D.C.), 4*(1), 43–63. https://doi.org/10.1037/scp0000125

Bittencourt, L. R., Silva, R. S., Santos, R. F., Pires, M. L., & Mello, M. T. (2005). Sonolência excessiva [Excessive daytime sleepiness]. *Revista brasileira de psiquiatria (Sao Paulo, Brazil: 1999), 27 Suppl 1*, 16–21. https://doi.org/10.1590/s1516-44462005000500004

Burlacu, A., Brinza, C., Brezulianu, A., & Covic, A. (2021). Accurate and early detection of sleepiness, fatigue and stress levels in drivers through heart rate variability parameters: A systematic review. *Reviews in Cardiovascular Medicine, 22*(3), 845–852. https://doi.org/10.31083/j.rcm2203090

Caldwell, J. A., Caldwell, J. L., Thompson, L. A., & Lieberman, H. R. (2019). Fatigue and its management in the workplace. *Neuroscience and Biobehavioral Reviews*, *96*, 272–289. https://doi.org/10.1016/j.neubiorev.2018.10.024

Canadian Centre for Occupational Health and Safety (2017). OSH Answers Fact Sheet: Fatigue. Updated August 2017; https://ccohs.ca/oshanswers/ psychosocial/fatigue.html.

Chaput J. P. (2010). A good night's sleep for a healthier population. *American Journal of Preventive Medicine*, *38*(3), 349. https://doi.org/10.1016/j.amepre.2009.10.043

Counted, V., Possamai, A., & Meade, T. (2018). Relational spirituality and quality of life 2007 to 2017: An integrative research review. *Health and Quality of Life Outcomes*, *16*(1), 75. https://doi.org/10.1186/s12955-018-0895-x

Devenney, L. E., Coyle, K. B., Roth, T., & Verster, J. C. (2019). Sleep after heavy alcohol consumption and physical activity levels during alcohol hangover. *Journal of Clinical Medicine*, *8*(5), 752. https://doi.org/10.3390/jcm8050752

Eriksen, W., & Bruusgaard, D. (2004). Do physical leisure time activities prevent fatigue? A 15 month prospective study of nurses' aides. *British Journal of Sports Medicine*, *38*(3), 331–336. https://doi.org/10.1136/bjsm.2002.004390

Flanagan, J. L., Simmons, P. A., Vehige, J., Willcox, M. D., & Garrett, Q. (2010). Role of carnitine in disease. *Nutrition & Metabolism*, *7*, 30. https://doi.org/10.1186/1743-7075-7-30

Gurubhagavatula, I., Barger, L. K., Barnes, C. M., Basner, M., Boivin, D. B., Dawson, D., Drake, C. L., Flynn-Evans, E. E., Mysliwiec, V., Patterson, P. D., Reid, K. J., Samuels, C., Shattuck, N. L., Kazmi, U., Carandang, G., Heald, J. L., & Van Dongen, H. (2021). Guiding principles for determining work shift duration and addressing the effects of work shift duration on performance, safety, and health: guidance from the American Academy of Sleep Medicine and the Sleep Research Society. *Journal of Clinical Sleep Medicine: JCSM: official publication of the American Academy of Sleep Medicine*, *17*(11), 2283–2306. https://doi.org/10.5664/jcsm.9512

Han, B. C., Butler, E. (2015). *The burnout society.* http://site.ebrary.com/id/11071027.

Jeklin, A. T., Perrotta, A. S., Davies, H. W., Bredin, S., Paul, D. A., & Warburton, D. (2021). The association between heart rate variability, reaction time, and indicators of work-place fatigue in wildland firefighters. *International Archives of Occupational and Environmental Health*, *94*(5), 823–831. https://doi.org/10.1007/s00420-020-01641-3

Johansson, S., Skjerbæk, A. G., Nørgaard, M., Boesen, F., Hvid, L. G., & Dalgas, U. (2021). Associations between fatigue impact and lifestyle factors in people with multiple sclerosis–The Danish MS hospitals rehabilitation study. *Multiple Sclerosis and Related Disorders*, *50*, 102799. https://doi.org/10.1016/j.msard.2021.102799

Johns, S. A., Brown, L. F., Beck-Coon, K., Talib, T. L., Monahan, P. O., Giesler, R. B., Tong, Y., Wilhelm, L., Carpenter, J. S., Von Ah, D., Wagner, C. D., de Groot, M., Schmidt, K., Monceski, D., Danh, M., Alyea, J. M., Miller, K. D., & Kroenke, K. (2016). Randomized controlled pilot trial of mindfulness-based stress reduction compared to psychoeducational support for persistently fatigued breast and colorectal cancer survivors. *Supportive Care in Cancer: official journal of the Multinational Association of Supportive Care in Cancer*, *24*(10), 4085–4096. https://doi.org/10.1007/s00520-016-3220-4

Kahraman, T., Ozdogar, A. T., Abasiyanik, Z., Ozakbas, S., & Multiple Sclerosis Research Group (2021). Associations between smoking and walking, fatigue, depression, and health-related quality of life in persons with multiple sclerosis. *Acta Neurologica Belgica*, *121*(5), 1199–1206. https://doi.org/10.1007/s13760-020-01341-2

Kuo, H. J., Huang, Y. C., & García, A. A. (2022). An integrative review of fatigue in adults with type 2 diabetes mellitus: Implications for self-management and quality of life. *Journal of Clinical Nursing*, *31*(11–12), 1409–1427. https://doi.org/10.1111/jocn.16058

Li, J., Liu, J., Liu, P., & Qi, Y. (2020a). Analysis of factors contributing to the severity of large truck crashes. *Entropy (Basel, Switzerland)*, *22*(11), 1191. https://doi.org/10.3390/e22111191

Li, X., Wang, X., Song, L., Tian, J., Ma, X., Mao, Q., Lin, H., & Zhang, Y. (2020b). Effects of Qigong, Tai Chi, acupuncture, and Tuina on cancer-related fatigue for breast cancer patients: A protocol of systematic review and meta-analysis. *Medicine*, *99*(45), e23016. https://doi.org/10.1097/MD.0000000000023016

Marqueze, E. C., Ulhôa, M. A., & Moreno, C. R. (2012). Irregular working times and metabolic disorders among truck drivers: A review. *Work (Reading, Mass.)*, *41 Suppl 1*, 3718–3725. https://doi.org/10.3233/WOR-2012-0085-3718

Martins, A. J., Martini, L. A., & Moreno, C. (2019). Prudent diet is associated with low sleepiness among short-haul truck drivers. *Nutrition (Burbank, Los Angeles County, Calif.)*, *63–64*, 61–68. https://doi.org/10.1016/j.nut.2018.11.023

Martins, A. J., Vasconcelos, S. P., Skene, D. J., Lowden, A., & de Castro Moreno, C. R. (2016). Effects of physical activity at work and life-style on sleep in workers from an Amazonian Extractivist Reserve. *Sleep Science (Sao Paulo, Brazil)*, *9*(4), 289–294. https://doi.org/10.1016/j.slsci.2016.10.001

Meeusen, R., & Decroix, L. (2018). Nutritional supplements and the brain. *International Journal of Sport Nutrition and Exercise Metabolism*, *28*(2), 200–211. https://doi.org/10.1123/ijsnem.2017-0314

Mohandas, H., Jaganathan, S. K., Mani, M. P., Ayyar, M., & Rohini Thevi, G. V. (2017). Cancer-related fatigue treatment: An overview. *Journal of Cancer Research and Therapeutics*, *13*(6), 916–929. https://doi.org/10.4103/jcrt.JCRT_50_17

Moreira-Almeida, A., Koenig, H. G., & Lucchetti, G. (2014). Clinical implications of spirituality to mental health: Review of evidence and practical guidelines. *Revista Brasileira de Psiquiatria*, 36 (2), 176–182.

Moreno, C. R., Louzada, F. M., Teixeira, L. R., Borges, F., & Lorenzi-Filho, G. (2006). Short sleep is associated with obesity among truck drivers. *Chronobiology International*, *23*(6), 1295–1303. https://doi.org/10.1080/07420520601089521

Moreno, C. R., Marqueze, E. C., Sargent, C., Wright Jr, K. P., Ferguson, S. A., & Tucker, P. (2019). Working Time Society consensus statements: Evidence-based effects of shift work on physical and mental health. *Industrial Health*, *57*(2), 139–157. https://doi.org/10.2486/indhealth.SW-1

Murillo-Rodríguez, E., Barciela Veras, A., Barbosa Rocha, N., Budde, H., & Machado, S. (2018). An overview of the clinical uses, pharmacology, and safety of modafinil. *ACS Chemical Neuroscience*, *9*(2), 151–158. https://doi.org/10.1021/acschemneuro.7b00374

Repantis, D., Bovy, L., Ohla, K., Kühn, S., & Dresler, M. (2021). Cognitive enhancement effects of stimulants: A randomized controlled trial testing methylphenidate, modafinil, and caffeine. *Psychopharmacology*, *238*(2), 441–451. https://doi.org/10.1007/s00213-020-05691-w

Robbins, R., Grandner, M. A., Buxton, O. M., Hale, L., Buysse, D. J., Knutson, K. L., Patel, S. R., Troxel, W. M., Youngstedt, S. D., Czeisler, C. A., & Jean-Louis, G. (2019). Sleep myths: An expert-led study to identify false beliefs about sleep that impinge upon population sleep health practices. *Sleep Health*, *5*(4), 409–417. https://doi.org/10.1016/j.sleh.2019.02.002

Rocha, F. P., Marqueze, E. C., Kecklund, G., & Moreno, C. (2022). Evaluation of truck driver rest locations and sleep quality. *Sleep Science (Sao Paulo, Brazil)*, *15*(1), 55–61. https://doi.org/10.5935/1984-0063.20210028

Rosa, H. (2013) *Social Acceleration: A New Theory of Modernity*. New York, Columbia University Press, 470 p.

Ruscitto, C., & Ogden, J. (2017). The impact of an implementation intention to improve mealtimes and reduce jet lag in long-haul cabin crew. *Psychology & Health, 32*(1), 61–77. https://doi.org/10.1080/08870446.2016.1240174

Sack R. L. (2010). Clinical practice. Jet lag. *The New England Journal of Medicine, 362*(5), 440–447. https://doi.org/10.1056/NEJMcp0909838

Sagah Zadeh, R., Shepley, M., Sadatsafavi, H., Owora, A. H., & Krieger, A. C. (2018). Alert workplace from healthcare workers' perspective: Behavioral and environmental strategies to improve vigilance and alertness in healthcare settings. *HERD, 11*(2), 72–88. https://doi.org/10.1177/1937586717729349

Schwartz, J. R., Roth, T., Hirshkowitz, M., & Wright, K. P. (2009). Recognition and management of excessive sleepiness in the primary care setting. *Primary Care Companion to the Journal of Clinical Psychiatry, 11*(5), 197–204. https://doi.org/10.4088/PCC.07r00545

Shockey, T. M., & Wheaton, A. G. (2017). Short sleep duration by occupation group–29 states, 2013–2014. *MMWR. Morbidity and Mortality Weekly Report, 66*(8), 207–213. https://doi.org/10.15585/mmwr.mm6608a2

Smith, L., Tanigawa, T., Takahashi, M., Mutou, K., Tachibana, N., Kage, Y., & Iso, H. (2005). Shiftwork locus of control, situational and behavioural effects on sleepiness and fatigue in shiftworkers. *Industrial Health, 43*(1), 151–170. https://doi.org/10.2486/indhealth.43.151

Taylor, A. H., & Dorn, L. (2006). Stress, fatigue, health, and risk of road traffic accidents among professional drivers: the contribution of physical inactivity. *Annual Review of Public Health, 27*, 371–391. https://doi.org/10.1146/annurev.publhealth.27.021405.102117

Ulhôa, M. A., Marqueze, E. C., Burgos, L. G., & Moreno, C. R. (2015). Shift work and endocrine disorders. *International Journal of Endocrinology, 2015*, 826249. https://doi.org/10.1155/2015/826249

Ulhôa, M. A., & Moreno, C. R. (2022). Circadian rhythm sleep-wake disorders: an overview. In C. Frange, F. Morgadinho, & S. Coelho (Eds.). *Sleep Medicine and Physical Therapy–A Comprehensive Guide for Practitioners*. New York: Springer Cham, pp. 103–113.

van Drongelen, A., Boot, C. R., Hlobil, H., Smid, T., & van der Beek, A. J. (2017). Risk factors for fatigue among airline pilots. *International Archives of Occupational and Environmental Health, 90*(1), 39–47. https://doi.org/10.1007/s00420-016-1170-2

Van Rensburg, D. C. C. J., Van Rensburg, A. J., Fowler, P., Fullagar, H., Stevens, D., Halson, S., Bender, A., Vincent, G., Claassen-Smithers, A., Dunican, I., Roach, G. D., Sargent, C., Lastella, M., & Cronje, T. (2020). How to manage travel fatigue and jet lag in athletes? A systematic review of interventions. *British Journal of Sports Medicine, 54*(16), 960–968. https://doi.org/10.1136/bjsports-2019-101635

Verster, J. C., Bervoets, A. C., de Klerk, S., Vreman, R. A., Olivier, B., Roth, T., & Brookhuis, K. A. (2014). Effects of alcohol hangover on simulated highway driving performance. *Psychopharmacology, 231*(15), 2999–3008. https://doi.org/10.1007/s00213-014-3474-9

Watson, P., Whale, A., Mears, S. A., Reyner, L. A., & Maughan, R. J. (2015). Mild hypohydration increases the frequency of driver errors during a prolonged, monotonous driving task. *Physiology & Behavior, 147*, 313–318.

Section 4

Managing Fatigue and
Promoting Alertness
in Transportation

4.1 Approaches to Fatigue Management

Where We Are and Where We're Going

Madeline Sprajcer, Matthew J. W. Thomas, and Drew Dawson

Appleton Institute, Central Queensland University, Adelaide, SA, Australia

CONTENTS

4.1.1 HISTORY OF REGULATORY APPROACHES TO FATIGUE MANAGEMENT

The advent of electricity allowed for the rise of 24/7 work operations in industrialised nations, which in turn brought about the need for hours of work to be managed. Hours of work limitations (e.g., shift duration, cumulative hours of work, breaks, etc.) were used not only in response to growing demands for fair work arrangements, but to manage fatigue (Moore-Ede, 1993). It was assumed that fatigue could be avoided (or at least minimised) if working time conformed to specified limitations.

This traditional approach to managing fatigue—hours of work limitations and other compliance requirements—would generally be described as prescriptive. In

DOI: 10.1201/9781003213154-23

many jurisdictions, this approach to fatigue management continues today, and reflects a long-standing approach to the management of safety in general, through both prescriptive regulation and organisational rule-based approaches to safety management (Reason et al., 1998). With respect to fatigue, regulatory bodies, or even individual organisations, develop certain limitations, within which workers are deemed to be 'safe' (i.e., not fatigued).

Across all modes of transport internationally, prescriptive approaches to fatigue management can be found in place today, from flight and duty time limitations set out by commercial aviation regulation, through to requirements for the frequency and duration of minimum rest periods for seafarers under the Standards of Training Certification and Watchkeeping for Seafarers (STCW) convention. Although considerable variation exists in prescriptive limits across transport industries worldwide, these limits typically pertain to factors such as (1) maximum hours of work in any work period, (2) maximum cumulative hours of work across a week or month, (3) minimum rest requirements between work periods, (4) maximum number of consecutive work periods prior to a day or days free of work, and (5) limitations relating to night work. In addition to these basic limitations, prescriptive regulation in the transport industries includes sector-specific limitations, such as rules around changes in the start times of work periods (such as lay-back and lift-up limitations in the rail industry which govern shift start and end times that are either earlier or later than originally scheduled,) and rules around extended rest periods after crossing multiple time zones in aviation.

The inherent assumption in prescriptive approaches to fatigue management is that compliance with set working hours rules equates to fatigue being effectively managed. Unfortunately, prescriptive systems do not consider that, due to a range of factors, it is possible for a worker to comply with these limitations (i.e., to operate within the 'prescriptive envelope') but still experience fatigue (and fatigue-related risk) (Honn et al., 2019).

With an increase in circadian and sleep research in the 1970s and 1980s came a greater understanding of the influence of individual sources of fatigue relating to circadian factors and an individual's prior sleep/wake history. Based on this growing field of research, researchers and industry professionals began to use this understanding to inform fatigue-related risk assessment, including modelling fatigue likelihood based on prior sleep and work (Åkerstedt et al., 2004; Fletcher & Dawson, 2001a, 2001b; Hursh et al., 2004). This information was used to help organisations make decisions regarding work schedule limitations and improve productivity (Dawson et al., 2017). In the mid-2000s, fatigue began to be conceptualised as a hazard—much like other hazards managed via organisational Safety Management Systems (SMS) (Dawson & McCulloch, 2005). With this perspective of fatigue as a workplace hazard, the approaches adopted to manage fatigue shifted alongside safety management more broadly, to adopt a risk-based approach to managing workplace fatigue. Within this context, a more sophisticated approach, beyond that of simple prescriptive hours of work rules, became warranted.

Risk-based approaches to fatigue management emphasise that simple rules around the duration of work and rest periods, or limitations set on cumulative totals of work, do not guarantee that an operator will not experience fatigue. As a result, risk-based fatigue management systems must also include strategies that identify and mitigate fatigue-related risk as it occurs in the workplace. Within transport operations, the risk-based approach to fatigue management typically includes the identification and mitigation of fatigue-related risk through three types of processes: (1) predictive, (2) proactive, and (3) reactive (Rangan et al., 2013).

First, *predictive* processes identify sources of fatigue in the design of work and include more sophisticated approaches to scheduling than can be achieved by simplistic rule sets (e.g., the use of bio-mathematical modelling rather than following rules such as 'no more than 72 hours can be worked across seven consecutive days'. Second, *proactive* processes focus on day-of-operations management, and include risk management strategies such as individual fitness for duty assessment or real-time operator monitoring. These processes are underpinned by training for individuals on the application of appropriate fatigue management strategies around sleep and health. Third, *reactive* processes respond to instances where an operator has experienced elevated levels of fatigue, and include risk management strategies such as reporting and investigation to address the causes of fatigue or fatigue-related incidents.

4.1.1.1 CONCEPTUALISING THE SPECTRUM OF APPROACHES TO FATIGUE MANAGEMENT

While broadly, prescriptive and risk-based fatigue management systems could be categorised as discrete categories—encompassing entirely different ways of managing fatigue in the workplace—we may alternatively conceptualise them as a spectrum. This spectrum ranges from prescriptive, compliance-based systems at one end to comprehensive risk-based systems, called fatigue risk management systems (FRMS), at the other end. Between these two poles exist fatigue management systems that include certain components from each. Fatigue management systems that fall between the prescriptive and risk-based approaches could be considered as employing a hybrid model of fatigue management (Figure 4.1.1).

4.1.2 STRENGTHS AND WEAKNESSES OF APPROACHES TO FATIGUE MANAGEMENT

There are a range of reasons industries and organisations may choose to implement certain fatigue management systems (i.e., compliance-based, risk-based, or hybrid).

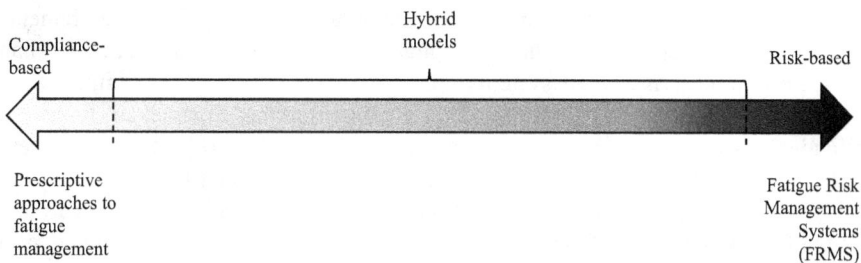

FIGURE 4.1.1 The spectrum of approaches to fatigue management.

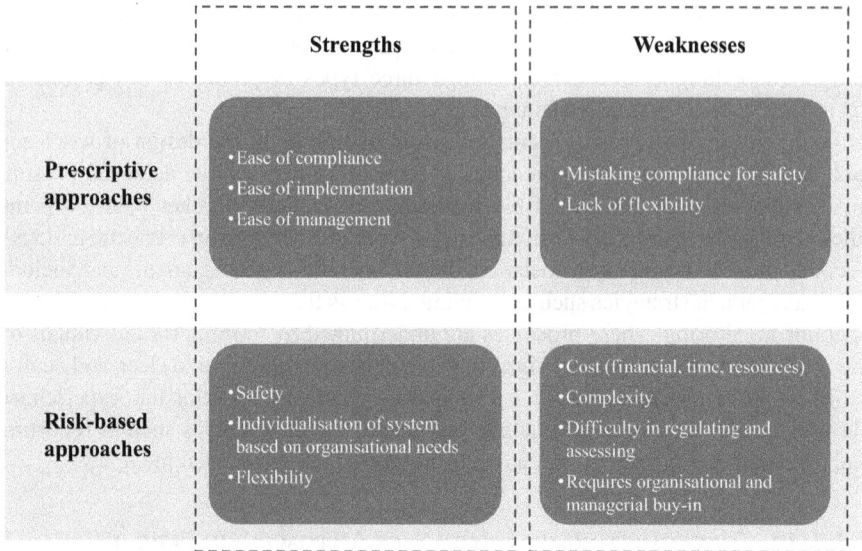

	Strengths	**Weaknesses**
Prescriptive approaches	• Ease of compliance • Ease of implementation • Ease of management	• Mistaking compliance for safety • Lack of flexibility
Risk-based approaches	• Safety • Individualisation of system based on organisational needs • Flexibility	• Cost (financial, time, resources) • Complexity • Difficulty in regulating and assessing • Requires organisational and managerial buy-in

FIGURE 4.1.2 Strengths and weaknesses of prescriptive and risk-based fatigue management systems.

Prior to an industry or organisation deciding how they might best manage fatigue, it is critical to be aware of the strengths and weaknesses of the different approaches to fatigue management. An overview of key strengths and weaknesses can be seen in Figure 4.1.2.

4.1.2.1 PRESCRIPTIVE APPROACHES TO FATIGUE MANAGEMENT: STRENGTHS

One of the key reasons industries and organisations may choose to rely on prescriptive approaches to fatigue management is simplicity. A prescriptive approach will generally outline limits for a range of activities (e.g., shift length, break duration and frequency, and time on task). As a result, determining whether workers have complied with these limitations is very straightforward, and for the regulator, it is therefore easy to determine compliance at an organisational level. Prescriptive approaches to fatigue management are also typically simple to implement—it is relatively straightforward to communicate this type of fatigue management requirements to workers and supervisors. Furthermore, ongoing management is also far easier than for more complex risk-based systems. For example, some Australian mines have a lockout function, whereby after working a certain number of (tracked) hours, an individual's swipe entry pass will be disabled, and they will no longer have access to the workplace—making it very simple to ensure compliance (though perhaps not safety). Similarly, given the interplay between the industrial and safety drivers around hours of work, managing fatigue through prescriptive limits has the advantage of a transparent, shared rule-set that can be negotiated and agreed upon in the industrial setting.

4.1.2.2   PRESCRIPTIVE APPROACHES TO FATIGUE MANAGEMENT: WEAKNESSES

While there are obvious benefits to implementing simple, prescriptive fatigue management systems, there are also a range of weaknesses that must be considered. The primary weakness of prescriptive approaches to fatigue management is the likelihood that compliance is mistaken for safety. That is, under prescriptive systems, compliance is used as an indirect proxy for safety. However, compliance may be an ineffective proxy in actuality—as prescriptive systems do not consider any factors that may impact fatigue other than hours of work. For example, prior sleep wake behaviour would not be considered, nor would the signs and symptoms of fatigue (Dawson & McCulloch, 2005). Furthermore, prescriptive systems make no allowance for non-work causes of fatigue. For example, an individual working night shifts may have their sleep impacted by neighbours performing home renovations during the day, being too hot to sleep comfortably, children who are at home during school holidays—or any number of other factors. Even if this individual was compliant with prescriptive hours of work rules, these non-work factors would likely result in poor sleep quality and/or duration (and subsequent fatigue). Under a prescriptive system, there is generally no mechanism to identify or manage any fatigue associated with these non-work-related factors that can affect sleep. As such, it is possible (and indeed likely) that at certain times, workers would experience uncontrolled fatigue (i.e., they would experience fatigue but would not have undertaken a risk assessment or implemented any control measures).

The other main weakness of prescriptive fatigue management systems is a lack of operational flexibility. In particular, the use of prescriptive management systems (generally underpinned by industry regulatory bodies) typically does not allow organisations to develop hours of work systems that meet their own operational needs. Any hours of work that are worked outside of the prescribed regulatory limitations would not be permitted outside of emergency circumstances. This has the potential to limit the organisation in terms of operational outcomes and/or service delivery. This can be problematic as many industries and organisations that use shift work can be impacted by a range of external (and often internal) factors likely to affect work scheduling (e.g., in the rail industry, train delays can significantly impact work hours). However, organisations may not be able to respond to non-emergency shift extension requirements (e.g., to make up for operational delays or to complete urgent work) under prescriptive fatigue management systems, as such changes may exceed permitted working time limitations.

4.1.2.3   RISK-BASED APPROACHES TO FATIGUE MANAGEMENT: STRENGTHS

In comparison to prescriptive fatigue management systems, risk-based approaches generally allow for far greater operational flexibility. Organisations are generally able to develop individualised systems based on their operational needs—as long as they are able to demonstrate to relevant regulatory bodies (or via the legal system in the event of an incident) that they are operating under a safe system of work. Risk-based approaches generally include the potential to implement longer hours of work than prescriptive systems—as it is the risk associated with these hours of work that is managed—rather than the hours of work themselves. Because they are based on the assessment (and subsequent management) of fatigue-related risk, risk-based systems are typically associated with a greater degree of worker safety. That is, fatigue is able to be identified, assessed, and managed during all work time—rather than operating under the assumption that under a certain threshold of work hours fatigue will not occur. Furthermore, non-work causes of fatigue can be identified and managed appropriately under risk-based fatigue management systems. That is, non-work factors are generally included within the risk assessment framework—which allows for appropriate countermeasures to be identified and implemented. Furthermore, risk-based approaches have the capacity to integrate technological solutions as part of fatigue management. For example, this may include the use of driver monitoring technology or wearables to identify fatigue during certain times and/or activities.

4.1.2.4   RISK-BASED APPROACHES TO FATIGUE MANAGEMENT: WEAKNESSES

Despite the clear benefits of risk-based fatigue management systems with regard to safety and flexibility, there are also weaknesses to consider. Critically for many organisations, the cost associated with developing, implementing, and managing a risk-based fatigue management system can be prohibitive. This is due not only to the time and resources involved with developing a tailored approach to fatigue management, but to the resources required for ongoing management (particularly given the key FRMS component of monitoring and evaluation). For many organisations, FRMS may require either the employment of additional staff and/or subject matter expert consultants—potentially associated with a significant cost.

The time and resources associated with the development and implementation of risk-based fatigue management systems reflect the level of complexity of this type of system. Risk-based approaches typically include a range of components designed to identify and manage fatigue that interact, resulting in more complex fatigue management systems than those simply based on compliance with clear rules. Furthermore, organisations may find internal regulation and assessment of risk-based fatigue management systems more difficult than simple prescriptive systems, given that in many cases there is no 'right answer'. Rather than measuring compliance, organisations would likely be required to measure both lead (e.g., outcomes of bio-mathematical modelling of rosters, sleep data gained from wearable devices) and lag (e.g., fatigue-related incidents, fatigue events detected by technology) indicators of fatigue, in addition to ensuring that assessment criteria and regulation are evidence-based and fit for purpose (Sprajcer et al., 2021). Risk-based fatigue management systems also require engagement from all levels of an organisation as fatigue is considered to be a shared responsibility. At the organisational and supervisory level, roles and responsibilities typically include, for example, provision of appropriate resources and support of a non-punitive organisational culture (when fatigue is reported). For workers, their responsibilities typically include ensuring they use time away from work to obtain adequate sleep, reporting if they are experiencing fatigue at work, and complying with relevant policies and procedures. Furthermore, converting an organisation from a traditional prescriptive system to using a risk-based approach is likely to involve a significant cultural shift—which requires both worker and organisational (and managerial) buy-in to be effective. As such, for some organisations (particularly smaller organisations without significant resources and/or large health and safety teams), risk-based fatigue management systems may be desirable but impractical.

4.1.3 FATIGUE RISK MANAGEMENT SYSTEMS

FRMS describes a set of data-driven fatigue management practices designed to identify and manage fatigue-related risk (Sprajcer et al., 2021). Key components of FRMS include policy and governance strategies, risk assessment and mitigation systems, training and education delivery, and continual improvement via monitoring and evaluation (Honn et al., 2019). Of note, FRMS consists of a risk-based approach to fatigue management, where the likelihood of fatigue during a given period is identified and used in conjunction with the potential consequences of a fatigue-related error to identify proportionate control measures. This system therefore can be used in place of traditional prescriptive approaches, as fatigue-related risk can be managed irrespective of hours of work. Therefore, increased operational flexibility is often afforded. Critically, FRMS also includes the ongoing monitoring and evaluation of safety data (e.g., fatigue-related incidents, hours worked), which is used to inform an organisation's fatigue management practices.

There are also some differences in the conceptualisation of risk, and interpretation of what a 'risk-based' system for fatigue management entails. For some organisations and regulatory bodies, 'FRMS' and 'risk-based fatigue management' have been appropriated as terms to describe prescriptive systems that 'manage risk' by limiting hours of work. However, risk-based approaches to fatigue management in fact refer to systems of work where fatigue is managed in a similar way to other hazards (e.g., ISO 31000) (Dawson & McCulloch, 2005). That is, risk assessment processes are used to identify fatigue-related risk and proportionate control measures. These control measures can be implemented to allow for the flexibility to operate outside of traditional prescriptive limits.

4.1.3.1 Cultural Differences in Approaches to Fatigue Management

Internationally, there are differing viewpoints on the best way to manage workplace fatigue, which are likely impacted by a range of cultural and economic factors. Typically, jurisdictions with individualist cultures (e.g., North America and Australia) are more likely to support fatigue management systems that allow for individualised system development and management (i.e., FRMS) (Gander et al., 2011). Comparatively, countries and jurisdictions with collectivist cultures (e.g., some areas in Europe) may be supportive of broad prescriptive approaches that apply to all organisations within an industry (or all industries) (European Commission, 2011). It must be acknowledged, however, that all authors of this chapter come from an individualist society and thus may be unaware of the nuances around safety-related decision-making that cultures and countries different from our own may consider. Furthermore, the size of a country also may impact fatigue management practices.

For example, medium sized countries such as Australia or New Zealand may be able to change regulatory practices far more quickly than larger countries, due to reduced bureaucratic processes and reduced lobbying power from interest groups. As a result of these factors, risk-based approaches to fatigue management (i.e., FRMS) have become more common in Australia, New Zealand, the United States, and Canada than in other areas.

In comparison to many Western countries, there is a relative recency in the formal management of fatigue in other parts of the world. As a result, fatigue management systems (including regulatory practices) may be less developed in these areas. Furthermore, fatigue management inspectorates can be costly to run–which may not be prioritised in some jurisdictions. There are also a range of transnational organisations responsible for providing guidance or regulation on the management of fatigue within certain industries. For many of these industries, there is also a trend towards the use of risk-based (FRMS) systems—which can be used to manage the vastly different operational environments seen globally. For example, transnational aviation management organisations (e.g., the International Civil Aviation Organisation) provide clear guidance on the use of FRMS, which have been adopted widely internationally.

4.1.4   EMERGING TRENDS IN FATIGUE MANAGEMENT

The adoption of risk-based approaches to fatigue management differs based on jurisdiction, industry, and even organisation. FRMS is now an option within many regulatory frameworks, but generally is not mandatory. As a result, for many industries worldwide, there is the potential for companies to implement the components of FRMS that suit their organisation (or that they can effectively manage) and leave the rest. This means that for many industries/organisations, fatigue management systems operate somewhere on the spectrum from prescriptive, compliance-based, through to risk-based or FRMS approaches. As noted above, these fatigue management systems that include both prescriptive and risk-based components could be characterised as a hybrid between the two systems.

Within a variety of industries internationally there is a growing trend towards the implementation of these hybrid models rather than either the prescriptive or risk-based model in isolation. These models generally include prescriptive maximum limitations (as seen within a standard prescriptive approach) but have the scope for extension where safe systems of work can be demonstrated. That is, where work can be performed within the prescriptive limitations, additional risk assessments and fatigue management strategies (as would be seen within FRMS or a similar system) are not required. However, if operational need requires workers to operate outside of the bounds of these initial prescriptive limitations, there are systems in place to assess and manage fatigue-related risk. Generally, this would be done via the use of a risk-based framework for managing fatigue. That is, a risk assessment would be performed to assess the likelihood of fatigue, the consequences of a fatigue-related error, and the associated risk. This would result in the implementation of proportionate control measures used to mitigate this risk while operating outside of the original prescriptive limitations. One example of this approach is the recent changes undergone within Canadian aviation regulations, which now permit safety cases to be developed for hours of work that are outside of established limits (Transport Canada, 2022).

There are a number of potential benefits of employing a hybrid model of fatigue management, which likely explains the increasing popularity of this approach in recent years. Key strengths and weaknesses of the hybrid model are presented in Figure 4.1.3. One strength of the hybrid model is a degree of accessibility and cost-effectiveness that is difficult to achieve when implementing a fully risk-based approach to fatigue management (i.e., FRMS). The implementation of a hybrid model generally requires far less time and cost investment due to the 'off the shelf' nature of much of the approach (i.e., the prescriptive components). Beyond that, a framework for managing work that is planned to exceed these limits is required but can usually be far simpler and faster to develop and implement. Moreover, the size of the cultural shift required to operate a risk-based system may be reduced—as deviation from traditional systems is minimal, and only occurs under specific circumstances. The reduction in required resources compared to fully risk-based approaches makes a hybrid model a much more attractive option for smaller or less well-resourced organisations. These organisations are able to obtain some of the benefits of a risk-based approach (i.e., increased flexibility), without the burden of high costs and a significant time investment. Furthermore, it is likely that hybrid models afford a greater degree of risk management (and therefore safety) at times when maximum limitations must be exceeded, as compared with prescriptive systems (where exceedances may occur despite the best efforts of organisations to comply with limits). Within a prescriptive system, where an emergency or unplanned situation occurs and working time limitations are exceeded, there are often no contingencies in place to manage the associated increased risk of fatigue. Hybrid models of fatigue management should also reduce the amount of involvement required from relevant regulatory bodies.

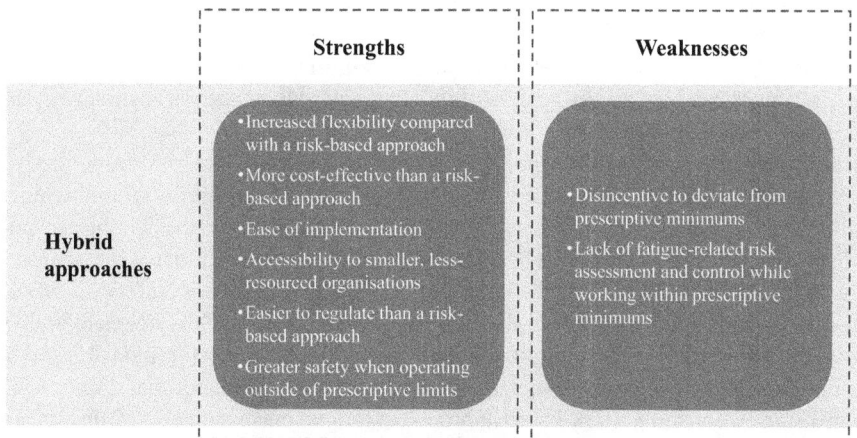

FIGURE 4.1.3   Strengths and weaknesses of a hybrid model of fatigue management.

A number of industries currently require all FRMS approaches (and any changes) to be comprehensively reviewed by the regulator (e.g., when greater flexibility than standard hours of work limits is desired by heavy vehicle operators in Australia, their safety case must be reviewed by the National Heavy Vehicle Regulator)—a time-consuming and costly undertaking. By using a combination of prescriptive and risk-based systems, the review process would likely be streamlined in many cases—as fewer tailored components need evaluation.

Despite the clear benefits of adopting a hybrid approach to fatigue management, there are also some potential drawbacks that must be considered. While hybrid approaches generally include provisions for increased flexibility, there may be a disincentive to utilise this flexibility because of the increased burden (i.e., to demonstrate that a safe system of work is in place). Given that much of the work performed with a hybrid model in place would not require this type of demonstrable safety regarding work practices, organisations may not be inclined to undertake the additional activities required to perform work outside of the prescriptive limits. This would likely be exacerbated by a lack of familiarity with this process (e.g., if increased flexibility is required infrequently, workers and/ or supervisors may be unfamiliar with risk assessment procedures). Furthermore, weaknesses of the prescriptive components of the hybrid model are similar to those described in relation to the prescriptive model itself. That is, workers may experience uncontrolled fatigue-related risk while working within the prescriptive envelope, where fatigue is not assessed.

For smaller organisations (i.e., those with a limited number of workers and/or financial resources), or organisations where operational flexibility is needed only occasionally or for a small number of workers or workgroups, hybrid models of fatigue management may be the ideal solution. These companies would be able to establish prescriptive rules under which the majority of their work could be performed—likely to have a small associated cost and requiring simple ongoing management. Where increased operational flexibility is required, they would then have the option to implement a risk-based approach to fatigue management—used to demonstrate a safe system of work for work falling outside of the prescriptive envelope. Conversely, a hybrid model may be less attractive for larger, better-resourced organisations, which have a greater need for operational flexibility and would likely be willing to invest the necessary time and resources.

Critically, the implementation of a hybrid model (or indeed any risk-based model) of fatigue management involves a shift in the burden of responsibility from the regulating body to the organisation. That is, where an organisation wishes to operate outside of standard limits, they must be able to prove that they can do so in a safe manner. This is in opposition to prescriptive systems, where the burden of 'safety' is on the regulatory body (that determines the limit under which all work is deemed 'safe'). Within a range of jurisdictions, there are some organisations (or industries) that would like the opportunity for increased operational flexibility, but that do not want to invest in establishing a risk-based approach to fatigue management (i.e., that do not want the responsibility of establishing safe systems of work). For these organisations, a hybrid model may be an effective compromise—where the 'burden' is only required under certain circumstances, and where operational flexibility is needed. An organisation that wishes to operate outside of this prescriptive envelope, but does not want to provide evidence of a safe system of work, is essentially admitting that their systems are not demonstrably safe.

4.1.5 FUTURE DIRECTIONS IN FATIGUE MANAGEMENT

Going forward, transport industries will need to consider how a range of technological advancements fit within their fatigue management systems. Currently, wearables (i.e., those that detect sleep and/or activity) and fatigue detection technologies (e.g., driver-facing cameras that detect eye closures, brain activity monitoring, etc.) have been integrated by some organisations as proactive fatigue countermeasures. As technology of all kinds develops, however, organisations will be faced with more options that will need integration into fatigue management systems. For example, the advent of self-driving vehicles (i.e., vehicles where an individual monitors the drive, but is not in control of the vehicle at all times) will present an interesting challenge for fatigue management (see also Chapter 6.1 of this book). In this case, the driver (or rather—the 'driver as passenger') may be required to respond in emergency situations. However, under most circumstances, this individual will undertake minimal active work (aside from monitoring)—which may increase the likelihood of inadvertent sleep episodes during the drive. This is just one example of the potential unintended consequences of technological advancement that will need consideration.

4.1.6 RESOURCES

For organisations wishing to implement risk-based approaches to fatigue management (i.e., FRMS), there are key resources available that can be used as a basis for policy development. National and international resources are available from a range of sources—some industry-specific and some general. For those interested in reading more about FRMS development, implementation, and management, we suggest the following resources as a starting point:

Civil Aviation Safety Authority (Australia). (2020). Fatigue Risk Management System Handbook. Available from: www.casa.gov.au/sites/default/files/2021-12/fatigue-risk-management-systems-handbook.pdf

Australian Pipelines and Gas Association. (2019). Fatigue Risk Management Guidelines. Available from: www.apga.org.au/sites/default/files/uploaded-content/website-content/apga_fatigue_management_guidelines_v1.2_.pdf

IPIECA (2019). Managing fatigue in the workplace: A guide for the oil and gas industry. Available from: www.ipieca.org/media/4729/managing_fatigue_2019.pdf

Queensland Government (Australia). (2009). Fatigue Risk Management System Resource Pack. Available from: www.yumpu.com/en/document/read/12949908/fatigue-risk-management-system-resource-pack

International Air Transport Association, International Federation of Air Line Pilots' Associations, International Civil Aviation Organisation. (2011). Fatigue Risk Management System (FRMS) Implementation Guide for Operators. Available from: www.icao.int/safety/fatiguemanagement/FRMS%20Tools/FRMS%20Implementation%20Guide%20for%20Operators%20July%202011.pdf

SUMMARY POINTS FOR PRACTITIONERS

- Fatigue management systems exist on a spectrum ranging from traditional prescriptive approaches to risk-based (FRMS) approaches.
- There are strengths and weaknesses of each of these approaches.
- There is a trend towards hybrid versions of fatigue management, which includes a 'prescriptive envelope' for standard operations combined with a risk-based approach to fatigue management where increased operational flexibility is desired.
- Hybrid approaches may be more appropriate for smaller organisations without the resources to implement a full FRMS.

REFERENCES

Åkerstedt, T., Folkard, S., & Portin, C. (2004). Predictions from the three-process model of alertness. *Aviation, Space, and Environmental Medicine*, *75*(3), A75–A83.

Dawson, D., Darwent, D., & Roach, G. D. (2017). How should a bio-mathematical model be used within a fatigue risk management system to determine whether or not a working time arrangement is safe? *Accident Analysis & Prevention*, *99*, 469–473.

Dawson, D., & McCulloch, K. (2005). Managing fatigue: It's about sleep. *Sleep Medicine Reviews*, *9*(5), 365–380.

European Commission. (2011). *European Working Time Directive (Directive 2003/88/EC)*. http://ec.europa.eu/social/main.jsp?catId=706&langId=en&intPageId=205#navItem-1

Fletcher, A., & Dawson, D. (2001a). Field-based validations of a work-related fatigue model based on hours of work. *Transportation Research Part F: Traffic Psychology and Behaviour*, *4*(1), 75–88.

Fletcher, A., & Dawson, D. (2001b). A quantitative model of work-related fatigue: Empirical evaluations. *Ergonomics*, *44*(5), 475–488.

Gander, P., Hartley, L., Powell, D., Cabon, P., Hitchcock, E., Mills, A., & Popkin, S. (2011). Fatigue risk management: Organizational factors at the regulatory and industry/company level. *Accident Analysis & Prevention*, *43*(2), 573–590.

Honn, K. A., van Dongen, H. P. A., & Dawson, D. (2019). Working time society consensus statements: Prescriptive rule sets and risk management-based approaches for the management of fatigue-related risk in working time arrangements. *Industrial Health*, *57*(2), 264–280.

Hursh, S. R., Balkin, T. J., Miller, J. C., & Eddy, D. R. (2004). The fatigue avoidance scheduling tool: Modeling to minimize the effects of fatigue on cognitive performance. *SAE Transactions*, 111–119.

Moore-Ede, M. (1993). *The Twenty-Four Hour Society: Understanding Human Limits in a World That Never Stops*. Addison-Wesley.

Rangan, S., Bowman, J. L., Hauser, W. J., McDonald, W. W., Lewis, R. A., & Van Dongen, H. P. (2013). Integrated fatigue modeling in crew rostering and operations. *Canadian Aeronautics and Space Journal*, *59*(01), 1–6.

Reason, J., Parker, D., & Lawton, R. (1998). Organizational controls and safety: The varieties of rule-related behaviour. *Journal of Occupational and Organizational Psychology*, *71*(4), 289–304.

Sprajcer, M., Thomas, M. J., Sargent, C., Crowther, M. E., Boivin, D. B., Wong, I. S., Smiley, A., & Dawson, D. (2021). How effective are fatigue risk management systems (FRMS)? A review. *Accident Analysis & Prevention*, 106398.

Transport Canada (2022). Advisory Circular (AC) No. 700-045: Exemption and Safety Case Process for Fatigue Risk Management Systems. Available at: https://tc.canada.ca/en/ aviation/reference-centre/advisory-circulars/advisory-circular-ac-no-700-045

4.2 Rules Resistance

The Inequitable Trade, Missing Logical Links, and Solutions to Surmount the Challenge

Clinton Marquardt

Sleep & Fatigue Specialist, PMI Inc., Ottawa, ON, Canada. www.SleepandDreams.com

CONTENTS

Parent: "Be home by 10:00 p.m."
Teenager: "Why?"
Parent: "Because I said so".
Teenager: "But all my friends can stay out until 11:00 p.m., it's not fair!"
Parent: "Too bad. I am the boss."

This age-old argument between parents and teenagers illustrates one of the biggest challenges you will encounter as a fatigue manager, getting your shift-workers to accept rules or regulations that dictate when they can work and when they must rest (from here onward referred to as *rules* or *work and rest rules*). It also hints at why they resist the rules. In my 30 years working in the field of sleep and fatigue, I have seen shift-workers resist rules for two main reasons. Like the teenager told to be home at 10:00 pm without any logic to support the rule, shift-workers are told to follow the rules even if they cannot see how the rules are linked to fatigue, they too are not provided with the logic behind the rules. I call this reason the *missing logical links*. The second reason concerns a trade. The teenager is not promised any personal benefit in exchange for obeying the rule. In fact, all he or she sees is a loss, missing the one extra hour of freedom. Shift-workers see rules similarly because, in exchange for accepting the rules, their compensation and consecutive off-duty days are usually reduced. The trade, they perceive, is an *inequitable trade*. Over my years of struggles with shift-worker resistance, I have developed strategies that can make your job as a fatigue manager a little easier when implementing rules. I will share these strategies and a little more background on the missing logical links and the inequitable trade in this chapter.

4.2.1 THE INEQUITABLE TRADE

Most shift-workers have never crashed a train, ditched an aircraft, smashed a vehicle, or grounded a ship because they were fatigued or worse, fell asleep. Most never will. Yet severe and low probability outcomes such as these are the ones that are often used as examples to support the need for science-based rules to manage fatigue. Such rules normally reduce the total hours of work and spread off-duty days out from being consecutive to interspersed across shift schedules to better manage fatigue. This reduces the compensation that shift-workers receive and the bulk periods of time they have available for leisure and personal activities such as hygiene, family responsibilities, etc. (leisure and personal activities are referred to collectively from here onward as *personal time*). Consequently, shift-workers tend to feel that they are giving up a lot to reduce the risk of severe outcomes like crashes, which are already very unlikely or rare. The trade does not seem fair.

Although shift-work occurs across many industries with very unique cultures, I have found that the perception of an inequitable trade is a universal shift-worker phenomenon. I have worked with clients in all modes of transportation, military and policing, healthcare, fire and rescue, engineering, forestry and manufacturing and every time I have been involved with implementing rules, the inequitable trade challenge surfaces. One approach I have found useful in improving acceptance of rules is to reduce the perception of inequity in the trade by raising awareness about the *hidden benefits* of sleep and improved fatigue management that can result from the rules. To do so, I first try to show shift-workers how they may already be experiencing negative outcomes that they are not aware of, such as safety incidents and financial losses, due to poor sleep and fatigue. I call these outcomes *hidden costs*. I then show them how the rules will allow more and better sleep, and less fatigue, all of which can result in hidden benefits such as improved safety, reductions in financial loss and personal benefits such as better short and long-term mental and physical health.

The stated intent of most rules is to positively influence safety. Showing shift-workers real-life examples of how the rules will likely reduce hidden negative safety outcomes that are less severe and more likely than crashes demonstrates how the rules will serve the exact purpose for which they were designed, that is, to improve safety. To illustrate this link, I first provide the shift-workers with general science-based information on the aspects of human performance, such as the ability to pay attention (e.g., Ingre et al. 2006), that can become impaired when people are fatigued but have not yet fallen asleep. Although many shift-workers have never fallen asleep at work, most can recall feeling fatigued at work and so, when presented with this science-based information, can at least conceive of the possibility that performance can be impaired due to fatigue. I then show how their fatigue-related performance impairments could have already contributed to some of their risky safety experiences at work.

Using vignettes from the organisation's own safety records can be helpful for this purpose because shift-workers can easily see that the safety incident was not fictitious and since it happened for their organisation once, it can happen again. For instance, perhaps an organisation keeps a record of speeding tickets issued to drivers of their vehicles. I would explain how speeding is a risky behaviour that can result from a common fatigue-related impairment, such as inattention, that causes a shift-worker to miss a reduced speed limit sign. It is important to also link the performance impairment–inattention–back to fatigue. To do this, I show how the shift-worker was likely fatigued at the time due to a lack of sleep and/or poor quality sleep related to the current, non-science-based rules. With this illustration process, shift-workers can usually see how many of the performance impairments, and less severe and higher probability safety incidents and near-misses, they have already experienced could have been due to fatigue resulting from current scheduling practices. To start correcting the shift-workers' perceptions that they are giving up a lot by accepting the rules, that is, to remedy the inequitable trade of giving up compensation and bulk personal time to reduce the risk of very unlikely severe outcomes, I demonstrate how the rules could have prevented the fatigue and subsequent inattention and even, possibly, the speeding ticket. In other words, I demonstrate how they will be trading compensation and bulk personal time to manage the hidden costs of fatigue (i.e., speeding tickets) by accepting the rules in exchange for hidden personal benefits that are much more likely, such as improved personal safety and improved bank account balances from fewer speeding tickets, than reducing the risk of severe outcomes like crashes.

Shift-workers often see improvements to safety solely as an organisational benefit, with good reason. If you follow the process I outlined above, it would be clear that safety would have been improved for the speeding shift-worker while operating a company vehicle during company time. Even if shift-workers understand how rules will reduce hidden costs (i.e., speeding tickets) and provide hidden benefits to safety (i.e., safer drivers abiding by speed limits), the trade does not seem equitable because what the shift-workers see is that in exchange for their personal losses (e.g., reductions in compensation and bulk off-duty time), the organisation receives the benefits (e.g., safer drivers at work and fewer speeding tickets paid by the company), while the shift-worker receives no benefit.

Repeating the above process using examples that show shift-workers how accepting the rules, and giving up compensation and bulk personal time, will lead to hidden personal benefits can make the perceived trade seem more equitable. Shift-workers know all too well how a really bad sleep makes them feel. But most are unaware of the hidden personal costs they may already be incurring from regularly sleeping a little less than required or repeatedly experiencing poor-quality sleep. If they are unaware of the hidden costs, they are also likely unaware of the hidden benefits they could be enjoying from improved sleep under a science-based set of rules. There is an abundance of research documenting the elevated risks of numerous negative physical and mental health outcomes for shift-workers, both short and long term (e.g., Brown et al., 2020; Costa, 1996). It would be difficult for shift-workers to argue that an improvement to their current health, like getting fewer colds (Prather et al., 2015), or a reduction in risk of developing a serious disease like cancer in the future (International Agency for Research on Cancer, 2010), does not offer some personal benefit. As a fatigue manager, if you can show your shift-workers how the rules will likely result in a relatively immediate personal health benefit or a reduced risk of a health cost in the future, they will be more likely to accept the new rules than if the benefits remain hidden.

Here is a summary of the steps you can follow to show your shift-workers that the trade is more equitable than they realise, and that by trading their compensation and bulk personal time, they can enjoy hidden personal benefits such as improved health:

1. Introduce the hidden health costs of insufficient sleep using science-based information.
2. Select a few negative health outcomes from the science-based information that are already occurring for some, or all, of your shift-workers.
3. Show how the current scheduling practices make it difficult to regularly obtain an adequate quantity of good-quality sleep and how this sleep impairment increases the likelihood of the negative health outcomes that workers are already experiencing (as prescribed in the previous step).
4. Demonstrate how the rules will allow shift-workers to sleep longer and better on a more regular basis and, subsequently, enjoy improved health.

To improve acceptance of the rules, I suggest repeating these steps for a couple of hidden benefits that are important to your shift-workers and where science supports the notion that improved sleep will result in this hidden benefit. For example, perhaps your shift-workers value athletic performance or intimate relationships. Research indicates that improving sleep quantity can improve athletic performance (Bonnar et al., 2018) and improving sleep quality can improve sexual life quality (Khastar et al., 2020). If your rules will allow more sleep and better sleep, then your shift-workers will likely enjoy these two hidden benefits in exchange for giving up some compensation and bulk personal time and will, hopefully, see that the trade is more equitable.

I would like to share one final note on the perceived inequitable trade discussion. It is much easier for shift-workers to trade valuable bulk personal time and financial compensation when they already believe in, and understand, the relationship between sleep and fatigue and its effects on hidden costs and benefits. If you are contemplating the design and implementation of your own rules or can foresee a future with rules being imposed by a governing body, start building awareness about sleep and fatigue well before you attempt to implement any rules. An early change in attitudes and behaviours can facilitate a later implementation of rules.

4.2.2   THE MISSING LOGICAL LINKS

When I started working in the area of sleep and fatigue almost 30 years ago, the rules governing hours of work I encountered did not incorporate any science concerning sleep or fatigue. They were designed simply to ensure that workers were fairly compensated for their time and that, if organisations operated 24/7, workers would be allowed to work at night. It was not uncommon to see a set of rules that would allow a worker to continue to work from day into night without a hard-stop point, provided that he or she was paid time-and-half and then double-time with increasing work hours. Of course, many occupational health and safety rules would allow the worker to refuse the work if it was deemed unsafe. However, I cannot recall ever hearing about a worker who actually put their hand up and said, "I have been awake too long, it is unsafe to continue and we need to shut this project down so we can all get some sleep." Now, admittedly, this was at a time well before science-based safety practitioners made industry aware of the risks associated with long duty days. Back then, an employee's decision to continue to work was based on sound logic for the era. That is, shift-workers made a lot of money for working 24/7 and overtime and this allowed organisations to continue their operations with a constantly available, and motivated, workforce.

In contrast, the trend today is to deal with the issue of fairly compensating workers for their time in a set of policies or collective agreements that are separate from those that address hours of work and rest. Specific rules governing hours of work and rest aimed at reducing fatigue risk are instead developed by applying the logic of sleep and fatigue science and taking operational requirements into consideration. While the rules are based on this new logic, they rarely, if ever, clearly state the logic. That is, the documents stating the rules do not describe how the rules will result in better fatigue management, the logical links are missing. This sets up an understandable resistance in shift-workers.

Consider again the parent–teenager argument from the beginning of this chapter. I suggest that, because the teenager asked for a reason for the 10:00 pm curfew, the parent could have reduced the teenager's resistance by providing a logical reason for the curfew. I think we can borrow from this suggestion and increase the likelihood that shift-workers will accept work and rest rules if we provide them with the logic behind the rules.

For shift-workers to understand the logic, they must first understand the relationship between fatigue, fatigue risk factors, and sleep requirements. We all need a certain amount of good-quality sleep on a daily basis. The normal range of daily sleep needed is between 6 and 9 hours (Anch et al., 1988; Hirshkowitz et al., 2015), with the average being around 8 hours. While "bad quality" sleep can be difficult to define because of the wide ranging tolerance to sleep disruptions, good-quality sleep is easier to define. The National Sleep Foundation's indicators for good sleep quality in adults (Ohayon et al., 2017) are:

- falling asleep in 15 minutes or less,
- one or less awakening of greater than 5 minutes per night,
- awake time of 20 minutes or less per night after falling asleep,
- sleep efficiency of 85% or greater (sleep efficiency = time spent asleep/time in bed),
- REM sleep duration of 21 to 30% of total sleep duration,
- stage 1 sleep duration of 5% or less of total sleep duration,
- stage 3 sleep duration of 16 to 20% of total sleep duration, and
- being able to get through the day without a nap.

What I refer to as *sleep-related fatigue* results from differences between the sleep a person obtains and the sleep a person requires. That is, if sleep does not approximate the quantity and quality parameters above, the risk of sleep-related fatigue is increased.

There are two related influences on the risk of sleep-related fatigue. The first influence concerns the ratios of sleep to hours of life and to hours of wakefulness. If we round off the average quantity of sleep needed every day to 8 hours, we can say that, for every 24 hours of life, you need 8 hours of sleep. With 8 hours of sleep we are left with 16 hours of wakefulness in a 24-hour period. You can think of this last ratio as a transaction, where 8 hours of sleep buys you 16 hours of wakefulness. After 16 hours, you will have used up your *purchased* wakefulness and if you stay awake longer, the risk of sleep-related fatigue will increase (e.g., Mulhall et al., 2019).

The second influence on the risk of sleep-related fatigue concerns the lower quantity and poor-quality sleep that most shift-workers experience during day sleep compared to night sleep (e.g., Tilly et al., 1982). One of the reasons day sleep is shorter and of poorer quality is that our biology is *programmed* for sleep at night and wakefulness during the day (see Chapter 3.1 for more on circadian rhythms and biological programming). This means that, even if shift-workers do obtain an adequate amount of sleep during the day, it usually does not match the National Sleep Foundation's indicators for good sleep quality and fatigue risk remains increased.

Differences between the sleep needed and sleep obtained are often categorised into fatigue risk factors. They are called risk factors because, although fatigue is not guaranteed to result, the probability of fatigue does increase because of these factors. Fatigue risk factors are discussed in greater detail in other chapters of this book—see Chapter 2.5 and 4.3, and all of Section 3, for example—and, although terminology may differ, the categorisations are usually consistent with these:

1. *Acute Sleep Disruption* = obtaining an inadequate quantity and/or quality of sleep in the short term, usually the immediately preceding 24 hours.
2. *Chronic Sleep Disruption* = obtaining an inadequate quantity and/or quality of sleep across a longer period of time than with acute sleep disruption; the

quantity and/or quality disruptions are not as significant in magnitude but occur more frequently than with acute sleep disruption.

3. *Continuous Wakefulness* = being awake for too long when compared to the amount of sleep obtained.
4. *Circadian Rhythm Effects*
   4.1. *Circadian Rhythm Timing* = being awake when biology is programmed to be asleep, this is normally at night.
   4.2. *Circadian Rhythm Desynchronisation* = when biological programming is out of synchronisation with external patterns like clock times, or when internal physiological patterns are out of synchronisation with each other.

4.2.3 THE LOGICAL LINKS BETWEEN THE FATIGUE RISK FACTORS AND THE RULES

There is a core set of rules that are normally used to address the fatigue risk factors. I will describe these rules below and provide the logic that fatigue managers must first understand themselves, and then share with their shift-workers to help them also understand the logical links between the rules and the fatigue risk factors. With this understanding, fatigue managers will, hopefully, see better acceptance of the rules from their shift-workers.

Every industry has unique operational requirements. Unfortunately, I do not know your unique requirements, and attempting to outline all the logical links between them and your work and rest rules would require at least an extra chapter. Please do keep in mind that if your rules have not incorporated all the science because of operational requirements, you will have to communicate this to your shift-workers as well. If you do not, and your shift-workers' knowledge of sleep and fatigue science is sufficiently advanced, they will likely see the areas where the rules neglect some of the science and, if they have been told that the rules are based solely on science, they will not understand the need for the divergence. For example, although your industry may require night shifts, your rules may not limit the number of consecutive night shifts. If shift-workers know the science-based link between the number of consecutive night shifts and the risk of fatigue, they may question why night shifts have not been limited. If a logical operational reason for the missing limit is not provided to the shift-workers, their acceptance of the rules will decrease. If, however, you provide logic by stating something like "historical data shows that no one has ever worked more than one-night shift, and, given that future operational requirements will be no different, a limit to the number of consecutive night shifts is not required", acceptance of the rules will be less likely to be compromised.

As with operational requirements, I do not know if your industry is taking a risk-averse or risk-tolerant approach to managing fatigue. Science provides us with acceptable ranges. For example, and as mentioned above, although normal daily sleep requirements range from 6 to 9 hours, the average is about 8 hours. If your industry is taking a risk-averse approach, the rules may attempt to ensure that all shift-workers, even the longer sleepers, have ample opportunity for sleep. This would mean providing greater than 9 hours off-duty as a minimum to allow for personal time, in addition to the 9 hour sleep period. However, if your industry is taking a risk-tolerant approach, perhaps because the tasks being performed are less susceptible to fatigue-related performance impairments, the rules may only cater to the average person's sleep duration of 8 hours. This would mean shorter off-duty periods compared with the risk-averse approach.

Due to my incomplete understanding of your industry's or organisation's operational needs and approach to managing fatigue, I am going to shy away from providing actual limits and requirements. Instead, I will focus on the logic behind each of the core rules.

4.2.3.1 Link between Daily Work Duration Rules, Acute and Chronic Sleep Disruption, and Continuous Wakefulness

Sufficiently limited daily work durations attempt to provide enough off-duty time for people to complete personal activities and obtain the requisite amount of sleep on a daily basis. Providing time for personal activities reduces the likelihood of acute and chronic disruptions to sleep quantity because, from what I have learned through years of discussions with shift-workers is that they will usually curtail their sleep to squeeze in personal activities rather than skip the activity to fit in the time for sleep.

There is a fine line between "sufficiently" and "insufficiently" limited. If there is ample time off-duty every day, then the likelihood of both fatigue risk factors, acute and chronic disruptions to sleep quantity, will be reduced. If, however, there is just a little bit less time off-duty than needed, shift-workers may sleep a little less than they need every day and, although this would not necessarily result in acute sleep disruption, it could lead to a chronic sleep disruption.

A third fatigue risk factor, continuous wakefulness, can also be managed by limiting daily work durations. Most core rule sets consider the transactional ratio of 8 hours of sleep buys 16 hours of wakefulness and limit daily work durations to much less than 16 hours. This helps to ensure that all work and personal activities with a critical safety component, such as driving to and from work, can be completed within the 16 hours of wakefulness.

4.2.3.2 LINK BETWEEN WEEKLY WORK HOURS RULES, CHRONIC SLEEP DISRUPTION, AND THE CIRCADIAN RHYTHM DESYNCHRONISATION EFFECT

Weekly work hour limitations are required because, in some situations, daily work duration limits can nevertheless allow long work durations that only ensure that the lower range of normal daily sleep quantity (i.e., 6 hours) can be obtained. On those days, shift-workers may find it difficult to get an adequate quantity of sleep. While the reduction in sleep quantity may not dramatically increase fatigue risk with a single occurrence, repeated occurrences without a period of recovery (see the discussion of recovery periods in sub-section 4.2.3.5) would result in chronic sleep disruption and increase the risk of fatigue.

For schedules without any full days off-duty, limiting the amount of work across a week effectively forces a secondary cap on daily work durations. For example, if the rules impose a 60-hour weekly limit, a shift-worker would only be able to work up to 8.6 hours per day if they were required to work every day. The secondary cap on daily work durations limits the shift-worker's exposure to a chronic disruption to sleep quantity by providing more time across the week to complete personal activities and sleep.

Although rules limiting weekly work hours provide more time for sleep, thereby reducing the risk of a chronic disruption to sleep quantity, they do not help with the risk of a chronic disruption to sleep quality resulting from repeatedly sleeping during the day. Repeatedly obtaining poorer quality sleep (a chronic disruption to sleep quality) increases the risk of fatigue even though sleep quantity may be adequate. What is needed to reduce the risk of fatigue resulting from chronic disruptions to sleep quantity and quality is a practice that allows shift-workers to obtain an adequate quantity of night-time sleep, in some form of regular basis.

Schedules with full days off-duty can sometimes fill this need. With this rule, off-duty time is imposed after the accumulation of a certain number of hours of work per week. For example, a rule may indicate that shift-workers must take one full off-duty day after working 50 hours in a week. During the off-duty day, shift-workers have more time for sleep than during on-duty days and can sleep longer and make up for some of the chronic disruption to sleep quantity that could have resulted from repeatedly curtailing sleep to accommodate personal activities. If the timing of the off-duty day permits the better quality night-time sleep, shift-workers can also make up for some of the chronic disruption to sleep quality that may have resulted from repeatedly sleeping during the day.

An additional benefit of off-duty time that permits night-time sleep is that it can reduce the circadian rhythm desynchronisation effect. This fatigue risk factor normally does not begin to manifest after one night shift. It can, however, begin to occur after a week of night shifts that expose shift-workers to influential biological time cues such as meals, sleep, light, and physical and social activity at biologically incompatible clock times. During off-duty time, shift-workers can experience these time cues at more appropriate clock times to resynchronise circadian rhythms and reduce the risk of fatigue.

4.2.3.3 Link between Night Shift Rules and the Circadian Rhythm Timing Effect

Science-based rules almost always address the greater risk of fatigue that occurs when shift-workers are awake at night. This circadian rhythm timing effect can be managed in two ways: reducing work hours during the riskiest period of the night, referred to as the circadian trough, and/or by requiring the use of extra precautions during night shifts. The former practice works best when operations can be halted for some duration during the circadian trough, removing the greatest period of risk. However, in continuous operations, if one shift-worker is not working during the circadian trough, another shift-worker is, and there is no net decrease in overall fatigue risk at the organisational level. In these situations, rules normally require extra precautions that science has shown to be effective as fatigue management strategies, such as increased communications between employees, increased oversight between supervisors and employees, tactical caffeine use, and controlled napping during night shifts to reduce the risk of fatigue associated with the circadian rhythm timing effect.

4.2.3.4 LINK BETWEEN OFF-DUTY PERIOD RULES AND ACUTE AND CHRONIC SLEEP DISRUPTION

While rules limiting the work hours across daily and weekly timeframes may force the occurrence of off-duty time, they do not specify the minimum duration of time free from duty in between consecutive shifts. For example, there may be a rule limiting on-duty time to 12 hours per calendar day. Although this would provide 12 hours off-duty per day, the 12 hours on-duty could be comprised of a number of consecutive shifts with limited time in between that would make it difficult to obtain enough good-quality sleep. This is one of the biggest complaints I have heard from shift-workers in the maritime industry where the watch-keeping schedule is to work for 6 hours and then be off for 6 hours constantly. Lacking a rule that specifies the minimum off-duty time in between shifts means there is no guarantee that shift-workers will have enough time for sleep and personal activities on a daily basis. For this reason, the core set of rules usually ensures a certain period of off-duty time in between shifts. If the off-duty period regularly allows for at least 8 hours of sleep, the likelihood of fatigue from acute and chronic disruptions to sleep quantity is reduced for the average shift-worker. Normally, to allow eight hours of sleep, the time in between shifts is set to at least nine hours. Logically this makes sense because it would be very difficult for a shift-worker to obtain 8 hours of sleep and attend to any personal needs such as eating, hygiene and preparation for bed and the next shift in less than 9 hours. Recall, however, that the normal range of sleep quantity is 6 to 9 hours. A risk-averse approach would, therefore, have to consider the longer, but still normal sleepers, and provide greater than 9 hours in between shifts.

4.2.3.5 LINK BETWEEN RECOVERY PERIOD RULES, ACUTE AND CHRONIC SLEEP DISRUPTION, AND THE CIRCADIAN RHYTHM DESYNCHRONISATION EFFECT

The rules providing off-duty periods greater than 9 hours may reduce the likelihood of acute and chronic sleep disruption, but they do not guarantee that these fatigue risk factors will be absent. Even the best sleepers occasionally sleep less than desired or have poor-quality sleep regardless of whether they are sleeping at night or during the day. This means it is likely that, at some point, regardless of the rules, acute and/or chronic sleep disruption will increase the risk of fatigue in your shift-workers. Rules will usually include mandatory recovery periods, sometimes referred to as *reset breaks*, to counteract naturally occurring sleep disruptions as well as those resulting from shift schedules. The logic here is that providing regularly occurring off-duty periods of sufficient duration allows the shift-worker to obtain enough good-quality sleep to essentially *cancel out* any fatigue accumulated through exposure to acute and chronic sleep disruption. The regularity is provided by requiring one recovery period after a number of calendar days, consecutive day and/or night duties, reaching the weekly work hours limits, or by requiring one recovery period within a certain period of time. For example, the Canadian Duty and Rest Period Rules for Railway Operating Employees (DRPR) requires freight railway companies to provide one 32-hour reset break that begins before the end of any consecutive seven-day period.

The duration of the recovery period is usually designed to allow for two consecutive night-time sleep periods. One night sleep period may be sufficient to offset the effects of acute and chronic sleep disruptions for some shift-workers, but if two nights are provided, the effects are more likely to be cancelled out for almost all shift-workers regardless of fatigue risk factor magnitudes (e.g., Gander, Graeber, & Belenky, 2011).

Recovery periods also serve to resynchronise circadian rhythms. Due to a combination of social pressure to be awake during the day and circadian rhythm influences, most shift-workers revert to sleeping at night and being active during the day on their full days off. Sleeping at night, twice, results in exposure to biological time cues (e.g., daylight, eating) at the appropriate clock times. Although this may not be enough exposure to reset all magnitudes of circadian rhythm desynchronisation, it can reduce the risk of fatigue associated with this risk factor. The DRPR is a good example of providing the opportunity for two nights of sleep to both cancel out the acute and chronic sleep disruptions and reduce the risk of circadian rhythm desynchronisation. These rules require that the reset break includes two periods of 8 hours undisturbed by the company that begin and end within the period between 10:00 pm and 8:00 am.

4.2.3.6   Link between Consecutive Night Shift Rules, Chronic Sleep Disruption, and the Circadian Rhythm Desynchronisation Effect

Some day shift patterns can lead to fatigue risk factors and some do not. For example, a shift-worker could theoretically work a 6-hour shift from 10:00 am to 4:00 pm every day for 30 days and not be exposed to any fatigue risk factors. Whereas only a few consecutive day shifts that start too early could cause acute and/or chronic sleep disruption in those shift-workers who are unable to initiate sleep earlier in the evenings. To be effective, a science-based rule for consecutive day shifts would have to address all permutations of day shifts. This would create a rule with too much complexity to be of practical value. This is the reason that the core set of rules I have described does not limit consecutive day shifts.

As a fatigue manager, lacking a limit to the number of consecutive day shifts should not be a cause for concern. Other rules within the core set effectively limit the number of consecutive day shifts. For example, if a mandatory recovery period is required once every seven days, and the daily work duration is limited to 12 hours and the required off-duty period is also set to 12 hours, the shift-worker could only work five consecutive 12-hour day shifts per week.

The situation is different for consecutive night shifts. Night shifts are more reliably associated with fatigue because they require daytime sleep, which, as mentioned, is normally insufficient in quantity and quality. It also exposes shift-workers to biological time cues at inappropriate times. Repeated exposure to these conditions results in fatigue from chronic sleep disruption and circadian rhythm desynchronisation. Limiting the number of night shifts in a row restricts the accumulation of fatigue due to these risk factors and this is the reason for which the core set of rules includes a limit to the number of consecutive night shifts.

As with the information about the personal benefits associated with better sleep and improved fatigue management as discussed in section 4.2.2, I suggest that you share the information about sleep requirements and fatigue risk factors with employees well before attempting to provide the logical links to the rules. A thorough understanding of this information gained earlier can make it easier for shift-workers to understand the logical links later.

4.2.4   CONCLUSIONS

Convincing a workforce to wilfully accept rules that will reduce their compensation and bulk periods of personal time with no obvious personal benefit is one of the greatest challenges encountered by fatigue managers. The perceived inequity in this trade can be reduced, however, by providing shift-workers with science-based information about the hidden benefits they will likely experience from more and better sleep, and less fatigue resulting from science-based rules that dictate when they can work and when they must rest. But this does not go far enough. Fatigue managers should also provide their shift-workers with the logical links between each rule and its intended effect on specific fatigue risk factors. Addressing the perceived inequitable trade and the missing logical links can improve shift-worker acceptance of the rules. It may not solve all your rules resistance issues as a fatigue manager, but, in my experience, it can be an effective strategy to, in the very least, improve acceptance.

SUMMARY POINTS FOR PRACTITIONERS

- One of your biggest challenges as a fatigue manager will be surmounting shift-worker resistance to work and rest rules.
- If you address the two main reasons for the resistance—(1) the inequitable trade and (2) the missing logical links—you can improve acceptance of work–rest rules.
- Demonstrating that work and rest rules result is an equitable trade of compensation and consecutive off-duty days in exchange for valued personal benefits can reduce shift-worker resistance to work and rest rules.
- Use science to show that more and better sleep and improved fatigue management results in valued personal benefits.
- Providing information about the logical links between work and rest rules and a reduction in the impact of fatigue risk factors can reduce shift-worker resistance to work and rest rules.
- Fatigue managers should start building awareness about sleep and fatigue, the benefits of regularly obtaining an adequate quantity of good-quality sleep, and sharing information about sleep requirements, the ratio of sleep to wakefulness, and circadian rhythms and their relationship to the risk of fatigue with their shift-workers well before implementing work and rest rules.

REFERENCES

Anch, A., Browman, C., Mitler, M., & Walsh, J. (1988). *Sleep: A Scientific Perspective.* Prentice-Hall.

Bonnar, D., Bartel, K., Kakoschke, N., & Lang, C. (2018). Sleep interventions designed to improve athletic performance and recovery: A systematic review of current approaches. *Sports Medicine, 48*, 683–703.

Brown, J. Martin, D., Nagaria, Z., Verceles, A., Jobe, S., & Wickwire, E. (2020). Mental health consequences of shift work: An updated review. *Current Psychiatry Reports, 22*(2), 7.

Costa, G. (1996). The impact of shift and night work on health. *Applied Ergonomics, 27*(1), 9–16.

Gander, P., Graeber, R., & Belenky, G. (2011). Fatigue risk management. In M. Kryger, T. Roth, & W. Dement (Eds.), *Principles and Practice of Sleep Medicine* (Fifth Edition, pp. 760–769). W.B. Saunders.

Hirshkowitz, M., Whiton, K., Albert, S., Alessi, C., Bruni, O., Don Carlos, L., Hazen, N., Herman, J., Katz., E., Kheirandish-Gozal, L., Neubauer, D., O'Donnell, A., Ohayon, M., Peever, J., Rawding, R., Sachdeva, R., Setters, B., Vitiello, M., Ware, J., & Hillard, P. (2015). National Sleep Foundation's sleep time duration recommendations: Methodology and results summary. *Sleep Health, 1*, 40–43.

Ingre, M., Åkerstedt, T., Peters, B., Anund, A. & Kecklund, G. (2006). Subjective sleepiness, simulated driving performance and blink duration: Examining individual differences. *Journal of Sleep Research, 15*, 47–53.

International Agency for Research on Cancer (2010). *Monographs on the Evaluation of Carcinogenic Risks to Humans: Painting, Firefighting and Shiftwork.* World Health Organization Press.

Khastar, H., Mirrezaie, S., Chashmi, N., & Jahanfar, S. (2020). Sleep improvement effect of sexual life quality among rotating female shift workers: A randomized controlled trial. *The Journal of Sexual Medicine, 17*(8), 1467–1475.

Mulhall, M., Sletten, T., Magee, M., Stone, J., Ganesan, S., Collins, A., Anderson, C., Lockley, S., Howard, M., & Rajaratnam, S. (2019). Sleepiness and driving events in shift workers: The impact of circadian and homeostatic factors. *Sleep, 42*(6), 1–13.

Ohayon, M., Wickwire, E., Hirshkowitz, M., Albert, S., Avidan, A., Daly, F., Dauvilliers, Y., Ferri, R., Fung, C., Gozal, D., Hazen, N., Krystal, N., Lichstein, K., Mallampalli, M., Plazzi, G., Rawding, R., Scheer, F., Somers, V., & Vitiello, M. (2017). National Sleep Foundation's sleep quality recommendations: First report. *Sleep Health, 3*, 6–19.

Prather, A., Janicki-Deverts, D., Hall, M., & Cohen, S. (2015). Behaviorally assessed sleep and susceptibility to the common cold. *Sleep, 38*(9), 1353–1359.

Tilley, A., Wilkinson, R., Warren, P., Watson, B., & Drud, M. (1982). The sleep and performance of shift workers. *Human Factors, 24*(6), 629–641.

4.3 Work Scheduling

Biomathematical Modelling for Fatigue Risk, and Its Role in Fatigue Risk Management Processes

Steven R. Hursh and Jaime K. Devine

Institutes for Behavior Resources, Inc., Baltimore, MD, USA

CONTENTS

4.3.1 INTRODUCTION

The term "biomathematics" refers to the use of mathematical equations or principles to describe observable biological processes. Alexander Borbély first published a description of a two-process conceptual model of sleep regulation using biomathematics in 1982. The two-process model asserts that sleep is regulated by a sleep-dependent process (Process S) and a circadian process (Process C) (Borbély, 1982). Circadian processes drive wakefulness during the day and sleepiness during the night in humans and other diurnal animals (Monk, 1990). The model asserted that sleep propensity and the duration of sleep were due to the combined action of time since the individual had last slept (Process S) and time of day (Process C). Inspired by Borbély's two-process model, the first biomathematical model dedicated to fatigue prediction added sleep inertia as a third factor and was aptly called the three-process model of alertness (TPM) by Folkard and Åkerstedt in 1987 (Folkard & Åkerstedt, 1987).

DOI: 10.1201/9781003213154-25

4.3.2 COMPONENTS OF THE THREE-PROCESS MODEL

The TPM predicts alertness and task performance based on three components known to affect fatigue. The first component is the circadian rhythm, or Process C in Borbély's two-process model. The human circadian clock regulates a biological concept of time based on environmental inputs, like daylight or food intake (Czeisler et al., 1986). The circadian rhythm is adaptable, meaning that phases can be shifted to align with a new schedule, seasonal variation in light, or travel to a new time zone after an adjustment period (Czeisler et al., 1986; Lamond et al., 2003). Activities occurring at inappropriate circadian phases (such as sleeping during the day or working during the night) result in decreased alertness and performance (Lamond et al., 2003; Monk, 1990).

The second component known to affect fatigue is homeostatic sleep regulation. Conceptualised in Borbély's two-process model as Process S, homeostatic pressure to sleep builds with increased time spent awake independently from time-of-day effects (Borb & Achermann, 1999; Borbély, 1982). Fatigue accumulates with excessive time spent awake. Sleep alleviates the homeostatic pressure up to a break point (Åkerstedt, Ingre, Kecklund, Folkard, & Axelsson, 2008), which is to say that no amount of sleep can completely eliminate the need for sleep at a later point in time. It has also been more recently recognised that long periods of sleep restriction can induce a change in the dynamics of the sleep homeostat that retards the recovery of full alertness, even after sleep is no longer restricted (Hursh et al., 2004; McCauley et al., 2013). This factor can have implications for modelling the impact and recovery from schedules that reduce opportunities for normal amounts of sleep and several models have incorporated a dynamic regulatory factor to account for these findings (McCauley et al., 2013).

The third component of the TPM is sleep inertia, also known as the "wake-up component" or Process W. As described in Chapter 3.2 of this book, sleep inertia refers to a temporary state of grogginess following the transition between sleep and wakefulness (Tassi & Muzet, 2000). Despite being short-lived, sleep inertia can have consequences for performance and alertness directly following an awakening (Hilditch & McHill, 2019).

Like the TPM, the majority of modern biomathematical models of fatigue (BMMFs) have been fundamentally influenced by Borbély's two-process model (Mallis, Mejdal, Nguyen, & Dinges, 2004; Van Dongen, 2010). Seven of these models were reviewed as part of the Fatigue and Performance Modelling Workshop held in Seattle, WA, on June 13 to 14, 2002 (Mallis et al., 2004). An overview of these seven reviewed models is included in Table 4.3.1. All the reviewed models were found to be based on homeostatic sleep regulation and the circadian rhythm (Mallis et al., 2004). It is important to note that more than these seven BMMFs exist and that models may have changed since 2002 (Kandelaars, Dorrian, Fletcher, Roach, & Dawson, 2005; Peng & Bouak, 2015). However, as of the writing of this chapter, the review done during the Fatigue and Performance Modelling Workshop remains the largest scale comparison of multiple established BMMFs.

BMMFs differ with respect to input requirements, output features, and how performance or fatigue is computed. One major difference between models is how sleep information is incorporated into fatigue predictions. Models can be categorised as

TABLE 4.3.1
Biomathematical Models Reviewed during the 2002 Fatigue and Performance Modelling Workshop

Model	Publication
Two-Process Model	Achermann, P. "The two-process model of sleep regulation revisited." *Aviation, Space, and Environmental Medicine* 75, no. 3 (2004): A37–A43.
Sleep/Wake Predictor Model	Åkerstedt, T, Folkard, S, and Portin, C. "Predictions from the three-process model of alertness." *Aviation, Space, and Environmental Medicine* 75, no. 3 (2004): A75–A83.
System for Aircrew Fatigue Evaluation (SAFE) Model	Belyavin, AJ, and Spencer, MB. "Modeling performance and alertness: The QinetiQ approach." *Aviation, Space, and Environmental Medicine* 75, no. 3 (2004): A93–A103.
Interactive Neurobehavioural Model	Jewett, ME, and Kronauer, RE. "Interactive mathematical models of subjective alertness and cognitive throughput in humans." *Journal of Biological Rhythms* 14, no. 6 (1999): 588–597.
Sleep, Activity, Fatigue, and Task Effectiveness (SAFTE) Model	Hursh, SR, Redmond, DP, Johnson, ML, Thorne, DR, Belenky, G, Balkin, TJ, Storm, WF, Miller, JC and Eddy, DR. "Fatigue models for applied research in warfighting." *Aviation, Space, and Environmental Medicine*, 75.3 (2004): A44–A53.
Fatigue Audit InterDyne (FAID) Model	Roach, GD, Fletcher, A, and Dawson, D. "A model to predict work-related fatigue based on hours of work." *Aviation, Space, and Environmental Medicine* 75, no. 3 (2004): A61–A69.
Circadian Alertness Simulator (CAS) Model	Moore-Ede M, Heitmann A, Guttkuhn, R, Trutschei, U, Aguirre, A and Croke D. "Circadian alertness simulator for fatigue risk assessment in transportation: Application to reduce frequency and severity of truck accidents." *Aviation, Space, and Environmental Medicine*, 75.3 (2004): A107–A118.

using either one-step or two-step approaches, shown graphically in Figure 4.3.1. A one-step model predicts performance from input data without an intermediary step. Input data could be work schedule information alone or schedule information in combination with sleep data. Estimates of sleep data can be used for a one-step model but generally sleep data is collected from volunteers or operators. One-step models have been found to produce similar fatigue and performance predictions to one another, though they all may underestimate fatigue resulting from chronic exposure to short sleep (Van Dongen, 2004).

If no actual sleep measurements are available, a two-step model will infer when and for how long sleep would be estimated to occur based on the work schedule data and other social or logistical limitations on sleep opportunities (Kandelaars et al., 2005). Two-step models first estimate sleep timing and duration and then use these resulting sleep estimations to predict fatigue (Kandelaars et al., 2005).

Two-step BMMFs that can estimate fatigue and performance based solely on work times are particularly useful for proactive evaluation of proposed schedules or in

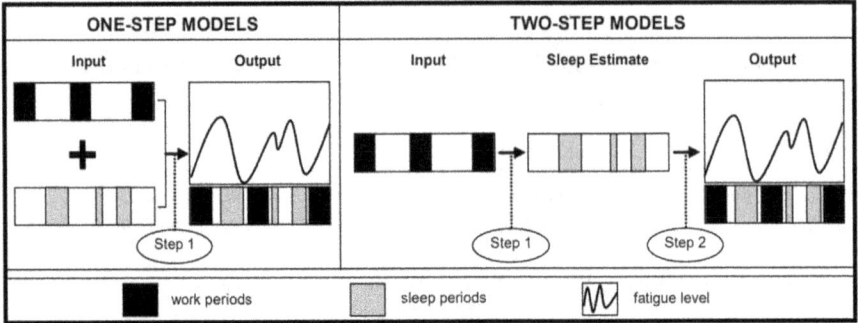

FIGURE 4.3.1 Classic overview of one-step model versus two-step model approach to modelling fatigue. A one-step model uses objective sleep data and work schedule data as input to predict fatigue risk. In the two-step model, sleep-wake behaviour is predicted from work schedule data in the first step. Fatigue risk or performance outputs are predicted in the second step. Reprinted from Kandelaars et al. (2005).

operational settings where collecting sleep data may not be convenient or feasible. The inputs required by each model can vary and should take industry-specific operational factors into consideration. For example, in the context of aviation, a two-step model should account for the impact of time zone changes greater than 3 hours when estimating sleep patterns. Other examples include accounting for the quality of a rest facility, whether workers have the ability to take a nap while on-shift, and how much time it takes to commute between work and home. BMMFs proactively evaluate work schedules to maximise efficiency while reducing risk exposure, so it is important that any sleep estimator used in a two-step model is tested for accuracy in addition to validating the model's fatigue or performance outputs.

Another factor that impacts fatigue on the job is workload. Workload is a very general term that can refer to the length of the duty day, the complexity of tasks performed, unexpected challenges during the duty day that add additional burden on the individual, and even the lack of experience of co-workers that can shift burden to more experienced personnel. Some workload factors can be predicted in a BMMF. For example, in flight operations, many workload factors are known in advance, like the number of flight segments in a flight duty period, the difficulty of the landing patterns into the airports, the usual congestion at a particular airport, and language difficulties in some regions of the world (Honn, Satterfield, McCauley, Caldwell, & Van Dongen, 2016).

4.3.3　RESEARCH AND VALIDATION OF BIOMATHEMATICAL MODELS

BMMFs are commonly used in the transportation and shiftwork industries to evaluate on-the-job performance or fatigue risk. Models are often geared towards use in a specific industry, which helps explain why models frequently differ with respect to input or output parameters. However, accuracy in fatigue prediction is the root goal of any

BMMF. For this reason, establishing validity of the model through laboratory and field research testing is of the utmost importance to model developers. Historically, it has been the developers of BMMF software packages, rather than regulators, who have undertaken validation efforts (Dawson, Darwent, & Roach, 2017; Fletcher & Dawson, 2001).

Validation testing for BMMFs falls into two categories: laboratory validation and operational validation. In laboratory validation studies, sleep and circadian parameters are experimentally manipulated in a controlled environment and the effects of resulting levels of fatigue are compared against model predictions. Importantly, operational validation establishes model accuracy in predicting fatigue that is specific to the target population during normal operations. A model which is optimised for predicting sleep and fatigue in aviation, for example, may not necessarily generalise to another operational population such as police officers (Riedy et al., 2020).

While there is no global guidance for what constitutes sufficient validation of a BMMF, common features of validation testing include collection of objective sleep data, performance testing such as using a psychomotor vigilance task (PVT), and/or subjective reports of sleep and fatigue (Fletcher & Dawson, 2001; Paul, Hursh, & Love, 2020; Tabak & Raslear, 2010). Some industries have set their own specific guidance for operational validation of a BMMF. For example, the United States Federal Railroad Administration (FRA) sets two criteria for model validity: (1) that the model documents sensitivity to circadian, sleep, and sleep inertia effects on a well-known behavioural or performance-based indicator of fatigue and (2) that the model demonstrates sensitivity to the risk of a human factors railroad accident caused by fatigue (https://railroads.dot.gov/elibrary/49-cfr-part-270-and-271-fatigue-risk-management-programs-certain-passenger-and-freight). The United States Fatigue Accident Validation (FAV) database is a central resource for confirming model sensitivity to rail accident risk (www.fra.dot.gov/rpd/policy/1975.shtml). The FRA then decides whether the model can be considered scientifically valid and may be used for the analysis of work schedules in the rail industry (Raslear, 2013).

The United States Federal Aviation Administration (FAA) has not suggested criteria for the evaluation of fatigue models but has sponsored work to validate one BMMF, the SAFTE-FAST model (Roma, Hursh et al., 2012). Furthermore, the FAA made extensive use of modelling during the development of the most recent flight and duty time regulations for scheduled airlines—14 CFR Parts 117, 119, and 121. In addition, the FAA has published guidance for fatigue risk management and includes modelling as a key element of the fatigue risk management system (FRMS) process (AC 120-103a), similar to the process chart depicted in Figure 4.3.2.

4.3.4 THE PLACE FOR MODELLING WITHIN FATIGUE RISK MANAGEMENT SYSTEMS

In safety-sensitive industries, BMMFs are frequently incorporated into a comprehensive FRMS as a way to prospectively assess fatigue risk associated with proposed work schedules (see Chapter 4.1 for further discussion on FRMS). A successful FRMS is a set of policies, procedures, and best practices developed by operational personnel in order to manage situations which are known to increase the risk of on-the-job

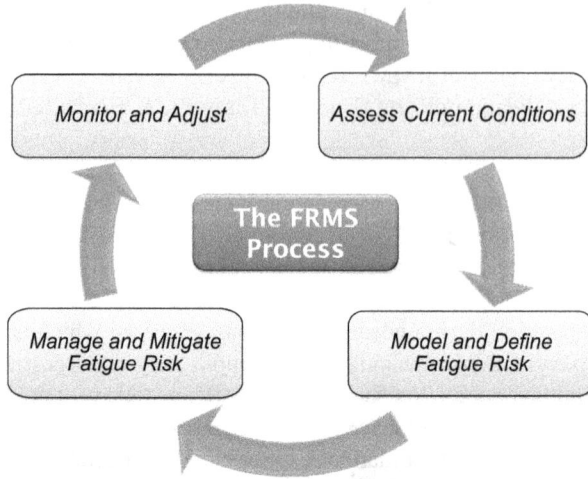

FIGURE 4.3.2   An outline of the Fatigue Risk Management System (FRMS) process. Model and Define Fatigue Risk is indicated in the lower right-hand corner of the cycle.

fatigue (Fourie, Holmes, Bourgeois-Bougrine, Hilditch, & Jackson, 2010). BMMFs are often incorporated into an FRMS as a way to predict potentially hazardous levels of fatigue as a result of schedules or rosters (Dawson et al., 2017; Gander et al., 2016). BMMFs are intended to be one component of a comprehensive, multi-layered FRMS (CASA, 2014).

4.3.5   APPLICATION OF MODELLING IN THE SCHEDULING PROCESS

Hypothetical schedule scenarios can be assessed with a BMMF to explore the impact of a proposed work schedule on fatigue risk. Regulators for some safety-sensitive industries have set standard criteria for BMMF estimations to ensure that proposed work patterns do not have operators working during a period of high fatigue risk. These criteria are termed "fatigue thresholds" because regulations state that any work schedule in which a fatigue prediction exceeds a set threshold of fatigue risk is considered unacceptable. It has been suggested that a more comparative approach could provide greater insight into the sources of fatigue risk or guidance for intervention than the use of fixed fatigue thresholds (Rangan & Van Dongen, 2013).

The danger of a fixed threshold is the assumption that all conditions that lead to the same level of some model output are comparable in terms of risk. Risk changes as a continuous process but a strict threshold implies that values just short of the threshold are fundamentally different from values just beyond the threshold. This can lead to scheduling decisions that drive all schedules to levels just short of the threshold, increasing aggregate fatigue risk. A better approach would examine the entire distribution of fatigue scores and make scheduling decisions that tend to move the entire distribution to better scores, rather than focussing on the region around some threshold.

One of the virtues of a BMMF is that it allows the user to experiment with different patterns and approaches to reduce fatigue and verify that the proposed changes will have the expected effects. It is not uncommon for a scheduling change to reduce fatigue on one shift but have an unintended ripple effect that increases fatigue on other shifts. Using a BMMF to prospectively model fatigue risk can help avoid such consequences in advance of actual operations. BMMFs can also be useful in operational settings as an educational tool to help explain the basic principles of sleep, circadian rhythms, and fatigue, or as a forensic tool to determine the potential role that fatigue may have played in the occurrence of an adverse event, accident, or injury (Dawson, Reynolds, Van Dongen, & Thomas, 2018).

4.3.6 EXAMPLES OF MODELLING IN DIFFERENT TRANSPORTATION MODES

BMMFs have been widely implemented in commercial, military, and general aviation to proactively manage fatigue risk, plan work/rest cycles, training, and safety investigations (CASA, 2014; DuBose, 2011; Paul et al., 2020; Rangan et al., 2020). Rail and maritime industries also use BMMFs regularly in their efforts to mitigate fatigue (Raslear, 2013; Register, 2011; Peng, Bouak, & Wang, 2021; van Leeuwen, Pekcan, Barnett, & Kecklund, 2021). Outside of the transportation industry, BMMFs have been used to predict fatigue in a number of shiftwork populations, including healthcare, law enforcement, and even simulated space missions (Flynn-Evans et al., 2020; Riedy et al., 2020; Sagherian et al., 2018; Schwartz et al., 2021).

4.3.7 FUTURE PERSPECTIVES ON MODELLING

BMMFs reflect our current scientific understanding of sleep and fatigue and should be expected to change as more information about these systems becomes available. Pertinent areas where models can be improved for use in the transportation industry include incorporating individual variability, workload, and accounting for the use of stimulants to counteract fatigue, to name a few (Ramakrishnan et al., 2016; Van Dongen, Baynard, Maislin, & Dinges, 2004; Vital-Lopez, Balkin, & Reifman, 2021).

Individuals differ with respect to vulnerability to sleep loss but BMMFs are designed for estimating group or organisational risk. It is therefore not currently appropriate to use BMMFs to evaluate fatigue for a specific individual or the validity of a fatigue report or accident investigation for a specific individual. As discussed in sub-section 4.3.2, some workload factors are known beforehand and can be incorporated into a fatigue prediction. However, many workload factors cannot be predicted, such as bad weather, equipment failures, and personnel issues. Stimulants—medications which promote feelings of wakefulness—are commonly used in the transportation industry to counteract the performance-impairing effects of fatigue (Ramakrishnan et al., 2016; Williamson, 2007). Incorporating an understanding of how stimulants influence on-the-job alertness and ability to sleep during recovery periods is an important next step towards superior understanding of fatigue risk in transportation industries.

4.3.8 BEST PRACTICES FOR FATIGUE MODELLING

All BMMFs are based on research studies and operational experience with a range of individuals. The models are tools with which operators can conduct proactive assessments of the fatigue potential of schedules in a relatively straightforward and inexpensive way, with little need of formal training or expertise. Analysis of data from BMMFs in transportation operations relies on certain specific assumptions, as summarised in Table 4.3.2.

Given these assumptions, BMMFs predict levels of performance during duties. These predictions are only estimates of risk based on average responses to the assumed conditions. Although modelling is a valuable tool for proactive and reactive assessment of conditions that could cause fatigue, BMMFs have important limitations acknowledged by those who invent models and those organisations that advocate modelling (IFMTF, 2015). Those limitations are described in Table 4.3.3.

It is important to acknowledge that fatigue modelling should not be used to pre- dict or assess the performance or accident risk of a specific individual. As a corollary

---

TABLE 4.3.2
Assumptions for the Analysis of BMMF Data in Transportation

---

1) Duties will be conducted as planned.
2) Operators will commute to the point of reporting with sufficient allowance of time to obtain adequate sleep prior to duty. *Commute times can be included in BMMFs, but do not account for individual differences in commute distances or time.*
3) Operators will have patterns of sleep typical of the average person with a need for eight hours of sleep per day.
4) For sleep opportunities while on duty, environmental conditions for sleep will be appropriate for the quality of rest facility defined in the schedule.
5) The operator will be fully rested at the beginning of the schedule and their circadian process is acclimated to the location at the start of the schedule.

TABLE 4.3.3
Limitations of BMMFs

BMMF Limitations

---

1) A BMMF is not a Fatigue Risk Management System (FRMS).
2) A model should not be used by individuals, operators, or regulators as a go/no-go decision tool.
3) The output of a model does not necessarily predict subjective measures of fatigue or sleepiness.
4) Model outputs represent the population average and may not be accurate for specific individuals.
5) Model sleep predictions may not reflect actual sleep, which is fundamental to the validity of the model's output.
6) Models may not consider the operational context and mitigations commonly used by operations to sustain attention.

of this limitation, fatigue modelling should also not be used to evaluate the validity of a fatigue report for a specific individual. Since BMMF outcomes are based on the expected performance of an average person, they should not be used to determine if a fatigue report from a specific person was valid or justified.

BMMFs have become valuable tools for fatigue risk management but have limitations that should be understood when they are applied by an organisation. All models are based on an evolving body of information about fatigue in the workplace. The accuracy of model predictions may differ relative to observations and a model may not be generalisable to novel sleep–wake–work scenarios. Operators must be mindful of the ongoing scientific process and inherent variability of results when interpreting the impact of predicted fatigue on operational risk.

SUMMARY POINTS FOR PRACTITIONERS

- BMMFs use mathematical equations to represent sleep need, circadian rhythms, and sleep inertia in order to predict fatigue risk, performance, or alertness.
- BMMFs can be used to predict population average fatigue risk, not individual risk.
- BMMFs should be evaluated in laboratory and field environments to establish the validity of their predicted outcomes.
- BMMFs should be used as part of a comprehensive FRMS in transportation.

REFERENCES

Åkerstedt, T., Ingre, M., Kecklund, G., Folkard, S., & Axelsson, J. (2008). Accounting for partial sleep deprivation and cumulative sleepiness in the three-process model of alertness regulation. *Chronobiology International, 25*(2), 309–319. doi:10.1080/07420520802110613

Borb, A. A., & Achermann, P. (1999). Sleep homeostasis and models of sleep regulation. *Journal of Biological Rhythms, 14*(6), 559–570.

Borbély, A. A. (1982). A two process model of sleep regulation. *Human Neurobiology, 1*(3), 195–204. Retrieved from www.ncbi.nlm.nih.gov/pubmed/7185792

CASA. (2014). Biomathematical fatigue models. Civil Aviation Safety Authority.

Czeisler, C. A., Allan, J. S., Strogatz, S. H., Ronda, J. M., Sánchez, R., Ríos, C. D.,... . Kronauer, R. E. (1986). Bright light resets the human circadian pacemaker independent of the timing of the sleep-wake cycle. *Science, 233*(4764), 667–671. doi:10.1126/science.3726555

Dawson, D., Darwent, D., & Roach, G. D. (2017). How should a bio-mathematical model be used within a fatigue risk management system to determine whether or not a working time arrangement is safe? *Accident Analysis & Prevention, 99,* 469–473.

Dawson, D., Reynolds, A. C., Van Dongen, H. P., & Thomas, M. J. (2018). Determining the likelihood that fatigue was present in a road accident: A theoretical review and suggested accident taxonomy. *Sleep Medicine Reviews, 42,* 202–210.

DuBose, N. N. (2011). Flightcrew member duty and rest requirements: Does the proposed legislation put to rest the concern over pilot fatigue. *Journal of Air Law and Commerce, 76,* 253.

Fletcher, A., & Dawson, D. (2001). Field-based validations of a work-related fatigue model based on hours of work. *Transportation Research Part F: Traffic Psychology and Behaviour, 4*(1), 75–88.

Flynn-Evans, E. E., Kirkley, C., Young, M., Bathurst, N., Gregory, K., Vogelpohl, V.,... . Marquez, J. J. (2020). Changes in performance and bio-mathematical model performance predictions during 45 days of sleep restriction in a simulated space mission. *Scientific Reports, 10*(1), 1–14.

Folkard, S., & Åkerstedt, T. (1987). Towards a model for the prediction of alertness and/or fatigue on different sleep/wake schedules in *Contemporary Advances in Shiftwork Research*, A. Oginski, J. Pokorski & J. Rutenfranz (Eds.). Medical Academy, Krakow, 231–240.

Fourie, C., Holmes, A., Bourgeois-Bougrine, S., Hilditch, C., & Jackson, P. (2010). Fatigue risk management systems: A review of the literature. *London, Department for Transport*, 20–25.

Gander, P. H., Wu, L. J., van den Berg, M., Lamp, A., Hoeg, L., & Belenky, G. (2016). Fatigue risk management systems. *Principles and Practice of Sleep Medicine* (6th ed.). Philadelphia, PA: Elsevier, 697–707.

Hilditch, C. J., & McHill, A. W. (2019). Sleep inertia: Current insights. *Nature and Science of Sleep, 11*, 155–165. doi:10.2147/NSS.S188911

Honn, K. A., Satterfield, B. C., McCauley, P., Caldwell, J. L., & Van Dongen, H. P. (2016). Fatiguing effect of multiple take-offs and landings in regional airline operations. *Accident Analysis and Prevention, 86*, 199–208. doi:10.1016/j.aap.2015.10.005

Hursh, S. R., Redmond, D. P., Johnson, M. L., Thorne, D. R., Belenky, G., Balkin, T. J.,... . Eddy, D. R. (2004). Fatigue models for applied research in warfighting. *Aviation, Space, and Environmental Medicine, 75*(3), A44–A53.

[IFMTF] IATA Fatigue Management Task Force. (2015). Uses and limitations of biomathematical fatigue models - White paper. International Air Transport Association. Retrieved from www.iata.org/contentassets/5f976bb3ca2446f3a40e88b18dd61fbb/uses-limitations-of-biomathematical-fatigue-models.pdf

Kandelaars, K. J., Dorrian, J., Fletcher, A., Roach, G. D., & Dawson, D. (2005). *A review of biomathematical fatigue models: Where to from here?* Sixth International Conference on Fatigue in Management in Transportation, Seattle, WA, September 11–15.

Lamond, N., Dorrian, J., Roach, G., McCulloch, K., Holmes, A., Burgess, H.,... . Dawson, D. (2003). The impact of a week of simulated night work on sleep, circadian phase, and performance. *Occupational and Environmental Medicine, 60*(11), e13–e13.

Mallis, M. M., Mejdal, S., Nguyen, T. T., & Dinges, D. F. (2004). Summary of the key features of seven biomathematical models of human fatigue and performance. *Aviation, Space, and Environmental Medicine, 75*(3 Suppl), A4–A14. Retrieved from www.ncbi.nlm.nih.gov/pubmed/15018262.

McCauley, P., Kalachev, L. V., Mollicone, D. J., Banks, S., Dinges, D. F., & Van Dongen, H. P. (2013). Dynamic circadian modulation in a biomathematical model for the effects of sleep and sleep loss on waking neurobehavioral performance. *Sleep, 36*(12), 1987–1997.

Monk, T. H. (1990). The relationship of chronobiology to sleep schedules and performance demands. *Work & Stress, 4*(3), 227–236. doi:10.1080/02678379008256985

Paul, M. A., Hursh, S. R., & Love, R. J. (2020). The importance of validating sleep behavior models for fatigue management software in military aviation. *Military Medicine, 185*(11–12), e1986–e1991. doi:10.1093/milmed/usaa210

Peng, H., & Bouak, F. (2015). Development of bio-mathematical models for human performance under fatigue. *DRDC Scientific Report, DRDC-RDDC-2015-R280.*

Peng, H., Bouak, F., & Wang, W. (2021). A comparison of performance prediction models for crew fatigue analyses. Defence Research and Development Canada Scientific Report No. DRDC-RDDC-2021-R066, April.

Ramakrishnan, S., Wesensten, N. J., Kamimori, G. H., Moon, J. E., Balkin, T. J., & Reifman, J. (2016). A unified model of performance for predicting the effects of sleep and caffeine. *Sleep, 39*(10), 1827–1841. doi:10.5665/sleep.6164

Rangan, S., Riedy, S. M., Bassett, R., Klinck, Z. A., Hagerty, P., Schek, E.,.... Van Dongen, H. P. A. (2020). Predictive and proactive fatigue risk management approaches in commercial aviation. *Chronobiology International, 37*(9–10), 1479–1482. doi:10.1080/07420528.2020.1803902

Rangan, S., & Van Dongen, H. P. (2013). Quantifying fatigue risk in model-based fatigue risk management. *Aviation, Space, and Environmental Medicine, 84*(2), 155–157. doi:10.3357/asem.3455.2013

Raslear, T. (2013). *Criteria and procedures for validating biomathematical models of human performance and fatigue: procedures for analysis of work schedules.* Retrieved from https://railroads.dot.gov/elibrary/criteria-and-procedures-validating-biomathematical-models-human-performance-and-fatigue

Register, F. (2011). *49 CFR Part 228; Hours of Service of Railroad Employees; Substantive Regulations for Train Employees Providing Commuter and Intercity Rail Passenger Transportation; Conforming Amendments to Recordkeeping Requirements; Final Rule. 76 FR 50359.* U.S. Government Publishing Office.

Riedy, S. M., Fekedulegn, D., Andrew, M., Vila, B., Dawson, D., & Violanti, J. (2020). Generalizability of a biomathematical model of fatigue's sleep predictions. *Chronobiology International, 37*(4), 564–572.

Sagherian, K., Zhu, S., Storr, C., Hinds, P. S., Derickson, D., & Geiger-Brown, J. (2018). Biomathematical fatigue models predict sickness absence in hospital nurses: An 18 months retrospective cohort study. *Applied Ergonomics, 73*, 42–47.

Schwartz, L. P., Devine, J. K., Hursh, S. R., Mosher, E., Schumacher, S., Boyle, L.,.... Fitzgibbons, S. C. (2021). Biomathematical modeling predicts fatigue risk in general surgery residents. *Journal of Surgical Education, 76*(6), 2094–2101.

Tabak, B., & Raslear, T. G. (2010). *Procedures for validation and calibration of human fatigue models: The Fatigue Audit InterDyne tool.* Retrieved from https://railroads.dot.gov/elibrary/procedures-validation-and-calibration-human-fatigue-models-fatigue-audit-interdyne-tool

Tassi, P., & Muzet, A. (2000). Sleep inertia. *Sleep Medicine Reviews, 4*(4), 341–353.

Van Dongen, H. (2004). Comparison of mathematical model predictions to experimental data of fatigue and performance. *Aviation, Space, and Environmental Medicine, 75*(3), A15–A36.

Van Dongen, H. P. (2010). Predicting sleep/wake behavior for model-based fatigue risk management. *Sleep, 33*(2), 144–145.

Van Dongen, H. P., Baynard, M. D., Maislin, G., & Dinges, D. F. (2004). Systematic interindividual differences in neurobehavioral impairment from sleep loss: Evidence of trait-like differential vulnerability. *Sleep, 27*(3), 423–433. Retrieved from www.ncbi.nlm.nih.gov/pubmed/15164894.

van Leeuwen, W. M., Pekcan, C., Barnett, M., & Kecklund, G. (2021). Mathematical modelling of sleep and sleepiness under various watch keeping schedules in the maritime industry. *Marine Policy, 130*, 104277.

Vital-Lopez, F. G., Balkin, T. J., & Reifman, J. (2021). Models for predicting sleep latency and sleep duration. *Sleep, 44*(5), zsaa263.

Williamson, A. (2007). Predictors of psychostimulant use by long-distance truck drivers. *American Journal of Epidemiology, 166*(11), 1320–1326.

4.4 Fatigue Risk Thresholds

Emily M. Moslener, Hans P. A. Van Dongen, and Kimberly A. Honn

Sleep and Performance Research Center & Department of Translational Medicine and Physiology, Washington State University, Spokane, WA, USA

CONTENTS

4.4.1 MANAGING RISKS IN THE WORKPLACE

Operating in any work environment is associated with a certain degree of risk, which may be multi-dimensional (e.g., financial and safety). To assess the various risk factors that may be present in a workplace, it is useful to consider two distinct aspects: likelihood and potential consequences (ISO 31000:2018; International Organization for Standardization, 2018). That is, the more likely a risk factor is to manifest itself, where likelihood can be seen as the product of probability (or frequency) and exposure (or duration), the greater the overall risk (Rangan & Van Dongen, 2013). Likewise, the more potentially consequential (or costly) a risk factor is, the greater the overall risk. For example, safety-related risks associated with road transportation tend to be greater in areas with dense traffic because that increases the likelihood of collisions. And safety-related risks also tend to be greater if hazardous materials are being transported, as the consequences of even a single accident could be severe. As this example implies, overall risk is a combination of likelihood and possible consequences, and this provides a scheme to classify overall risk from low to very high.

The same scheme can also guide the management of risk by minimising the likelihood of a risk factor and/or by mitigating its potential consequences. Thus, to continue the example, overall road transportation risk may be managed by building a bigger road system and thereby reducing traffic density, so as to reduce the likelihood of collisions. Overall road transportation risk may also be managed by separating hazardous materials transport from other traffic and thereby mitigating the expected severity of an accident, so as to reduce the potential consequences. This latter approach also limits exposure to dense traffic, so it reduces overall risk through both aspects: likelihood and possible consequences.

DOI: 10.1201/9781003213154-26

Risk management aids such as risk matrices (Kovačević et al., 2019) can be used to illustrate that risks may be diminished by reducing the likelihood and/or mitigating the potential consequences of an incident (e.g., see Dixon, 2016). Although widely used as a conceptual framework, risk matrices leave unanswered the question of what constitutes an acceptable level of risk. A relatively novel perspective on this question is to cast it in terms of risk appetite, that is, "the amount and type of risk that an organisation is willing to pursue or retain" (ISO 73:2009; International Organization for Standardization, 2009). However, most industries currently cast it in terms of "risk tolerance," that is, the readiness of an organisation to bear the *managed* risk in order to achieve its objectives (adapted from ISO 73:2009; International Organization for Standardization, 2009). This effectively reduces the question of what an acceptable level of risk is to establishing what risk level, for any of the multiple risk factors that may be present in the work environment, the organisation (and its stakeholders) can endure—i.e., a *risk threshold*. This chapter is concerned with establishing acceptable risk thresholds, in particular as they pertain to risks originating from human fatigue.

A risk threshold determines an organisation's needed efforts to manage risk factors and what degree of risk reduction should be accomplished. Establishing a risk threshold often includes consideration of a variety of risk factors associated with humans in the workplace, who are essential for an organisation's success but at times may be limited in availability (e.g., absenteeism and staff shortages), capability (e.g., poorly equipped and insufficiently trained), or reliability (e.g., distracted and fatigued). In the field of human factors and ergonomics, extensive research has been devoted to curbing human-related risks by reducing the likelihood and potential consequences of human error. This quest took on a whole new dimension from about the middle of the previous century, when work hours started to extend into the night and the 24/7 economy began to take shape (Honn et al., 2019). Specifically, humans become mentally fatigued when work hours are extended and/or placed at night (Van Dongen et al., 2022), and that makes them more prone to error and accidents (Marcus & Rosekind, 2017).

Although incidents related to human error are stochastic in nature (Reason, 1990), the extent to which they are more likely to occur as a consequence of fatigue is predictable (Raslear et al., 2011). This means that the overall risk related to fatigue is at least partially predictable as well, and therefore amenable to the establishment of a risk threshold—i.e., a *fatigue risk threshold*. In safety management and regulatory settings, much debate has been devoted to setting appropriate fatigue risk thresholds, which is increasingly informed by scientific evidence (Gurubhagavatula et al., 2021). Fatigue risk thresholds are the focus of this chapter.

4.4.2 HUMAN FATIGUE

Many industries require employees to work extended, night-time, or irregular hours in order to meet 24/7 demand (Burke & Cooper, 2008). Such work hours are inconsistent with biological constraints on alertness (Åkerstedt, 2000), which stem from the interaction of the circadian and homeostatic processes of sleep/wake regulation (Daan et al., 1984). The circadian process reflects the brain's internal, biological clock, which tracks time of day, and the homeostatic process reflects the need for sleep by tracking prior sleep and wakefulness (Borbély, 1982). In healthy individuals, the interplay of these two processes is such that when daily sleep is both sufficiently long (~7 hours or more for the average adult; Watson et al., 2015) and timed appropriately (i.e., at night; Dijk & Czeisler, 1994), alertness is stable and optimal through the day, and fatigue is limited to that which results specifically from task-related fatigue (e.g., extended time on task; Mackworth, 1964). However, when work or other demands for wakefulness reduce or displace sleep, the two processes become misaligned in time and the stability of alert wakefulness is disrupted. This leads to a state of fatigue, which is amplified by wake extension and peaks in the late night and early morning hours (Van Dongen & Dinges, 2005). This condition of misalignment between the circadian and homeostatic processes also exacerbates task-related fatigue (Wesensten et al., 2004), and furthermore accumulates across days with insufficient sleep (Van Dongen et al., 2003).

Fatigue may be defined as a state of reduced mental or physical performance capability, resulting from sleep loss or extended wakefulness, circadian rhythmicity, workload, or other factors (IATA et al., 2011). Fatigue has multiple facets, with physical fatigue manifesting as degraded physical performance and mental fatigue manifesting as degraded cognitive performance (Gurubhagavatula et al., 2021). Fatigue also has physiological and subjective correlates (Oonk et al., 2008), and a plethora of tools are available to detect evidence of fatigue (Abe et al., 2014). Furthermore, the biological processes that drive human fatigue vary systematically over time, and their dynamics are well understood (Muck et al., 2022). This means that changes over time in the likelihood of a worker experiencing a fatigue-related incident are trackable and predictable, and fatigue and its associated risks can thus be assessed and anticipated. This provides a foundation for the establishment of fatigue risk thresholds and the management of fatigue risks.

4.4.3 LIMITING WORK HOURS TO MANAGE FATIGUE RISK

Before the Second World War, when work was often physical in nature and physical fatigue was a dominant fatigue risk factor, the relationship between work hours and fatigue was more or less linear—longer work hours were associated with greater fatigue. A good way to manage fatigue risk, therefore, was to cap the amount of time spent on the work floor. Hours of service regulations and rules that prescribe maximum work durations and minimum rest durations between work episodes are based on this idea.

During and after the Second World War, the demand for work spread across all hours of the day and increasing levels of mechanisation and automation shifted the emphasis of human involvement in the workplace from mostly physical to mostly mental in nature (Wong et al., 2019). Nonetheless, the primary approach to managing fatigue risk has continued to be through work duration restrictions and hours of service regulations, and to some extent this makes sense. That is, a cap on work hours curbs exposure to workplace risks from fatigue. Furthermore, as misalignment between the circadian and homeostatic processes from reduced and displaced sleep drives fatigue, requiring sufficient time for rest between work episodes protects opportunities for recuperative (night-time) sleep and helps to limit the development of excessive fatigue. As such, within the framework of hours of service, establishing fatigue risk thresholds involves setting boundaries on work hours (as a proxy for the build-up of fatigue and fatigue risk) and time off (as a proxy for the dissipation of fatigue and fatigue risk; Gurubhagavatula et al., 2021).

However, with respect to mental fatigue in a 24/7 setting, the relationship with work hours is highly non-linear (Åkerstedt, 1995). For instance, night shift workers typically experience the greatest level of fatigue in the morning hours at the end of their shift (Wilson et al., 2019), with a concomitant increase in accident risk during the commute home (Lee et al., 2016). Yet, because of how the circadian and homeostatic processes interact, extending wakefulness into the subsequent afternoon would, paradoxically, be associated with a reduction in fatigue (Van Dongen & Dinges, 2005). Therefore, the correspondence between limitations on work hours and success in curbing overall fatigue risk can break down, and create incongruence between adherence to the prescribed working time arrangements and risk mitigation outcomes (Honn et al., 2019). As illustrated in Figure 4.4.1, this can lead to a false sense of security, needless loss of productivity, and/or non-compliance with the work hour limitations to avoid such consequences. Setting the work hours limitation(s) at a level that is too permissive would allow for too much exposure to excessive fatigue risk (Figure 4.4.1, top left), but setting them at a level that is too restrictive causes loss of potential for productivity and possibly also loss of flexibility in work scheduling (Figure 4.4.1, top right).

As is also evident from Figure 4.4.1, regardless of what exactly is considered an "acceptable" level of fatigue risk for the operation at hand, establishing fatigue risk thresholds based on work hours requires striking a balance between being too restrictive and too permissive. That is, the work hour limitation(s) should rule out most of the work schedules that exceed the acceptable risk level, but not at the cost of too many work schedules that could have longer work hours without appreciable increase in risk (Honn et al., 2019). However, even when a balance can be identified between overly restrictive or permissive work hour limitations, because of incongruence between work hour durations and fatigue risk, there remains a subset of shifts that are allowed despite their excessive risk, and a subset of shifts that are prohibited, despite their acceptable risk (Figure 4.4.1, bottom left).

The challenges in balancing acceptable work hours and limiting risk do not mean, however, that managing fatigue risk in 24/7 operations by means of work hour limitations is a hopeless endeavour. Work hour limitations, such as hours of service regulations, can be crafted to require and account for the use of fatigue mitigation strategies. The possibilities are manifold, ranging from planned on-the-job nap opportunities (Sallinen et al., 1998) to the use of fatigue detection and warning systems (Sparrow et al., 2019) and from mandating access to caffeine (Temple et al., 2018) to implementation of a wide range of "fatigue proofing" strategies (Dawson et al., 2012). As illustrated in Figure 4.4.1 (bottom right), the advantages of this approach are twofold. That is, the threshold for *managed* risk can be more permissive than when not accounting for fatigue risk management, and the link between work duration and expected fatigue risk tightens. Hence, the distinction between work schedules with acceptable versus unacceptable risk tends to be less ambiguous, such

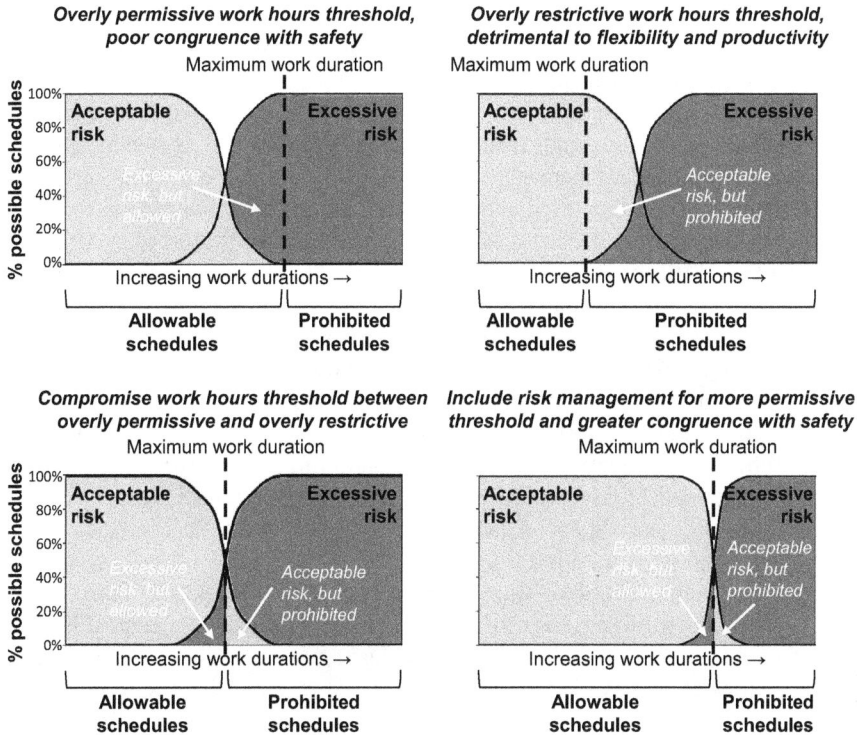

FIGURE 4.4.1 Illustration of the challenges of limiting work hours to manage fatigue risk. Each panel shows an example threshold rule for maximum work hours and the implications for fatigue risk versus adherence to the rule. In each panel, the light grey area represents schedules that would have acceptable risk, and the dark grey area represents schedules that would have excessive risk. A dashed vertical line represents the maximum work duration that is set in each example, with allowable schedules (i.e., not exceeding the maximum work duration) to the left and prohibited schedules to the right.

that it is less challenging to strike a good balance that rules out most of the work schedules with excessive risk while retaining most of the work schedules with acceptable risk. Guiding principles for deciding on work hour limitations with the objective of managing fatigue risk have recently been published (Gurubhagavatula et al., 2021).

4.4.4 MEASURING AND LIMITING FATIGUE TO MANAGE FATIGUE RISK

Regulating working time as an approach to managing fatigue risk is relatively easy to apply and enforce, and is implemented in industries around the world. However, setting risk thresholds based on work and rest time involves an implicit, but incorrect, assumption that fatigue risk increases steadily with working time and decreases steadily with rest. Because fatigue—in particular, mental fatigue—depends on a variety of factors including time of day (through the biological clock) and sleep insufficiency (e.g., from a sleep disorder), this assumption is not always met.

Although work and rest durations are key drivers of work-related fatigue risk that can be controlled, this does not mean that the way fatigue risk is managed has to focus on working time arrangements *per se*. The efficacy of working arrangements can be enhanced by adding provisions for the management of fatigue more directly (Gurubhagavatula et al., 2021), such as the inclusion of fatigue proofing strategies (Dawson et al., 2012) or provisions for on-the-job napping (Sallinen et al., 1998). As illustrated in Figure 4.4.1 (bottom right), this can yield benefits in terms of productivity and scheduling flexibility without incurring excessive risk. Moreover, it can help to improve congruence between adherence to working time rules and effective management of fatigue risk, with attendant benefits for compliance and risk outcomes.

To take this idea a step further, in addition to—or even in lieu of—tracking work and rest times, fatigue may be managed by quantifying fatigue risk through measurement (or methodical prediction) and comparing that to a threshold specifying an acceptable level of risk. In this paradigm, work is not, or not necessarily, stopped when a maximum work duration is exceeded, but rather work must be discontinued when the maximum allowable fatigue risk is exceeded (or work may then only be continued with appropriate mitigations in place). This approach is appealing because it manages fatigue risk directly, without relying solely on a tenuous link between work/rest times and fatigue, and it has the potential to avoid the risk incongruence issues of relying on work time restrictions to manage fatigue risk as illustrated in Figure 4.4.1.

While work and rest hours are comparatively straightforward to assess and regulate, how to estimate fatigue risk is less obvious. Adverse fatigue risk outcomes (i.e., accidents) and fatigue-related incidents (e.g., safety-critical events) are used to estimate fatigue risk in road and rail transportation and in aviation (see Chapter 4.3 of this book). Aggregated across whole industries, such data sets can be sufficiently rich to show meaningful trends and illuminate situations that lead to elevated fatigue risk (Hursh et al., 2006). Yet, accidents and fatigue-related incidents may be too rare and/ or sporadic, or too much confounded by risk factors other than fatigue, to serve as a reliable index of fatigue risk. Also, accidents and incidents are lagging risk indicators; when they occur, the fatigue risk may well already be too high.

Leading risk indicators, on the other hand, can flag impending fatigue risk before it becomes unacceptably high, allowing for timely intervention. Leading indicator measurement modalities applied in operational settings usually seek to quantify fatigue rather than the associated risk, because fatigue is a more concrete measurement target and high levels of fatigue imply at least the possibility of high risk. Leading indicator measurement modalities include subjective (i.e., self-reported) assessments of fatigue (sleepiness) and objective (i.e., task-based) assessments of performance impairment, as well as real-time monitoring of physiological (e.g., cardiac or ocular) indicators of fatigue. Finally, scientific advances in understanding the quantitative relationship between sleep/wake/work schedules and the patterns of fatigue they produce have led to the development of biomathematical models that can predict fatigue without a need to take measurements (see Chapter 4.3 of this book). Each of these methods has advantages and disadvantages and specific considerations with regard to setting fatigue risk thresholds.

Three important criteria should be considered when establishing fatigue risk thresholds:

1. *Implementation*: a meaningful and measurable or estimable outcome must be available to which the threshold pertains.
2. *Differentiation*: the threshold must clearly distinguish acceptable levels of fatigue from unacceptable levels of fatigue.
3. *Effectiveness*: there should be a high degree of real-world congruence between adherence to the threshold (i.e., compliance) and avoiding fatigue risk; and between non-adherence to the threshold (i.e., non-compliance) and incurring fatigue risk.

For each of the measurement/prediction modalities mentioned above—accidents, safety-critical events, subjective and objective assessments of fatigue, real-time fatigue monitoring, and biomathematical model predictions—the extent to which they presently meet the three criteria above is shown in Table 4.4.1.

Each measure for setting a fatigue risk threshold has key benefits and uses for managing fatigue risk, although no single measure fully satisfies the *implementation, differentiation,* and *effectiveness* criteria. The available measures also approach the issue of fatigue risk from different angles, including different viewpoints for application (i.e., prospective, on-the-job, and retrospective). For a comprehensive approach to managing fatigue with the help of fatigue risk thresholds, any or all of the described

TABLE 4.4.1
Criteria to Be Considered in Establishing Appropriate Fatigue Risk Thresholds for Operational Settings

Measure Used for Threshold	Basis for Threshold	Viewpoint for Application	Criterion 1: Implementation	Criterion 2: Differentiation	Criterion 3: Effectiveness
Accidents	Safety	Retrospective	No	Yes	Yes
Safety-critical events	Risk	On-the-job or retrospective	Yes	No	Yes
Subjective and objective fatigue assessments	Fatigue	On-the-job	Yes	Partly	Partly
Real-time fatigue monitoring	Physiological correlates of fatigue	On-the-job	Partly	Partly	Unknown
Biomathematical model predictions	Biology-based expected fatigue	Prospective or retrospective	Yes	Yes	Unknown

measures can be used in combination. For example, biomathematical models can be used prospectively to predict fatigue in planned schedules to ensure they do not *a priori* exceed a fatigue risk threshold. Then, during the work periods, subjective and/ or objective fatigue assessments, or real-time fatigue monitoring systems, can be used to verify that fatigue stays below the threshold. Retrospective analyses of accidents and safety-critical events, with or without the help of a biomathematical model, can identify patterns or elements of work shifts (e.g., routes and tasks) that carry excessive fatigue risk. Fatigue risk management systems (FRMS) present a formalised framework for using multiple complementary methods and thresholds to manage fatigue in an operation (Lerman et al., 2012).

4.4.5 SETTING A THRESHOLD LEVEL

Regardless of the fatigue risk measurement tools selected for use in an operation, setting the right fatigue risk threshold is critical for efficacy. One way to do this is through evidence-based and stakeholder-informed decision-making. Guiding principles have been published in the context of work duration thresholds (Gurubhagavatula et al., 2021), and this method would be equally applicable to fatigue risk thresholds. When shifting the focus from work hours to fatigue levels, however, additional approaches become possible based on comparisons with known standards, historical records, or prior evidence of acceptable risk under similar circumstances.

An example of comparing fatigue risk with a known (and accepted) standard comes from the road safety domain. With regard to automobile driving, research has shown that a comparison can be made between risks associated with fatigue and risks associated with alcohol intoxication (Dawson & Reid, 1997). Although the effects of fatigue and alcohol on driving are qualitatively different, they show quantitatively comparable effects on fatigue assessment tools (Williamson & Feyer, 2000). Based on this equivalence, it would be reasonable to set a fatigue risk threshold at the level where the fatigue measurement associated with the threshold (say, performance on an objective fatigue assessment tool, such as a driving simulator) shows the same level of impairment as what is observed for alcohol at the legally allowed level of intoxication (typically 0.05% or 0.08% blood alcohol concentration). The central argument for setting a fatigue risk threshold this way is the concept of *equivalent level of safety* or, more broadly, *equivalent level of risk*—when scenario A can be shown to be no more risky than scenario B, and the risk associated with scenario B has already been deemed to be acceptable for a given risk threshold, then by implication the same holds for scenario A.

The example based on comparing fatigue with alcohol serves well to illustrate the concept of equivalent level of risk, but a stronger case for equivalence may be made based on comparing fatigue in one scenario with fatigue in another, similar scenario for which the acceptability of risk has already been established (Van Dongen & Belenky, 2012). As such, the safety record of past operations can be used to establish an inherently valid fatigue risk threshold for a particular operational environment.

Figure 4.4.2 illustrates the use of existing safety data from commercial aviation operations to perform a preliminary evaluation of the safety of alternative

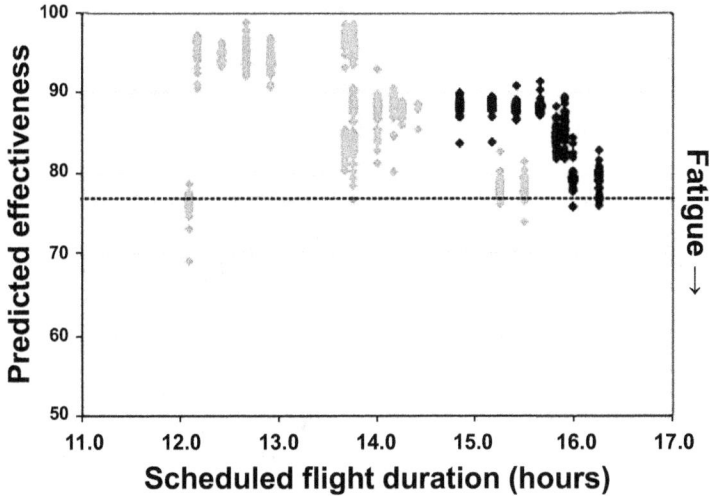

FIGURE 4.4.2 Illustration of the establishment of a fatigue risk threshold based on the proven safety record of a similar operation. Fatigue predictions from a biomathematical model are shown for a set of augmented (four-pilot) long-range flights (grey) and hypothetically scheduled, augmented (four-pilot) ultra-long-range flights (black), plotted as a function of scheduled flight duration against predicted effectiveness for the landing phase of flight, where greater effectiveness scores correspond to less fatigue (Hursh et al., 2004). Comparing the hypothetical ultra-long-range flights to a threshold established with the historically safe long-range flights (dotted line at predicted effectiveness of 77) showed that almost all of the hypothetical flights would have predicted effectiveness scores above the threshold, implying an acceptable degree of fatigue risk. Figure adapted from Van Dongen and Belenky (2012).

flight schedules as predicted by means of a biomathematical model. In this case, the historical safety records of a relatively large sample of long-range flight operations with flight durations below 16 hours, all of which had been operated without fatigue-related accidents, were first analysed with the model. The analysis showed that 95% of these flights had a predicted effectiveness score greater than 77 (where greater effectiveness corresponds to less fatigue). This threshold (dotted line in Figure 4.4.2) could be considered to reflect acceptable risk and could thus be used to establish a generalised fatigue risk threshold. Subsequently, this specific threshold was used for the main objective of the preliminary investigation; that is, to evaluate whether hypothetical ultra-long-range flights with flight durations anticipated to exceed 16 hours in more than 10% of cases would be associated with greater levels of risk than the long-range flights. A formal statistical comparison, taking the form of equivalence testing or non-inferiority testing, confirmed that the fatigue risk of the hypothetical flights would not exceed the established fatigue risk threshold. Strengthened by the use of a real-world scenario with a historical record of safety to set the fatigue risk threshold, the result of this preliminary investigation provided one piece of evidence towards a safety case (Gander et al., 2017) that ultimately led to regulatory acceptance of ultra-long-range flight operations in the United States.

It should be noted that reference data used to establish a risk threshold may be context-dependent, subject to the assessment or opinion of others and specific to the setting and historical context. That is, what is deemed an acceptable level of risk is at least partially determined by the risk tolerance of stakeholders from industry, labour, government, and society. Thus, fatigue risk thresholds are inherently context-dependent (Van Dongen & Belenky, 2012) and should be re-evaluated when circumstances change or when applied in a novel setting.

4.4.6 CONCLUSIONS

Workplace fatigue increases the likelihood of errors and incidents and constitutes a threat to safety and productivity. Across a wide range of industries and operations, this puts a premium on managing risks associated with fatigue, while protecting productivity and preserving the integrity of an operation. Overall fatigue risk is proportional to both the likelihood and the potential consequences of fatigue, and both may vary considerably over time. However, while adverse outcomes related to fatigue tend to be stochastic in nature, fatigue makes them more likely in a way that is driven by biological processes that are well understood and predictable. This provides a basis for managing fatigue risk through working time arrangements to curb the build-up of fatigue and/or through fatigue measurement or prediction to detect (and mitigate) excessive fatigue or risk. Regardless of the approach taken, though, questions arise about what is an appropriate fatigue risk threshold.

There are no one-size-fits-all answers. The degree of exposure to fatigue and the potential consequences of fatigue and other risk factors vary substantially across industries, employee roles, and job tasks. Moreover, what is considered an acceptable level of risk (i.e., risk tolerance) in any particular industry may differ based on the perspective (e.g., as seen by industry, labour, regulator, or the public). Thus, fatigue risk thresholds are inherently context-dependent (Van Dongen & Belenky, 2012). To build on guidance from Gurubhagavatula et al. (2021, abstract, p. 1), a science-based approach to managing fatigue risks requires (1) recognition and understanding of key factors that contribute to fatigue and fatigue-related risks, (2) understanding of available mitigation strategies for fatigue and/or fatigue-related risks, and (3) evidence-based and stakeholder-informed decision-making processes for setting fatigue risk thresholds. This and other chapters in this book should help to provide the knowledge base needed to pursue this worthy endeavour, which may save resources and contribute to productivity while also improving worker safety, health, and satisfaction.

SUMMARY POINTS FOR PRACTITIONERS

- For managing fatigue risk, working time restrictions are only partially effective.
- An alternative or complementary strategy involves comparing measured or predicted fatigue to a fatigue risk threshold.
- A fatigue risk threshold can be established on the basis of a variety of different metrics, each with their own advantages, disadvantages, and specific uses.

- A fatigue risk threshold is dependent on context and risk tolerance.
- Setting an appropriate fatigue risk threshold can be done based on pre-established standards, historical records, or previously collected evidence of acceptable risk under similar circumstances.

REFERENCES

Abe, T., Mollicone, D., Basner, M., & Dinges, D.F. (2014). Sleepiness and safety: Where biology needs technology. *Sleep and Biological Rhythms*, 12(2), 74–84.

Åkerstedt, T. (1995). Work hours, sleepiness and the underlying mechanisms. *Journal of Sleep Research*, 4(S2), 15–22.

Åkerstedt, T. (2000). Consensus statement: fatigue and accidents in transport operations. *Journal of Sleep Research*, 9(4), 395.

Borbély, A.A. (1982). A two process model of sleep regulation. *Human Neurobiology*, 1, 195–204.

Burke, R.J., & Cooper, C.L. (Eds.). (2008). *Long Work Hours Culture: Causes, Consequences and Choices*. Bingley: Emerald Group Publishing.

Daan, S., Beersma, D.G., & Borbély, A.A. (1984). Timing of human sleep: Recovery process gated by a circadian pacemaker. *American Journal of Physiology–Regulatory, Integrative and Comparative Physiology*, 246(2), R161–R183.

Dawson, D., Chapman, J., & Thomas, M.J. (2012). Fatigue-proofing: A new approach to reducing fatigue-related risk using the principles of error management. *Sleep Medicine Reviews*, 16(2), 167–175.

Dawson, D., & Reid, K. (1997). Fatigue, alcohol and performance impairment. *Nature*, 388 (6639), 235–237.

Dijk, D.J., & Czeisler, C.A. (1994). Paradoxical timing of the circadian rhythm of sleep propensity serves to consolidate sleep and wakefulness in humans. *Neuroscience Letters*, 166(1), 63–68.

Dixon, J. (2016). *Work Health and Safety Procedures 2016*. Sydney: University of Sydney.

Gander, P., Mangie, J., Wu, L., van den Berg, M.J., Signal, L., & Phillips, A. (2017). Preparing safety cases for operating outside prescriptive fatigue risk management regulations. *Aerospace Medicine and Human Performance*, 88(7), 688–696.

Gurubhagavatula, I., Barger, L.K., Barnes, C.M., Basner, M., Boivin, D.B., Dawson, D., Drake, C.L., Flynn-Evans, E.E., Mysliwiec, V., Patterson, P.D., Reid, K.J., Samuels, C., Shattuck, N.L., Kazmi, U., Carandang, G., Heald, J.L., & Van Dongen, H.P.A. (2021). Guiding principles for determining work shift duration and addressing the effects of work shift duration on performance, safety, and health: Guidance from the American Academy of Sleep Medicine and the Sleep Research Society. *Sleep*, 44(11), zsab16.

Honn, K.A., Van Dongen, H.P.A., & Dawson, D. (2019). Working Time Society consensus statements: Prescriptive rule sets and risk management-based approaches for the management of fatigue-related risk in working time arrangements. *Industrial Health*, 57(2), 264–280.

Hursh, S.R., Raslear, T.G., Kaye, A.S., & Fanzone, J.F. (2006). Validation and calibration of a fatigue assessment tool for railroad work schedules, summary report. Report No. DOT/FRA/ORD-06/21. Washington, DC: Federal Railroad Administration.

Hursh, S.R., Redmond, D.P., Johnson, M.L., Thorne, D.R., Belenky, G., Balkin, T.J., Storm, W.F., Miller, J.C., & Eddy, D.R. (2004). Fatigue models for applied research in warfighting. *Aviation, Space and Environmental Medicine,* 75(3 Suppl.), A44–A53.

IATA, ICAO, IFALPA. (2011). *Fatigue Risk Management Systems Implementation Guide for Operators*, 1st ed.

International Organization for Standardization. (2009*). Risk Management–Vocabulary (ISO Guide 73:2009)*. Geneva: ISO Copyright Office.

International Organization for Standardization. (2018). *Risk Management–Guidelines, 2nd ed. (ISO Standard No. 31000:2018)*. Geneva: ISO Copyright Office.

Kovačević, N., Stojiljković, A., & Kovač, M. (2019). Application of the matrix approach in risk assessment. *Operational Research in Engineering Sciences: Theory and Applications,* 2(3), 55–64.

Lee, M.L., Howard, M.E., Horrey, W.J., Liang, Y., Anderson, C., Shreeve, M.S., O'Brien, C.S., & Czeisler, C.A. (2016). High risk of near-crash driving events following night-shift work. *Proceedings of the National Academy of Sciences of the United States of America*, 113(1), 176–181.

Lerman, S.E., Eskin, E., Flower, D.J., George, E.C., Gerson, B., Hartenbaum, N., Hursh, S.R., & Moore-Ede, M. (2012). Fatigue risk management in the workplace. *Journal of Occupational and Environmental Medicine*, 54(2), 231–258.

Mackworth, J.F. (1964). Performance decrement in vigilance, threshold, and high-speed perceptual motor tasks. *Canadian Journal of Psychology,* 18(3), 209–223.

Marcus, J.H., & Rosekind, M.R. (2017). Fatigue in transportation: NTSB investigations and safety recommendations. *Injury Prevention,* 23(4), 232–238.

Muck, R.A., Hudson, A.N., Honn, K.A., Gaddameedhi, S., & Van Dongen, H.P.A. (2022). Working around the clock: Is a person's endogenous circadian timing for optimal neurobehavioral functioning inherently task-dependent? *Clocks & Sleep,* 4(1), 23–36.

Oonk, M., Tucker, A.M., Belenky, G., & Van Dongen, H.P.A. (2008). Excessive sleepiness: Determinants, outcomes, and context. *International Journal of Sleep and Wakefulness*, 1, 141–147.

Rangan, S., & Van Dongen, H.P.A. (2013). Quantifying fatigue risk in model-based fatigue risk management. *Aviation, Space, and Environmental Medicine,* 84(2), 155–157.

Raslear, T.G., Hursh, S.R., & Van Dongen, H.P.A. (2011). Predicting cognitive impairment and accident risk. *Progress in Brain Research*, 190, 155–167.

Reason, J. (1990). *Human Error.* New York: Cambridge University Press.

Sallinen, M., Härmä, M., Åkerstedt, T., Rosa, R., & Lillqvist, O. (1998). Promoting alertness with a short nap during a night shift. *Journal of Sleep Research*, 7(4), 240–247.

Sparrow, A.R., LaJambe, C.M., & Van Dongen, H.P.A. (2019). Drowsiness measures for commercial motor vehicle operations. *Accident Analysis and Prevention*, 126, 146–159.

Temple, J.L., Hostler, D., Martin-Gill, C., Moore, C.G., Weiss, P.M., Sequeria, D.J., Condle, J.P., Lang, E.S., Higgins, J.S., & Patterson, P.D. (2018). Systematic review and meta-analysis of the effects of caffeine in fatigued shift workers: Implications for Emergency Medical Services personnel. *Prehospital Emergency Care*, 22(Suppl. 1), 37–46.

Van Dongen, H.P.A., Balkin, T.J., Hursh, S.R., & Dorrian, J. (2022). Performance deficits during sleep loss and their operational consequences. Kryger, M., Roth, T., Goldstein, C.A., Dement, W.C., Eds., *Principles and Practice of Sleep Medicine,* 7th ed., 742–749.

Van Dongen, H.P.A., & Belenky, G. (2012). Model-based fatigue risk management. In Matthews, G., Desmond, P.A., Neubauer, C., & Hancock, P.A., Eds. *The Handbook of Operator Fatigue.* Farnham: Ashgate, 487–506.

Van Dongen, H.P.A., & Dinges, D.F. (2005). Sleep, circadian rhythms, and psychomotor vigilance. *Clinics in Sports Medicine*, 24(2), 237–249.

Van Dongen, H.P.A., Maislin, M.S., Mullington, J.M., & Dinges, D.F. (2003). The cumulative cost of additional wakefulness: Dose-response effects on neurobehavioral functions and sleep physiology from chronic sleep restriction and total sleep deprivation. *Sleep*, 26(2), 117–126.

Watson, N.F., Badr, M.S., Belenky, G., Bliwise, D.L., Buxton, O.M., Buysse, D., Dinges, D.F., Gangwisch, J., Grandner, M.A., Kushida, C., Malhotra, R.K., Martin, J.L., Patel, S.R., Quan, S.F., & Tasali, E. (2015). Recommended amount of sleep for a healthy adult: a joint consensus statement of the American Academy of Sleep Medicine and Sleep Research Society. *Sleep*, 38(6), 843–844.

Wesensten, N.J., Belenky, G., Thorne, D.R., Kautz, M.A., & Balkin, T.J. (2004). Modafinil vs. caffeine: Effects on fatigue during sleep deprivation. *Aviation, Space and Environmental Medicine*, 75(6), 520–525.

Williamson, A.M., & Feyer, A.M. (2000). Moderate sleep deprivation produces impairments in cognitive and motor performance equivalent to legally prescribed levels of alcohol intoxication. *Occupational and Environmental Medicine*, 57(10), 649–655.

Wilson, M., Permito, R., English, A., Albritton, S., Coogle, C., & Van Dongen, H.P.A. (2019). Performance and sleepiness in nurses working 12-h day shifts or night shifts in a community hospital. *Accident Analysis and Prevention*, 126, 43–46.

Wong, I.S., Popkin, S., & Folkard, S. (2019). Working Time Society consensus statements: A multi-level approach to managing occupational sleep-related fatigue. *Industrial Health*, 57(2), 228–244.

4.5 Fatigue Profiling

An Approach to Understand Occurrence, Causes, and Effects of Fatigue in People Working in Different Transport Sectors

Ross O. Phillips

Norwegian Centre for Transport Research (TØI),
Oslo, Norway

CONTENTS

4.5.1   INTRODUCTION

Fatigue is thought to contribute to a substantial number of serious collisions and dangerous incidents in different transport sectors (Marcus & Rosekind, 2017). Despite this, we know relatively little about the progress of fatigue shaped by work constraints in different transport settings (Phillips, 2014; Sallinen & Hublin, 2015). At the same time, new technologies and automation threaten to increase the monotonous aspects of work performed by operators in transport and increase the complexity of surrounding systems. One result of this will be that the causes of operator fatigue will increase in complexity and become more difficult to manage (Woods et al., 2016). An understanding of the consequences for operators of vehicles and vessels in different types of operation of the transport sector would be helped if we knew more about the occurrence, causes and effects of different sorts of fatigue in these workers (Hancock, 2019; Hancock et al., 2020). Given this, there is a surprising lack of comparative data on transport operator fatigue. This is in part due to lack of agreement on how to operationalise fatigue and lack of consistent guidance on how to map fatigue in ways that are amenable to organisational safety management (Phillips, 2015; Skau et al., 2021).

The current chapter hopes to inform about how the situation might be addressed by describing a survey of people operating different forms of vehicles and vessels on the occurrence, causes, and effects of different sorts of fatigue. Operators surveyed work in different branches of the Norwegian road, rail, and maritime sectors. For each operator type, standard measures are used to build a fatigue profile, which allows for comparative fatigue assessments that will be useful to safety managers in different sectors.

4.5.2   WHAT IS FATIGUE PROFILING?

To help safety managers assess and mitigate the risks associated with human operation of a transport form, it is useful to build a fatigue profile for each operator role. A fatigue profile is a description of the various causes and signs of fatigue, and any fatigue-related errors or near miss incidents that are typical for a group of people operating a vehicle or vessel in a given work context. One way to structure a fatigue profile is to use Dawson and McCulloch's Fatigue Risk Trajectory to consider fatigue at the following hazard levels (Dawson & McCulloch, 2005; Phillips et al., 2017):

0. framework conditions and fatigue-awareness culture
1. work characteristics
2. recovery from work
3. fatigue-related symptoms
4. fatigue-related errors
5. fatigue-related collisions and incidents

Each of the above hazard levels is a level of defence that can reduce the possibility of a fatigue-related collision or incident (Dawson & McCulloch, 2005). To be optimally effective, transport safety management systems should therefore include the monitoring and mitigation of fatigue risks at each hazard level (see also Chapter 1.2 of this book). Here is an illustrative example: Level 1 describes risks from work that can cause fatigue, such as the limited opportunity for quality sleep that shift schedules can create. Opportunities for improving schedules to reduce fatigue might be limited by management awareness of fatigue problems, regulations, or the industrial or social context in which work is organised. The latter are Level 0 fatigue risks. Even if it is possible to design schedules that give operators ample opportunity for sleep, other aspects of life or work such as psychosocial stress or an uncomfortable sleeping environment, can make it difficult to sleep. We should also measure and control the actual sleep obtained (Level 2 risks). Even operators that have slept enough can display fatigue symptoms (e.g., in circadian lows, due to poor health or chronic sleep deficit), so we should also monitor for fatigue while the operator is operating (Level 3). Any fatigue-related errors that still manifest themselves should be assessed (Level 4), and we should try to monitor and learn from fatigue-related incidents that may still occur (Level 5). By monitoring and controlling fatigue risks at all levels of the safety trajectory, we have a robust, multi-layered defence against fatigue-related collisions. Full descriptions of each hazard level are available in the literature (Dawson & McCulloch, 2005; Phillips, 2016; Phillips et al., 2017). Measures for assessing risks at each hazard level are summarised in Table 4.5.1.

4.5.3 COMPARING FATIGUE PROFILES FOR PEOPLE OPERATING VEHICLES AND VESSELS IN SEA, RAIL, AND ROAD SECTORS

To illustrate the usefulness of fatigue profiling, our group has generated fatigue profiles for different types of land - and sea-based operator (Phillips et al., 2015). The results illustrate how safety managers might go about assessing fatigue risks in their own operations, as the basis of measures for multi-layered mitigation (Phillips et al., 2017). The results also inform managers about causes of fatigue that are particular to their sector.

To generate the fatigue profiles, transport operators in Norway were surveyed in two waves. In the first survey wave, we included questions about framework conditions and culture, general work characteristics, recovery from work, fatigue levels for the preceding three months, workload (NASA Task Load Index; Hart & Staveland, 1988), job demands/resources and fatigue (Epworth Sleepiness Scale, Checklist Individual Strength (see Table 4.5.1). The second survey wave asked operators to report on sleep and fatigue for their most recent operating period, and included ratings on the Karolinska Sleepiness (KSS) scale. We received a total of 1,776 valid responses to the first survey wave, from maritime watch officers working on a range of vessel types (n=794); train operators (n=155); and professional drivers of trucks, buses, and taxis (n=917). About one-third of operators participating in the first wave also participated in the second wave (Phillips et al., 2015). To illustrate the findings, we compare fatigue risks at each hazard level for the different sorts of operator surveyed.

4.5.3.1 LEVEL 0—FRAMEWORK CONDITIONS AND FATIGUE AWARENESS CULTURE

Fatigue risks embedded in framework conditions appeared to be higher for operators working at sea than for those working on land. Twenty-three per cent of maritime watch officers said they had to work even though they were too exhausted to do so—a proportion that was substantially higher than for land-based officers. Maritime officers also rated pay, violations, training, and planning as worse. Between 20 and 38 per cent of maritime watch officers also reported violating working time regulations at least once a week, depending on the type of maritime operation they worked in. In comparison, 11 per cent of truck drivers reported exceeding the driving and resting

TABLE 4.5.1
Description of Fatigue Hazard Levels

Fatigue Hazard Level		Description	Example of Measures
0	Framework conditions and fatigue awareness culture	Social organisation, power of supply chain actors to set demands, aspects of transport infrastructure (e.g., resting places), freedom to choose or change schedule, management commitment to reduce fatigue, colleague attitude to fatigue.	Fatigue awareness culture Organisational and branch conditions
1	Work characteristics	Sort of work one does and when and how long one does it for. Important aspects of work content are physical and psychological overload and underload. Important aspects of work timing are time of day at which work done, length of work or time on task, time awake since last sleep, length of time and time of day for recovery from work. Shift patterns should also be considered.	Workload, e.g., NASA-TLX Job demands and resources Work timing Shifts: Fatigue Risk Index
2	Recovery from work	Sleep length and quality, timing of sleep, work–home interference, psychological detachment from work.	Sleep quantity and quality Psychological detachment Work–home interference
3	Fatigue symptoms	Sleepiness, acute fatigue, chronic fatigue, burnout, physical exertion, lack of motivation.	Broader acute fatigue Sleepiness Physical exertion Generalised fatigue Burnout Checklist Individual Strength
4	Fatigue-related errors	Occupation-specific slips, errors, errors of perception, planning or communication problems caused by lack of focus or irritability.	Driver behaviour questionnaire
5	Fatigue-related incidents and collisions	Near misses, collisions, other unsafe practice causing work-related injury (especially ships), but also health outcomes can be considered.	Accident analyses Injury data, reporting systems Sickness absence

regulations at least once a week. Very few of the rail operators reported working time violations.

Despite the poorer framework conditions, maritime watch officers rated culture for fatigue awareness more positively than land-based operators. Relatively higher proportions of maritime watch officers reported telling someone when they felt fatigued, and many told their line manager. A culture for fatigue-awareness was less prevalent in the rail sector, where cargo operators agreed less than any other type of operator that their employer treated fatigue as a serious risk.

4.5.3.2 LEVEL 1—WORK CHARACTERISTICS

Almost all rail operators worked irregular hours (rosters), and a high proportion reported that they worked shifts known to be associated with elevated levels of fatigue. However, rail operators worked fewer total working hours than any of the other operators surveyed, with an average workday of 8.9 hours, of which 6.5 hours was spent operating the train. The work of a rail operator was characterised by a high level of mental demand, probably linked to the need to maintain vigilance to railway signals outside the cabin for much of the time spent operating the train. Rail operators also reported having little control over how the work was done. Relative to others, rail operators reported that they most often experienced physical discomfort from poor air or temperature; cargo rail operators reported the most frequent discomfort from noise and vibrations.

Road operators drove for 6.8 hours on a typical workday lasting on average 9.4 hours. Of the road operators, truck drivers worked the most, reporting an average workday lasting 10.6 hours. Many truck drivers reported spending considerable time on physical tasks in addition to driving. Apart from driving, the main activity of taxi owner-drivers was waiting. Taxi owner-drivers reported working the most hours per week of all land-based operators, with half of them working six or seven days a week. Despite working so many days a week, the length of the average working day was reported as 9.9 hours. The main challenges for local bus drivers were working early starts and split shifts (typically two 3 to 4 hour shifts with a break in the middle of the day), and experiencing high psychological demands with low job support with little say about how their work is done.

Bridge watch was the main activity reported by maritime watch officers, and paperwork appeared to be the main secondary activity for many. At least one in two officers in several types of operation said that they are often alone on the bridge during a watch. While there was variation according to maritime branch worked in, overall job demands (cognitive demands, goal conflicts) were higher for maritime officers than for operators in land-based sectors. Watch officers reported spending an average of 11.1 hours on watch and working 12.6 hours on a normal working day. The 6-on/6-off watch system is the most prevalent, even though researchers regard it as one of the more fatiguing (Phillips, 2014).

4.5.3.3 LEVEL 2—RECOVERY FROM WORK

Sleep debt is the sleep duration you need minus the sleep duration that you get. Respondents were asked to estimate the average number of hours of sleep they obtained during a typical 24-hour period encompassing a working day, during the three months prior to the survey. To estimate sleep debt respondents were also asked how much sleep they felt they needed. Rail operators reported an average of 1.23 hours of sleep debt on a typical workday, road operators reported 1.16 hours, and watch officers 1.04 hours (Figure 4.5.1).

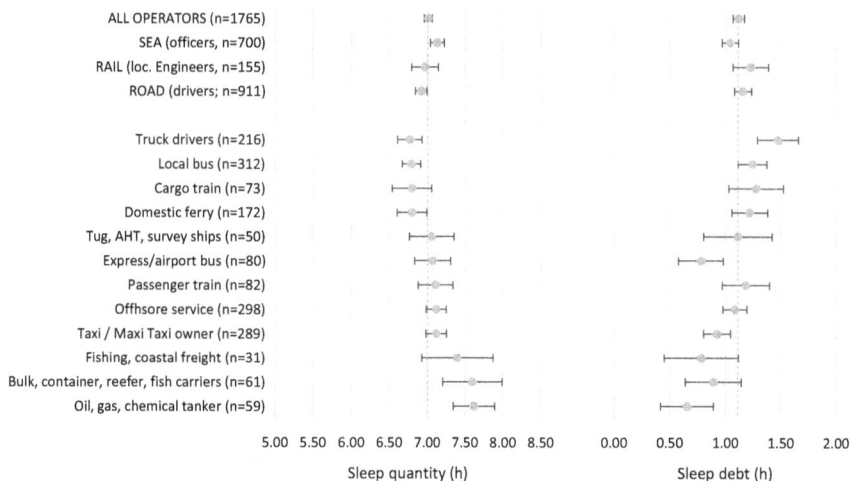

FIGURE 4.5.1   The amount of sleep that operators reported getting on typical workdays over the three months prior to the survey, relative to their sleep debt. Reproduced with permission from Phillips et al. (2015).

Rail operators also reported poorer sleep quality (12.96 out of possible 20 using items taken from the Karolinska Sleep Questionnaire; Åkerstedt et al., 2008) than road operators (13.92 out of 20). Sleep quality in rail cargo was especially poor. Relative to other road operators, truck drivers reported the highest sleep debt (1.47 h) and the poorest sleep quality. Maritime watch officers were least able to detach psychologically from work during non-work time.

4.5.3.4   Level 3—Fatigue-Related Symptoms

Our survey of fatigue-related symptoms included the use of KSS, where scores over 6 are associated with impaired operator performance (Åkerstedt, 2014):

1. Extremely alert
2. Very alert
3. Alert
4. Rather alert
5. Neither alert nor sleepy
6. Some signs of sleepiness
7. Sleepy, no great effort to stay awake
8. Sleepy, but some effort to keep awake
9. Very sleepy, great effort to keep awake, fighting sleep

Rather than ask operators to rate average sleepiness over the past month, three months or year, we asked about the most recent work period (Diependaele, 2015). People have been shown to be rather good at estimating variations in momentary sleepiness across the course of a recent period using retrospective ratings (Folkard, Spelten et al., 1995). In our survey, rail operators reported the highest retrospective ratings of fatigue. The average sleepiness for the final hour of operating was 5.7 on the nine-point KSS scale, versus 5.1 for watch officers and 4.3 for road operators (see Figure 4.5.2).

Prevalence of severe sleepiness (proportion in each group scoring KSS 8 or 9) for the final operating hour was 16 per cent for rail operators, 10 per cent for watch officers, and 4 per cent for road operators.

It is also informative to compare sleepiness across work periods for different types of operator (Figure 4.5.3). To do this, respondents were asked to indicate how they felt "before", during the "first hour", "middle hour", and "last hour", and "after" their last operating period. A curve for each group was then constructed from group average KSS scores on these five time points (Figure 4.5.3).

A closer inspection of curves by safety managers can inform them about potential performance-impairing effects of fatigue from sleep inertia or during other challenging periods in the course of a shift. On inspecting the curves, they should consider normal biorhythms and any local contextual effects on KSS ratings (e.g., level of physical activity and light exposure). For night workers, a steep increase in KSS ratings over the course of the shift, often ending above 6, is expected. For instance,

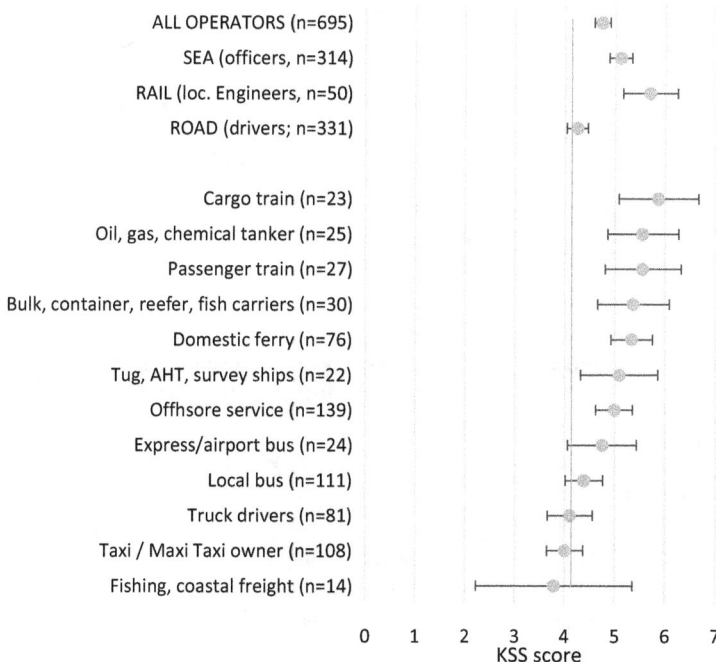

FIGURE 4.5.2 Average KSS scores for final hour of last driving or watch period, with 95% confidence intervals. The vertical line indicates the mean for all operators. Reproduced with permission from Phillips et al. (2015).

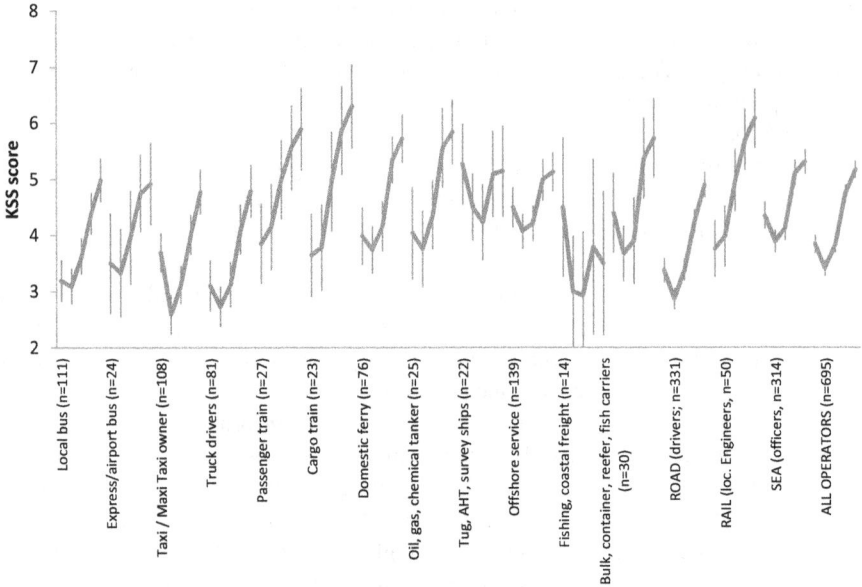

FIGURE 4.5.3 Average KSS scores during the last driving or watch period, with 95% confidence intervals. Reproduced with permission from Phillips et al. (2015).

cargo train operators tend to work more nights than passenger train operators, and the steeper increase in KSS curve for cargo train operators is consistent with this pattern.

4.5.3.5 LEVEL 4—FATIGUE-RELATED ERRORS

In our study, falling asleep while operating, over a three-month period (leading up to the survey) was used as a proxy for fatigue-related errors, but this measure would be usefully supplemented by measures capturing safety-critical errors specific to individual operator types (e.g., signal approach at too high speed for rail operators and red light missed by car drivers).

Figure 4.5.4 gives prevalence rates of sleeping while operating for different types of vehicle operators.

Rail operators reported the highest prevalence of sleeping while operating, with 63 per cent of cargo and 52 per cent of passenger train operators having nodded off or slept at least once in the three months preceding the survey. The corresponding proportion for maritime watch officers was 29 per cent, and for bus and truck drivers it was 26 per cent.

4.5.3.6 LEVEL 5—FATIGUE-RELATED COLLISIONS

The number of fatigue-related collisions reported is often too low to be useful for comparison, and this was the case in our survey. Indeed, an advantage of a multi-layered

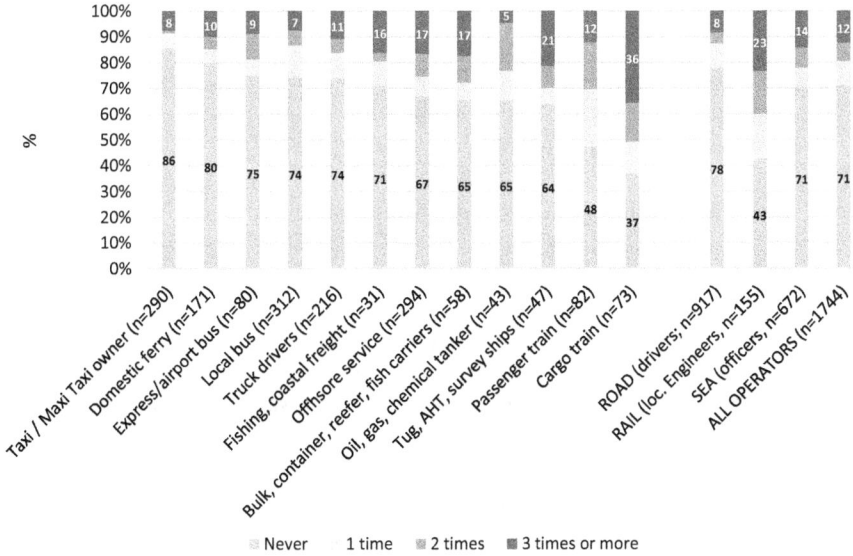

FIGURE 4.5.4 Operator response to "During the last 3 months, how many times have you slept (or dropped off for a moment) while you were driving at work/on watch?". Reproduced with permission from Phillips et al. (2015).

approach to fatigue risk management is that causes and signs of fatigue, which are far more abundant, can be monitored and mitigated as necessary to further prevent collisions from occurring.

4.5.4 PROFILE SUMMARIES

Based on the analysis of survey findings, we can summarise for each operator type the main fatigue risks across hazard levels. To illustrate, we summarise the main fatigue risks for each transport sector surveyed. Note how useful it is to compare by sector or other operator types.

Rail
- Culture in which there is relatively low awareness of fatigue as a risk.
- Framework conditions are relatively positive and low proportions of drivers report that they have to drive when exhausted.
- Work is dominated by a sustained vigilance task, little task variety, low levels of control. The time of day of the work task and sleep opportunity are more problematic than the amount of work.
- Relatively high sleep debt and poor sleep quality may impede recovery from work and may be associated with signs of slightly elevated general fatigue.
- Levels of acute sleepiness towards the end of an operating period are higher than for other operators.

- Highest reported prevalence of sleeping while operating.
- Highest reported acute fatigue levels while operating even though fewer say they have to operate when exhausted—implies that acute fatigue experienced by rail operators is sudden and unpredictable.

Road

- Framework conditions rated less positively than in the rail sector. A greater proportion of road vehicle operators than train operators need to drive when they are too exhausted to do so.
- A higher proportion of road vehicle operators also report violating laws designed to limit time spent driving and working.
- Both the nature of fatigue-related work challenges, and the extent to which irregular hours and challenging shifts are worked, vary widely according to the type of operation.
- Job support is low overall.
- Truck drivers reported the highest levels of sleep debt and lowest levels of sleep quality; more drivers slept away from home when working.
- Fatigue in truck drivers is more physical than cognitive or emotional in nature.
- A relatively high proportion of bus drivers reported that they lack energy after work.
- Relative to the maritime and rail operators in this study, the incidence of sleep reported by road vehicle operators was low, but no less concerning given that the chance of having a collision due to drowsy operating is higher when driving a road vehicle than when driving a train or maritime vessel.

Sea

- Framework conditions, including working time violations and having to work while exhausted, are worse for maritime officers than for land-based operators.
- Operators work the longest hours day after day (although most have extended periods to recover from tours at sea).
- Many often work alone on the bridge and work at night.
- Many watch systems curtail sleep length and require operators to sleep at times of day when sleeping is most difficult.
- Cognitive job demands are high.
- Acute sleepiness levels towards end of a watch can approach those of rail operators in some types of operation.
- Marine officers scored higher on concentration fatigue and burnout than did road operators.
- Relative to road operators, incidence of falling asleep while operating (on watch) is high.

To make visible the course of fatigue across the hazard "trajectory", it is also possible to produce more detailed summary tables for each operator type (see Tables 4.5.2 to 4.5.4). Such tables are useful for safety managers.

TABLE 4.5.2
Fatigue Risk Profile for Train Operators

Hazard Level	Description	Fatigue Risk Factors for Train Operators
4	Fatigue-related errors (proxy measure)	• 52 per cent of passenger and 63 per cent of cargo train operators report sleeping or nodding off at least once while operating during the 3 months preceding the survey. • 36 per cent of cargo operators report doing this at least three times.
3	Fatigue symptoms	• Train operators report higher levels of fatigue and sleepiness for the final hour of operating than any other operator. • Average sleepiness for the last hour of operating is 5.7 on a 9-point scale (KSS). • 16 per cent report severe sleepiness (KSS 8 or 9) for the last hour of operating. • Fatigue symptoms are generally worse for cargo than passenger operators. • Fatigue after work is characterised by low energy, lack of motivation, and sleepiness. • Broader fatigue, but not sleepiness, may generalise to life beyond work. • One in four cargo operators reports excessive daytime sleepiness (ESS>10).
2	Recovery from work	• Train operators sleep for an average of 6.97 hours on a workday, and have an average 1.23 hours of sleep debt. • Eight per cent of road operators obtained less than 5 hours sleep in the 24 hours preceding their last operating period. • 14 per cent obtained less than 12 hours sleep in the 48 hours preceding their last operating period. • Sleep quality (rated at 12.96 out of 20) is poor relative to that of road operators (13.92 out of 20). • 75 per cent of cargo operators report that their main sleep is split into two bouts. • 90 per cent of cargo operators say that it is not unusual to sleep away from home while working. • Work–home interference is high for cargo operators.
1	Work characteristics	• Main challenge from sustained demand of vigilance task. • Little task variety or control over how work is done. • Relatively high levels of discomfort from physical work environment, especially in cargo transport. • The timing of work is more problematic than the amount of work. • 56 per cent of passenger operators work early shifts at least once a week. • 80 per cent of cargo operators work nightshifts at least once a week. • Almost all work irregular hours.
0	Framework conditions and fatigue awareness culture	• Ten per cent often have to drive when too exhausted. • Less than half report when they feel too exhausted to operate. • Cargo operators are half as likely as passenger to inform line manager or operative centre. • Relative to other operators, fewer rail operators agree that drivers understand and are aware of fatigue. • Cargo operators agree less than any other operator in any other sector that employers treat fatigue as a serious risk.

TABLE 4.5.3
Fatigue Risk Profile for Professional Drivers of Road Vehicles

Hazard Level	Description	Fatigue Risk Factors for Road Operators
4	Fatigue-related errors (proxy measure)	• 25 per cent of bus and truck drivers report nodding off or sleeping while driving at least once during the three months preceding the survey. • 7–10 per cent of all road operators report nodding off or sleeping while driving at least three times during the preceding three months.
3	Fatigue symptoms	• Drivers report a sharp decrease in alertness over the course of an operating period. • Average sleepiness for the last hour is 4.3 on a 9-point scale (KSS). • Four per cent of all road operators report levels of severe sleepiness in the last hour of driving. • Local bus drivers lack more energy and report greater physical discomfort after work; truck drivers report greater physical discomfort. • 27–28 per cent of bus and truck drivers report excessive daytime sleepiness. • Truck drivers report higher levels of burnout.
2	Recovery from work	• Road operators obtain an average of 6.92 hour sleep on a work day, with an average sleep debt of 1.16 hours. • Sleep debt is 1.47 hours for truck drivers—higher than for any other operator. Truck drivers also report poorer sleep quality (13.44 out of 20) than bus or taxi operators. 40 per cent of truck drivers say it is normal to sleep in the truck (as well as at home) on work days, which may be linked to higher reported work–home interference. • Five per cent of road operators obtained less than 5 hours sleep in the 24 hours preceding their last operating period. • 16 per cent obtained less than 12 hours sleep in the 48 hours preceding their last operating period.
1	Work characteristics	• Driving is the main operator task for all road operators. All road operators report driving between 6.7 and 6.9 hours on a typical day at work. 58–85 per cent of road operators work irregular hours, and many find out at short notice what hours they will work. Overall, road operators receive low levels of job support relative to rail and maritime operators. • Truck drivers: Truck drivers say they work most—10.6 hours on a work day on average. 59 per cent of truck drivers spend over 20 per cent of work time on physical tasks, and physical demands are rated as equal to mental demands overall. There are relatively high levels of effort and frustration, but drivers also report a certain degree of freedom and higher performance achievement. • Taxi owner-drivers: Half of taxi owner-drivers work six or seven days a week, and the average reported daily working hour for taxi owner-drivers is 9.9 hours. 45 per cent of taxi owner-drivers work a nightshift at least once a week. Other demanding shifts are also common. 39 per cent spend over 40 per cent of work time waiting for jobs, at ranks etc. Emotional demands are higher than for any other operator.

TABLE 4.5.3 (Continued)
Fatigue Risk Profile for Professional Drivers of Road Vehicles

Hazard Level	Description	Fatigue Risk Factors for Road Operators
		• Local bus drivers: Rate time pressure, frustration, emotional and cognitive job demands and goal conflicts as higher than do most other drivers in road transport; yet performance achievement is lower. Report that they have least say in how they do their work. Also experience more discomfort from noise, vibration, and air quality. Half of local bus drivers also work split shifts and backwardly rotating shifts at least once a week.
0	Framework conditions and fatigue awareness culture	• 18–19 per cent of truck and local bus drivers often have to drive when they are too exhausted.
		• When this happens, ca. 40 per cent tell a line manager (of those who have them). Drivers' ratings of framework conditions (violations, pay, training, etc.) are less positive than in the rail sector but more positive than in the maritime sector.
		• 11 per cent of truck drivers and 6–9 per cent of bus drivers say they violate regulations designed to limit operating time at least once a week.
		• Drivers rate employers as taking fatigue relatively seriously.
		• Truck drivers rate shipping agents as taking fatigue less seriously.

4.5.5 DISCUSSION

Fatigue profiling of operator groups can help inform safety managers about the risks that people they manage face, and thus where action is needed most. Fatigue profiling is a multi-layered approach, in which fatigue risks that have the potential to cascade through successive hazard levels can be caught early and mitigated (Phillips et al., 2017). The results presented in this chapter illustrate one way that fatigue profiling can be done, but managers can choose from many other measures of fatigue risk at each hazard level to create their profiles. That said, one value of the profiling approach is that it allows fatigue risks faced by people in different roles and industries to be compared with those faced by others; therefore, the use of standard measures should be agreed at sector level, and their widespread use should be encouraged.

Safety managers may face constraints when attempting to survey their workforce, not least in terms of participation levels. This problem may be limited in companies with open reporting cultures, especially if the advantages to that monitoring fatigue has for the individual worker are explained. If managers are more aware of when and how fatigue arises, they can implement measures to reduce fatigue levels in their work force. This in turn will lower the risk of accident involvement and any fatigue-related health issues that might arise in the shorter or longer term. On a related point, however, managers should consider that the approach described here considers only how constraints shared by a group of operators can combine to produce fatigue. It does not consider any individual-level causes of fatigue. While individual-level risks can be mitigated during recruitment and training (i.e., Level 0 mitigation), life changes, other illnesses, or other individual-level events can also occur and cause fatigue in the individual.

TABLE 4.5.4
Fatigue Risk Profile for Maritime Watch Officers (Including Captains)

Hazard Level	Description	Fatigue Risk Factors for Watch Officers at Sea
4	Fatigue-related errors (proxy)	• 29 per cent have nodded off at least once on watch in the three months preceding the survey. • 14 per cent report doing so at least three times.
3	Fatigue symptoms	• Officers generally become more sleepy as the watch progresses, but officers on offshore service and tug/AHT/survey ships get less sleepy towards the middle of a watch. • Average sleepiness for last hour of watch is 5.1 on a nine-point scale (KSS). • Ten per cent report severe sleepiness for the last hour of watch. • Officers on domestic ferries are more fatigued after their watch than officers on other vessels (SOFI). • 23 per cent of all watch officers report excessive daytime sleepiness. • Maritime officers score higher on concentration fatigue and burnout than road operators overall.
2	Recovery from work	• Maritime officers get 7.13 hours of sleep on a work day on average, and the sleep debt is slightly lower than average (1.04 hours). • Domestic ferry officers get only 6.80 hours on average (sleep debt 1.22 hours). • Four per cent of all officers had slept less than 5 hours in the 24 hours preceding their watch. • 12 per cent had slept less than 12 hours in the 24 hours preceding their watch. • Sleep quality (13.21 out of 20) is worse for maritime officers than for road operators (13.92 out of 20), and split sleeps are common (as dictated by watch systems). • Psychological detachment from work during free time is relatively poor, apart from domestic ferry officers. • Work–home interference is reported as high by offshore service officers.
1	Work characteristics	• Bridge watch is the main activity in most types of operation. • On tankers, paperwork takes more time than watch activity. One in four officers in other types of operation spends at least 40 per cent of work time on paperwork (does not include fishing/coastal freight). • One in four offshore service officers and at least one in two of the other officers said they were often alone on the bridge during a watch. • Mental demand levels appear to reflect the extent to which sustained vigilance is required on watch. Otherwise workload varies by the type of operation, e.g., fishing/coastal freight officers rate physical demands as relatively high, whereas domestic ferry officers rate time pressure demands as relatively high.

TABLE 4.5.4 (Continued)
Fatigue Risk Profile for Maritime Watch Officers (Including Captains)

Hazard Level	Description	Fatigue Risk Factors for Watch Officers at Sea
0	Framework conditions and fatigue awareness culture	• Job demands (cognitive, emotional demands, and goal conflict) are overall higher in the maritime sector than in the road and rail sectors. • Overall colleague and manager support is rated highly relative to some land-based types of operation. • Operating position is the most frequent source of physical discomfort at work, more so than noise or vibration. • In terms of days worked in the last 90 days, tanker and offshore service officers work the most, and domestic ferry officers the least. • Maritime officers spend on average 11.1 hours on watch and 12.6 hours working on a normal working day. • 42 per cent of respondents work 6–6, the most prevalent watch system. Watch systems vary with the type of operation. • Watch officers rate framework conditions (pay, violations, and training) as poor relative to land-based operators. • 20–38 per cent of officers violate working time regulations at least once a week, depending on the type of operation (does not include domestic ferry). • 23 per cent overall say that they often have to work when they are too exhausted (higher than for land-based operators). • Rates of reporting fatigue to others are high relative to road and rail sectors. 22 per cent said they tell usually someone, most often colleagues, but 30–51 per cent tell line managers. • Slight lack of agreement that there is a culture of fatigue awareness, but officers rate this more positively than land-based operators do.

The reader will note that we have profiled fatigue risks for land- and sea-based transport operators, mainly at levels 0, 1, 2, and 3 of the Fatigue Risk Trajectory. Safety managers will have access to objective data, from incident reports, or from fatigue or driver monitoring technology, that can be used to "fill in" levels 4 and 5, and/ or supplement self-report data. The reader might also note that our survey data was exclusively based on self-reports, which is vulnerable to response bias and the extent to which respondents represent the workforce they are intended to represent. Moreover, modern data collection methods can make it difficult to determine response rates (e.g., not everyone reads their e-mail, and addresses on e-mail lists are often outdated; how many people read a Facebook page?). In this survey the minimum response rate was estimated to be between around 20 and 35 per cent, depending on operator group.

When considering such challenges, the promise of fatigue profiling should be borne in mind. To explore this, potential studies are needed that use fatigue profiling to assess the relative importance of different types of "latent" factors (i.e., factors at earlier levels of the trajectory) by studying their relative contribution to risk factors at later levels. If done well, such studies could lead to job redesign that improves working conditions for many operators. For instance, we may find that sleep quality (level 2) is a main risk for sleeping on watch and groundings for maritime officers working on tankers; or we may find that cognitive job demands are a main predictor of burnout and poor safety performance for local bus drivers. Similar studies could also help establish the importance for safety of broader and longer-term fatigue relative to acute sleepiness or mental exhaustion.

It would also be useful to compare scores on several of the standard measures used here with scores for transport operators and other workers found in other studies. This is needed to gain a better perspective on the size of the fatigue problem for different types of Norwegian operator. We have in other words only compared road, rail, and maritime sectors in Norway with each other. Without a systematic comparison with international studies, it is difficult to make conclusions about the absolute size of the fatigue problems measured here. Despite their limitations, the studies we describe show that different types of transport operation have a unique fatigue risk profile and, in doing so, underline the need for fatigue to be managed as part of a Safety Management System that can be adapted to different branch contexts.

SUMMARY POINTS FOR PRACTITIONERS

- To manage the risks to safety posed by fatigue, there is a need to understand how fatigue is shaped by the different contexts that transport operators work in.
- One way to do this is to generate fatigue profiles for groups of operators in similar work settings.
- One way to generate a fatigue profile is to measure fatigue causes shaped by framework conditions, organisational culture, work characteristics and recovery from work through to actual fatigue-related incidents.
- Using this approach to compare sea- and land-based transport operators generates useful knowledge about particular fatigue outcomes and causes faced by different sorts of transport operators.
- Fatigue profiling can provide useful and comprehensive information to fatigue risk management as part of a safety management system.

REFERENCES

Åkerstedt, T., Ingre, M., Kecklund, G., Folkard, S., & Axelsson, J. (2008). Accounting for partial sleep deprivation and cumulative sleepiness in the three process model of alertness regulation. *Chronobiology International, 25*(2&3), 309–319.

Dawson, D., & McCulloch, K. (2005). Managing fatigue: It's about sleep. *Sleep Medicine Reviews, 9*(5), 365–380. http://dx.doi.org/10.1016/j.smrv.2005.03.002

Diependaele, K. (2015). Sleepy at the wheel. Analysis of the extent and characteristics of sleepiness among Belgian car drivers. Belgian Road Safety Institute -- Knowledge Centre Road Safety. Research report nr. 2015-R-06-EN.

Folkard, S., Spelten, E., Totterdell, P., Barton, J., & Smith, L. (1995). The use of survey measures to assess circadian variations in alertness. *Sleep, 18*(5), 355–361.

Hancock, P. A. (2019). Some pitfalls in the promises of automated and autonomous vehicles. *Ergonomics, 62*(4), 479–495. https://doi.org/10.1080/00140139.2018.1498136

Hancock, P. A., Kajaks, T., Caird, J. K., Chignell, M. H., Mizobuchi, S., Burns, P. C., Feng, J., Fernie, G. R., Lavallière, M., Noy, I. Y., Redelmeier, D. A., & Vrkljan, B. H. (2020). Challenges to human drivers in increasingly automated vehicles. *Human Factors*, *62*(2), 310–328. https://doi.org/10.1177/0018720819900402

Hart, S. G., & Staveland, L. E. (1988). Development of NASA-TLX (Task Load Index): Results of empirical and theoretical research. *Advances in Psychology, 52*, 139–183.

Marcus, J., & Rosekind, M. R. (2017). Fatigue in transportation: NTSB investigations and safety recommendations. *Injury Prevention*, *23*, 232–238.

Phillips, R. O. (2014). *An assessment of studies of human fatigue in land and sea transport. Fatigue in Transport Report II.* (No. 1354/2014; TØI Reports). Institute of Transport Economics (TØI).

Phillips, R. O. (2015). A review of definitions of fatigue–and a step towards a whole definition. *Transport Research–Part F*, *29*, 48–56.

Phillips, R. O. (2016). *Countermeasures for use in fatigue risk management.* No. 1488/2016 TØI Reports. Institute of Transport Economics (TØI).

Phillips, R. O., Kecklund, G., Anund, A., & Sallinen, M. (2017). Fatigue in transport: A review of exposure, risks, checks and controls. *Transport Reviews*, *37*(6), 742–766. https://doi.org/10.1080/01441647.2017.1349844

Phillips, R. O., Sagberg, F., & Bjørnskau, T. (2015). *Fatigue in operators of land–and sea-based transport forms in Norway. Risk Profiles Fatigue in Transport Report IV.* No. 1440/2015 TØI Reports. Institute of Transport Economics (TØI).

Sallinen, M., & Hublin, C. (2015). Fatigue-inducing factors in transportation operators. *Reviews of Human Factors and Ergonomics*, *10*(1), 138–173. https://doi.org/10.1177/1557234X15574828

Skau, S., Sundberg, K., & Kuhn, H.-G. (2021). A proposal for a unifying set of definitions of fatigue. *Frontiers in Psychology*, *12*, 4680. https://doi.org/10.3389/fpsyg.2021.739764

Woods, D. D., Dekker, S., Cook, R. I., Johannesen, L., & Sarter, N. B. (2016). *Behind Human Error* (2nd edn.). Taylor & Francis.

4.6 Fatigue Detection Technology

Clémentine François and Jérôme Wertz

Tobii AB, Liège, Belgium

CONTENTS

4.6.1 INTRODUCTION

Sleepiness is a physiological and uncontrollable need to sleep, which can occur at any time during the day, with a greater prevalence during the night (Bérubé, 1991). It induces hypo-vigilance in individuals and an alteration of their capacity to process information and execute a task correctly, and can lead to disastrous crashes, especially in transportation (Klauer, Dingus, Neale, Sudweeks, & Ramsey, 2006). To help mitigate and manage the operational risk of operator fatigue[1], fatigue risk management systems (FRMS) are widely used in transport. However, FRMS still remain a challenge to implement in a real-world application as many factors have an impact on fatigue.

Therefore, developing technologies to monitor an operator's[2] fatigue in real time is of paramount importance to improve safety for all transport applications despite the increasing autonomy of vehicles. Indeed, since the widespread adoption of autonomous vehicles may in some cases still take several decades, monitoring the operator's fatigue will remain a necessity. This is made more likely because, by progressively replacing the continuous and stimulating activity of operating a vehicle with a passive monitoring activity, the risk of fatigue may even be increased by the monotony of the automated task (El Khatib, Ou, & Karray, 2020).

To improve road safety and to establish the legal framework for the approval of automated and fully driverless vehicles in the European Union (EU), the European Parliament and EU Member States adopted a new General Safety Regulation in 2019

DOI: 10.1201/9781003213154-28

introducing a range of mandatory advanced driver assistant systems that can help to reduce crashes (General Safety Regulation, 2021). This regulation notably imposes attention warning technology in case of driver fatigue or distraction.

Characterising fatigue, monitoring its level, and determining the times when it reaches a dangerous level thus constitute an important and valuable endeavour in the area of public health and safety. Expectations are therefore high regarding the benefits of fatigue detection technologies, but it is also important to be aware of the many challenges that are associated with the development, adoption, and use of these technologies by operators.

4.6.2 FATIGUE DETECTION: CHALLENGES AND REQUIREMENTS

The development of a fatigue detection technology must consider quite a large and diverse set of technical, environmental, and human factors. This technology must effectively capture the moment when an operator's fatigue reaches a level that is too dangerous to continue operating safely, while at the same time not distracting the operator, being secure, respecting privacy, and being robust to several noise variables.

To maintain safe control of the vehicle and normal operator behaviour, fatigue detection technologies should indeed not tend to intrude on the operator's privacy or be a disturbing factor for the operator that could lead to unnatural or unsafe behaviour. Disturbing technology may indeed be poorly perceived and may end up having effects that are opposite to those intended, for example, it may distract the operator and thus add a risk for safety.

Privacy is also increasingly considered and regulated all over the world. This is especially the case in Europe, with the recent introduction of the General Data Protection Regulation (GDPR). Regarding fatigue detection technologies, the new EU safety regulation for motor vehicles includes the following provision:

> Drowsiness detection technology shall be designed in such a way that it does not continuously record nor retain any data other than what is necessary in relation to the purposes for which they were collected or otherwise processed within the closed-loop system.

General Safety Regulation, 2021

This means that any data collected by fatigue detection technologies should only be used for the purpose for which it is designed and should not be accessible for other reasons.

Another major challenge for fatigue detection technologies is robustness with respect to the diversity across the population (e.g., physiognomy) and conditions in which they must operate (e.g., environment).

Moreover, fatigue is not binary, it is a progressive state. So, providing a warning at the appropriate time, that is, early enough to enable the operator to react but without providing too many false alerts, is a real challenge. Indeed, too many false alerts may be seen as a nuisance, could cause distraction, and reduce acceptance of the technology.

In addition to this, there is no single, fully objective, and universally accepted reference measure (i.e., ground truth) that can be used to characterise the operator's fatigue state. Therefore, developing fatigue detection technology and being able to evaluate its performance can be very complex.

The validation process indeed requires (1) setting up an appropriate data collection method in a relevant environment that induces several operator fatigue states of differing severity while ensuring their safety, (2) determining the reference measure of fatigue to be used, and (3) determining the metrics for evaluating performance. The approach to performance evaluation of the technology therefore requires a multidisciplinary expertise beyond engineering skills.

However, since fatigue detection technologies for road vehicles are becoming mandatory in Europe, the process to standardardise evaluation protocols has been initiated. The type of fatigue detection technology is not specified in the EU regulation, but certain performance requirements are stipulated for vehicles to be homologated. This standardisation process will be iterative and is currently subjected to limitations, notably because of the lack of a widely accepted, objective reference.

The regulation applies to Europe at present, but similar regulations are currently being developed in other regions of the world, such as in China with the GB/T for advanced driver assistance systems (GB/T 39263-2020, s.d.). The EuroNCAP safety rating programme, which determines the safety level of a vehicle, also includes some consideration of fatigue detection systems in its assessment protocol (Euro NCAP–Occupant Status Monitoring, s.d.).

Depending on the sector and the use of the technology, it is often necessary for the provider of fatigue detection solution to demonstrate that its solution complies with one or several standards. This is important to know at the beginning of the development process, as it usually requires defining a specific development methodology/process including defining technology requirements, functionalities, design, testing and evaluation methods, as well as some coding rules that the technology needs to fulfil.

Another big challenge with fatigue detection technologies is whether and how users will adopt them. Indeed, even if the technology is mandated in the vehicle, it is important that the user (the operator) trusts and feels comfortable with the technology. Several design aspects must therefore be considered while developing, integrating, and marketing fatigue detection solutions. These include, for example, minimising false alarms, designing a well-adapted interface, and communicating clear messages on how the data collected by these technologies are used. In some use cases, the latter helps to ensure that the operators do not feel they are being monitored with bad intentions.

4.6.3 SEVERAL APPROACHES TO FATIGUE DETECTION

Fatigue is a physiological state that cannot be measured directly in a fully objective way. Rather, it must be estimated using indicators. This is an important distinction to understand, as no technology advertised as measuring fatigue is actually measuring fatigue; in all cases, regardless of technology or method, indicators of fatigue are measured, and fatigue level is imputed. If we focus on the traditional indicators and approaches to characterise the real-time fatigue level of an individual, we can define several categories that depend mainly on the type of indicators, as discussed next.

4.6.3.1 SUBJECTIVE INDICATORS

There are different subjective scales for the assessment of fatigue, the most used of which is the Karolinska Sleepiness Scale (KSS), a nine-point Likert scale (Åkerstedt & Gillberg, 1990). The principle is simple. People must self-assess their condition and determine the level of fatigue they are at using the scale and the description provided for each level on the scale. This type of scale enables a quick, easy, and very affordable assessment of fatigue but has several disadvantages: It is not a continuous assessment of the operator's state, it becomes less reliable after several hours of monotonous driving, it requires operator participation and therefore inevitably disturbs the natural behaviour of the operator, and, finally, the operator's self-assessment can be influenced by several factors and is not (by definition) an objective measure of state (Brown, 1997). Nevertheless, its wide use by the scientific community, its validation via several different techniques, and its ease of use have, since the introduction of the new EU regulation, made it the reference measure for the validation of fatigue detection technologies in the European automotive industry (General Safety Regulation, 2021).

4.6.3.2 INDIVIDUAL PERFORMANCE INDICATORS

If we focus our efforts on improving safety, the key question is how risky the current performance of the operator is. The performance reflects the effects of several factors—such as fatigue—on the ability of the individual to perform the task. There are various methods for measuring an individual's performance while executing a task: For example, one might ask the person to respond to a stimulus as quickly as possible and measure their reaction time (Dinges & Powell, 1985). However, while these types of tests are very useful in assessing an individual's fatigue state in lab, they constitute a distraction from the main task (i.e., driving) and cannot provide a continuous measure of the individual's state in real conditions. Another approach is to focus on indicators related to the performance of the primary task, that is, operating the vehicle. In the case of road driving, for example, one could focus on, for example, steering wheel movements, vehicle position on the road, vehicle speed, and speed deviation (Liu, Hosking, & Lenné, 2009). This approach is useful with an aim to avoid crashes and has the advantage of being non-intrusive. However, even if there is a link between these indicators and fatigue, their measurement does not represent a direct estimate of the state of fatigue, as the indicators can be influenced by many factors other than fatigue (e.g., distraction, experience, weather conditions, etc.). In addition, in case of semi-autonomous vehicles, these indicators are often useless as the operator is supervising the vehicle behaviour rather than directly controlling it.

4.6.3.3 Body Behavioural Indicators

Indicators based on body behaviour include data extracted from head, face, eye, mouth, and body movements, and are recognised as relevant for detecting the fatigue of a person in an operational context such as driving a vehicle (Chen & Ji, 2012). Several types of sensors can extract information about the operator's behaviour, for example, accelerometer, pressure sensors, radars, etc. The most used at present is a camera placed in front of the operator and that enables to collect several signals/features (e.g., head pose, opening of the eye, mouth movements, facial expressions, body pose, etc.) in real time and in a continuous way. Further analysis of these signals enables a system to determine several indicators (e.g., duration of blinks, number of yawns, etc.) which can then be used to determine and provide estimated levels of fatigue.

Among these indicators, the measurement of ocular activity is the most relevant and appropriate method to estimating fatigue. The activity of the eyes indeed reflects the activity of the brain (eye activity is often also considered to be a physiological indicator) and several ocular parameters are recognised as very reliable indicators of fatigue (Schleicher, Galley, Briest, & Galley, 2008). The best known of these is the PERcentage of eye CLOSure (PERCLOS) (Dinges & Grace, 1998).

The reliability of the measurement of fatigue using the body behaviour indicators depends strongly on the specifications of the sensor, the operating conditions, as well as on the quality and performance of the data processing steps. Moreover, when based on a single sensor (e.g., a camera), these indicators present a risk of data loss (e.g., due to occlusions) or low-quality data but this can be mitigated by combining multiple sensors.

This body behavioural approach is considered as the most relevant for a transport application as it presents many advantages: It is a continuous, non-intrusive, and real-time measurement of the symptoms (indicators) of a fatigued state, and several studies have shown that this approach can reliably detect fatigue (Jacobé de Naurois, Bourdin, Stratulat, Diaz, & Vercher, 2019).

4.6.3.4 Physiological Indicators

Fatigue is a physiological state corresponding to a "deactivation" of our central nervous system (CNS). Moving towards a physiological approach that provides information about the state of activation of our CNS seems therefore to make a lot of sense. Moreover, physiological indicators represent an objective, continuous, and more direct estimate of the state of fatigue. In this category, there are several sources of information, mainly brain, cardiac, and electrodermal activities.

The gold standard, considered by many experts, is brain activity, which can be measured via an electroencephalogram (EEG), and it is the most direct indicator of CNS activity (Gillberg, Kecklund, & Åkerstedt, 1996). Brain activity is in fact the standard indicator for the scoring of sleep stages, including a fatigue stage (American Association of Sleep Medicine (AASM, 2020). Indicators of fatigue in the EEG are related to the presence of brain waves oscillating in specific frequency bands (i.e., alpha [8 to 12] Hz and theta [4 to 7] Hz). However, this technique requires electrodes to be placed on the scalp, the signals obtained are very sensitive to noise (disturbance in the signal) and even if some automatic scoring algorithms exist, most of the time, experts are required to manually score fatigue by interpreting the signals. The brain activity approach is therefore not currently feasible for the monitoring of fatigue in most of operational context.

Heart rate variability is related to the autonomic nervous system, which controls our cognitive states including fatigue (Vicente, Laguna, Bartra, & Bailón, 2016). Indeed, when operators are fatigued, heart rate decreases and its variability increases. Heart rate variability refers to the changes in heart rate from one beat to the next and can be analysed in both the time and frequency domain. Cardiac activity can be measured via a variety of different techniques, including (1) electrocardiography (ECG) — for instance, with electrodes placed on the torso, (2) photoplethysmography (PPG) sensors—that are now frequently found in connected smartwatches, for example, (3) ballistocardiography(BCG)—for instance, with radar sensors, etc. However, heart rate is also influenced by other factors than fatigue, such as age, health conditions, and body movement, which can make interpretation of the signal difficult.

Skin conductance, also known as electrodermal activity or galvanic skin response (GSR), is a measure of the electrical resistance between two electrodes placed on the skin surface. This resistance varies according to perspiration, which is also controlled by the autonomic nervous system. Skin conductance is therefore an indicator of fatigue and can be easily measured by electrodes placed on the skin. However, it has the disadvantage of being influenced by external factors such as the weather, especially temperature and humidity, and by other cognitive states such as stress and anxiety (Michael, Passmann, & Becker, 2012).

All of these physiological methods can therefore give a good indication of whether a person is awake or fatigued, but they are all associated with limitations as they can vary with many other external and internal factors, including other emotional and cognitive states. Combined, these physiological activities could be very relevant for the detection of fatigue but capturing them accurately and synchronously in an operational environment is still a challenge and would require several sensors.

4.6.4 VALIDATION OF FATIGUE DETECTION TECHNOLOGIES

Assessing the performance and the reliability of a fatigue detection technology is crucial to ensure that it meets the requirements set to improve safety as well as to ensure its adoption by users. To carry out this validation of a fatigue detection technology, the process to be implemented is rather complex.

Firstly, data is needed. This data must represent the target population for the technology, be collected in the target environment, and must contain both awake and fatigue states.

Fatigue indicators cannot be artificially produced in a relevant way by a human being. The data collection protocol thus must induce real fatigue in people in the most naturalistic way as possible, for example, by using sleep deprivation, or requiring participants to engage in a long task duration. To do so, driving simulation tasks are often used in data collection protocols to lower the risk (Soares, Ferreira, & Couto, 2020).

To validate that the technology produces the expected result in the real operational conditions, it is also necessary to consider as many conditions and factors as possible that may influence the functioning and the performance of the technology, from collection of raw data to final determination of fatigue level, and to verify that the technology is providing a reliable level of fatigue in these conditions. However, when collecting validation data for fatigue, it is important to select only those conditions and factors that have a real impact on the detection of the state of fatigue. It is indeed laborious and time-consuming to collect fatigue data and one can verify the proper functioning of the technology for the other conditions and factors with awake data, which is easier to collect. The process can therefore be simplified using modularity and seeing the overall fatigue detection technology as a set of modules that can each be evaluated independently. If one takes the example of a camera-based fatigue detection technology, one can separate the sensor, the software layer that processes the images to extract facial and body features, and the software layer that determines fatigue. Each of these modules is indeed influenced by different factors and can be validated independently and accordingly. This modular approach enables to globally optimise the validation process.

Secondly, to validate a fatigue detection technology, key performance indicators (KPIs) are needed. However, there is no single reliable reference measure to characterise the fatigue state of an individual. Several approaches and methods for characterising fatigue can be used, but none fulfil all requirements to be used as a unique, fully objective, direct, and non-disturbing reference measure for fatigue. Therefore, it is important to consider the use case, the associated constraints, and the requirements of the global solution to select the best reference measure to use. When possible, it is ideal to combine several reference measures as this increases the objectivity and the reliability of the validation.

Moreover, fatigue is not a binary state; rather, it is progressive. For instance, before an operator falls asleep, in general, he will be in a state that is somewhere between being fully awake and being asleep. Considering this, and the fact that there is no way of characterising fatigue in a fully objective manner using a single reliable reference measure, it is therefore quite challenging to define KPIs and to determine metrics (e.g., sensitivity and specificity) to use for assessing the performance and the reliability of fatigue detection technologies. False positive and negative rates are often used as metrics as they give a good indication of the reliability of the fatigue detection technology and can be used as representative indirect measures of user experience and safety.

In addition to these considerations, the validation process generally also depends on the technology's application, the use case, and the level of expertise of the team in charge of the development or the assessment of the technology. For instance, assessment guidelines and protocols for mandatory fatigue detection system in EU (General Safety Regulation, 2021) are developed with the help of experts in both fatigue detection and use case. At present, these experts recommend the use of the subjectively scored KSS, assessed every 5 minutes, as a reference measure, and they impose a certain target of true positive rate (i.e., also called sensitivity) for the technology to be approved and integrated into road vehicles. These protocols will continue to evolve in future and according to use cases. However, as not all validation requirements are defined within the regulation, this will inevitably lead to variation among validation approaches for different fatigue detection technologies, depending on the expertise within their individual development or assessment teams.

4.6.5 CONCLUSIONS

Fatigue detection technologies represent a true asset that, depending on their implementation, can improve safety across all transport applications. They can effectively supplement FRMS by providing continuous, objective, and real-time estimation of an operator's state, and can, therefore, act directly (by providing warnings or assistance) to reduce the risk of errors and accidents.

The development of fatigue detection technologies raises several challenges to ensure the expected benefits. It involves understanding the human brain and behaviour, considering environmental and application constraints, and focusing efforts on technology that is non-disturbing, that complies with standards and regulation, and that reliably estimates the fatigue state of the operator. It is important to address and consider all these elements to develop a technology that meets the safety objective and that is well adopted by operators.

Fatigue cannot be measured directly. Several approaches exist to estimate the state of fatigue of an individual, but few are applicable in operational conditions while ensuring good reliability and performance. Technologies based on body behavioural indicators (mainly eye-related data, also considered as physiological data) currently seem to be the most appropriate, but the approach chosen depends mainly on the use case and its constraints. Moreover, progress is adding more indicators sources and is fusing existing indicators to improve the robustness and reliability of these technologies.

Evaluating the performance of fatigue detection technologies can be very complex. It is a process that must consider a large and diverse set of technical and human factors while coping with a lack of unique, fully objective, and universally agreed reference measure. One way to optimise this process and to make it more accessible is to opt for a modular approach. In addition, a process of standardisation of assessment protocols of fatigue detection technology is underway in the automotive industry and could therefore serve as a basis for all other use cases in the future.

SUMMARY POINTS FOR PRACTITIONERS

- Fatigue detection technologies provide warnings or assistance to reduce the risk of errors and accidents.
- Fatigue detection technologies can effectively supplement FRMS by providing continuous, objective, and real-time estimation of an operator's state.
- The development of fatigue detection technologies raises several challenges that are important to address to ensure their adoption by users and the improvement of safety.
- Fatigue cannot be measured directly. Several approaches exist to estimate the state of fatigue of an operator, and technologies based on behavioural (mainly eye-related) data currently seem to be the most appropriate.

- Evaluating the performance of fatigue detection technologies can be very complex. One way to optimise this process and to make it more accessible is to opt for a modular approach. A process of standardisation of assessment protocols of fatigue detection technology is underway in the automotive industry and could serve as a basis for all transport applications in the future.

NOTES

1 For the sake of consistency, the term "fatigue" is used in this chapter as a synonym for "sleepiness/drowsiness".
2 In this chapter, the term "operator" means any individual interacting with an equipment (e.g., pilot, driver, air controller).

REFERENCES

Åkerstedt, T., & Gillberg, M. (1990). Subjective and objective sleepiness in the active individual. *International Journal of Neuroscience*, 52(1–2), 29–37.

American Association of Sleep Medicine (AASM). (2020). *The AASM manual for the scoring of sleep and associated events.*

Bérubé, L. (1991). *Terminologie de neuropsychologie et de neurologie du comportement.* Montréal: Éditions de la Chenelière.

Brown, I. D. (1997). Prospects for technological countermeasures against driver fatigue. *Accident Analysis & Prevention*, 29(4), 525–531.

Chen, J., & Ji, Q. (2012). *Drowsy driver posture, facial, and eye monitoring methods.* In A. Eskandarian (Ed.) Handbook of intelligent vehicles, London: Springer, pp. 913–940.

Dinges, D., & Grace, R. (1998). *PERCLOS: A valid psychophysiological measure of alertness as assessed by psychomotor vigilance.* US Department of Transportation, Federal Highway Administration, Report Number FHWA-MCRT-98-006.

Dinges, D. F., & Powell, J. W. (1985). Microcomputer analyses of performance on a portable, simple visual RT task during sustained operations. *Behavior Research Methods, Instruments, & Computers*, 17, 652–655.

El Khatib, A., Ou, C., & Karray, F. (2020). Driver inattention detection in the context of next-generation autonomous vehicles design: A survey. *IEEE Transactions on Intelligent Transportation Systems*, 21(11), 4483–4496.

Euro NCAP–Occupant Status Monitoring. (s.d.). From www.euroncap.com/en/vehicle-safety/the-ratings-explained/safety-assist/occupant-status-monitoring/.

GB/T 39263-2020. (s.d.). From www.chinesestandard.net/PDF.aspx/GBT39263-2020.

General Safety Regulation. (2021, April 23). From https://eur-lex.europa.eu/legal-content/EN/TXT/?uri=CELEX%3A32021R1341&qid=1634047801787.

Gillberg, M., Kecklund, G., & Åkerstedt, T. (1996). Sleepiness and performance of professional drivers in a truck simulator–Comparisons between day and night driving. *Journal of Sleep Research*, 5, 12–15.

Jacobé de Naurois, C., Bourdin, C., Stratulat, A., Diaz, E., & Vercher, J.-L. (2019). Detection and prediction of driver drowsiness using artificial neural network models. *Accident Analysis & Prevention*, 126, 95–104.

Klauer, S. G., Dingus, T. A., Neale, V. L., Sudweeks, J. D., & Ramsey, D. J. (2006). *The impact of driver inattention on near crash/crash risk: An analysis using the 100-car naturalistic driving study data.* US Department of Transportation Report No. DOT HS 810 594.

Liu, C. C., Hosking, S. G., & Lenné, M. G. (2009). Predicting driver drowsiness using vehicle measures: Recent insights and future challenges. *Journal of Safety Research*, 40(4), 239–245.

Michael, L., Passmann, S., & Becker, R. (2012). Electrodermal lability as an indicator for subjective sleepiness during total sleep deprivation. *Journal of Sleep Research*, 21(4), 470–478.

Schleicher, R., Galley, N., Briest, S., & Galley, L. (2008). Blinks and saccades as indicators of fatigue in sleepiness warnings: Looking tired? *Ergonomics*, 51(7), 982–1010.

Soares, S., Ferreira, S., & Couto, A. (2020). Driving simulator experiments to study drowsiness: A systematic review. *Traffic Injury Prevention*, 21(1), 29–37.

Vicente, J., Laguna, P., Bartra, A., & Bailón, R. (2016). Drowsiness detection using heart rate variability. *Medical and Biological Engineering and Computing*, 54(6_), 927–937.

4.7 Individual Countermeasures to Fatigue

Fran Pilkington-Cheney

Psychology Department, School of Social Sciences,
Nottingham Trent University, Nottingham, UK

CONTENTS

4.7.1 INTRODUCTION

One approach to reducing fatigue risk and managing fatigue is the use of individual countermeasures, defined as strategies individuals can use to manage fatigue. Generally, there are two main types of countermeasures: operational and individual. While the focus of this chapter is individual countermeasures to fatigue, it should be recognised that operational countermeasures (such as fatigue risk management systems, scheduling, hours of work and duty times, and education) can directly or indirectly influence individual countermeasure use. Nevertheless, individual countermeasures are a key consideration in fatigue management. Many operational countermeasures are out of the control of workers themselves. Vehicle operators may, however, be able to implement certain strategies to manage their fatigue and therefore need to know what is effective. It is important to note that the countermeasures discussed in this chapter are short-term strategies used to manage mild fatigue. If vehicle operators are severely fatigued, then it is important that they stop and do not continue to operate.

4.7.2 EFFECTIVE COUNTERMEASURES

It is vital to understand the cause of fatigue before deciding on an appropriate countermeasure, as this may impact the effectiveness (defined as countermeasures that have objectively been shown to alleviate fatigue). In May and Baldwin's (2009) model of fatigue causation (shown in Chapter 2.5), contributing factors have been categorised into sleep-related and task-related fatigue. The defining feature of this model is the distinction between the types of fatigue, and it is this distinction that is important when considering effective strategies to counteract fatigue. The appropriate countermeasure for someone who is sleepy would be different to the one for someone who is mentally overloaded due to increased task demand. Although May and Baldwin's model was designed for driver fatigue, the information is relevant to all workplace fatigue.

4.7.2.1 TASK-RELATED FATIGUE COUNTERMEASURES

The main countermeasure for task-related fatigue, both active and passive, is to ensure that regular breaks are taken. Rest breaks can help to break up the monotony of tedious tasks and are temporarily beneficial, being suggested as a countermeasure strategy for workplace fatigue (Caldwell et al., 2019). The research for other countermeasures to task-related fatigue is less certain. It follows that if someone is experiencing fatigue through overload, then minimising additional distractions could aid performance and concentration until a break can be obtained. Conversely, to combat underload, secondary tasks could therefore be effective for mitigating passive fatigue if they do not result in distraction. However, due to the nature of the task, this could be less achievable and more dangerous when driving. Although the most effective countermeasure for task-related fatigue is taking a break, importantly, taking a break without sleep is not effective for sleep-related fatigue. Most of the countermeasure research focuses on sleep-related fatigue, possibly due to the severe consequences of falling asleep during a safety critical task. Therefore, counteracting sleep-related fatigue will be the focus going forward.

4.7.2.2 SLEEP-RELATED FATIGUE COUNTERMEASURES

The only effective countermeasures to sleep-related fatigue (apart from adequate sleep and only working at times of peak alertness) are napping and caffeine. Although these are promoted as evidence-based mitigation strategies, it is important to recognise that they are not intended to be relied upon or to compensate for regular short or poor-quality sleep. In addition, they should not be promoted at the expense of operational measures, but rather as an addition, to be used strategically when required.

Napping

Napping has been shown to reduce physiological and subjective effects of fatigue on driving performance (Horne & Reyner, 1996; Watling, Smith, & Horswill, 2014). Naps of approximately 30 minutes reduce sleep-related fatigue for 1 to 2 hours post nap (Horne & Reyner, 1996), with daytime naps between 10 and 20 minutes showing decreases in subjective sleepiness, increases in objective alertness, and improvements in cognitive performance (Hilditch et al., 2017). However, napping requires time and facilities, which are not always accessible to individuals. There is also the issue of "readiness to sleep", as people may struggle to nap "on cue". Perception may be another barrier, associating napping with "sleeping on the job" or with an inability to cope with the work, which is linked to workplace culture. The benefit of a nap depends to some extent on the time of day it is taken, and the level of fatigue experienced. For example, a 10-minute nap following a day without sleep offered limited benefit to driving performance following a night shift (Hilditch et al., 2017).

Napping can result in instances of sleep inertia, resulting in reduced alertness and performance decrements. Severe symptoms can last 15 to 30 minutes after sleep but can take over an hour for full recovery (Hilditch & McHill, 2019). The length and timing of a nap influences sleep inertia, with performance decrements being exacerbated by previous sleep loss and time of day (Hilditch & McHill, 2019). For instance, a 10-minute nap at night, although not as effective as during the day, produced minimal sleep inertia and helped to mitigate some short-term impairments to performance during a simulated night shift (Hilditch et al., 2016), whereas a 30-minute night-time nap resulted in sleep inertia. Caffeine before a short nap reduces subsequent sleep inertia (Centofanti et al., 2020; Horne & Reyner, 1996); however, the inclusion of caffeine requires additional planning. It is important that fatigue education discusses napping and awareness of sleep inertia to ensure individuals allow sufficient recovery time (~20 to 30 minutes, up to an hour in severe cases) before continuing.

Caffeine

Caffeine is one of the most researched and established countermeasures in Western society for sleep-related fatigue. Caffeine is effective as it has a physiological effect on the brain, promoting wakefulness by blocking adenosine receptors. It can be found in a variety of forms such as coffee, tea, energy drinks, and tablets; however, the caffeine content can vary, as shown in Table 4.7.1. It is worth noting that certain products have fixed amounts of caffeine in them (e.g., energy drinks, tablets), whereas some products will have an approximated amount that will vary depending on various factors (e.g., bean, brewing time, size of drink).

TABLE 4.7.1
Approximate Caffeine Content of Regularly Consumed Products (UK)

Product	Approximate Caffeine Content (U.K.)
Instant coffee (2 g serve)	50 mg–90 mg
Energy Drink (250 ml)	80 mg
Coffee shop drink (large latte, cappuccino, flat white)	66 mg
Caffeinated tablet (per tablet)	50 mg
Cup of tea (1 bag)	30 mg–50 mg
Carbonated soft drink (330 ml)	32 mg
Chocolate (milk; dark, 50 g)	< 10 mg; < 25 mg

It is well established that caffeine counteracts sleepiness, with low to moderate doses effectively reducing the impact of sleep loss on alertness, vigilance, and cognitive performance (McLellan et al., 2016). A recent review of the effects of caffeine consumption found improvements in response time and accuracy on attention tests and information processing tasks, improvements in executive function and enhancements to certain vehicle measures in driving tests, concluding caffeine to be an effective countermeasure to the cognitive and physical impairments associated with sleep loss (Irwin et al., 2020). Driving simulator studies have shown that alertness is increased, and performance improved 20 minutes following caffeine consumption (e.g., Horne & Reyner, 1996; Reyner & Horne, 2002), with ongoing benefits to performance and sleepiness during prolonged driving (Mets et al., 2011). Repeated doses of caffeine (in the form of chewing gum) have also been shown to mitigate fatigue-related driving performance impairments, reducing drowsiness and the impact on driving errors (Aidman et al., 2018). Caffeine therefore has been suggested as an effective fatigue countermeasure, with reports of increased use in workers who experience disruptions to sleep or increased sleep-related fatigue, such as truck drivers (Filtness et al., 2020; Pylkkönen et al., 2015).

However, it is difficult to determine the effectiveness of caffeine as a driver sleepiness countermeasure for habitually high caffeine consumers. High caffeine consumers become accustomed and therefore likely need increased amounts to maintain alertness. There is little research exploring the influence of a caffeinated countermeasure for habitual caffeine use. However, self-report truck driver data indicates that high caffeine consumers are associated with poor health behaviours and report more crashes and worse driving safety indicators compared to low caffeine consumers (Filtness et al., 2020). There are also differences for individuals in terms of sensitivity to the effects of caffeine (e.g., effectiveness as a fatigue countermeasure) as well as sensitivity in terms of tolerance to caffeine (which can impact sleep quality and duration). Increased caffeine consumption can also result in increased need for facilities, which can be a barrier to its use (Pilkington-Cheney et al., 2020).

4.7.3 INEFFECTIVE COUNTERMEASURE USE

Caffeine and napping are not always the preferred strategies for fatigue management. Below is a list of commonly reported strategies which have little or limited evidence of effectiveness for sleep-related fatigue:

- Cold air/fresh air/air conditioning
- Turning up music/radio
- Talking to someone (passenger, or the phone)/singing to self
- Splashing cold water on the face
- Changing driving position/stretching/going for a walk/taking a break
- Sugar

A large questionnaire study of the Swedish public found that the most used countermeasures to increase alertness when driving were to take a walk (54%), turn on the radio (52%), open a window (47%), drink coffee (45%), and converse with a passenger (35%) (Anund et al., 2008). Of this list, only drinking caffeinated coffee would offer any benefit to sleep-related fatigue. Research exploring the effectiveness of countermeasures following 5-hour sleep restriction during extended, monotonous simulated driving found that cold air to the face and listening to the radio provided no significant benefit in terms of driving incidents or participant sleepiness (Reyner & Horne, 1998). However, subjectively, listening to the radio resulted in lower sleepiness reports for most of the drive. A more recent real-road driving study (both day and night driving) found no effect of opening a window, and minor acute effects of listening to music on subjective sleepiness and blink duration, concluding that these measures have little practical relevance in counteracting the effects of night driving or driving duration, and therefore driver sleepiness (Schwarz et al., 2012). Taking a break without a nap also provides no benefit to sleepy drivers (Horne & Reyner, 1999), or if any benefit is gained, it is short-lived (Phipps-Nelson et al., 2011). Despite reports of use by drivers to manage fatigue (Pilkington-Cheney et al., 2020), the evidence surrounding the efficacy of sugar as a countermeasure is inconsistent, with reports of sleepiness worsening over time following consumption, particularly during afternoon simulated driving (Horne & Baulk, 2004).

A lack of association has been found between effective sleepiness countermeasures such as stopping, taking a nap, utilising caffeine, and swapping drivers, with reports of driving while sleepy (Watling, Armstrong, Obst, et al., 2014). Despite knowing these countermeasures to be effective (Anund et al., 2008), they are used less often than ineffective strategies (e.g., opening a window or turning on the radio) or alongside effective strategies (Pylkkönen et al., 2015). It may be that the use of ineffective strategies to counteract sleepiness is due to convenience or accessibility, as well as some expectation of an alerting effect.

Differences have been noted between professional and non-professional drivers in relation to countermeasures (Gershon et al., 2011). Listening to the radio and opening a window were frequently used and perceived as highly effective strategies by both groups. However, more tactical countermeasures were reported by some professional drivers such as planning for rest stops and using napping and caffeine. Interestingly, most professional respondents were truck drivers (52%), who have also been reported to use both napping and rest breaks to counteract sleep-related fatigue (Pylkkönen et al., 2015). Within aviation, strategic use of caffeine and napping are frequently used to increase alertness (Sallinen et al., 2017), with pilots using controlled rest (in seat, on the flight deck) and bunk rest (in a designated crew rest facility) to manage fatigue. In comparison, tram drivers report the use of light meals and talking to others during rest breaks to manage fatigue (Onninen et al., 2020). Outside of rest breaks, caffeine and "self-activation" strategies (e.g., moving around, opening a window, changing driver behaviour or position, and talking to self) are commonly used by tram drivers, with similar strategies being reported by train drivers (Filtness & Naweed et al., 2017). Similarly, in a recent study with city bus drivers (Pilkington-Cheney et al., 2020), although caffeine and napping were occasionally used, strategies which have limited evidence of effectiveness were also heavily relied upon, such as opening a window, stretching, singing, talking, and using forms of sugar. It is possible that constraints of the workplace (e.g., scheduling, break location, facilities, and sole driver) inadvertently encourage the use of ineffective strategies which are less influenced by workplace constraints.

The use of ineffective strategies (or strategies with limited evidence of effectiveness) alongside or instead of effective countermeasures highlights the importance of education, both in terms of effectiveness of countermeasures but also in understanding the cause of fatigue. It is vital that for individual fatigue countermeasures to work, vehicle operators know what is effective. Importantly, individuals will use what is available to them to manage fatigue, or what they think will work. Therefore, there is a need for education and discussion around countermeasure effectiveness, and accessibility to effective strategies, so that vehicle operators can make informed choices on what to do when fatigued.

4.7.4 INFLUENCE OF OTHER FACTORS

The decision to use a fatigue countermeasure is a complex process which involves a chain of decisions (see Figure 1.5.3 in Chapter 1.5), all of which need to be met to result in appropriate countermeasure use. Firstly, a vehicle operator must be able to recognise that they are fatigued. There has been debate relating to the extent individuals can accurately identify their sleepiness. For example, during experimental research, participants are frequently asked to report on their state, alerting them to their increasing sleepiness levels, which may be different from real-world driving. However, a recent systematic review concluded that drivers are aware of sleepiness when driving (Cai et al., 2021). Despite this, individuals continue to drive. This relates to the next step in the chain of decisions, that is, individuals need to be motivated to act on this feeling. Individuals can be motivated to act by using a countermeasure, or they may be motivated to continue driving, which may be exacerbated by pressure to continue working or the urge to get home following work, overriding acknowledgement of increasing sleepiness. Additionally, individuals are not able to predict the exact moment that they will fall asleep. Related to this, drivers must be aware of the consequences and risks of continuing to drive while fatigued. There are questions as to whether drivers acknowledge the risk of sleepiness, with research suggesting that sleepy driving is considered a risky behaviour, but not as risky as other driving behaviours, for example, speeding (Watling, Armstrong, Smith & Obst, 2016). Thinking back to May and Baldwin's model of fatigue causation (2009), individuals must also understand the cause of fatigue and be aware of the appropriate strategies to counteract this. Finally, vehicle operators must not be prevented to act, for example, by barriers or restrictions, such as limited access to facilities, incorrect knowledge, or workplace culture.

As individual countermeasures are, by definition, strategies that individuals themselves choose to use (or not use) to reduce fatigue, education relating to effective countermeasures is essential, as it has the potential to inform decisions. Educating about the importance of adequate sleep and the risks and dangers of fatigue, as well as the availability of scientifically supported strategies to promote sleep and increase alertness, is cited as a necessary component of workplace fatigue management (Caldwell et al., 2019). It is vital that individuals know how to recognise and understand the cause of fatigue, when to act (e.g., when to use an appropriate countermeasure and when to stop) and what to do when they are fatigued, and this can be facilitated by educational interventions and operator support. All workers within the transportation industry would benefit from education informing people about the basics of sleep health, and importantly, what is and what is not effective at reducing fatigue. It is clear from the research that individuals do *something* to manage their fatigue, and it is therefore essential that they know and understand the effectiveness of *what* they are using.

However, although education is important, it is not enough to mitigate fatigue as a stand-alone intervention. Any education must consider environment and accessibility, as restrictions may prevent individuals from using effective strategies. Education will not be effective if individuals are prevented from implementing knowledge gained. Access to facilities is key for individuals to be able to engage with effective strategies such as caffeine and napping, both requiring adequate facilities, and time. Workers are reliant on their organisation for access. Therefore, even if individuals have been educated in effective strategies to reduce fatigue, if access to adequate facilities (e.g., canteens, toilets and napping areas) are not provided, then that knowledge cannot be used. Similarly, private drivers are reliant on access to safe places to stop to engage with strategies (e.g., service stations), with personal safety being an important consideration in terms of napping.

In relation to environment, certain professional groups have been shown to use caffeine and napping and this is likely influenced by their workplace. For example, truck drivers face fewer restrictions than public transport service providers, as, although they typically drive alone with restrictions on work hours and driving time, they can plan stops to engage with countermeasures. Private car drivers are also likely to be in control of their schedule and choosing when and where to stop. However, other transport drivers experience additional barriers to countermeasure use. Public service providers (e.g., bus, train, and tram drivers) are often the sole driver on duty responsible for their vehicle and are typically not in control of the timing or location of their rest breaks. These factors impact the use of countermeasures for both sleep -and task-related fatigue and could explain reliance on less effective strategies to manage fatigue (as reported above in sub-section 4.7.3).

A final consideration, but arguably one of the most important, is workplace culture. As discussed in Chapter 1.5, an open/just safety culture is a key feature of successful fatigue management. In terms of countermeasures, decisions to use caffeine and napping strategies may be influenced by organisational perception, resulting in less engagement with effective measures even if there is adequate access to them. Open culture needs to be established to help facilitate conversations about fatigue and encourage engagement with effective countermeasures and educational interventions. However, as culture change takes time, other measures could be introduced to help alleviate fatigue risk (e.g., education) while working towards an open safety culture. Taking the time to develop this culture should lead to fatigue being discussed openly between workers and managers, resulting in honest conversations and increased incidence reporting. This is vital, as individual fatigue countermeasures should only be used in the short term, with the longer-term goal of addressing the root cause of any fatigue-related problems being the main aim.

It is important to recognise that restrictions and barriers will likely lead individuals away from effective countermeasures, encouraging reliance on ineffective strategies that are less influenced by, for example, workplace constraints, or result in a lack of engagement with countermeasures at all (e.g., not taking any action to alleviate fatigue). This highlights the complex issue of individual countermeasure use, and the importance of a holistic approach.

4.7.5 CONCLUSIONS

The use of individual countermeasures is an important issue in the management of fatigue, with a need for effective strategies that vehicle operators can use before, during, and after duty. However, these should be used strategically as short-term measures for mild fatigue and not relied upon. It is vital that increasing the uptake of effective countermeasures does not lead to overuse or encourage individuals to continue working when they are excessively fatigued. Individuals need to be educated about the use of countermeasures and have the ability and opportunity to use this knowledge when needed. Barriers that may restrict effective countermeasure use or encourage the use of ineffective measures need to be recognised and addressed. Importantly, there is a need to develop a culture whereby the management of fatigue, including effective countermeasures, can be discussed openly, ultimately reducing fatigue risk.

SUMMARY POINTS FOR PRACTITIONERS

- It is important to understand the cause of fatigue to be able to use an appropriate countermeasure. This will require education.
- Caffeine and napping strategies can be effective as short-term countermeasures to sleep-related fatigue. Taking regular breaks can be effective for task-related fatigue.
- Restrictions impact countermeasure use, for example, adequate access. Facilities should be reviewed and, where possible, provided, and initiatives should be introduced to enable workers to engage with effective countermeasures.
- Initiatives relating to individual countermeasures should not be provided in isolation, but as part of operational fatigue management, supported by an open safety culture.

REFERENCES

Aidman, E., Johnson, K., Paech, G. M., Della Vedova, C., Pajcin, M., Grant, C., Kamimori, G., Mitchelson, E., Hoggan, B. L., Fidock, J., & Banks, S. (2018). Caffeine reduces the impact of drowsiness on driving errors. *Transportation Research Part F: Traffic Psychology and Behaviour, 54*, 236–247.

Anund, A., Kecklund, G., Peters, B., & Åkerstedt, T. (2008). Driver sleepiness and individual differences in preferences for countermeasures. *Journal of Sleep Research, 17*(1), 16–22.

Cai, A. W., Manousakis, J. E., Lo, T. Y., Horne, J. A., Howard, M. E., & Anderson, C. (2021). I think I'm sleepy, therefore I am–Awareness of sleepiness while driving: A systematic review. *Sleep Medicine Reviews, 60*, 101533.

Caldwell, J. A., Caldwell, J. L., Thompson, L. A., & Lieberman, H. R. (2019). Fatigue and its management in the workplace. *Neuroscience & Biobehavioral Reviews, 96*, 272–289.

Centofanti, S., Banks, S., Coussens, S., Gray, D., Munro, E., Nielsen, J., & Dorrian, J. (2020). A pilot study investigating the impact of a caffeine-nap on alertness during a simulated night shift. *Chronobiology International, 37*(9–10), 1469–1473.

Filtness, A. J., Hickman, J. S., Mabry, J. E., Glenn, L., Mao, H., Camden, M., & Hanowski, R. J. (2020). Associations between high caffeine consumption, driving safety indicators, sleep and health behaviours in truck drivers. *Safety Science, 126*, 104664.

Filtness, A. J., & Naweed, A. (2017). Causes, consequences and countermeasures to driver fatigue in the rail industry: The train driver perspective. *Applied Ergonomics, 60*, 12–21.

Gershon, P., Shinar, D., Oron-Gilad, T., Parmet, Y., & Ronen, A. (2011). Usage and perceived effectiveness of fatigue countermeasures for professional and nonprofessional drivers. *Accident Analysis & Prevention, 43*(3), 797–803.

Hilditch, C. J., Centofanti, S. A., Dorrian, J., & Banks, S. (2016). A 30-minute, but not a 10-minute nighttime nap is associated with sleep inertia. *Sleep, 39*(3), 675–685.

Hilditch, C. J., Dorrian, J., Centofanti, S. A., Van Dongen, H. P. A., & Banks, S. (2017). Sleep inertia associated with a 10-min nap before the commute home following a night shift: A laboratory simulation study. *Accident Analysis & Prevention, 99*(Part B), 411–415.

Hilditch, C. J., & McHill, A. W. (2019). Sleep inertia: Current insights. *Nature and Science of Sleep, 11*, 155–165.

Horne, J. A., & Baulk, S. D. (2004). Awareness of sleepiness when driving. *Psychophysiology, 41*(1), 161–165.

Horne, J. A., & Reyner, L. A. (1996). Counteracting driver sleepiness: Effects of napping, caffeine and placebo. *Psychophysiology, 33*(3), 306–309.

Horne, J. A., & Reyner, L. A. (1999). Vehicle accidents related to sleep: A review. *Occupational and Environmental Medicine, 56*(5), 289–294.

Irwin, C., Khalesi, S., Desbrow, B., & McCartney, D. (2020). Effects of acute caffeine consumption following sleep loss on cognitive, physical, occupational and driving performance: A systematic review and meta-analysis. *Neuroscience & Biobehavioral Reviews, 108*, 877–888.

May, J. F., & Baldwin, C. L. (2009). Driver fatigue: The importance of identifying causal factors of fatigue when considering detection and countermeasure technologies. *Transportation Research Part F: Traffic Psychology and Behaviour, 12*(3), 218–224.

McLellan, T. M., Caldwell, J. A., & Lieberman, H. R. (2016). A review of caffeine's effects on cognitive, physical and occupational performance. *Neuroscience & Biobehavioral Reviews, 71*, 294–312.

Mets, M. A., Ketzer, S., Blom, C., Van Gerven, M. H., Van Willigenburg, G. M., Olivier, B., & Verster, J. C. (2011). Positive effects of Red Bull® Energy Drink on driving performance during prolonged driving. *Psychopharmacology, 214*(3), 737–745.

Onninen, J., Hakola, T., Puttonen, S., Tolvanen, A., Virkkala, J., & Sallinen, M. (2020). Sleep and sleepiness in shift-working tram drivers. *Applied Ergonomics, 88*, 103153.

Phipps-Nelson, J., Redman, J. R., & Rajaratnam, S. M. (2011). Temporal profile of prolonged, night-time driving performance: Breaks from driving temporarily reduce time-on-task fatigue but not sleepiness. *Journal of Sleep Research, 20*(3), 404–415.

Pilkington-Cheney, F., Filtness, A. J., & Haslam C. (2020). A qualitative study exploring how city bus drivers manage sleepiness and fatigue. *Chronobiology International, 37*(9–10), 1502–1512.

Pylkkönen, M., Sihvola, M., Hyvärinen, H. K., Puttonen, S., Hublin, C., & Sallinen, M. (2015). Sleepiness, sleep, and use of sleepiness countermeasures in shift-working long-haul truck drivers. *Accident Analysis & Prevention, 80*, 201–210.

Reyner, L. A., & Horne, J. A. (1998). Evaluation of 'in-car' countermeasures to sleepiness: Cold air and radio. *Sleep, 21*(1), 46–51.

Reyner, L. A., & Horne, J. A. (2002). Efficacy of a "functional energy drink" in counteracting driver sleepiness. *Physiology & Behavior, 75*(3), 331–335.

Sallinen, M., Sihvola, M., Puttonen, S., Ketola, K., Tuori, A., Härmä, M., Kecklund, G., & Åkerstedt, T. (2017). Sleep, alertness and alertness management among commercial airline pilots on short-haul and long-haul flights. *Accident Analysis & Prevention, 98*, 320–329.

Schwarz, J. F. A., Ingre, M., Fors, C., Anund, A., Kecklund, G., Taillard, J., Philip, P., & Åkerstedt, T. (2012). In-car countermeasures open window and music revisited on the real road: Popular but hardly effective against driver sleepiness. *Journal of Sleep Research, 21*(5), 595–599.

Watling, C. N., Armstrong, K. A., Obst, P. L., & Smith, S. S. (2014). Continuing to drive while sleepy: The influence of sleepiness countermeasures, motivation for driving sleepy, and risk perception. *Accident Analysis & Prevention, 73*, 262–268.

Watling, C. N., Armstrong, K. A., Smith, S. S., & Obst, P. L. (2016). Crash risk perception of sleepy driving and its comparisons with drink driving and speeding: Which behavior is perceived as the riskiest? *Traffic Injury Prevention, 17*(4), 400–405.

Watling, C. N., Smith, S. S., & Horswill, M. S. (2014). Stop and revive? The effectiveness of nap and active rest breaks for reducing driver sleepiness. *Psychophysiology, 51*(11), 1131–1138.

4.8 Light as a Countermeasure to Sleepiness and Its Potential for Use in the Transport Industry

Shamsi Shekari Soleimanloo and Simon Smith

Institute for Social Science Research (ISSR), The University of Queensland, Brisbane, Qld, Australia

CONTENTS

4.8.1 INTRODUCTION: FATIGUE, A CHALLENGE FOR THE TRANSPORT INDUSTRY

Road injuries kill 1.35 million people worldwide (World Health Organization (WHO), 2018) and are expected to cost the global economy $1.8 trillion (2010 US$) between 2015 and 2030 (Chen et al., 2019). Driver fatigue and sleepiness are closely-related issues in the transportation industry and contribute to 20 to 30% of road crashes globally (Tefft, 2014).

Sleepiness and *fatigue* are intertwined constructs but may be distinguished by contributing factors. Driver fatigue stems primarily from sleep-related sources (mainly inadequate sleep duration, regularity, timing, and quality) and other contributing factors. Sleep-related sources of driver fatigue encompass total or partial sleep loss, fragmentation of sleep, extended wake periods (Lowden et al., 2009), poor sleep quality, short break durations, and circadian (body clock) misalignment (Lowden et al., 2009; Wilson et al., 2010). Other contributing factors to fatigue include long shift duration (Anund et al., 2015), work demands, the presence of sleep disorders, and other causes of increased sleep propensity (Williamson et al., 2011). This chapter uses *fatigue* to refer to the interchangeably used terms *fatigue* and *sleepiness* due to inadequate sleep (duration, regularity, timing, and quality) and time-on-task.

Alertness is not considered the exact opposite of sleepiness but refers to a state of wakefulness that generally follows a circadian rhythm and an increased readiness to respond to external stimuli (Sturm & Willmes, 2001). Optimum alertness is essential in retaining performance and safe decision-making in complex road environments (Schweizer et al., 2013).

In the current 24-hour society, it is not always feasible to schedule transportation operations optimally for driver alertness. Although sufficient prior sleep remains the best mitigation strategy, drivers typically take reactive and sometimes arbitrary approaches to maintain their alertness (Wesensten et al., 2015) (see Chapter 4.7). Therefore, it is critical to identify pragmatic technologies to maintain or improve driver alertness while on the road. Light can improve neurophysiological, subjective, and behavioural outcomes of alertness in specific contexts and has promise as a technology to improve driver alertness.

This chapter summarises the mechanisms behind the alerting effects of light, the current evidence for alerting effects of light in driving and other settings, current lighting technologies and their transferability to the transport industry, and the limitations of current knowledge and future research direction.

4.8.2 MECHANISMS OF ALERTING EFFECTS OF LIGHT

Light induces its alerting effects through the human eye's photoreceptors in the retina [rods, cons and the intrinsically photosensitive retinal ganglion cells (ipRGCs)]. Rods and cones mainly exert light's visual effects but can also mediate human alertness (Xu & Lang, 2018). The ipRGCs called melanopsin receptors induce human alertness through melatonin-dependent or independent pathways (Figure 4.8.1). Melatonin is a hormone the pineal gland expresses in response to darkness that signals sleep onset at multiple sites within the body.

The ipRGCs–SCN–RHT pathway is a *melatonin-dependent* pathway that involves ipRGCs projecting to the suprachiasmatic nuclei (SCN) in the hypothalamus through the retinohypothalamic tract (RHT) (Lok et al., 2018). The SCN is the principal circadian clock that can effectively suppress the expression of melatonin and promote alertness in response to light.

Several *melatonin-independent* pathways induce acute alerting effects of light and improve human attention via the projection of ipRGCs to either (a) the ventral lateral preoptic area (VLPO) in the anterior hypothalamus; (b) the locus coeruleus (LC) in

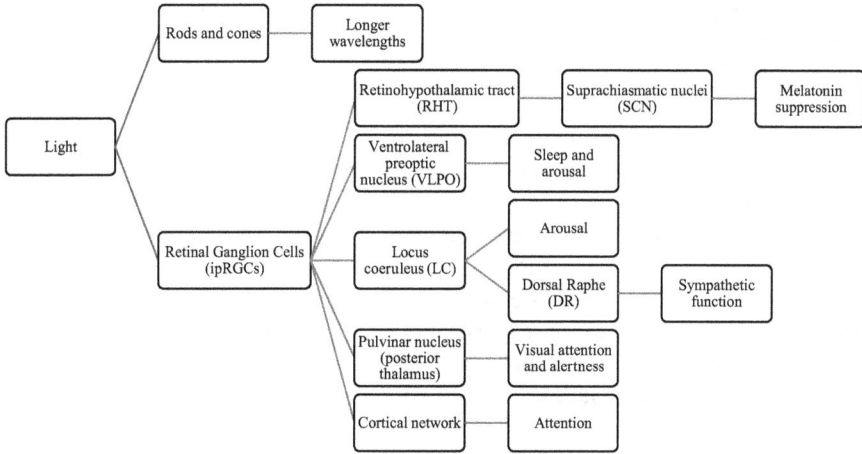

FIGURE 4.8.1 Pathways of alerting effects of light based on Cajochen (2007) and Lok et al. (2018).

the brainstem; (c) dorsal raphe nucleus in the brainstem; (d) pulvinar nucleus in the posterior thalamus, and (e) brain cortical network. The activation of the ipRGCs–VLPO pathway acts as a "switch" for sleep by inhibiting arousal. Conversely, the inactivation of these neurotransmitter systems promotes alertness (Cajochen, 2007). The ipRGCs–LC pathway increases arousal after the excitement of the neuropeptide orexin within the LC (Cajochen, 2007). The ipRGCs–C–DR pathway involves the activation of the Dorsal Raphe nucleus in the brainstem (innervated by projections from the LC) that promotes alertness by altering sympathetic function (Lok et al., 2018). The ipRGCs–PN pathway regulates visual attention and alertness via activation of the pulvinar nucleus in the posterior thalamus. Finally, the ipRGCs–CN pathway activates an extensive cortical network engaged in attention (Cajochen, 2007). In short, light increases alertness and attention via several direct and indirect neural pathways.

4.8.2.1 FACTORS CONTRIBUTING TO ALERTING EFFECTS OF LIGHT

The alerting effects of light are determined by light's physical characteristics (intensity, spectrum, colour temperature, and photon density) and their interplay with the time of day, lighting duration, the viewer's photic history, and individual differences (Vetter et al., 2021), as described below.

Light intensity: There is a positive dose–response relationship between light intensity and its alerting effects, increasing alertness with higher light intensities (Cajochen, 2007).

Wavelength and colour temperature: Light wavelength also has a dose–response relationship with its alerting effects, with shorter (more blue) wavelengths typically having more significant alerting effects than longer (redder) wavelengths (Cajochen, 2007) due to the higher sensitivity of the melanopsin receptors (ipRGCs) to blue light. Additionally, light with higher correlated colour temperatures (CCT) or narrowband light with higher short-wavelength energy is more alertness-inducing than warmer lights or light with attenuated short-wavelength energy (Souman et al., 2018).

Time of day: Ambient light varies by time of day, and thus the type of photoreceptors involved in modulating alertness. The artificial light at night contains more blue light stimulating the melanopsin receptors (ipRGCs), whereas daylight contains longer wavelengths (e.g., green light) mediated by rods and cones (Xu & Lang, 2018).

Duration: The length of one's exposure to light appears to change aspects of the alerting response. For instance, exposure to blue light (wavelength = 460 nm) for 2 hours suppresses melatonin and improves autonomous indicators of alertness, while exposure for over 6 hours improves neurophysiological measures of alertness (Cajochen, 2007).

Photic history: The photic history refers to a person's light exposure prior to the lighting condition of interest. One's photic history increases the baseline levels of alertness before exposure to the desired light. Therefore, with previous exposure to light in the real world, much higher light levels are typically required to elicit a specific alerting response compared to the light levels in laboratory settings with controlled photic history (Vetter et al., 2021).

Individual differences: Individual differences (e.g., in genotype, chronotype, pupillary dilation, photoreceptor sensitivity and distribution) interact with features of light exposure, including spectrum and time of day (Xu & Lang, 2018).

4.8.3   MEASURES OF HUMAN FATIGUE AND ALERTNESS

Absolute levels of fatigue and alertness are complicated to measure. Evidence suggests that subjective sleepiness, neurophysiological indices, behavioural indices, and objective driving performance can quantify critical dimensions of driver fatigue. The alerting effects of light can be quantified by changes in the magnitude and direction of these measures of fatigue.

Neurophysiological measures: Fatigue increases electroencephalographic (EEG) theta (4 to 8 Hz) activity, EEG alpha bursts (Kecklund & Åkerstedt, 1993), electrooculographic (EOG) slow rolling eye movements (Cajochen, 2007), and eye-blink duration (Cori et al., 2019), but decreases blink frequency and eyelid movements (Shekari Soleimanloo et al., 2019), heart rate variability (Lok et al., 2018), and heart rate (Borghini et al., 2014).

Behavioural measures: Fatigue increases reaction time and attentional lapses and impairs other cognitive measures (Jackson et al., 2013).

Self-reported sleepiness: Fatigue increases perceived sleepiness measured by brief subjective instruments such as the Karolinska Sleepiness Scale.

Driving performance: Fatigue impairs a range of driving performance outcomes. For instance, it increases the standard deviation of lane position (or lateral lane variability (Forsman et al., 2013), steering wheel variability (Forsman et al., 2013), and lane departures (Anund et al., 2015).

4.8.4   ALERTING EFFECTS OF LIGHT IN NON-DRIVING SETTINGS

Laboratory studies and applied work have characterised the effects of various light profiles on neurophysiological, subjective, and behavioural outcomes of alertness.

A review of 19 studies assessing the alerting effects of *daytime* exposure to *polychromatic white light* (comprised of several wavelengths) concluded that 15 minutes to 24 hours of exposure to high intensities ranging from 300 lx to > 7000 lx improved sustained attention, subjective sleepiness, EEG and ECG activities when compared with lower intensities (ranging from 0.01 lx to 400 lx). Of ten studies reporting sustained attention and 18 reporting subjective sleepiness, five reported improvements in reaction times and 14 reported less sleepiness. Of seven EEG and seven autonomic activity studies (including heart rate and heart rate variability), four and three reported positive improvements in EEG measures and autonomic activity, respectively. Six studies reporting changes in both EEG and subjective measures of sleepiness suggested a higher sensitivity of EEG-related outcomes to light than to subjective sleepiness (Lok et al., 2018).

A systematic review of 24 studies examining the acute alerting effects of various intensities and wavelengths of light found improved EEG-based measures by blue light. Of six examined alerting effects of monochromatic light (comprised of one specific wavelength), four reported acute alerting effects of blue light on EEG-based measures (Xu & Lang, 2018).

Another systematic review of 68 studies assessing the effects of light wavelength, intensity, or correlated colour temperatures (CCT) on subjective sleepiness and objective performance (reaction time and attention lapses) reported reduced sleepiness and faster reaction times on a simple reaction time task (Souman et al., 2018). Of 45 studies of various polychromatic white light intensity (100 to 10000 lx at the eye vs. dim light from <1 to 1411 lx at the eye) and 15 studies of white light with a high CCT, reductions in subjective sleepiness were confirmed in 28 and 4 studies, respectively. However, there were no clear patterns of subjective sleepiness in response to time or exposure duration. Of 14 studies comparing the effects of various wavelengths of monochromatic light, only four studies reported less sleepiness with blue light (470 nm) compared to either red (630 nm) or green (555 nm) lights (Souman et al., 2018). Of 16 studies examining the effects of polychromatic light on objective performance, only two reported faster reaction time on simple reaction time tasks under higher intensities of polychromatic light. Similarly, from five studies of white light with a high CCT, only one confirmed reduced reaction time but no reduction in attention lapses. Conversely, five of eight monochromatic-light studies reported faster reaction times (Souman et al., 2018).

In summary, polychromatic light improves physiological outcomes of alertness and subjective alertness compared to monochromatic light. However, there also appears to be a robust positive association between monochromatic blue light and physiological measures of alertness. The evidence supports faster reaction times with monochromatic blue light than with polychromatic white light. There are mixed findings for times of day during which polychromatic or monochromatic light has robust effects.

4.8.5 ALERTING EFFECTS OF LIGHT IN DRIVING SETTINGS

Studies on the effects of light on driver alertness are scarce, with no available systematic reviews. The inconclusive findings of six driving studies described below reflect the impact of versatile light intensities, light spectrums, bandwidths, dominant wavelengths, photon densities, times of day, durations of exposure, frequencies of exposure (continuous or temporary), and photic histories on small sample sizes, primarily male participants.

In a nocturnal simulated driving study, effects of randomised blue (460 nm, 1.1 lx), red (640 nm, ~1 lx), or ambient broadband (~0.2 lx) lights on subjective and objective performance of eight drivers were examined. The blue and red lights were projected by an LED light source panel (13 cm × 45 cm), located behind the steering wheel at a 49-cm distance from the eye, whereas the ambient light was sourced by the simulator and the EEG monitor screens. A 6-hour exposure to blue light attenuated EEG delta (1.0 to 4.5 Hz) and theta (4.5 to 8 Hz) activity, slowed eye movement events, and improved simple reaction times compared to the ambient broadband light. Still, it did not change subjective sleepiness and driving performance outcomes. A delayed measurement of outcomes 4 hours post-intervention revealed sustainability of the reduction of delta and theta activities and slow eye movements with blue light (Phipps-Nelson et al., 2009).

A daytime simulated-driving study in 19 drivers assessed the alerting effects of exposure to 44 minutes of bright light (5600 lx at the eye) in randomly sleep-deprived or well-rested drivers compared to the effects of ambient dim light (35 lx) in sleep-deprived drivers. The bright light was provided within a cubicle with three fluorescent light units (one 4100-K light facing the subject at ~18 cm from the driver's eyes in the seated position and two 5000-K lights on the sides of the cubicle). While exposure to bright light did not improve reaction time, it improved subjective sleepiness and several driving performance indicators (reduced terminal crashes, lateral lane variability, and steering wheel variability) (Weisgerber et al., 2017).

Another daytime simulated driving study in 17 drivers examined the effects of blue-enriched polychromatic white light (with a maximum peak of spectral irradiance at 440 nm, 469 lx at the eye) on driving performance, auditory reaction time, and subjective sleepiness. A 40-W LED lamp, located between the driver's eyes and the screen at a 60-cm distance from the participants' left eye, projected the light. Exposure to blue-enriched white light improved the reaction time but not subjective sleepiness. Surprisingly, blue-enriched white light degraded the accuracy of lane-keeping measures (Rodríguez-Morilla et al., 2018).

A nocturnal naturalistic driving study compared the subjective sleepiness of six truck drivers after 30-minute exposure to one of three counterbalanced conditions during a 45-minute break halfway into the drive; a 1000-lx bright light, a 600-lx UV and red-light-attenuated light or a control condition. The bright light was projected by four full-colour miniature lights within a lightbox (50 cm x 40 cm x 10 cm) on the steering wheel, whereas a hat-like light visor projected the modified light. The same lightbox created the control condition with no light. None of these three lighting conditions improved subjective sleepiness compared to the control condition (Landström et al., 2004).

Another naturalistic driving study assessed the effects of nocturnal blue light on the driving performance of 40 non-professional drivers. Drivers received randomised blue light, caffeine (400 mg), or placebo condition (no light, placebo caffeine) before and during the 15-min break. An LED light source (placed on the dashboard at a 75-cm distance from the driver's eyes) produced the blue light (468 nm, with an order of 20 lx at the eye). Blue light improved driving performance (reduced inappropriate line crossings and lateral lane variability) compared to the placebo condition (Taillard et al., 2012).

In a recent naturalistic driving study, the effects of blue-enriched white light on EEG alpha activity, reaction time on a simple reaction time task, and subjective sleepiness were compared to a placebo condition in 37 individuals when driving a test car twice a day (morning vs. evening). The in-vehicle daylight-supplementing system comprised 18 blue LEDs (40 lm, peak wavelength: 471 nm) and 36 white LEDs (25 lm, 2700 K), placed on the car's roof at a 20-cm distance from the driver's eyes. The daylight system was connected to a digital ambient photosensor and generated an additional light (33 to 1320 lx at the cornea) for respective measured ambient light 25 to >2000 lx at the windshield. Participant exposure to light did not improve subjective sleepiness or reaction time in the morning or afternoon sessions but increased EEG-based alertness (reduced alpha activity) in the morning drive (Canazei et al., 2021).

To summarise, the limited evidence from these driving studies highlights that nocturnal exposure to blue light *can* improve EEG-related outcomes of alertness and reduce reaction time or unsafe driving indicators (inappropriate line crossings and lateral lane variability), but not subjective sleepiness. Daytime administration of high-intensity polychromatic bright light reduces unsafe driving indicators (reduce terminal crashes, lateral lane variability, and steering wheel variability) and subjective sleepiness, but not reaction time. Conversely, daytime blue-enriched light can improve EEG-based alertness outcomes but not subjective sleepiness.

4.8.6 CHALLENGES OF TRANSFERABILITY OF THE LIGHTING SETUPS TO THE TRANSPORT INDUSTRY

There are some considerable challenges to transferring the research-based lighting setups to the transport industry, as described in the following:

1. The current lighting standards primarily address the visual effects of light for built environments, including roadways, rather than nonvisual responses to light (Stefani & Cajochen, 2021). No specific regulations or standards exist for the shape, size, or placement of lighting setups when used as an alerting stimulant. The available studies on alerting effects of light have typically adopted purpose-built lighting setups, which vary in type, shape, size, placement in the car, and adaptability to ambient light. For instance, lightboxes placed on the steering wheel (Landström et al., 2004), commercial light visors worn on the head (Landström et al., 2004), and blue or red light LED source panels located behind the steering wheel (Phipps-Nelson et al., 2009) or in the middle of the dashboard (Taillard et al., 2012), adaptive blue-enriched white light LED

sources mounted on the ceiling (Canazei et al., 2021), and fluorescent bright light cubicles (Weisgerber et al., 2017). The versatile characteristics of these studies limit the validity and generalisability of findings to the real world.

2. Acute alerting effects of lighting setups in driving settings have been mainly derived from research undertaken in laboratory conditions while controlling for confounding factors such as photic history. Therefore, the magnitude of the carryover effect of individuals' photic history in real-world settings is not evident.

3. Driving studies reflect non-professional drivers mostly, with a lower prevalence of sleep apnoea, circadian rhythm disorder, shift work and consecutive night shifts than professional drivers.

4. There is a potential for light to exert undesired side effects (e.g., contrast effects, uncomfortable spectral distributions, eye discomfort and irritation) (Lowden & Kecklund, 2021; Sunde et al., 2020), which could challenge the transferability of these lighting setups to the real world to enhance human alertness. For instance, a study among shift workers found a significant increase in irritability and blurred vision at midnight or early morning compared to 11 pm under both blue-enriched (106 lx, 17,000 K) or longer-wavelength (43 lx, 4,000 K) lighting setups (Sunde et al., 2020), although with lesser eye discomfort, eye fatigue and irritation with blue-enriched light compared to a traditional longer-wavelength lighting setup. Likewise, two driving studies (Anund et al., 2011; Taillard et al., 2012) reported the withdrawal of 14 to 16% of drivers due to dazzling nocturnal blue light. Another naturalistic driving study acknowledged the potential for their custom-made in-vehicle lighting system to induce glare in the morning or evening and adopted a sun visor to eliminate the glare (Canazei et al., 2021).

5. The available evidence does not provide any information on the potential distraction of drivers by the in-vehicle lighting setup or interaction of the lighting system with the light from oncoming traffic during night-time drivers.

Given the limitations mentioned above, the findings of driving-related studies are likely to apply to transport operations; however, the specifics may vary.

4.8.7   FUTURE IN-VEHICLE LIGHTING SETUPS AND RESEARCH DIRECTION

The available research-based evidence provides rough guidance on characteristics of the future adaptive in-vehicle lighting systems in driving settings to be effective in reducing driver fatigue, as follows:

1. For the lighting setup to make the driver alert, the driver should initially be of low alertness (e.g., sleep-deprived or circadian-misaligned) (Canazei et al., 2021).

2. The lighting system should manipulate the light intensity and wavelength in response to the time of day. Lower light intensities at night are required due to stronger circadian drive and higher sleep pressure. In contrast, a driver's photic history (previous exposure to light) during the day increases their baseline alertness and requires higher light intensities to elicit the desired alerting effect (Xu & Lang, 2018).
3. The lighting system should consider light's possible delayed alerting effects when adjusting the wavelength and duration (Xu & Lang, 2018).
4. The lighting device should be an unintrusive (in-vehicle) system with no visual discomfort (glare, dazzling, irritation, eyestrain, headache, and nausea) (Anund et al., 2011).
5. The duration, frequency, and timing of a driver's exposure to light should be based on the light's spectrum, intensity, side effects, and the driver's work–rest schedule (Vetter et al., 2021).
6. The light should neither distract the driver nor interfere with the visibility of upcoming traffic lights, particularly at night.

Future research should be tailored towards the large-scale naturalistic driving settings for developing an ideal in-vehicle adaptive lighting system that meets visual standards, provides sufficient alerting effects while adapting to inter-individual differences, and maintains driver comfort and safety.

SUMMARY POINTS FOR PRACTITIONERS

- The physical characteristics of light (intensity, spectrum, colour temperature, and photon density) and their interplay with the time of day, lighting duration, previous light exposure and individual differences inform the magnitude and stability of alerting effects.
- Blue light *can* reduce risky driving indicators (e.g., inappropriate line crossings and lateral lane position variability) and improve physiological and behavioural alertness measures (brain activity on EEG and simple reaction time) during night-time drives.
- High-intensity white light can reduce risky driving indicators (terminal crashes, lateral lane position variability, and steering wheel variability) and subjective sleepiness during daytime drives.
- Large-scale naturalistic driving studies are required to transfer versatile lighting setups to the transport industry with no discomfort or distraction to drivers.

NOTE

This research work was partially supported by the Australian Government through the Australian Research Council's Centre of Excellence for Children and Families over the Life Course (Project ID CE200100025).

REFERENCES

Anund, A., Fors, C., Kecklund, G., Leeuwen, W. van, & Åkerstedt, T. (2015). *Countermeasures for fatigue in transportation: A review of existing methods for drivers on road, rail, sea and in aviation.* http://urn.kb.se/resolve?urn=urn:nbn:se:vti:diva-7823

Anund, A., Kecklund, G., & Åkerstedt, T. (2011). *Sleepiness, crashes and the effectiveness of countermeasures Consolidated report within ERANET node 15.* www.vti.se/publications

Borghini, G., Astolfi, L., Vecchiato, G., Mattia, D., & Babiloni, F. (2014). Measuring neurophysiological signals in aircraft pilots and car drivers for the assessment of mental workload, fatigue and drowsiness. *Neuroscience and Biobehavioral Reviews, 44,* 58–75.

Cajochen, C. (2007). Alerting effects of light. *Sleep Medicine Reviews, 11*(6), 453–464. www.smrv-journal.com/article/S1087-0792(07)00100-1/fulltext

Canazei, M., Staggl, S., Pohl, W., Schüler, S., Betz, D., Ottersbach, J., & Popp, R. (2021). Feasibility and acute alerting effects of a daylight-supplementing in-vehicle lighting system–Results from two randomised controlled field studies during dawn and dusk. *Lighting Research and Technology, 0.* https://doi.org/10.1177/1477153520982371

Chen, S., Kuhn, M., Prettner, K., & Bloom, D. E. (2019). The global macroeconomic burden of road injuries: Estimates and projections for 166 countries. *The Lancet Planetary Health, 3*(9), e390–e398. https://doi.org/10.1016/S2542-5196(19)30170-6

Cori, J. M. M., Anderson, C., Soleimanloo, S. S., Jackson, M. L. L., Howard, M. E. E., Shekari Soleimanloo, S., Jackson, M. L. L., & Howard, M. E. E. (2019). Narrative review: Do spontaneous eye blink parameters provide a useful assessment of state drowsiness? *Sleep Medicine Reviews, 45,* 95–104. https://doi.org/https://doi.org/10.1016/j.smrv.2019.03.004

Forsman, P. M., Vila, B. J., Short, R. A., Mott, C. G., & Van Dongen, H. P. (2013). Efficient driver drowsiness detection at moderate levels of drowsiness. *Accident Analysis and Prevention, 50,* 341–350.

Jackson, M. L., Croft, R. J., Kennedy, G. A., Owens, K., & Howard, M. E. (2013). Cognitive components of simulated driving performance: Sleep loss effects and predictors. *Accident Analysis and Prevention, 50,* 438–444.

Kecklund, G., & Åkerstedt, T. (1993). Sleepiness in long distance truck driving: An ambulatory EEG study of night driving. *Ergonomics, 36*(9), 1007–1017.

Landström, U., Åkerstedt, T., Byström, M., Nordström, B., & Wibom, R. (2004). Effect on truck drivers' alertness of a 30-min. exposure to bright light: A field study. *Perceptual and Motor Skills, 98*(3 I), 770–776. https://doi.org/10.2466/pms.98.3.770-776

Lok, R., Smolders, K. C. H. J., Beersma, D. G. M., & de Kort, Y. A. W. (2018). Light, alertness, and alerting effects of white light: A literature overview. *Journal of Biological Rhythms, 33*(6), 589–601. https://doi.org/10.1177/0748730418796443

Lowden, A., Anund, A., Kecklund, G., Peters, B., & Åkerstedt, T. (2009). Wakefulness in young and elderly subjects driving at night in a car simulator. *Accident Analysis and Prevention, 41*(5), 1001–1007.

Lowden, A., & Kecklund, G. (2021). Considerations on how to light the night-shift. *53*(5), 437–452. https://doi.org/10.1177/14771535211012251

Phipps-Nelson, J., Redman, J. R., Schlangen, L. J. M., & Rajaratnam, S. M. W. W. (2009). Blue light exposure reduces objective measures of sleepiness during prolonged nighttime performance testing. *Chronobiology International, 26*(5), 891–912. https://doi.org/10.1080/07420520903044364

Rodríguez-Morilla, B., Madrid, J. A., Molina, E., Pérez-Navarro, J., & Correa, Á. (2018). Blue-enriched light enhances alertness but impairs accurate performance in evening chronotypes driving in the morning. *Frontiers in Psychology, 9*(MAY), 688. https://doi.org/10.3389/FPSYG.2018.00688/BIBTEX

Schweizer, T. A., Kan, K., Hung, Y., Tam, F., Naglie, G., & Graham, S. (2013). Brain activity during driving with distraction: an immersive fMRI study. *Frontiers in Human Neuroscience, 7*(FEB). https://doi.org/10.3389/FNHUM.2013.00053

Shekari Soleimanloo, S., Wilkinson, V. E. E., Cori, J. M. M., Westlake, J., Stevens, B., Downey, L. A. A., Shiferaw, B. A. A., Rajaratnam, S. M. W. M. W., & Howard, M. E. E. (2019). Eye-blink parameters detect on-road track-driving impairment following severe sleep deprivation. *Journal of Clinical Sleep Medicine, 15*(9). https://doi.org/10.5664/jcsm.7918

Souman, J. L., Tinga, A. M., te Pas, S. F., van Ee, R., & Vlaskamp, B. N. S. (2018). Acute alerting effects of light: A systematic literature review. In *Behavioural Brain Research* (Vol. 337, pp. 228–239). Elsevier BV. https://doi.org/10.1016/j.bbr.2017.09.016

Stefani, O., & Cajochen, C. (2021). Should we re-think regulations and standards for lighting at workplaces? A practice review on existing lighting recommendations. *Frontiers in Psychiatry, 12*, 671. https://doi.org/10.3389/FPSYT.2021.652161/BIBTEX

Sturm, W., & Willmes, K. (2001). On the functional neuroanatomy of intrinsic and phasic alertness. *NeuroImage, 14*(1), S76–S84. https://doi.org/10.1006/NIMG.2001.0839

Sunde, E., Pedersen, T., Mrdalj, J., Thun, E., Grønli, J., Harris, A., Bjorvatn, B., Waage, S., Skene, D. J., & Pallesen, S. (2020). Alerting and circadian effects of short-wavelength vs. long-wavelength narrow-bandwidth light during a simulated night shift. *Clocks & Sleep 2020, Vol. 2, Pages 502–522, 2*(4), 502–522. https://doi.org/10.3390/CLOCKSSLEEP2040037

Taillard, J., Capelli, A., Sagaspe, P., Anund, A., Åkerstedt, T., & Philip, P. (2012). In-car nocturnal blue light exposure improves motorway driving: a randomised controlled trial. *PloS One, 7*(10), e46750. https://doi.org/10.1371/journal.pone.0046750

Tefft, B. C. (2014). Prevalence of motor vehicle crashes involving drowsy drivers, United States, 2009–2013. *AAA Foundation for Traffic Safety*, 1–8.

Vetter, C., Pattison, P. M., Houser, K., Herf, M., Phillips, A. J. K., Wright, K. P., Skene, D. J., Brainard, G. C., Boivin, D. B., & Glickman, G. (2021). A Review of human physiological responses to light: Implications for the development of integrative lighting solutions. https://doi.org/10.1080/15502724.2021.1872383

Weisgerber, D., Nikol, M., & Medicine, R. M.-S. (2017). Driving home from the night shift: a bright light intervention study. *Sleep Medicine, 30*, 171–179. https://doi.org/https://doi.org/10.1016/j.sleep.2016.09.010

Wesensten, N. J., Balkin, T. J., & Belenky, G. (2015). Countermeasures for mitigating fatigue in motor vehicle operators. *Reviews of Human Factors and Ergonomics, 10*(1), 115–137. https://doi.org/10.1177/1557234X15574827

Williamson, A., Lombardi, D. A., Folkard, S., Stutts, J., Courtney, T. K., & Connor, J. (2011). The link between fatigue and safety. *Accident Analysis and Prevention, 43*, 498–515. https://doi.org/10.1016/j.aap.2009.11.011

Wilson, M., Chattington, M., & Marple-Horvat, D. E. (2010). Eye movements drive steering: reduced eye movement distribution impairs steering and driving performance. *40*(3), 190–202. https://doi.org/10.3200/JMBR.40.3.190-202

World Health Organization (WHO). (2018). *Global status report on road safety 2018*. www.who.int/publications/i/item/9789241565684

Xu, Q., & Lang, C. P. (2018). Revisiting the alerting effect of light: A systematic review. *Sleep Medicine Reviews, 41*, 39–49. https://doi.org/10.1016/J.SMRV.2017.12.001

4.9 It Takes Two

Health Management and Its Interface with Fatigue

Anjum Naweed[1], Janine Chapman[1], and Amy C. Reynolds[2]

[1]Central Queensland University, Appleton Institute for Behavioural Science, , Adelaide, SA, Australia
[2]Flinders University, Adelaide Institute for Sleep Health, Adelaide, SA,Australia

CONTENTS

4.9.1   INTRODUCTION

This chapter considers health management and its intersection with fatigue in three transport industries: rail, road (bus, trucking, and taxiing), and tourism. By health management, we refer to approaches taken by employers to devise effective legislation, programmes, policies, and supports to protect and promote worker health as well as to prevent disease.

An overview of the industries and the work-related burden of disease in relation to productivity and safety is presented, alongside factors contributing to ill health within the transport sector. This is followed by evidence demonstrating the link between fatigue and key health conditions. We consider current approaches to health management under the broader safety management system, drawing attention to how this sits alongside fatigue risk management.

Finally, we bring together commonalities from these industries to identify gaps in current approaches, and put forward recommendations for holistic health management policy and practice. A conceptual simple causal loop diagram is presented (Figure 4.9.2) to illustrate these ideas. Although emphasis is on the Australian context,

DOI: 10.1201/9781003213154-31

these findings are broadly generalisable and comparable to industries in developed countries worldwide.

4.9.2 BACKGROUND OF RAIL, ROAD, AND REEF TOURISM INDUSTRIES

Rail, bus, commercial truck, taxi, and the (Great Barrier) reef tourism industries are all examples of service industries that transport people and/or goods to serve an important economic role. They rely on optimising efficiency, performance, and flow. Operating vehicles or vessels in a complex and dynamic service industry context is highly skilled and pressured work, often requiring shift work and long, irregular hours. In addition to certification and commercial licensing, there is a requirement for technical (e.g., use of technologies) and non-technical (e.g., teamworking, communication) knowledge. All of the operations run at high intensities, nearly all are affected by peak/off-peak capacity changes, and all but one operates 24/7 year-round (reef tourism is seasonalised). This intensity, coupled with the public interface, creates an imperative to manage safety. Further, these industries suffer from worker shortage, high turnover, and looming future demand (Australasian Railway Association 2018; Dalton et al., 2021; McLeay, 2022; Queensland Government, 2021; Shipway, 2021; Wearn, 2021), making workers particularly susceptible to fatigue.

While one or more people are required to physically operate vehicles/vessels in these industries, each can only function as part of a broader distributed system. Rail is centralised through network control (Naweed, 2020), bus and commercial reef tourism operations rely on traffic control centres, and fleet activities in commercial trucking and taxiing are usually monitored and controlled by central dispatch offices.

Rail and bus operate government-owned and private company/franchise models with workers typically employed directly by the organisation running the services. Reef tourism operates a private company/franchise model with workers employed by the company, but also utilise volunteer and transient workers (e.g., working holiday visa holders) (Pabel et al., 2020), making implementation of industry-wide health and safety policies more challenging. The employer in the taxi industry is often ambiguous (Machin & De Souza, 2004) as drivers can lease vehicles or provision their own (e.g., as gig economy workers) (Leighton, 2016). All these factors carry implications for fatigue management.

4.9.3 POOR HEALTH AND FATIGUE IN TRANSPORT

Given the responsibility vested in transport operators, there is a need to effectively manage the health of those operating/crewing the vehicles/vessels. Chronic health conditions are linked to fatigue in transport workers and should be a critical consideration when managing fatigue. Globally, transport workers are disproportionately impacted by specific health conditions and risk factors, affecting their well-being and fitness for work. Rates of these chronic health conditions vary across transport industries, but are often more prevalent than rates in other occupational groups, and the general population. These include diabetes (Carlsson et al., 2020; Sieber et al.,

2014), cardiovascular disease (Howard et al., 2020; Yook et al., 2018), sleep disorders (Huhta et al., 2021; Yusoff et al., 2010), musculoskeletal and chronic pain conditions (Naweed et al., 2020, 2022), and mental health problems (Crizzle et al., 2020; Pyzyk, 2020; Ruiz-Grosso et al., 2014; van Vreden et al., 2020).

The most common sleep disorders in transport are obstructive sleep apnoea (OSA) and insomnia, which frequently co-occur (Sweetman et al., 2021). Although sleep disorders are highly prevalent, they are commonly undiagnosed (Kales & Straubel 2014). In drivers (truck and professional), rates of OSA are thought to be as high as 40% (Huhta et al., 2021; Yusoff et al., 2010), with insomnia closer to 27% (Garbarino et al., 2017). OSA estimates are even higher in some studies of rail employees. Rates of either sleep disorder have not been established in the reef tourism industry to date. However, true prevalence rates may be underestimated in some industries, which rely on self-report of risk factors, particularly if workers perceive a threat to their employment as a consequence of reporting (Lechat et al., 2021; Naweed et al., 2018; Sweetman et al., 2021).

Fatigue is also a common symptom in patients living with diabetes and cardiovascular diseases (Ekmann et al., 2012; Lindeberg et al., 2012). The same is true for musculoskeletal conditions (Christensen et al., 2013); the interplay between pain and mood states likely contributes to the reported increases in fatigue in these workers (Feuerstein et al., 1987). Disturbances to sleep while experiencing pain may further exacerbate fatigue levels and contribute to altered mood states. Medications for pain can also have sedating effects which may further enhance experiences of fatigue (Leung, 2011).

Poor mental health is also linked to fatigue. In undiagnosed and untreated patients, this may be partly explained by sleep disturbances commonly co-occurring with mental health conditions. Some medications used to treat mental health concerns can also exacerbate fatigue symptoms (Targum & Fava, 2011). Chronic fatigue in patients with depression may contribute to recurrence of major depressive episodes (Lam et al., 2013), further impacting worker well-being and safety. Prevalent health concerns affecting transport workers are often interrelated, and influence fatigue either directly or indirectly via consequences of treatment (e.g., impact of medications). There is a strong need for comprehensive, holistic approaches to support health, fitness for work, and safety priorities in the transport industry.

4.9.4 FACTORS CONTRIBUTING TO POOR HEALTH AT WORK

The factors impacting worker health are complex and multifaceted. Factors at the individual, job design, organisation, and industry levels subsequently influence poor health in the transport workplace across the lifespan, contributing to the higher rates of chronic health conditions in workers. Figure 4.9.1 shows an overview of these potential factors.

The prevalence of chronic conditions is impacted at the individual level, including age, life stage and gender, family demands (Mackie, 2008; Naweed, Chapman, et al., 2017), and lifestyle factors (Brodie et al., 2021; Chapman & Naweed, 2015; Mina & Casolin, 2007; Naweed et al., 2018). The work environment and schedule of drivers

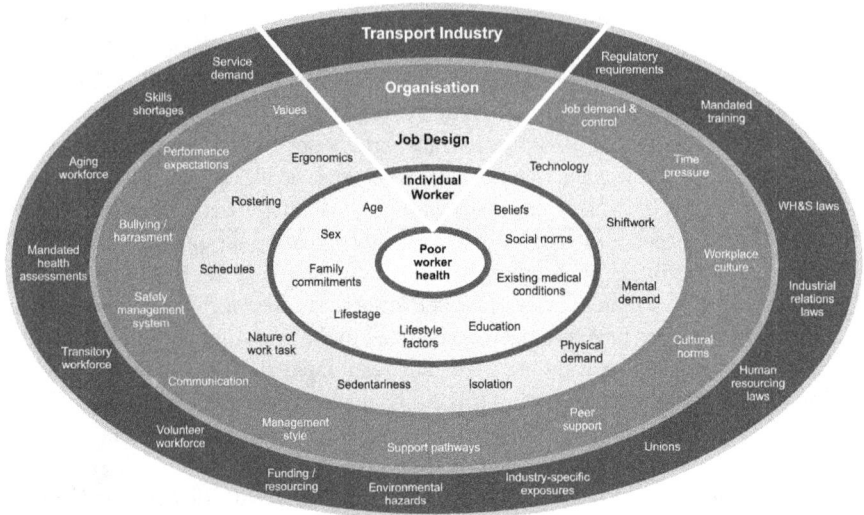

FIGURE 4.9.1 Conceptual overview of factors at various system levels that may directly and/or indirectly impact poor health of transport workers.

are rarely conducive to healthy eating preparation or accessibility, or opportunity for regular physical activity (Apostolopoulos et al., 2011; French et al., 2010). It is also common for shift workers to use alcohol and other substances as a way of managing sleep (Dorrian et al., 2017). Thus, work conditions contribute to higher prevalence of risky lifestyle factors, which by extension can contribute to chronic disease and fatigue.

A range of transport-related job design and organisational factors are also associated with poor health outcomes and chronic conditions, including shift work schedules, insufficient sleep, and inflexible or irregular work schedules (Brum et al., 2015; Kecklund & Axelsson, 2016; Liu et al., 2018). Sedentary job roles (Ford & Caspersen, 2012) and ergonomic factors (e.g., poor cab design) similarly have negative impacts on physical health (Anderson, 1992; Naweed et al., 2020; Naweed & Moody, 2015) and can influence physical fatigue. Hazardous workplace conditions, particularly those with stressors including high job demands, low job support, and exposure to distressing events (Chavda, 2016; Theorell et al., 1992) are associated with increased risk for poor health (Landsbergis et al., 2015; Machin & De Souza, 2004; Parslow et al., 2004; Sorensen et al., 2011).

4.9.5 CURRENT APPROACHES TO FATIGUE IN HEALTH MANAGEMENT

For most transport service industries, worker health management is viewed through a safety lens. Consequently, the focus tends to be on mitigating health-related issues which could impact immediate safety, such as fatigue and cardiac risk leading to sudden incapacity. This is particularly true for rail, the largest carrier of passengers, and the most physically restrictive transport industry covered in this chapter. The challenge here is that management of worker health tends to emphasise the responsibility of the worker, rather than recognising the role of industry and employers for improving health as a pathway to managing fatigue. This also varies by country, provider, and even individual workplace sites

Developed in response to 2003's Waterfall rail disaster (Hocking, 2006), the Australian National Standard for Health Assessment of Rail Safety Workers (National Transport Commission, 2017) requires periodic individual mental and physical health assessment for rail safety workers. Guidelines for categorisation as "fit" (ranging from unconditional to subject to review) or "unfit" (temporarily/permanently) for duty are determined accordingly. As the health of rail workers forms part of the industry's own safety management system, different classes of workers are categorised based on the level of risk incumbent in their role and public responsibility (Naweed et al., 2018). Thus, a different approach is taken for trams (lower speed) and freight trains with two drivers because they are deemed lower risk. Biomathematical modelling or other fatigue management systems are considered separately in roster design (Filtness & Naweed, 2017).

The piecemeal nature of organisational level approaches means that motivated workers take responsibility for their own health management (Naweed, Trigg, et al., 2017), for example, by creative planning around uncertain/irregular rostering and using sick leave to manage fatigue (Filtness & Naweed, 2017). To address the lack of coordinated or mandated health management, the Australian rail industry has recently developed research-informed guidelines to help organisations develop work processes in ways that recognise the importance of health management and to proactively reduce chronic disease risks (Rail Industry Safety & Standards Board, 2019).

The Australian road industry is prioritised for risk prevention because of a high number of work-related fatalities, injuries, and illnesses (Safe Work Australia, 2020). Professional drivers are prone to cardiovascular disease and musculoskeletal disorders (Safe Work Australia, 2018). Despite this, prevention of chronic disease is not a key focus in national strategy (Brodie et al., 2021). For bus drivers, there is no mandated legislation around chronic disease risk factor management and health management remains underdeveloped in the bus industry. General guidelines and tool kits are available (Brodie et al., 2021), and bus associations have put together calls to implement a health, wellness, and safety strategy (Bus Association Vic., 2013). This guidance advises organisations to establish commitment and leadership support; proactively analyse their operations; develop KPIs; embed health and well-being into policies and practices; and provide ongoing monitoring, review/adjustment, and risk management (Bus Association Vic., 2013).

Heavy vehicle national law and regulation (National Heavy Vehicle Regulator, 2022) emphasise fatigue management for the truck industry, and prescribe maximum work and minimum rest requirements. In Australia, emphasis has traditionally been placed on long-haul heavy vehicle drivers, though there is increasing acknowledgement of the risk to short-haul drivers and the impact of fatigue on driver health and well-being (National Transport Commission, 2021). Like the rail and bus industries, health management is not mandated beyond the safety lens, and individual health and well-being is typically championed through advocacy (e.g., roadmap strategy for improving psychological safety) and guidance (e.g., toolbox talks, education) (Australian Trucking Association, 2021).

Based on OHS regulations for the maritime industry (Australian Government, 1995; 2003), reef operators are required to utilise approaches that allow workers to perform their work in a way that is safe and without risk to their health, providing information, instruction, training, and supervision. The emphasis is placed on physical hazards and certificates of competency. There is, however, an exemption that allows some domestic commercial vessels to operate without these requirements (Australian Maritime Safety Authority, 2020); a lack of mandated health management, and limited awareness of formal fatigue risk management (Pabel et al., 2020; Reynolds et al., 2021). More cohesive organisational approaches are constrained by utilisation of a part-volunteer workforce, primary emphasis on performance and customer satisfaction (Pabel et al., 2020), and potentially limited unionisation of the workforce.

Health management in the taxi industry is distinct due to daily fluctuations in work hours and income, exposure to specific hazards towards drivers (e.g., assault, verbal abuse), and ambiguous employment (Machin & De Souza, 2004). The default is general work health and safety law, with emphasis on vehicle roadworthiness, installation of safety equipment with technical knowledge and awareness of it, and safety procedures (Department of Justice and Attorney-General, 2012). Fatigue management takes the form of compliance with a chain of responsibility across booking companies, operators, and drivers (Department of Transport and Main Roads, 2021), with fatigue guidance based around its causal factors and recommended maximum work hours and minimum continuous rest periods (Commercial Passenger Vehicles Victoria, 2019). Compliance with work health and safety are agreed with the taxi operator along with responsibility to take reasonable care for one's own health and safety (Department of Justice and Attorney-General, 2012).

4.9.6 GAPS IN CURRENT APPROACHES: WHAT ARE WE MISSING?

The focus on health management in transport is typically piecemeal and ad hoc unless the industry features a pressing safety imperative, which drives both health and fatigue management approaches. The link between chronic health conditions and more acute risk factors such as fatigue is rarely recognised, and as such, they are viewed in isolation as separate issues. Responsibility for worker health tends to lie with the individual worker in current approaches, which is unsustainable and fails to consider the broader context. Taking coordinated and comprehensive steps to improve worker health and well-being also improves fatigue, and thus, can support mitigation of the acute safety risk arising from fatigue.

Within the transport sector, specific aspects which require a greater focus at the system and organisation level include mental health (Naweed et al., 2018; Rail Safety and Standards Board, 2021; van Vreden et al., 2020), workplace-led prevention of chronic conditions rather than individually focussed interventions (Naweed, Chapman, et al., 2017), and initiatives to drive change in organisational culture and provide confidential support pathways. The current approaches to health management drive workers to either conceal or self-manage health to receive fitness for work status. In our work with industry, we have heard stories of drivers buying equipment to manage sleep apnoea independently at home, because they are fearful of being "found out" by their organisation (Naweed et al., 2018). Without a mature, proactive culture, and ongoing, non-punitive health support pathways in place, such issues may inadvertently pose an even greater risk to safety.

4.9.7   WHERE TO FROM HERE?

The importance of comprehensive health management for worker and community safety cannot be understated. While some transport industries endeavour to manage chronic health conditions, there is still considerable opportunity to increase both the breadth of management for conditions which contribute to fatigue, and the number of sectors within the transport industries which actively screen for, and support health. The safety imperative in transport drives fatigue risk management to such an extent that it obscures the link between health management and fatigue, and eclipses the importance of a holistic, "whole-of-workplace" approach for managing both fatigue and health.

To give an example of how a holistic approach could operate, Figure 4.9.2 conceptualises whole-of-workplace targeted policy and procedure for reducing fatigue as a simple causal loop diagram (Naweed et al., 2022; Sterman, 2000). Health management is a central node where whole-of-workplace, multilevel initiatives (e.g., job redesign, improved rostering, work-life policies, and help-seeking pathways) and resulting changes in worker behaviour drive reductions in fatigue, with reduced fatigue then having the potential effect of further driving improved physical and mental health and reinforcing this loop. In the absence or deficiency of whole-of-workplace initiatives, and a lack of focus in physical and mental health management, optimal fatigue management remains a challenge. Multi-layered health conditions have multi-layered causal factors, with change required at all levels for sustainable benefit. This means moving away from individual-level solutions which are unsustainable without change at the organisational level and developing a better understanding of the role of safety management systems.

A safety management system, of which fatigue risk management is just one element, should not be confused with taking a systems perspective of the workplace. A systems perspective is an understanding of the holistic and interconnection of system elements, with appreciation that they may interact unpredictably and change over time. In comparison, a safety management system has a legislative focus and seeks to protect workers from work-related risk by implementing policies and procedures designed to address these risks. A legislative focus may also create emphasis for policies and procedures that focus on safety at the expense of a rich and broader system view (Karanikas et al., 2020), invariably bypassing those required for adopting a whole-of-workplace approach.

Change in factors at an industry level (see Figure 4.9.1) is typically provoked by major events driving political will and capital for paradigmatic shifts. In the

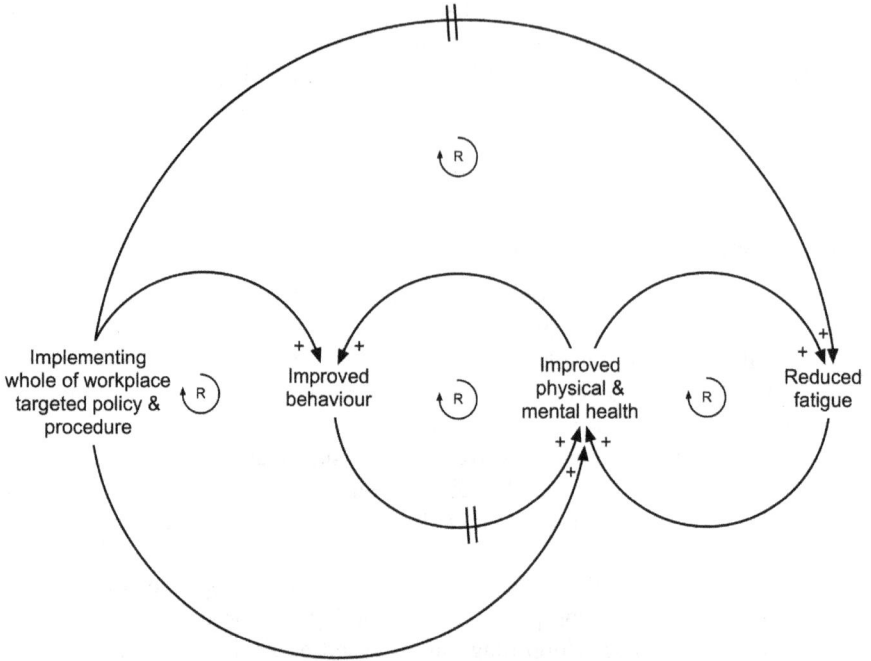

FIGURE 4.9.2 Conceptual simple causal loop diagram in the context of health management in the workplace, depicting the central role of improving physical and mental health and implementing whole of workplace change for driving reduced fatigue. *R* = reinforcing loops ("R") with positive polarity (+). Delay marks ("‖") indicate that it takes time for this effect to occur.

absence of influencing change at an industry level, the question becomes "how can organisations manage issues at more local (i.e., organisation, job design) levels?" To work towards improved health and fatigue management in transport industries, the following recommendations are offered.

First, organisations must take a proactive stance to prioritise long-term health rather than place sole focus on acute safety risk. It is also essential to prioritise mental health, particularly during periods of high workforce pressure (e.g., major events, or pandemic conditions). A whole-of-workplace approach is multipronged and includes management initiatives beyond biomathematical modelling, rostering, and fatigue risk management systems, which target just one system level. They may include concurrent initiatives to facilitate good physical health through work, via job redesign to increase opportunity for movement; the introduction of work–life policies; availability and access to healthy food alongside education around managing shift worker dietary needs; confidential support pathways and health advice for mental and physical health needs; improving staffing; fostering mature organisational cultures; and actively monitoring for and addressing signs of mental strain and poor coping. Inviting worker participation and input are critical for trust building. Ongoing evaluation and refinement are required for recognising and dealing with unpredictable impacts and fluctuating organisational needs.

Finally, enlightened health management recognises that the health benefits arising from such initiatives accrue over time (depicted through delay marks in Figure 4.9.2), therefore relying on sustained organisational commitment and proactivity. To create more fully informed whole-of-workplace targeted policy and procedures, it is critical to view the worker holistically. Neither health, fatigue, nor its management occur in a vacuum; they are inseparable and intrinsic to complex human functioning, and the broader context in which the worker is embedded.

SUMMARY POINTS FOR PRACTITIONERS

- Fatigue is closely linked with poor health in transport industries.
- Individual, job design, organisational and industry-level factors contribute to poor health.
- Current management of health and fatigue focus on safety imperatives and worker responsibility.
- Mature, pro-active cultures and ongoing, non-punitive supports are required.
- A holistic, whole-of-workplace approach to health management is recommended to reduce fatigue at the systems level.

REFERENCES

Anderson, R. (1992). The back pain of bus drivers. Prevalence in an urban area of California. *Spine, 17*(12), 1481–1488.

Apostolopoulos, Y., Sönmez, S., Shattell, M., Haldeman, L., Strack, R., & Jones, V. (2011). Barriers to truck drivers' healthy eating: Environmental influences and health promotion strategies. *Journal of Workplace Behavioral Health, 26*(2), 122–143.

Australasian Railway Association. (2018). Skills crisis: A call to action. Retrieved, Jan 15, 2022, from https://ara.net.au/wp-content/uploads/ARA-Skills-Capability-Study.pdf.

Australian Trucking Association. (2021). Healthy Heads in Trucks & Sheds–Toolbox Talk 1. Retrieved Jan 13, 2022, from www.trucksafe.com.au/alerts/healthy-heads-in-trucks-sheds-toolbox-talk-1/.

Brodie, A., Pavey, T., Newton, C., & Sendall, M. C. (2021). Australian bus drivers' modifiable and contextual risk factors for chronic disease: A workplace study. *PloS One, 16*(7), e0255225.

Brum, M. C. B., Filho, F. F. D., Schnorr, C. C., Bottega, G. B., & Rodrigues, T. C. (2015). Shift work and its association with metabolic disorders. *Diabetology & Metabolic Syndrome, 7*, 45. https://doi.org/10.1186/s13098-015-0041-4

Bus Association Vic. (2013). Making health and wellness a strategic priority: A guide for operators and leaders. Retrieved, Jan 13, 2022, from www.busvic.asn.au/resources/bus-industry-wellness.

Carlsson, S., Andersson, T., Talbäck, M., & Feychting, M. (2020). Incidence and prevalence of type 2 diabetes by occupation: Results from all Swedish employees. *Diabetologia, 63*(1), 95–103.

Chapman, J., & Naweed, A. (2015). Health initiatives to target obesity in surface transport industries: Review and implications for action. *Evidence Base, 2*, 1–32.

Chavda, S. (2016). Sickness absence of LU train drivers after track incidents. *Occupational Medicine, 66*(7), 571–575.

Christensen, A., Petersen, F., Soret, S., & Spencer-Hwang, R. (2013). The Association between low back pain and fatigue among commercial drivers. *Occupational Medicine & Health Affairs, 1*(101), 1–4.

Commercial Passenger Vehicles Victoria. (2019). Fatigue management guidelines. Retrieved, Jan 13, 2022, from https://cpv.vic.gov.au/__data/assets/pdf_file/0006/19365/Fatigue-management-guidelines.pdf.

Crizzle, A. M., McLean, M., & Malkin, J. (2020). Risk factors for depressive symptoms in long-haul truck drivers. *International Journal of Environmental Research and Public Health, 17*(11), 3764.

Dalton, T., Parker, F., & Delahunt, E. (2021). Driver shortage, heavy compliance making life hard for trucking companies. *ABC News.* www.abc.net.au/news/2021-11-12/driver-short age-hard-for-victorian-trucking-companies/100611784.

Department of Justice and Attorney-General. (2012). Work health and safety for taxi drivers and operators. Retrieved, Jan 13, 2022, from www.worksafe.qld.gov.au/__data/assets/pdf_file/0027/15786/whs-taxi-drivers.pdf.

Department of Transport and Main Roads. (2021). Chain of responsibility. Retrieved Jan 13, 2022, from www.tmr.qld.gov.au/business-industry/Taxi-and-limousine/Industry-info rmation/Industry-regulations/Chain-of-responsibility.

Dorrian, J., Heath, G., Sargent, C., Banks, S., & Coates, A. (2017). Alcohol use in shiftworkers. *Accid Anal Prev, 99*(Pt B), 395–400.

Ekmann, A., Osler, M., & Avlund, K. (2012). The predictive value of fatigue for nonfatal ischemic heart disease and all-cause mortality. *Psychosomatic Medicine, 74*(5), 464–470.

Exemption 17—Marine Safety (Great Barrier Reef Region and Torres Strait zone) (2020).

Feuerstein, M., Carter, R. L., & Papciak, A. S. (1987). A prospective analysis of stress and fatigue in recurrent low back pain. *Pain, 31*(3), 333–344.

Filtness, A., & Naweed, A. (2017). Causes, consequences and countermeasures to driver fatigue in the rail industry: The train driver perspective. *Applied Ergonomics, 60*, 12–21.

Ford, E. S., & Caspersen, C. J. (2012). Sedentary behaviour and cardiovascular disease: a review of prospective studies. *International Journal of Epidemiology, 41*(5), 1338–1353.

French, S. A., Hannan, P. J., Harnack, L. J., Mitchell, N. R., Toomey, T. L., & Gerlach, A. (2010). Pricing and availability intervention in vending machines at four bus garages. *J Occup Environ Med, 52 Suppl 1*(Suppl 1), S29–S33.

Garbarino, S., Magnavita, N., Guglielmi, O., Maestri, M., Dini, G., Bersi, F. M.,.... Durando, P. (2017). Insomnia is associated with road accidents. Further evidence from a study on truck drivers. *PloS One, 12*(10), e0187256.

Howard, M. E., Wolkow, A. P., Wilkinson, V., Swann, P., Jordan, A. S., O'Donoghue, F. J.,.... Hare, D. L. (2020). Feasibility of cardiovascular risk and sleep health screening in the transport industry. *Journal of Transport & Health, 18*, 100878.

Huhta, R., Hirvonen, K., & Partinen, M. (2021). Prevalence of sleep apnea and daytime sleepi-ness in professional truck drivers. *Sleep Medicine, 81*, 136–143.

Kales, S. N., & Straubel, M. (2014). Obstructive sleep apnea in North American commercial drivers. *Industrial Health, 52*(1), 13–24.

Karanikas, N., Popovich, A., Steele, S., Horswill, N., Laddrak, V., & Roberts, T. (2020). Symbiotic types of systems thinking with systematic management in occupational health & safety. *Safety Science, 128*, 104752.

Kecklund, G., & Axelsson, J. (2016). Health consequences of shift work and insufficient sleep. *BMJ, 355*, i5210.

Lam, R. W., Malhi, G. S., McIntyre, R. S., Demyttenaere, K., Gorwood, P., Michalak, E. E., & Hegerl, U. (2013). Fatigue and occupational functioning in major depressive disorder. *Australian & New Zealand Journal of Psychiatry, 47*(11), 989–991.

Landsbergis, P. A., Diez-Roux, A. V., Fujishiro, K., Baron, S., Kaufman, J. D., Meyer, J. D.,…. Szklo, M. (2015). Job strain, occupational category, systolic blood pressure, and hypertension prevalence: The multi-ethnic study of atherosclerosis. *J Occup Environ Med, 57*(11), 1178–1184.

Lechat, B., Appleton, S., Melaku, Y. A., Hansen, K., McEvoy, R. D., Adams, R.,…. Sweetman, A. (2021). Co-morbid insomnia and obstructive sleep apnoea is associated with all-cause mortality. *European Respiratory Journal*, 2101958.

Leighton, P. (2016). Professional self-employment, new power and the sharing economy: Some cautionary tales from Uber. *Journal of Management & Organization, 22*(6), 859–874.

Leung, S. Y. (2011). Benzodiazepines, opioids and driving: An overview of the experimental research. *Drug and Alcohol Review, 30*(3), 281–286.

Lindeberg, S. I., Rosvall, M., & Östergren, P.-O. (2012). Exhaustion predicts coronary heart disease independently of symptoms of depression and anxiety in men but not in women. *Journal of Psychosomatic Research, 72*(1), 17–21.

Liu, Q., Shi, J., Duan, P., Liu, B., Li, T., Wang, C.,…. Lu, Z. (2018). Is shift work associated with a higher risk of overweight or obesity? A systematic review of observational studies with meta-analysis. *International Journal of Epidemiology, 47*(6), 1956–1971.

Machin, M. A., & De Souza, J. M. D. (2004). Predicting health outcomes and safety behaviour in taxi drivers. *Transportation Research Part F: Traffic Psychology and Behaviour, 7*(4), 257–270.

Mackie, H. (2008). The health and fitness of log truck drivers: An evaluation of the industry and recommendations for action. Retrieved, Jan 15, 2022, from www.ternz.co.nz/Publi cations/The%20Health%20and%20Fitness%20of%20Log%20Truck%20Drivers.pdf.

McLeay, P. (2022). Truck driver workforce shortages: A perfect storm. Retrieved, Jan 15, 2022, from www.labourforce.com.au/cms/files/LF_Truck-Driver-Shortages_Web.pdf.

Mina, R., & Casolin, A. (2007). National standard for health assessment of rail safety workers: The first year. *Medical Journal of Australia, 187*(7), 394–397.

National Heavy Vehicle Regulator. (2022). Heavy Vehicle National Law and Regulations. Retrieved Jan 13, 2022, from www.nhvr.gov.au/law-policies/heavy-vehicle-national-law-and-regulations.

National Transport Commission. (2017). *National Standard for Health Assessment of Rail Safety Workers* (2017 edition). Melbourne, VIC: Author.

National Transport Commission. (2021). Industry input welcome to safely manage truck driver fatigue. Retrieved Jan 13, 2022, from www.ntc.gov.au/news/industry-input-welcome-truck-driver-fatigue.

Naweed, A. (2020). Getting mixed signals: Connotations of teamwork as performance shaping factors in network controller and rail driver relationship dynamics. *Applied Ergonomics, 82*, 102976.

Naweed, A., Bowditch, L., Trigg, J., & Unsworth, C. (2020). Out on a limb: Applying the person-environment-occupation-performance model to examine injury-linked factors among light rail drivers. *Safety Science, 127*, 104696.

Naweed, A., Bowditch, L., Trigg, J., & Unsworth, C. (2022). Injury by design: A thematic networks and system dynamics analysis of work-related musculoskeletal disorders in tram drivers. *Applied Ergonomics, 100*, 103644.

Naweed, A., Chapman, J., Allan, M., & Trigg, J. (2017). It comes with the job: Work organizational, job design, and self-regulatory barriers to improving the health status of train drivers. *Journal of Occupational and Environmental Medicine, 59*(3), 264–273.

Naweed, A., Chapman, J., & Trigg, J. (2018). "Tell them what they want to hear and get back to work": Insights into the utility of current occupational health assessments from the perspectives of train drivers. *Transportation Research Part A: Policy and Practice, 118*, 234–244.

Naweed, A., & Moody, H. (2015). A streetcar undesired: Investigating ergonomics and human factors issues in the driver–cab interface of Australian trams. *Urban Rail Transit, 1*(3), 149–158.

Naweed, A., Trigg, J., Allan, M., & Chapman, J. (2017). Working around it. *International Journal of Workplace Health Management, 10*(6), 475–490.

Occupational Health and Safety (Maritime Industry) Act 1993 (1995).

Occupational Health and Safety (Maritime Industry) Act 1993 (2003).

Pabel, A., Naweed, A., Ferguson, S. A., & Reynolds, A. (2020). Crack a smile: The causes and consequences of emotional labour dysregulation in Australian reef tourism. *Current Issues in Tourism, 23*(13), 1598–1612.

Parslow, R. A., Jorm, A. F., Christensen, H., Rodgers, B., Strazdins, L., & D'Souza, R. M. (2004). The associations between work stress and mental health: A comparison of organizationally employed and self-employed workers. *Work & Stress, 18*(3), 231–244.

Pyzyk, K. (2020). Fleets can support drivers' mental health through awareness, communication. *Transport Topics News*. www.ttnews.com/articles/fleets-can-support-drivers-mental-health-through-awareness-communication.

Queensland Government. (2021). Premier calls on Australians to "Work in Paradise" with new tourism campaign. *The Queensland Cabinet and Ministerial Directory*. https://statements.qld.gov.au/statements/92144.

Rail Industry Safety & Standards Board. (2019). Good practice in the management of rail driver health and wellbeing. Retrieved, Jan 13, 2022, from www.rissb.com.au/products/good-practice-in-the-management-of-rail-driver-health-and-wellbeing/.

Rail Safety and Standards Board. (2021). How is the mental health of rail employees? Retrieved Jan 15, 2022, from www.rssb.co.uk/what-we-do/key-industry-topics/health-and-wellbeing/mental-wellbeing/how-is-the-mental-health-of-rail-employees.

Reynolds, A. C., Pabel, A., Ferguson, S. A., & Naweed, A. (2021). Causes and consequences of sleep loss and fatigue: The worker perspective in the coral reef tourism industry. *Annals of Tourism Research, 88*, 103160.

Ruiz-Grosso, P., Ramos, M., Samalvides, F., Vega-Dienstmaier, J., & Kruger, H. (2014). Common mental disorders in public transportation drivers in Lima, Peru. *PloS One, 9*(6), e101066.

Safe Work Australia. (2018). Priority industry snapshot: Road transport. Retrieved, Jan 13, 2022, from www.safeworkaustralia.gov.au/system/files/documents/1903/road-transport-priority-industry-snapshot-2018.pdf.

Safe Work Australia. (2020). Australian Work Health and Safety Strategy 2012–2022. Retrieved, Jan 13, 2022, from www.safeworkaustralia.gov.au/resources-and-publications/corporate-publications/australian-work-health-and-safety-strategy-2012-2022.

Shipway, G. (2021). 'Not only is becoming a bus driver a rewarding job, it's also a long-term career opportunity': Buslink driver shortage spurs recruitment push. *The West Australian*. https://thewest.com.au/business/not-only-is-becoming-a-bus-driver-a-rewarding-job-its-also-a-long-term-career-opportunity-buslink-driver-shortage-spurs-recruitment-push-c-2584601.

Sieber, W. K., Robinson, C. F., Birdsey, J., Chen, G. X., Hitchcock, E. M., Lincoln, J. E.,... . Sweeney, M. H. (2014). Obesity and other risk factors: The national survey of US long-haul truck driver health and injury. *American Journal of Industrial Medicine, 57*(6), 615–626.

Sorensen, G., Landsbergis, P., Hammer, L., Amick III, B. C., Linnan, L., Yancey, A.,... . Pratt, C. (2011). Preventing chronic disease in the workplace: A workshop report and recommendations. *American Journal of Public Health, 101*(S1), S196–S207.

Sterman, J. (2000). *Business Dynamics: Systems Thinking and Modeling for a Complex World.* Boston: Irwin McGraw-Hill.

Sweetman, A., Melaku, Y. A., Lack, L., Reynolds, A., Gill, T. K., Adams, R., & Appleton, S. (2021). Prevalence and associations of co-morbid insomnia and sleep apnoea in an Australian population-based sample. *Sleep Medicine, 82*, 9–17.

Targum, S. D., & Fava, M. (2011). Fatigue as a residual symptom of depression. *Innovations in Clinical Neuroscience, 8*(10), 40–43.

Theorell, T., Leymann, H., Jodko, M., Konarski, K., Norbeck, H. E., & Eneroth, P. (1992). " Person under train" incidents: medical consequences for subway drivers. *Psychosomatic Medicine,54*(4), 480–488.

van Vreden, C., Xia, T., Pritchard, E., Collie, A., Newnam, S., Rajaratnam, S.,.... Iles, R. (2020). *Driving Health Study Report No 6: Survey of the physical and mental health of Australian professional drivers.* Victoria, Australia: Insurance Work and Health Group, Faculty of Medicine Nursing and Health Sciences, Monash University.

Wearn, R. (2021). Taxi driver shortage prompts public safety fears. *BBC News.* www.bbc.com/news/business-59158230.

Yook, J.-H., Lee, D.-W., Kim, M.-S., & Hong, Y.-C. (2018). Cardiovascular disease risk differences between bus company employees and general workers according to the Korean National Health Insurance Data. *Annals of Occupational and Environmental Medicine, 30*, 32–32.

Yusoff, M. F. M., Baki, M. M., Mohamed, N., Mohamed, A. S., Yunus, M. R. M., Ami, M.,... . Ishak, A. I. (2010). Obstructive sleep apnea among express bus drivers in Malaysia: Important indicators for screening. *Traffic Injury Prevention, 11*(6), 594–599.

4.10 Aircrew Fatigue and Scheduling

A Summary of Some Recent Studies Using the Same Outcome Measure

Torbjörn Åkerstedt[1] and Mikael Sallinen[2]

[1]Karolinska institute and Stockholm University, Stockholm, Sweden
[2]Finnish Institute of Occupational Health, Helsinki, Finland

CONTENTS

4.10.1 INTRODUCTION

Fatigue is a major cause of accidents in transport work, including aviation (Marcus & Rosekind, 2017), and fatigue risk management has become a key safety concept in aviation (Rangan et al., 2020). There is no consensus definition of fatigue, but in aviation research it has a connotation of sleepiness (Caldwell et al., 2009; Weiland et al., 2013), which refers to a drive towards sleep (Dement & Carskadon, 1982). Fatigue in aviation shows a pronounced link with sleep loss, time awake, and time of day (circadian low) (Gander et al., 2013; Hartzler, 2014; Powell, Spencer, Holland, & Petrie,

DOI: 10.1201/9781003213154-32

2008). These are also the factors that have been identified as fatigue determinants in laboratory studies (Dijk, Duffy, & Czeisler, 1992; Folkard & Åkerstedt, 1991). Air crew scheduling will sometimes be in conflict with the fatigue determinants. This occurs with night flights, that is, flights that encroach on the window of circadian low (WOCL, the period between 02:00 and 05:59 hours), increased duration of the flight duty period (FDP, period from reporting for duty to the end of the last sector of that duty), duty time (flight + other duties during a day) (Vejvoda et al., 2014), as well as increased number of sectors ("flights", or "legs") (Powell, 2007). Sleep duration is another factor (Gander et al., 2014), but is not technically "scheduled" by the carrier, even if scheduling may affect sleep hours. The total number of work hours per week is another variable of interest, since it seems to be of importance in industrial work (Wagstaff & Lie, 2011), although very little work has focused on aviation.

To minimise fatigue, authorities attempt to prevent fatigue through flight time limitations (FTL). The European Aviation Safety Agency (EASA) identifies night-time (02:00 to 04:59 hours), early morning start (05:00 to 05:59 hours or 05:00 to 06:59 hours, depending on the country), extended duration (>13 hours during day-time, or >10 hours during night-time), and a high number of sectors within a duty (> 6) as scheduling characteristics contributing to aircrew fatigue (EU, 2014). Night FDPs are subject to several restrictions with respect to scheduling according to the European FTL (EU, 2014). Thus, FDPs that do not encroach on the WOCL permit 13 hours of flying if only one or two sectors are involved. With increasing encroachment on the WOCL, the permissible FDP time is reduced, down to a lowest value at 9 hours. In addition to restrictions pertaining to the 24 hours window, the European FTL also restricts the total number of hours worked (duty time, i.e., both flight and non-flight hours) in any consecutive 7 days to 60 hours. EASA has started to investigate the efficacy of the present FTL, searching for possible improvement.

The purpose of the present chapter is to update the knowledge regarding aircrew scheduling and fatigue, based on five relatively recent studies that use the same measure of subjective fatigue. In particular, the interest is focused on whether the present FTL protects against high fatigue, or if high fatigue occurs despite regulatory efforts.

The review is based on studies on:

- fatigue during long-haul (LH) FDPs (Study 1) (Sallinen et al., 2017);
- fatigue during short-haul (SH) FDPs (Study 1) (Sallinen et al., 2017);
- fatigue and simultaneous effects of major scheduling factors (Study 2) (Sallinen et al., 2021);
- fatigue and number of ultra-short-haul sectors (Study 3) (Åkerstedt et al., 2021);
- cumulative fatigue across duty days (Study 3) (Åkerstedt et al., 2021);
- individual differences in fatigue and scheduling factors (Study 4) (Sallinen et al., 2018);
- self-reported causes of fatigue (Study 5) (Sallinen et al., 2021).

The outcome measure in the studies on subjective fatigue is the Karolinska Sleepiness Scale (KSS) (Åkerstedt & Gillberg, 1990), which is rated at least at top of descent, where the planned descent to final approach altitude is initiated in all studies. The scale has the following anchor points: 1 = extremely alert, 2 = very alert, 3= alert, 4 = rather alert, 5 = neither alert, nor sleepy, 6 = some signs of sleepiness, 7 = sleepy but no effort to keep awake, 8 = sleepy, some effort to keep awake, and 9 = very sleepy, great effort to keep awake, fighting sleep. The scale has been validated against line crossings in real road driving studies and crashes in driving simulators (Åkerstedt, Anund, Axelsson, & Kecklund, 2014). Increased risk starts around KSS = 7 and rises rapidly, with crashes in simulators starting to occur around 8, and line crossing on real roads at 7. For practical purposes, values ≥7 are considered high fatigue, and values ≥8 are considered very high fatigue.

4.10.2 FATIGUE DURING LONG-HAUL FDPS (STUDY 1) (SALLINEN ET AL., 2017)

To obtain an overall impression of fatigue in aircrew scheduling, we conducted a comprehensive study of both LH and SH pilots (Sallinen et al., 2017). This was a field study of a representative sample of pilots of an intermediate-sized airline. A total of 86 pilots (29 flying LH routes only (scheduled flight time > 6 hours, operated by wide body aircraft), 29 flying SH routes only (scheduled flight time ≤ 6 hours, operated by narrow body aircrafts), and 28 flying both types) completed the measurements. Two months of data was provided by each pilot, including 965 SH flight duty periods (FDPs) and 627 LH FDPs. Fatigue was measured through a diary asking for KSS ratings in all flight phases (at Blocks off / start, Top of climb (ToC), at least once during cruising phase, at Top of descent (ToD), and at Blocks on ("parking")). Sleep was measured through actigraphs. SH FDPs usually contain more than one sector ("flight"), while LH FDPs contain only one sector.

In this section we present the LH part of the project. We selected LH FDP routes outbound from Helsinki to East Asia (HA) starting at 22:45 hours, and inbound (return) from East Asia to Helsinki (AH) starting at 03:30 hours. We also selected the route Helsinki–New York, outbound (HN), starting at 13:05 hours from Helsinki and inbound (NH) starting 23:30 hours from New York. Please note that all start times are given in Helsinki time.

Figure 4.10.1 shows, for the LH flights (HN; NH; HA; AH), a significant pattern of subjective fatigue with high values during the night and the early morning, reaching a mean KSS = 6.54 during the cruise phase for the outbound flight from Helsinki to East Asia, slightly lower for the inbound flight, and with low levels during the daytime portions of the flights. The standard deviation (SD) for the peak at 6.54 is 1.22, meaning that the upper SD value reaches 7.76, well into the range of high fatigue. For outbound FDPs to New York (HN), mean fatigue was low (KSS = 3 to 4), but for homebound flights (NH), high peak fatigue (6.32) is reached during the cruise phase. The outbound flight to New York (HN) showed a significantly lower mean KSS than the other flights. The inbound flights from New York (NH) did not differ from the inbound flight from East Asia (AH). Thus, the direction of flight was of no consequence, at least for the inbound flights.

The burden of fatigue may be exposed more clearly by computing the percentage of flights producing at least one KSS rating ≥7. For the outbound flight from Helsinki

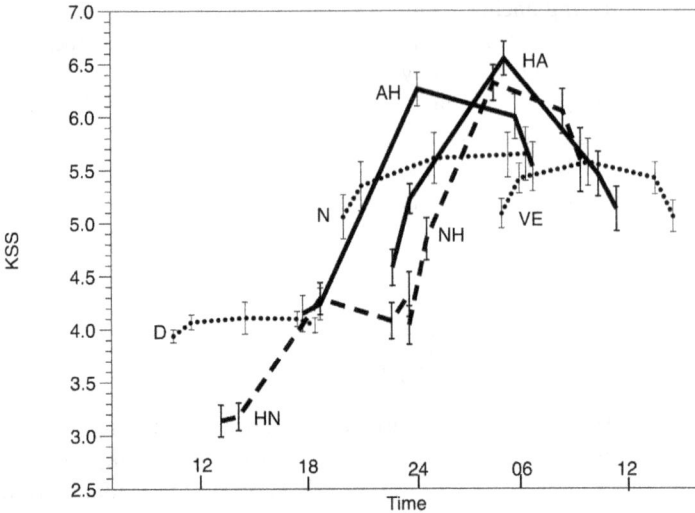

FIGURE 4.10.1 Average subjective fatigue ratings (KSS ± se) during blocks off, top of climb, cruising, top of descent, blocks on for long-haul and short-haul flight duty periods (FDPs), plotted at home base time. Short-haul (dotted lines): D= day FDP, N= night FDP, VE= very early FDP. Long-haul (dashed lines): HN = Helsinki–New York. NH = New York–Helsinki. Long-haul (solid lines), HA = Helsinki–East Asia. AH = East Asia–Helsinki.

to East Asia (HA), 82.8% of the flights contain at least one rating ≥7, with the inbound flight from New York to Helsinki (NH) almost as high (77.5%). For the outbound flight Helsinki-New York (HN), the corresponding figure was 4%. The rest of the LH flights showed intermediate levels. Again, the Helsinki-New York flight (HN) differed significantly from the other LH flights.

The impression from the data is that night/early morning is associated with increased fatigue, and peak levels reach into the region of very high fatigue as defined in previous work (Åkerstedt et al., 2014) and agree well with other studies of air-crew fatigue (Gander et al., 2013; Hartzler, 2014; Powell et al., 2008). Subjective fatigue results are in line with those found in studies of night driving on real roads, or in simulators, while daytime fatigue levels are low (Åkerstedt et al., 2014), and are also similar to many other field studies of fatigue in different types of transport work (Åkerstedt, 2019). The results also agree with established factors behind sleepiness/alertness regulation, such as effects of the circadian low, sleep loss, **and** time awake (Dijk et al., 1992; Folkard & Åkerstedt, 1991).

4.10.3 FATIGUE DURING SHORT-HAUL FDPS (STUDY 1) (SALLINEN ET AL., 2017)

The SH routes included outbound and inbound flights between Helsinki and a number of airports mainly in Europe. Figure 4.10.1 shows similar patterns of KSS ratings for SH FDPs (D; N; VE) as for LH FDPs (HN; NH; HA; AH), with a peak of KSS ≈ 5.4 to

5.6 occurring during very early (VE) (03:00 < start time ≤ 05:59) and night (N) (start time > 15:00, end time ≥ 03:00) SH FDPs (even if 15:00 hours is not "night" the latter part of the flight is). However, the level of fatigue during SH night FDPs (N) does not seem to reach as high as during the LH night FDPs (HN; NH; HA; AH). This difference may be due to a longer cruise phase and duty time during the LH FDPs. It may be that the SH FDPs require more active flying since the FDPs contain several sectors, involving more take-offs and landings. The higher levels of activity may prevent high levels of fatigue from manifesting. On the other hand, high fatigue (using the Samn–Perelli scale) has been reported for ToD as a function of number of sectors, as well as time on task (Powell et al., 2008). The latter study was, however, based on retrospective reports of fatigue given at blocks on. The retrospective approach may have confounded any masking effect of activity on fatigue during flying.

4.10.4 FATIGUE AND SIMULTANEOUS EFFECTS OF MAJOR SCHEDULING FACTORS (STUDY 2) (SALLINEN ET AL., 2020)

Study 1 clearly indicated that the timing of FDPs was a major determinant of aircrew fatigue; in particular, FDPs that cover normal sleep hours seem important. However, such flights are also associated with sleep loss and increased time awake, which were identified in the introduction as major determinants of fatigue. Also, the number of sectors in SH flights may be of importance. In addition, FDP duration may be important, but is often correlated with time spent awake. All these scheduling factors need to be taken into account simultaneously.

In a study (financed by EASA) aimed at testing the efficacy of the present FTL rules, we examined aircrew fatigue associated with several scheduling factors simultaneously. The latter included night FDPs longer than 10 hours, FDPs typical of disruptive schedules (i.e., early starts, late finishes, and night FDPs), as well as FDP duration, and number of sectors. An alternative way of classifying night FDPs was also examined to determine if there were additional subcategories that would warrant special attention.

A total of 392 aircrew members (96 females) representing 24 airlines participated in a study in which their fatigue was measured using KSS levels (correlation with Samn–Perelli ratings was $r = 0.87$ ($p<.001$)), using an app on a smartphone, across 14 consecutive days. The KSS ratings, given at ToD, served as the main outcome variable.

The analysis of FDP duration showed that the probability of high fatigue (KSS ≥ 7) being reported at ToD was 0.41 (i.e., 41% of the FDPs included KSS≥7 at ToD) and 0.32 during long (> 10 hours) and short (≤ 10 hours) night FDPs (including the WOCL, 02:00 to 05:59 hours), respectively, the difference not being statistically significant (the mean KSS rating for both categories was 5.4). The corresponding probability was 0.19 for early starts (05:00 to 06:59 hours), 0.31 for late finishes (23:00 to 01:59 hours), 0.34 for night FDPs (encroaching on the WOCL), and $p = 0.15$ for day FDPs ($p<0.001$)

The multiple logistic regression analysis showed that the significant predictors of high fatigue among day and night FDPs were those that encroached on the

WOCL and short prior sleep. Interestingly in the simple (unadjusted) analysis also time awake and start time were highly significant predictors. Fatigue in late finishing and day FDPs was predicted by FDP end time, FDP duration, and number of time zones crossed from west to east. In the simple analysis also time awake was highly significant. Note that prior sleep duration was not significant in the simple regression. Fatigue in early and day FDPs were predicted only by start time (no multivariable analysis carried out). Notably, the number of sectors was not significant in any of the analyses. The largest previous study on air-crew fatigue on SH flights (Powell et al., 2008) arrived at similar results, with respect to night flying and FDP duration as the main predictors, but not number of sectors. Since the number of sectors in the present study rarely exceeded 4, the lack of effect may be due to restriction of range.

In a separate analysis we tested the differences in fatigue between night FDPs that ended in, started in, or encompassed the WOCL. This indicated a significant difference with highest fatigue in the latter group, and lowest fatigue in the FDPs that ended in the WOCL. We assume that the reason is the amount of sleep loss involved.

Based on the results from the study presented above, we suggested a change of classification of FDPs, from early, day, late, and night FDPs to very early (02:00 to 04:59 hours), early (05:00 to 06:59 hours), day, late (23:00 to 01:59 hours), night (ending 00:00 to 05:59 hours), and "deep" night (starting <01:59 and ending ≥06:00) FDPs (the term "deep" is here used tentatively). Deep night would include the WOCL and morning hours. The very early flights were previously considered night flights, since they encroached on the period of 02:00 to 04:59. Figure 4.10.2 shows the probability of high fatigue for the different types of FDPs, placing "deep night" at the top. That type includes wakefulness during the normal sleep hours (sleep loss) and exposure to the circadian trough. The figure indicates which types of FDPs deserve special attention with respect to fatigue mitigation.

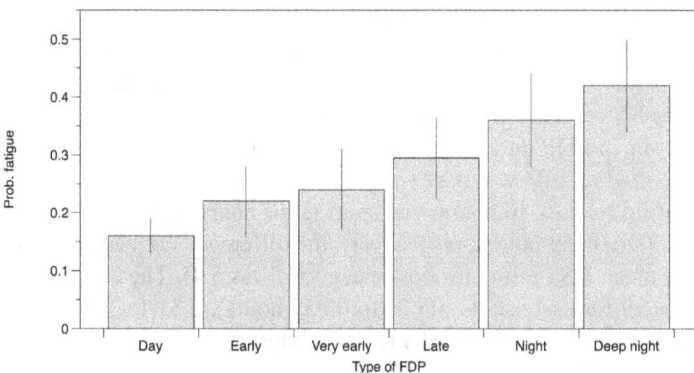

FIGURE 4.10.2 Probability (±se) of high fatigue for suggested FDP types (see text for explanation).

4.10.5 FATIGUE AND NUMBER OF ULTRA-SHORT-HAUL SECTORS (STUDY 3) (ÅKERSTEDT ET AL., 2021)

In Study 2 above, the number of sectors flown was rather modest, which seems to be the case for most air carriers. However, shuttle-type flights do occur on particular routes. To investigate the associations of many short sectors with fatigue, we (Åkerstedt et al., 2021) embarked on a further study of ultra-short-haul FDPs. A total of 106 aircrew (14% cabin crew) participated, rated fatigue on the KSS three times per FDP for four 7-day work periods, with up to 7 days off between work periods. Mixed model regression was applied to the data. Note that we here computed "duty time" (flight time plus other work) since the FTL uses that term for the limit (60 hours/any consecutive 7 days).

In the multivariable model that was generated, more sleep was associated with lower fatigue ratings ($p<0.001$), corresponding to 0.26 KSS units less per hour of sleep. Very early (starting 02:00 to 04:49 hours), early (starting 05:00 to 06:59 hours), and late (ending 23:00 to 01:59 hours) as well as duty time were also associated with higher fatigue, similar to what was seen in Study 3 and in Powell et al. (2008). However, number of sectors was not associated with fatigue in the multivariable analysis of the present study, although it was highly significant as a single predictor. Apparently, duty time (flight–plus other duty) accounted for the significant contribution of number of sectors. The lack of effect of number of sectors in the multivariable analysis disagrees with the significant contribution to fatigue in the study by Powell et al. (Powell, Spencer, Holland, Broadbent, & Petrie, 2007), but it might be that the finding was confounded by duty time.

The results suggest that sleep, duty time, and early starts are important predictors of fatigue in the 24 hours window.

4.10.6 CUMULATIVE FATIGUE ACROSS DUTY DAYS (STUDY 3) (ÅKERSTEDT ET AL., 2021)

In the study of number of sectors (Study 3) above, we also analysed the change in subjective fatigue across the seven days of the working week, followed by one week off (Åkerstedt et al., 2021). This was done through a mixed model analysis across the 7 days.

In the simple (unadjusted) analysis, no change in fatigue across the 7 days was seen for accumulation of duty, for block time ($\approx$FDP), or for days of work, and mean KSS remained = 4.2±2 across the seven days. Nor was any effect seen for accumulation of number of sectors. However, there were effects for accumulation of early, and very early, duties. For the latter, the regression across the week showed an increase from 4.2 to 6.2 KSS units (standard error (se) for the regression = 0.05). Fatigue *decreased* strongly with accumulation of day duties (by 0.11 KSS units per day duty). Fatigue also decreased with accumulation of sleep hours.

The multivariable analysis showed that fatigue decreased with accumulation of sleep duration (largest effect) and accumulated number of day duties, while it increased with accumulation of duty time (second largest), very early type of duty, block time ($\approx$ FDP), and number of sectors.

The results suggest that long working weeks up to ≈ 64 hours, where hours of work fall mostly during the day, do not seem to cause increased fatigue; however, disruptive duties are associated with increased ratings of fatigue, probably due to their negative influence on the number of sleep hours.

4.10.7 INDIVIDUAL DIFFERENCES IN FATIGUE AND SCHEDULING FACTORS (STUDY 4) (SALLINEN ET AL., 2018)

In the studies described above, it was observed that fatigue occurred more often in some pilots than in others. To confirm if this was, indeed, a recurrent phenomenon and, if confirmed, what might be associated with such an observation, the data reported earlier by Sallinen et al. (2017) were analysed from these angles.

The data from a total of 51 pilots who flew from Helsinki to East Asia, and back at least twice during the study, were selected for analysis (Sallinen et al., 2018). The east-west outbound and west-east inbound were selected because both directions resulted in similar and high KSS levels (the New York flights differed considerably in KSS levels because of the non-involvement of the WOCL in the outbound flight). The KSS levels were reported in a diary, and sleep was monitored through actigraphy. Pilots who rated KSS≥7 on each, some, or none of the flights were classified as fatigued "regularly", "sometimes", or "never", respectively.

On the outbound flights, 24% of pilots were classified as regularly fatigued, 54% as sometimes fatigued, and 22% as never fatigued. For the inbound flights, the distribution was 27%, 48%, and 25%. On the outbound flight, the "regularly fatigued" group reached a peak of KSS = 6.7±.2 (mean±SE) at ToD. The SD was 1.4, meaning that the highest SD value for KSS reached 8.1, well into the very high level of fatigue. The "never fatigued" group reached a maximum of 5.2±.2, which occurred an hour later than ToD, at blocks on. At the start of the flight from Helsinki all three groups had KSS values of 3.4 to 3.8±.2, which is quite alert. On the return flight, the differences among the groups were slightly larger.

The main difference among the groups, apart from subjective fatigue, concerned sleep duration prior to flight. The "never fatigued" group slept 54 minutes longer before the outbound flight, and 1 hour 23 minutes longer before the inbound return flight, than the "regularly fatigued" group ($p<0.05$ and $p<0.001$ across groups for the two directions of flights). Self-rated sleep quality and amount of napping did not affect the results, nor did amount of time awake. The "never fatigued" group also slept longer during days off, which suggests a lower sleep pressure in this group. The results agree with the findings of Gander et al. (2015), showing that shorter pre-flight sleep duration was related to sleepiness during FDPs . Possible contributing causes may include differences in factors like reduced commute time or a more comfortable room standard during layover; however, such information was not collected. The results indicate the importance of getting sufficient amounts of good-quality sleep before flights.

4.10.8 SELF-REPORTED CAUSES OF FATIGUE (STUDY 5) (SALLINEN ET AL., 2021)

While the causes of fatigue were seen in our studies as due mainly to time of day and lack of sleep, it is of interest to understand if pilots themselves attribute their fatigue to the same, or other causes. We used the data of the 87 pilots with SH and LH flights, described above (Sallinen et al., 2021). KSS ratings were collected as described, above, and causes of fatigue were rated at the end of each FDP (not at ToD).

The results showed that FDP timing (19% for SH pilots, 77% for LH pilots) and inadequate sleep (32% for SH pilots, 54% for LH) were listed most frequently as causes of fatigue. Extended time on task (7% for SH pilots, 23% for LH pilots), flight arrangements (≤ 10% for both), cockpit condition (3% for both), and visibility (2% for both) were less frequently listed causes. Those who listed the most frequent causes for fatigue also showed higher odds ratios (≈"probability") for high fatigue ratings. Such ratings were also mainly found in FDPs with an early morning start and those encroaching on night-time sleep. The results suggest that pilots' judgement of fatigue-inducing factors agree well with impressions from the field studies described above. The identification of FDP timing and inadequate sleep also agrees with previous studies (Bourgeois-Bougrine, Carbon, Gounelle, Mollard, & Coblentz, 2003), although that study also identified the number of sectors as a contributor.

4.10.9 DISCUSSION

Taken together, the results indicate that high fatigue is particularly common during night FDPs that cover the WOCL and FDPs that start in the WOCL (early and very early morning flights that start between 02:00 and 05:59 hours). The causes of increased fatigue appear to be exposure to the circadian trough through encroaching on the WOCL, and sleep loss due to early morning or night FDPs. It should also be emphasised that habitual sleep behaviour and sleep immediately before a flight may be significant contributors to fatigue if sleep durations are compromised. Also, duty time (flight time plus other work) contributed to increases in ratings of fatigue in several studies. The importance of number of sectors to fatigue remains to be determined; its effects may be confounded by its association with longer flight duty periods. A proper evaluation of the effect of number of sectors would require a study with FDP duration kept constant, as well as the time of day.

It should be remembered that European FTLs have maxima for the duration of FDPs, with 13 hours for day FDPs, 10 hours for night FDPs (with possibilities of some exceptions). Thus, we lack data on extreme durations. Similarly, the number of sectors has a maximum of 6. Furthermore, the FTL includes tables that reduce FDP duration for combinations of start times and number of sectors. Thus, the range of some key factors behind fatigue are restricted, which limits the associations with fatigue, which is positive in the real-life perspective. Still, the results above clearly indicate that, under the present FTL, quite high fatigue may be reached. Based on the collective results of the studies described in this chapter, mitigating efforts should be directed towards night and very early morning FDPs. One obvious countermeasure against fatigue on LH flights is "controlled rest" that is presently used in case of unpredicted high fatigue, as opposed to in-flight rest that is planned already before FDP start.

SUMMARY POINTS FOR PRACTITIONERS

- Flights that interfere with normal sleep hours, including night and early morning flights, are associated with highest fatigue and therefore need special consideration.
- Also, the duration of flight duty period seems to be a relatively important contributing factor to fatigue.
- Sleep duration (and quality) before flights is associated with in-flight fatigue. Proper sleep behaviour and sufficient sleep duration are important.
- Number of sectors seems to be of limited importance to the development of fatigue.
- Number of accumulated flight duty hours across a week seems to be of no importance under the present European FTL restrictions.

REFERENCES

Åkerstedt, T. (2019). Shift work–sleepiness and sleep in transport. *Sleep Medicine Clinics, 14*(4), 413–421. doi:10.1016/j.jsmc.2019.07.003

Åkerstedt, T., Anund, A., Axelsson, J., & Kecklund, G. (2014). Subjective sleepiness is a sensitive indicator of insufficient sleep and impaired waking function. *Journal of Sleep Research, 23*(3), 240–252. doi:10.1111/jsr.12158

Åkerstedt, T., & Gillberg, M. (1990). Subjective and objective sleepiness in the active individual. *International Journal of Neuroscience, 52,* 29–37.

Åkerstedt, T., Klemets, T., Karlsson, D., Habel, H., Widman, L., & Sallinen, M. (2021). Acute and cumulative effects of scheduling on aircrew fatigue in ultra-short-haul operations. *Journal of Sleep Research,* e13305. doi:10.1111/jsr.13305

Bourgeois-Bougrine, S., Carbon, P., Gounelle, C., Mollard, R., & Coblentz, A. (2003). Perceived fatigue for short–and long-haul flights: A survey of 739 airline pilots. *Aviation, Space and Environmental Medicine, 74*(10), 1072–1077.

Caldwell, J. A., Mallis, M. M., Caldwell, J. L., Paul, M. A., Miller, J. C., Neri, D. F.; Aerospace Medical Association Fatigue Countermeasures Subcommittee of the Aerospace Human Factors Committee. (2009). Fatigue countermeasures in aviation. *Aviation, Space and Environmental Medicine, 80*(1), 29–59.

Dement, W. C., & Carskadon, M. A. (1982). Current perspectives on daytime sleepiness: The issues. *Sleep, 5,* 56–66.

Dijk, D. J., Duffy, J. F., & Czeisler, C. A. (1992). Circadian and sleep-wake dependent aspects of subjective alertness and cognitive performance. *Journal of Sleep Research, 1,* 112–117.

[EU] European Union. (2014). Commission regulation No 83/2014. *Official Journal of the European Union.* Retrieved from https://eur-lex.europa.eu/LexUriServ/LexUriServ.do?uri=OJ:L:2014:028:0017:0029:EN:PDF.

Folkard, S., & Åkerstedt, T. (1991). A three process model of the regulation of alertness and sleepiness. In R. Ogilvie & R. Broughton (Eds.), *Sleep, Arousal and Performance: Problems and Promises* (pp. 11–26). Boston: Birkhäuser.

Gander, P. H., Mulrine, H. M., van den Berg, M. J., Smith, A. A., Signal, T. L., Wu, L. J., & Belenky, G. (2015). Effects of sleep/wake history and circadian phase on proposed pilot fatigue safety performance indicators. *Journal of Sleep Research, 24*(1), 110–119. doi:10.1111/jsr.12197

Gander, P. H., Signal, T. L., van den Berg, M. J., Mulrine, H. M., Jay, S. M., & Jim Mangie, C. (2013). In-flight sleep, pilot fatigue and psychomotor vigilance task performance on ultra-long range versus long range flights. *Journal of Sleep Research, 22*(6), 697–706. doi:10.1111/jsr.12071

Hartzler, B. M. (2014). Fatigue on the flight deck: The consequences of sleep loss and the benefits of napping. *Accident Analysis and Prevention, 62*, 309–318. doi:10.1016/j.aap.2013.10.010

Marcus, J.H., & Rosekind, M.R. (2017). Fatigue in transportation: NTSB investigations and safety recommendations. *Injury Prevention, 23*(4), 232–238.

Powell, D. M., Spencer, M. B., Holland, D., Broadbent, E., & Petrie, K. J. (2007). Pilot fatigue in short-haul operations: Effects of number of sectors, duty length, and time of day. *Aviation, Space and Environmental Medicine, 78*(7), 698–701.

Powell, D. M., Spencer, M. B., Holland, D., & Petrie, K. J. (2008). Fatigue in two-pilot operations: Implications for flight and duty time limitations. *Aviation, Space and Environmental Medicine, 79*(11), 1047–1050. doi:10.3357/asem.2362.2008

Rangan, S., Riedy, S. M., Bassett, R., Klinck, Z. A., Hagerty, P., Schek, E.,.... Van Dongen, H. P. A. (2020). Predictive and proactive fatigue risk management approaches in commercial aviation. *Chronobiology International*, 1–4. doi:10.1080/07420528.2020.1803902

Sallinen, M., Åkerstedt, T., Harma, M., Henelius, A., Ketola, K., Leinikka, M.,.... Puttonen, S. (2018). Recurrent on-duty sleepiness and alertness management strategies in long-haul airline pilots. *Aerospace Medicine and Human Performance, 89*(7), 601–608. doi:10.3357/AMHP.5092.2018

Sallinen, M., Onninen, J., Ketola, K., Puttonen, S., Tuori, A., Virkkala, J., & Åkerstedt, T. (2021). Self-reported reasons for on-duty sleepiness among commercial airline pilots. *Chronobiology International*, 1–11. doi:10.1080/07420528.2021.1927071

Sallinen, M., Sihvola, M., Puttonen, S., Ketola, K., Tuori, A., Härmä, M., Kecklund, G., & Åkerstedt, T. (2017). Sleep, alertness and alertness management among commercial airline pilots on short-haul and long-haul flights. *Accident Analysis and Prevention, 98*, 320–329. doi: 10.1016/j.aap.2016.10.029

Sallinen M, van Dijk H, Aeschbach D, Maij A, Åkerstedt T. (2020). A large-scale European Union study of aircrew fatigue during long night and disruptive duties. *Aerospace Medicine and Human Performance, 91*(8), 628-635. doi: 10.3357/AMHP.5561.2020.

Vejvoda, M., Elmenhorst, E. M., Pennig, S., Plath, G., Maass, H., Tritschler, K.,.... Aeschbach, D. (2014). Significance of time awake for predicting pilots' fatigue on short-haul flights: Implications for flight duty time regulations. *Journal of Sleep Research, 23*(5), 564–567. doi:10.1111/jsr.12186

Wagstaff, A. S., & Lie, J. A. S. (2011). Shift and night work and long working hours–a systematic review of safety implications. *Scandinavian Journal of Work Environment & Health, 37*(3), 173–185. doi: 10.5271/Sjweh.3146

Weiland, M., Nesthus, T., Compatore, C., Popkin, S., Mangie, J., Thomas, L. C., & Flynn-Evans, E. (2013). *Aviation fatigue: Issues in developing fatigue risk management systems.* Paper presented at the Proceedings of the Human Factors and Ergonomic Society 57th Annual Meeting.

4.11 Fatigue Management Education for Young Novice Drivers

Ashleigh J. Filtness, Sally Maynard, Rachel Talbot, Claire Quigley, and Evita Papazikou

Transport Safety Research Centre, Loughborough University, Loughborough, UK

CONTENTS

4.11.1 WHY IS THIS IMPORTANT?

Reducing driver fatigue requires instigating a behaviour change. Every person sleeps, therefore, every person has the potential to experience fatigue. It is not enough to advise someone not to drive when sleepy, rather it is preferable to address their underlying sleep health and behavioural beliefs to reduce the chance that a person may drive when fatigued. It is hypothesised that an educational programme addressing driver fatigue and the mechanisms underlying them aimed specifically at young drivers has the potential to change behaviour. Changing health behaviours can be difficult, as many factors feed into a person's readiness and willingness to change. However, it is possible to make a difference as behaviour change has previously been

DOI: 10.1201/9781003213154-33 **389**

seen in this age group around other high-risk behaviours, for instance, drugs and drinking alcohol.

4.11.2 WHO IS THIS CHAPTER FOR?

This chapter will be of utmost interest to anyone who regulates, engages with, or supports young people in learning to drive and would like to develop an education programme to reduce driver fatigue. For example, policymakers, driver fatigue campaign developers, driving instructors, teachers/education providers, parents/guardians, transport industry employing younger drivers, and police community officers. It provides advice about how to include driver fatigue and sleep health information related to safe driving within driver education. As such, this chapter may also be of interest for employers who have a driver fatigue education programme. This chapter summarises the main findings from this work; those interested in the full guidance report may contact the chapter authors directly.

Awareness and mitigation of driver fatigue is a higher order skill (beyond vehicle manoeuvring) that is necessary for safe driving. Within the "Goals for Driver Education" (GDE) matrix (Driver Metrics, 2022), this would relate to self-evaluation and awareness skills (Hatakka et al., 2002). The GDE is a framework which considers all the knowledge and skills a driver needs. Such higher order skills as self-evaluation and awareness are vital for road safety but unfortunately often receive lower priority in the learning to drive process than the practical vehicle handling skills.

4.11.3 HOW WAS THE INFORMATION IN THIS CHAPTER DEVELOPED?

The information presented in this chapter was developed by researchers at the Transport Safety Research Centre (TSRC), Loughborough University, UK, supported by a Road Safety Grant from the Department for Transport (DfT). The information collected was from UK participants and so applies most closely to that region; however, the overall findings and advice drawn from them are potentially generalisable to other jurisdictions internationally. The content of the chapter was informed by seven online focus groups with 35 participants (15 males and 20 females) who were either learner or novice (licenced within the previous two years) drivers. Participants were 18 to 24 years of age. Eight were still learning to drive; 27 were licenced drivers. The guided focus group discussions aimed to investigate motivations and situations that might lead to driver sleepiness, identify what is known about sleep and where this information is received from, and consider what education delivery mechanisms might be appropriate for this younger driver target group. A total of around five and a half hours of recordings were transcribed and thematically coded using a bottom-up approach, whereby the transcripts were used as a starting point to identify common themes. Two researchers first coded the same focus group transcript independently; through discussion and comparison of codes, a common coding dictionary was developed. The same two researchers coded the remaining six focus groups, each independently analysing three sessions.

Additionally, six one-to-one interviews were completed. Five of the interviews were with people who regularly interact with young novice drivers (for driving or non-driving-related reasons) in a manner that has potential to influence behaviour. The interviewees were a:

- driving instructor (male);
- youth group leader (female);
- sixth form (students aged 16 to 18 years) teacher (female);
- police community educator (male);
- progress coach at an FE College (students aged 16+) (female).

Participants were aged 35 to 50 years and had worked in their current role for between 3 and 12 years, although some had previously worked with young people in other capacities (e.g., the driving instructor was a former teacher). All participants completed the same structured interview, which asked them to consider their experience of engaging with young people in order to influence behaviour. Participants were asked about the following: effective education delivery, their experience of delivering sleep health education or seeing it delivered by someone else and who would be appropriate to deliver education relating to driver fatigue.

Although the focus was driver sleepiness, participants were asked to draw on their experience more broadly about influencing young adult behaviour. Two of the participants had direct experience of engaging with young drivers on the topic of driver sleepiness. The final interview was with a representative from the Driver Vehicle Standards Agency (DVSA). Over five and a half hours of recordings were transcribed and thematically coded using a bottom-up approach. Two researchers each coded the first interview transcript independently; through discussion and comparison of codes a common coding dictionary was developed. The same two researchers coded the remaining four interviews independently, with one analysing a further three interviews and the other researcher analysing the remaining one.

These findings were further expanded by a review of scientific literature addressing the main causes of driver sleepiness and features of successful education to reduce driver fatigue. Draft guidance was produced and reviewed by six academics who are recognised as experts in the fields of:

- driver sleepiness and fatigue research (2 females);
- sleep intervention and driver fatigue research with young adults (1 male);
- novice driver training research (1 female);
- behaviour change intervention research for transport workers (1 female);
- application of storytelling to support public engagement (1 male).

Following the review, comments were addressed, and the guidance was updated.

This chapter presents the combination of findings from the literature review, focus groups, interviews, and expert review. Findings informed by scientific literature include the relevant references; references are absent if the findings result from the primary data collection activities of the study.

The information presented in the following sections is a suggested guidance for best practice. Note that there is very little scientific research into how best to change sleep health behaviour to reduce driver fatigue in young people. This guidance is based on research evidence available at the time of the completed work (March, 2021); none of the proposed techniques have been evaluated. More research is needed to further enhance this guidance in the future.

4.11.3.1 WHY ARE YOUNG NOVICE DRIVERS AN IMPORTANT TARGET GROUP FOR FATIGUE MANAGEMENT?

Road crashes are the greatest killer of 15 to 24-year-olds in developed countries (OECD, 2006), with young drivers at a disproportionately greater crash risk compared with all other groups of drivers (Mayhew et al., 2003). Young drivers are overrepresented in sleep-related crashes (Blazejewski et al., 2012), with young (aged 17 to 24) drivers who report sleeping six or fewer hours per night at greater risk of crashing than those who sleep for longer (Martiniuk et al., 2013). This is of particular concern as fatigue crashes are associated with a higher risk of death and severe injury than other crashes (Horne & Reyner, 1995; Filtness et al., 2017).

A novice driver is considered here to be a person within two years of obtaining their licence. The overrepresentation of young novice drivers in crashes is recognised as one of the most challenging road safety problems to solve (Elvik, 2010). The vulnerability of these early years of learning to drive has been recognised internationally, with several jurisdictions mandating a graduated driver licencing system (GDL) (Bates et al., 2014). However, even with the support from GDL, those who are at a young age (15 to 24 years) when they first start to drive will also experience added pressure from physiological and psychological immaturity. It is these immaturities that put young drivers at greater risk of driver fatigue.

The adolescent brain is not yet physiologically mature and needs to sleep a lot, in a similar way to that of a child (Carskadon, 2011). However, adolescent lifestyle is more aligned to that of an adult, which creates a mismatch between the amount of sleep obtained and the amount of sleep needed. During this stage of physiological development, teenagers and young adults experience an increased preference for later bedtimes, caused by a shift in their circadian rhythm resulting in delayed sleep onset (Carskadon, 1990, 2011). The circadian rhythm is the regular oscillation of body systems which controls the sleep/wake cycle (our "body clock"). However, societal norms (e.g., college/work start times) mean that young adults still need to wake up earlier than they would like. Coinciding with this physiological change is a social change, whereby young adults are exposed to increasing education, work and social pressures, which often impact their sleep habits (Owens, 2014; Lund et al., 2010). Obtaining sufficient sleep is further hampered by recent trends in increased evening computer game and mobile phone use (Thomee et al., 2011) and the use of daytime stimulants (such as energy drinks), which can make it harder to fall asleep at night (Taylor & Bramowelth, 2012). The convergence of these factors results in an entire subsection of the population that is chronically sleep deprived. Ironically, it is at this vulnerable time that society first allows individuals to engage in the potentially dangerous task of driving.

In response to these risks, it is suggested that targeting driver fatigue education towards young novice drivers and pre-drivers may be beneficial for reducing fatigue crashes. Including pre-drivers as well as learner/novice drivers provides an opportunity to embed safe choices and beliefs prior to the period when actually learning to drive. It would then be more likely that such safe choices and beliefs will be acted upon once young drivers obtain their licence.

4.11.4   HOW CAN YOUNG NOVICE DRIVERS BEST BE ENGAGED IN AN EDUCATION PROGRAMME TO REDUCE DRIVER FATIGUE?

Behaviour change is most likely to occur when instigated within a supportive network, for example, through involvement of family, schools, local councils, government agencies, and similar organisations.

4.11.4.1   WHO SHOULD DELIVER THE EDUCATION?

Although all young novice drivers are at risk of driver fatigue, it may be beneficial to target those most likely to experience driver sleepiness: Males, those with higher trait sleepiness, those with high risk-taking tendency, and those with lifestyle factors which increase risk, for example, night workers (Filtness et al., 2017). Those interviewed as part of this work reported that targeting content to make it directly relevant for this age group will increase the chance of engagement. Existing settings where an education programme could be delivered include driver education programmes, within a driving school lesson, while being supervised by parents and as a classroom activity.

Young novice drivers reported in focus groups that accredited driving instructors are their most trusted source of information about driver fatigue. However, both focus groups and interviewees recognised that driver fatigue education programmes may be appropriately delivered from a variety of role holders, including youth group leader, school teacher, police community educator, and school/college progress coach. Additionally, parents are highly influential in safe driving behaviours (Bates et al., 2014) because drivers who have grown up observing safe driving behaviour are more likely to exhibit such behaviour themselves. Parents can also play a role in enforcing safe driving practice, for example, refusing to lend their vehicle to a young novice driver during night-time hours. Lastly, parents can enforce good sleep health and driver behaviour by adopting safe behaviours themselves, initiating discussions, challenging young drivers when necessary, and making discussions about driver sleepiness the norm.

4.11.4.2   WHAT IS THE BEST MECHANISM FOR ENGAGEMENT?

The interviewees reported that a mixed approach of both theoretical and practical exercises/examples would be most beneficial, for example, by combining expert views and personal peer experience. Theoretical components may include written information such as facts about sleep health, practical examples may include personal reflections of those who have had a sleep-related crash, and practical exercises may include controlled exposure to driver sleepiness. Such narratives and peer experience have the potential to be used within official printed documentation (e.g., the UK Highway Code), as online digital stories, as in-person storytelling within training/education workshops, or as a resource for trainers and instructors to use. Most important is the need to provide a variety of voices and different ways of communicating.

Repeated exposure to information about driver fatigue from multiple sources is likely to have most impact. A flexible outlook to delivery will likely benefit more people reflective of differing needs. Young drivers expressed a preference for short, quick exposure content suggesting that this style would be the most likely to produce engagement. However, aiming for short content requires a prioritisation of what information to deliver. Given this limitation of time, it is thought that the most impact is likely to be derived from challenging the belief that driver sleepiness is unavoidable and contesting normalisation of driver sleepiness. This derives from the focus group finding that many young novice drivers are already aware of the characteristics of good sleep habits and safe driving, but they do not necessarily act on this knowledge.

4.11.4.3 What Are the Biggest Barriers and How Can These Be Overcome to Ensure Effective Driver Fatigue Education?

The interviewees reported that the major barrier to the effectiveness of any engagement they have with young people is the need to generate the initial buy-in. It is necessary for participants to be engaged with an education programme for it to work. Dedicated techniques to increase engagement early on were reported to be beneficial. These could include the use of technology, interactive activities, and personalised approaches. If education is not easy to engage with or lacks interactive elements, then engagement is unlikely.

Another important barrier to be overcome is the belief, observed in the focus groups, that driver fatigue is unavoidable. While many young novice drivers recognise that it might be dangerous, this risk is often seen as worth taking in order to complete a journey. Therefore, it is necessary to challenge the notion that driving when sleepy is "normal" and unavoidable. Indeed, promoting the fact that sleepiness is "entirely predictable" (i.e., if you do not have enough sleep, you will be tired) was recommended by experts as something that could be stressed through open conversation about sleep including duration norms, frequency of difficulties, and potential countermeasures to fatigue. Young drivers' frequent experience of driver fatigue can give the impression that this is to be expected. Embedding right at the start of their driving education that this is not "normal" may help to change behaviour.

Providing evidence of the link to consequences of driver fatigue (while making them relatable to everyday life and driving performance) may be beneficial to increase buy-in to the education approach. However, this should be achieved without moralising, which would likely distance young adults.

Sleep, fatigue, and sleep health are not always talked about openly or honestly. Breaking down this barrier will promote conversation, and the more conversation they have about sleep, the more likely new drivers will be to challenge a perceived time urgency versus the safety trade-off and see sleep in a positive light. This may particularly involve engagement with parents and peers—if young drivers see others driving following little sleep with no consequences, or boasting that they did not get much sleep but still drove, this might be more likely to become normalised behaviour.

Another significant barrier to ensuring effective driver fatigue education is the required time investment, that is, many initiatives will take time to implement and engage with, particularly if they are potentially industry-wide (e.g., additions to driving instruction or theory tests), a step necessary to achieve repeated exposure. There is also a time element in asking young drivers, their peers, parents, educators, and instructors to engage with this information, which may be in the context of existing busy circumstances and commitments. This was of notable concern for those involved in the interviews. It will be important to encourage individuals to consider driver sleepiness and the importance of good sleep habits so that they are able to make time for it.

Including positive role modelling, such as involving a person considered by young adults to be a role model, within a social media campaign designed to promote the discussion and consideration of driver fatigue might further increase the uptake on education programmes in this area and break down barriers.

4.11.4.4 What Are the Most Important Topics to Cover in an Education Programme to Reduce Novice Driver Fatigue?

In designing any approach to reduce driver fatigue, it must be relevant for all and consider a range of fatigue exposures, from those who occasionally experience day-time sleepiness through to those who regularly drive when fatigued. This section includes suggested topic areas which should be covered in an education programme and why that topic is important. The selection of topic areas was informed by the biggest barriers to overcome as identified in the literature review and in the focus groups and interviews. It is a first step towards building such an education. All aspects would need to be developed and evaluated as part of future work.

Challenge the Belief that Driver Fatigue Is Unavoidable

This is likely to be the most important topic to cover. Even if a person has effective knowledge of good sleep habits and the risks of driver sleepiness, they may still drive when fatigued if they do not feel culpable for the behaviour, that it is "not their fault" as it is unavoidable. This might include challenging the thinking that sleep is wasted time, or that sleep should be sacrificed for other pursuits. Example content aimed at challenging the belief that driver fatigue is unavoidable is presented in Table 4.11.1.

TABLE 4.11.1
Example of Content to Include in a driver Fatigue Education for Young Novice Drivers that Will Challenge the Belief that Driver Fatigue Is Unavoidable

Example Content

Unpack the relationship between risk and reward. Provide detail about the risk of crashing, death, and injury to self, passengers, and others in attempts to personalise the potential outcome. Considering what the reward actually is, how much benefit there is to arriving quickly when fatigued and question, "is this truly worth the risk?"

Challenge the belief that short journeys are safe when sleepy. Provide evidence that fatigue-related crashes occur in town as well as on motorways and demonstrate the high severity of fatigue-related crashes compared to non-fatigue-related crashes regardless of journey length (Filtness et al., 2017). Explain that fatigue can be present without a long journey time. Highlight that people cannot foresee immediate sleep onset (although they can recognise increasing sleepiness (Cai et al., 2021)) and also that the more sleepy they feel, the higher the risk of localised microsleeps within parts of the brain, an event about which a person will be unaware, but that may cause major problems if it happens while driving (Ahlström, Jansson & Anund, 2017).

Demonstrate that fatigued people make poor decisions. If you are trying to decide about whether or not to drive at the point that you are already fatigued, you will be less able to accurately assess the risk. Provide advice on pre-planning to avoid being fatigued prior to starting driving.

Give personal examples of people who have driven fatigued and been in trouble with the police, demonstrating that within the legal system fatigue is considered the driver's fault. Provide the link to consequences.

Emphasise accountability. Be clear about what you are accountable for as a driver and provide a practical check list approach to confirming own fitness to drive. Assist young novice drivers to recognise the legal and social/moral accountability of being fit and healthy when driving. Stress personal control and responsibility.

Highlight the connection between lack of sleep and the risk of illness and its adverse effect on appearance, exploiting young people's normal interest in their looks.

Challenge the Normalisation of Driver Fatigue

The frequent experience of driver fatigue and regular observation of this in others may lead to a desensitisation to potential risk. It is important to cover this topic in order to challenge this perspective. The more times a person who is fatigued drives without crashing, the less risky it will seem. This can therefore mean that the risk of driving while fatigued will no longer be accurately perceived by that driver. In addition, driving is likely to be one of the first safety critical tasks with which young people engage. If individuals have experienced the impact of fatigue mainly at school, they will recognise their lack of attention there; however, the risks related to safety in that environment would be much lower than when driving. As a result, young drivers might continue to engage in similar behaviours (late bedtimes, use of electronics in bedroom and before bed, etc.) without equating it to increased risk when driving. Example content aimed at challenging the normalisation of driver fatigue is presented in Table 4.11.2.

TABLE 4.11.2
Example of Content to Include in a Driver Fatigue Education for Young Novice Drivers that Will Challenge the Normalisation of Driver Fatigue

Example Content

Personal interviews with drivers who previously held this belief, and subsequently had a fatigue-related crash. Explaining the consequences and the change in those drivers' subsequent perception of driver fatigue.

Give a comprehensive picture of the situation (i.e., all factors that lead to driver fatigue) with practical examples of how to take control. For example, driving in the early hours of the morning and late bedtimes may lead to driver fatigue and countermeasures can be introduced. This should then provide evidence that these factors are not "normal" but controllable and avoidable.

Facilitate discussion around the influence of media and how it challenges or promotes driver fatigue to increase awareness of its influence. Encourage participants to form their own views rather than being influenced by others.

For young adults, social norms are very influential. Challenging negative norms may be necessary for positive behaviour change. Encourage young people to protect themselves, their family and friends regardless of peer perception. For example, by being a good passenger if you believe your driver to be fatigued and suggesting stopping for a coffee. Consider using experience on social norms related to drunk driving as this is generally perceived negatively by young people.

Emphasise responsibility of being alert when driving; much like a licence, insurance, and having air in your tyres, it is also a requirement.

Promote the Wider Benefits of Good Sleep

Recognising wider benefits (beyond driving) of sleep could enhance motivation to prioritise and protect sleep, for example, through enhancing mental health and well-being. Regardless of the reason for the motivation, obtaining more sleep, at the right time of the day, in general would then reduce the risk of driver fatigue. Providing motivational factors beyond driving safety is likely to increase the range of participants with whom impact can be made. Example content to promote the wider benefits of good sleep is presented in Table 4.11.3.

Promote Effective Driver Fatigue Mitigation

It is essential for drivers to have a basic knowledge of what to do if they feel sleepy when driving. Since many young novice drivers will already have good basic knowledge, this area is potentially less important than those which relate more to implementing the knowledge and motivation for safe behaviour in relation to feeling sleepy. Nevertheless, it is important to cover best practice to ensure that all young novice drivers have this basic information. Example content to promote effective driver fatigue mitigation is presented in Table 4.11.4.

Provide an Understanding of Risk Factors Which Can Lead to Driver Fatigue and How to Avoid Them

Highlighting the main risk factors which can lead to a situation of driver fatigue could help people recognise when they may be at risk. If risks are identified, then

TABLE 4.11.3

Example of Content to Include in a Driver Fatigue Education for Young Novice Drivers that Will Promote the Wider Benefits of Good Sleep

Example Content

Demonstrate links between sleep and poor mental health.

Demonstrate the impaired function due to sleepiness, for example, poor mood, decision-making, reaction time, poor sport performance, and poor exam performance.

Discuss the benefits of good sleep on physical health, particularly the links between short sleep and weight gain.

Explain differences between chronic and acute sleep loss and their implications.

Demonstrate that impairment can occur from a one-off episode of minimal sleep loss.

Explain the circadian drive for wakefulness, sleep pressure, and sleep inertia.

Focus on motivation for change, and how lifestyle can be beneficial for sleep.

TABLE 4.11.4

Example of Content to Include in a Driver Fatigue Education for Young Novice Drivers that Will Promote Effective Driver Fatigue Mitigation

Example Content

Be clear to participants, if you feel sleepy when driving you should stop, have a caffeinated drink followed by a 20-minute nap. You may then be fit to drive for up to 90 minutes to get to a safe place for adequate sleep.

Advocate taking a break from driving every 2 hours.

Develop a strategy for checking on yourself and assess your own fatigue level. For example, if driving on a motorway in UK, use the "Tiredness kills Take a break" sign as your cue to self-evaluate fatigue.

Discuss behaviours and strategies which are frequently employed by young drivers, but which are not effective in alleviating sleepiness, for example, opening a window, turning up the music.

Emphasise that countermeasures are temporary solutions to get you to somewhere safe to stop driving.

Provide hints and tips on how to change sleep behaviour, for example, going to bed at a regular time, leaving phone downstairs.

knowing what to do can empower a young novice driver to take their own mitigating actions. In a similar way to promoting effective fatigue mitigation, it is likely that much of this advice will already be known. It is important to cover the basics, but also likely that most impact will be made by covering content in earlier sections related to implementing the knowledge and motivation. Example content aiming to provide a better understanding of the risk factors which can lead to driver fatigue and how to avoid them is presented in Table 4.11.5.

TABLE 4.11.5

Example of Content to Include in a Driver Fatigue Education for Young Novice Drivers that Will Provide an Understanding of Risk Factors that Can Lead to Driver Fatigue and How to Avoid Them

Example Content

Explain how to calculate an Epworth Sleepiness Scale (ESS) score (Johns, 1991), recognising that an ESS score of ≥12 indicates excessive sleepiness, and advising to contact their doctor and seek medical review in cases of extreme sleepiness. (This is recommended as ESS is the most widely used screening tool, however, its accuracy in identifying fatigue has been questioned (Kendzerska et al., 2014).)

Demonstrate the inverse relationship of how driving can be beneficial to sleep by reducing journey/commute times compared to public transport and, therefore, increasing opportunity for sleep.

Give advice on night-time driving risk. Include practical rules on when it is most risky and how to predict the time of day one is most likely to be sleepy.

Highlight that there are individual differences in sleep need. It is important to know yourself and know your limits.

Encourage the evaluation of lifestyle decisions and how these choices can influence risk, for example, when to go to bed, how to commute, etc. In particular, encourage young drivers not to drive at night.

Give examples of future and everyday situations which can be risk factors for increased sleepiness, for example, shift work, jet lag, looking after babies and small children whose own disturbed sleep is likely to disrupt that of their caregivers. This could highlight that learning from the education now and implementing good sleep habits will be of benefit in the future.

4.11.5 CONCLUSIONS

Young novice drivers are overrepresented in fatigue-related crashes (Blazejewski et al., 2012). The experience of fatigue is different for this age group compared to that of older, more experienced drivers because of an immaturity in physiological development leading to a high sleep need. Additionally, novice driving skills are still in development and may more easily be adversely impacted by fatigue than would be the case in experienced drivers. For any education programme on driver fatigue to be effective, it is essential that participants are engaged with the programme to feel motivated to enact the required changes in behaviour. Through consultation with young drivers, a selection of people who engage with young people and with academic experts, it is apparent that a series of barriers must be overcome as part of the education. These include the need to:

- generate initial buy-in;
- challenge the belief that driver fatigue is unavoidable;
- provide evidence that there are consequences to driver fatigue;
- create an environment in which people feel happy to be open and honest about fatigue;

- allow time for investment in the programme;
- provide evidence that it is acceptable to care about this topic, for example, using positive role modelling.

An effective education programme will likely be of short duration, use a mix of theoretical and practical exercises/examples and require repeat exposure to materials by participants. Having a short programme requires prioritising content. In this context, the academic experts were asked to suggest which elements/approaches should be prioritised as being most likely to have an impact. They were as follows (in no particular order):

- sleep–wake stability (consistent sleep and wake time across the week);
- causes of sleepiness;
- reasons why good sleep is important;
- challenging the normalisation of driver sleepiness (i.e., that it is unavoidable);
- consequences of driving when sleepy;
- ensuring adequate opportunity for sleep in terms of duration;
- reinforcing the idea not to start a drive when sleepy or if likely to become sleepy;
- how to avoid driver sleepiness;
- the dangers of driver sleepiness.

Part of the difficulty in educating novice drivers on driver fatigue is a lack of ownership as to who would be accountable for this education. From the focus groups, the young novice drivers were clear that their driving instructor is considered the greatest authority on driver fatigue. The Driver Vehicle Standards Agency (DVSA) interview confirmed that it is within the remit of DVSA to educate young people on driver sleepiness, but they recognise that there is variability among teaching practices of driving instructors, in that they may not all cover topics related to risks about driver fatigue. The interviewed driving instructor also recognised that driver fatigue is a topic they may cover, but it is one among many and perhaps educational settings are better placed to deliver this type of knowledge than instructors. However, the teacher interviewed felt similarly that, while it is a topic that could be covered in schools, it is one of many and would likely not be a priority. Consequently, driver fatigue education for young novice drivers in the UK does not, currently, have a clear home. Although these findings were from UK participants, it is likely that the guidance will be applicable to other jurisdictions. The guidance was informed by literature from a range of countries including the USA, Australia, and India, where young drivers are commonly reported as being overrepresented in fatigue crashes. Without prioritisation, driver fatigue will unfortunately remain an issue for this at-risk group.

ACKNOWLEDGEMENT

Funded through Road Safety Research Grant Support from Department for Transport, UK.

SUMMARY POINTS FOR PRACTITIONERS

- Young novice drivers are at increased risk of driver fatigue due to their sleep need being greater than the amount of sleep they get.
- Targeting education at 16 to 24-year-olds will provide opportunity to embed safe choices and beliefs at the start of learning to drive.
- Tailoring education specifically for this age group will increase engagement. For example, providing evidence that it is acceptable to care about this topic, and using positive role modelling.
- An effective education programme will likely be of short duration, use a mix of theoretical and practical exercises/examples, and require repeat exposure to materials.
- Prioritise topics that are most likely to have impact, including the importance of sleep more broadly beyond driver safety.

REFERENCES

Ahlström, C., Jansson, S., & Anund, A. (2017). Local changes in the wake electroencephalogram precedes lane departures. *Journal of Sleep Research*, *26*(6), 816–819.

Bates, L. J., Allen, S., Armstrong, K., Watson, B., King, M. J., & Davey, J. (2014). Graduated driver licensing: An international review. *Sultan Qaboos University Medical Journal*, *14*(4), e432.

Blazejewski, S., Girodet, P. O., Orriols, L., Capelli, A., Moore, N., & CESIR Group. (2012). Factors associated with serious traffic crashes: A prospective study in southwest France. *Archives of Internal Medicine*, *172*(13), 1039–1041.

Cai, A. W., Manousakis, J. E., Lo, T., Horne, J. A., Howard, M. E., & Anderson, C. (2021). I think I'm sleepy, therefore I am–Awareness of sleepiness while driving: A systematic review. *Sleep Medicine Reviews*, 101533.

Carskadon, M. A. (1990). Patterns of sleep and sleepiness in adolescents. *Pediatrician*, *17*(1), 5–12.

Carskadon, M. A. (2011). Sleep in adolescents: The perfect storm. *Pediatric Clinics*, *58*(3), 637–647.

Driver Metrics (2022). Driver beliefs and the goals for driver education matrix. Available from www.drivermetrics.com.

Elvik, R. (2010). Why some road safety problems are more difficult to solve than others. *Accident Analysis & Prevention*, *42*(4), 1089–1096.

Filtness, A. J., Armstrong, K. A., Watson, A., & Smith, S. S. (2017). Sleep-related vehicle crashes on low speed roads. *Accident Analysis & Prevention*, *99*, 279–286.

Hatakka, M., Keskinen, E., Gregersen, N. P., Glad, A., & Hernetkoski, K. (2002). From control of the vehicle to personal self-control; broadening the perspectives to driver education. *Transportation Research Part F: Traffic Psychology and Behaviour*, *5*(3), 201–215.

Horne, J. A., & Reyner, L. A. (1995). Sleep related vehicle accidents. *BMJ*, *310*(6979), 565–567.

Johns, M. W. (1991). A new method for measuring daytime sleepiness: The Epworth sleepiness scale. *Sleep*, *14*(6), 540–545.

Kendzerska, T. B, Smith, T. B., Brignardello-Petersin, R., Leung, R. S., & Tomlinson, G. A. (2014). Evaluation of the measurement properties of the Epworth Sleepiness Scale: A systematic review. *Sleep Medicine Reviews*, *18*(4), 321–331.

Lund, H. G., Reider, B. D., Whiting, A. B., & Prichard, J. R. (2010). Sleep patterns and predictors of disturbed sleep in a large population of college students. *Journal of Adolescent Health, 46*(2), 124–132.

Martiniuk, A. L., Senserrick, T., Lo, S., Williamson, A., Du, W., Grunstein, R. R., ... & Ivers, R. Q. (2013). Sleep-deprived young drivers and the risk for crash: The DRIVE prospective cohort study. *JAMA Pediatrics, 167*(7), 647–655.

Mayhew, D. R., Simpson, H. M., & Pak, A. (2003). Changes in collision rates among novice drivers during the first months of driving. *Accident Analysis & Prevention, 35*(5), 683–691.

[OECD] Organisation for Economic Co-Operation and Development . (2006). *Young drivers: The road to safety.* 772006011p4.indd (oecd.org)

Owens, J., Adolescent Sleep Working Group, Committee on Adolescence, Au, R., Carskadon, M., Millman, R., ... & O'Brien, R. F. (2014). Insufficient sleep in adolescents and young adults: An update on causes and consequences. *Pediatrics, 134*(3), e921–e932.

Taylor, D. J., & Bramoweth, A. D. (2010). Patterns and consequences of inadequate sleep in college students: Substance use and motor vehicle accidents. *Journal of Adolescent Health, 46*(6), 610–612.

Thomée, S., Härenstam, A., & Hagberg, M. (2011). Mobile phone use and stress, sleep disturbances, and symptoms of depression among young adults—a prospective cohort study. *BMC Public Health, 11*(1), 1–11.

Section 5

Transportation Fatigue Risk Management in Practice

5.1 Tram Operations Limited

Insights from Our Journey to Improve Fatigue and Wellness Management

Jackie Townsend, Cynthia Spencer, Andy Wallace, Bradley Jennings, and Ben Groome

Tram Operations Limited, Croydon, UK

CONTENTS

5.1.1 INTRODUCTION

This chapter presents a real-world case study based on the experience of Tram Operations Limited (TOL) and their Fatigue Management journey.

As operator of the Tramlink service in South London and Croydon on behalf of Transport for London, TOL is deeply embedded in the local communities they serve. Engagement and a high operational performance are essential to ensure that

DOI: 10.1201/9781003213154-35

communities can connect across the south region; for some, trams are their only mode of transport. Many TOL staff live within the communities where the tram service runs.

Managing fatigue is a complex set of activities, actions, and responsibilities. Whilst all individuals may experience fatigue, how they react to different scenarios may not be the same. There are different schools of thought on who has responsibility for managing fatigue. Is it the employer, or is it the employee, or is it both? Another layer of complexity is the industry itself, how is fatigue and well-being managed and what forms of guidance and tools are available? Fatigue information and guidance often vary between sectors.

As an employer, TOL has a duty of care for their safety critical staff. TOL took the approach of joint responsibility between themselves as employer and the individual driver.

5.1.2 THE CHALLENGE

In May 2017 we carried out an internal audit of our Fatigue Risk Management (FRM) arrangements. The audit served two purposes—the first to check compliance against our Fatigue Management Procedure; and the second, to test our Fatigue Management Procedure for currency and effectiveness against the UK Office of Rail and Road's (ORR) Good Practice Guide on Managing Rail Staff Fatigue (ORR,2013; 2021) and Health and Safety England's (HSE) guidance on Managing Shiftwork (HSE, 2006).

Up until that point our maximum working hour principles were more akin to a bus operation than a light rail system where rules relating to maximum working hours are less restrictive than those applicable to driving in railway settings, and where different risks arising from repetition, shift design, and route characteristics exist. The key tool we, as well as many other companies, used at the time was the European Working Directive (EU, 2003), which came into force in the UK under the Working Time Regulations (UK, 1998) as a safety measure, because of the recognised negative effects on health and safety of excessively long working hours. The European Working Directive (EU, 2003) provided for statutory minimum rest-break entitlements, annual leave, and working arrangements for night workers.

The challenge we had was wanting to know more about the relationship between work and home life and how people's behaviour, unknown medical conditions and lifestyle management could impact fatigue and alertness and, consequently, the number of incidents where fatigue may have played a role, whilst at work in a safety critical role.

We hoped that by having this in-depth understanding of the factors that influence fatigue and alertness would result in a more competent, safer workforce.

Our first step was to look to others in the light rail industry for assistance and goals to assist in managing fatigue. Historically, fatigue management practices within the light rail industry evolved from bus operating rules; today, the industry is influenced by a largely outdated and ineffective set of maximum working hours criteria that were initially used in heavy rail.

Case studies, fatigue tools, and specific guidance available about managing fatigue in operating trams were limited.

For our journey to improved fatigue management we used the ORR (2013; 2021) Good practice guidelines–Fatigue Factors. The benefit to the business was seen at a very high level; however, we were also looking for specific fatigue tools and guidance at an operational level.

5.1.3   THE APPROACH

The key steps in our approach included a review of our existing practices, which were current and compliant. As we learned more about the subject, we quickly discovered that we had a desire to move beyond a compliance-based system. Consultation with staff identified a shared wish to take a more holistic approach to our existing fatigue and well-being arrangements as such, a more innovative approach was needed.

We believed that fatigue and wellness management should go beyond simply implementing work rosters that meet an industry minimum standard. Our work encompassed wider health and welfare support for staff and their families; ensuring a deeper understanding of fatigue, its causes and how it could be better controlled. Our arrangements have been fully consulted internally and with trade unions, which gave us support at all levels of the organisation.

We looked for expert guidance from outside of our industry, partnering with Clockwork Research Ltd ("Clockwork"), which brought experience from aviation, petrochemical, and heavy mining.

Our innovative approach included fatigue and distraction detection technology (Seeing Machines Guardian device), real data analysis, and good practice taken from a wide range of high-risk industries.

The result was a bespoke Fatigue and Wellness Management Programme. The unique elements included using in-cab alertness monitoring data and staff fatigue self-reports to inform "fatigue-friendly" work patterns. These new work patterns were supplemented by enhanced fatigue and wellness training that was individually tailored to each staff member's role. A staff welfare programme with effective fatigue management at its core…this was a UK transport industry first!

This all-inclusive approach has seen us become industry leaders in our own right and one of the first UK passenger transport operators to implement a staff welfare programme with fatigue management that is based on real data and reports from our driving staff.

5.1.4   ACTION PLAN AND TIMELINE

The below timeline shows how, starting in May 2017, we looked in detail at our fatigue management and worked with Clockwork on the initial phases during the first 20 months (see Figure 5.1.1).

Following the internal audit of our FRM arrangements, we worked closely with Clockwork and our health and safety representatives to analyse the effectiveness of our existing FRM controls, bearing in mind that our starting point was our maximum working hour principles, which were based on a bus operation rather than a light rail system.

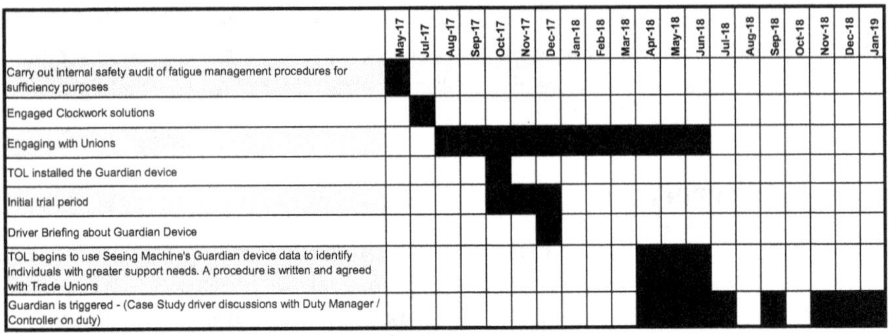

	May-17	Jul-17	Aug-17	Sep-17	Oct-17	Nov-17	Dec-17	Jan-18	Feb-18	Mar-18	Apr-18	May-18	Jun-18	Jul-18	Aug-18	Sep-18	Oct-18	Nov-18	Dec-18	Jan-19
Carry out internal safety audit of fatigue management procedures for sufficiency purposes	■																			
Engaged Clockwork solutions	■																			
Engaging with Unions			■	■	■															
TOL installed the Guardian device					■															
Initial trial period					■	■	■													
Driver Briefing about Guardian Device							■													
TOL begins to use Seeing Machine's Guardian device data to identify individuals with greater support needs. A procedure is written and agreed with Trade Unions													■	■						
Guardian is triggered - (Case Study driver discussions with Duty Manager / Controller on duty)														■		■				

FIGURE 5.1.1 Tram Operations Limited (TOL) fatigue project timeline.

Part of this work with Clockwork was to carry out a fatigue monitoring study which took place in 2017. Using the HSE Fatigue Index, which was subsequently revised and updated to the Fatigue Risk Index (FRI) (HSE 2006), and Sleep, Activity Fatigue and Task Effectiveness Model and associated Fatigue Avoidance Scheduling Tool (SAFTE-FAST), the study considered objective data: outputs of biomathematical modelling, real-time fatigue reporting data provided by the Fatigue Monitoring System ("Guardian"), and subjective data using feedback from staff that drive trams, gathered during a series of fatigue workshops.

5.1.4.1 THE FATIGUE RISK INDEX (FRI)

The FRI is a revised and updated version of the HSE Fatigue Index (HSE, 2006). It is designed primarily for comparing different work schedules, or for examining the potential impact of a change to one feature of a given work schedule (e.g., shift change-over times). It can also be used to identify the fatigue or risk associated with any particular shift within a given schedule that may be of concern.

Extensive changes were made to the previous version of the tool, incorporating recent information on issues including cumulative fatigue, time of day, shift length, the effect of breaks and the recovery from a sequence of shifts. An additional review was carried out of the trends in the risk of accidents and injuries related to different features of work schedules, which enabled the final version of the FRI to incorporate two separate indices, one related to fatigue (Fatigue Index) and the other to risk (Risk Index).

The objective of the FRI is to compare different shift schedules on the probability of high levels of sleepiness (the Fatigue score), and on the relative risk of an error that might result in an accident/injury (the Risk score).

The main applications of the FRI are in comparing work schedules, examining the impact of specific changes to work schedules, and identifying the fatigue risk associated with given shift schedules. The Fatigue Index is expressed in terms of the estimated average probability of employees experiencing a value of seven or more on the nine-point Karolinska Sleepiness Scale (KSS). The Risk Index is expressed in terms of an estimate of the relative risk of making an error that could contribute to an injury or accident. The two outputs are not simple transformations of one another, and hence the two predictions may differ substantially for some work schedules. The Fatigue and Risk Indices each provide an average value for every duty period.

5.1.4.2 SAFTE-FAST

SAFTE is a biomathematical model of the factors that contribute to fatigue. It is designed to simulate the underlying physiological system that causes degradations in cognitive performance. FAST implements the SAFTE biomathematical model of performance and fatigue to generate estimates of performance degradation owing to the individual's level of fatigue (SAFTE-FAST, 2022).

The purpose of the SAFTE-FAST system is to provide operators with prospective forecasts of expected fatigue risk so that proactive mitigations can be implemented to eliminate excessive fatigue risk. Retrospective and real-time assessments are also supported.

The primary application of the model is to aid operator scheduling by using work schedule information to estimate cognitive effectiveness. FAST can be used to examine specific schedules to determine vulnerabilities, to select optimal schedules and to plan napping and recovery sleep strategies.

The model provides a number of performance metrics (e.g., percent change in cognitive speed, lapse likelihood, reaction time) and sleep-wake metrics (e.g., sleep reservoir, circadian phase). The outputs of the model are a Manager Table, Summary File, and Visual FAST Graphic, all of which provide measurements of duty time below an adjustable criterion line.

Outputs were considered during the subsequent review of our driving rosters and were used to inform where breaks and rest days could be best employed to minimise the risk of fatigue. Staff feedback was additionally considered in development of our fatigue training materials and is reflected in the process we used to manage staff that reported as being too fatigued to carry out safety critical work.

No pre-change evaluation work was specifically undertaken by us, principally because the company's approach, at that time, to staff becoming fatigued was to grant them leave to cover the period of absence, or for the staff member to report as being sick. Post-evaluation, we implemented processes to record and monitor instances of fatigue.

A fatigue action plan of areas we wanted to improve upon was developed. This plan was fully discussed with our trade union colleagues throughout, incorporated into our wider company business planning arrangements, and tracked to completion using existing governance channels.

The areas that we focused on were tram driving and control room activities, all of which involved shift work and safety critical work that can be associated with high fatigue risk. We also reviewed existing and implemented new fatigue management controls for safety critical workers. Our approach was developed using the principles outlined in the UK ORR's good practice guide on managing rail staff fatigue (ORR, 2013; 2021).

Our **action plan** consisted of the following 11 actions:

1. Review our Fatigue Risk Management System (FRMS).
2. Use the initial fatigue data collated by Clockwork to identify ongoing fatigue data streams and our safety performance indicators.
3. Update our fatigue policy detailing our intent which was implemented as our Fatigue procedure.
4. Make any adjustments to our base rota.
5. Develop more appropriate fatigue education and training.
6. Establish a fatigue safety action group (FSAG).
7. Establish a fatigue reporting system.
8. Develop fatigue safety assurance/validation.
9. Develop a fatigue communication process.
10. Demonstrate senior management commitment.
11. Establish an effective safety culture based upon just culture principles.

The action plan was broken into three phases of work:

Phase 1—Situational Analysis

Working with Clockwork, we carried out a review of our current situation and looked for any gaps:

- Concluded that current Fatigue Risk Management System (FRMS) was compliance based.
- Used focus groups and roster analysis to determine specific causes of fatigue in drivers
- Reviewed our fatigue principles, using ORR best practice guidance. This involved assessing likely fatigue from a working pattern and comparing the work pattern against good practice guidelines, to identify potentially fatiguing features.
- Conducted a gap analysis against the ORR's "ROGS" (Railways and Other Guided Transport Systems (Safety) Regulations) nine-stage approach to managing rail staff fatigue (for more on ROGS, see ORR, 2022).
- Collected data from current roster analysis, conducted focus groups for process/ procedure, and identified mitigations to control operational fatigue.
- Wrote new fatigue policy to set out the processes and procedures workers are required to follow to limit the risk of fatigue.
- Reviewed existing fatigue education and training materials.

Phase 2—Building In-house Fatigue Risk Management Capability

Our existing FRMS covered all staff grades and built upon the ROGS nine-stage fatigue management approach outlined in the ORR's guidance for managing rail staff fatigue (ORR, 2013; 2021). We used both subjective and objective data to define bespoke work patterns and maximum working hours criteria that were unique to our operation:

- Reviewed our fatigue management policy.
- Established our FSAG.
- Used our FSAG to consult with safety critical workers on fatigue risk management arrangements.
- Trained key personnel in fatigue factors.
- Developed a bespoke online fatigue training package.
- Improved our staff families' awareness of fatigue management strategies.

Once both phases above were completed, we carried out a review and made further refinements to suit those changes identified in our risk profile.

The risk management procedure at the time (2017 to 2018) required investigation and review of all instances of fatigue, and ongoing monitoring of each fatigue support plan to conclusion. Strategic overview of the effectiveness of these measures was undertaken by our FSAG that met every 6 months.

Phase 3—Integration of Fatigue Risk Management Data

This phase was managed taking a **Plan, Do, Check, Act** approach to fatigue risk management (Table 5.1.1).

TABLE 5.1.1
Plan, Do, Check, Act Approach to Fatigue Risk Management

PLAN
- Review of the company's fatigue risk management procedure that describes our Fatigue Risk Management System (FRMS).

DO
- Gap analysis against ROGS regulation and other high-risk industries.
- Integrate any arrangements identified from the gap analysis into driving rosters.
- Determine maximum hours on shift and optimum number/duration of breaks.
- Review/analyse fatigue monitoring system data.
- Hold driver and controller workshops.
- Use output data to devise rosters.
- Consult with our safety representatives.

CHECK
- Perform regular review of fatigue plans for individuals.
- Make any changes to rosters.
- Carry out annual review of our FRM procedure.

ACT
- Regular check and review of the fatigue monitoring system data and our arrangements for fatigue, including the effect of fatigue on rosters and the number of instances.
- Review the effectiveness of our arrangements for monitoring fatigue at FSAG meetings.
- Develop individual fatigue plans, where required.
- Produce reports.
- Consult with staff and safety representatives on any trends identified from our fatigue monitoring and arrangements and on any subsequent changes to working patterns and rosters that may be required.

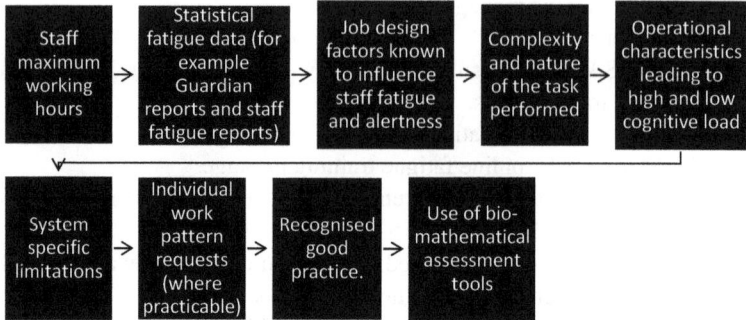

FIGURE 5.1.2   Our standards and work patterns.

This phase included a review of our standards and work patterns, as shown in Figure 5.1.2.

At the same time as carrying out our FRM review, we refocused our company culture to be based on the principles of a "Just/Open Culture" and demonstrated an improvement in our Safety culture. Most Just Cultures will take around 5 years to embed into a business. We focused on changing our Just Culture in less time using two key strands: proactive encouragement of staff self-reporting when they were fatigued and the introduction of error and violation principles.

This emphasis supported and reduced the likelihood of incidents and made compliance with health and safety legislation easier. It helped to promote a willingness to think and do things in a safe way. A key component to see the change in behaviour was to reinforce and encourage staff to self-report any near misses with no disciplinary consequences.

We used the method of support and learning rather than disciplinary as seen in our newly developed "Error and Violation" policy. We worked closely with our safety and operations teams and the safety representatives from the unions to jointly agree and implement this policy.

As part of our enhanced focus, we targeted four areas (see Table 5.1.2).

The electronic Competence Management system has been well received by staff, as they can access it, using their new tablets, to see their own competence records, completed assessments, and when the next one is due and to look at any knowledge gaps requiring further training.

We recognise and reward drivers through safe driving awards using Road Operators Safety Council (ROSCO). These awards are designed to provide an opportunity to recognise excellence and encourage safe driving amongst UK bus/tram operators. Drivers who have complied with the conditions of the scheme each year are entitled to awards in recognition.

Our fatigue enhancements were further supported with active internal promotion of two confidential reporting tools, whereby staff could anonymously share any safety concerns that they may have. We used Confidential Reporting for Safety (CIRAS), the industry tool for anonymous reporting of safety issues, and our parent company's confidential reporting system.

TABLE 5.1.2
Four Key Areas of Refocus of Company Safety Culture

Policy and Procedures
- Redefined our FRMS policy
- Reviewed our HR policies for absenteeism, grievance and disciplinary to align with our FRMS policy
- Developed principles for our Error and Violation policy with trade unions and safety representatives
- Reviewed our Equality and Dignity policy.

Engagement
- Proactively met more regularly with company safety representatives in an open and listening environment
- Ensured routine consultation with staff on any proposed changes
- Introduced two new staff communication channels–"The Loop" and "Tramlines".
- Managing Director carried one-to-one meetings with all safety critical staff.

Training and Assessment
- Introduced safety and training days for our safety critical staff
- Introduced a new electronic "Competence Management" system, to track the competence requirements of TOL and identify any remaining gaps for individual staff.

Behaviour Change
- Introduced a developmental approach to our competence management
- Recognised and rewarded positive safety behaviour amongst staff
- Proactively encouraged self-reporting for fatigue events, incidents, and near misses
- Conducted performance appraisals that included safety values
- Introduced our Error and Violation policy.

5.1.5 TOOLS FOR FATIGUE MANAGEMENT

We developed several key tools to help manage fatigue.

5.1.5.1 FATIGUE MANAGEMENT TRAINING

We enhanced our staff fatigue training and completely re-designed our staff fatigue training materials to improve its validity and relevance to staff.

Training was delivered in two stages (see Table 5.1.3).

The aim of our fatigue training was to provide all staff including Executive Team and Senior Leaders with a baseline knowledge of the factors that can affect fatigue and well-being and then provide targeted specialist knowledge relevant to each individual's company role. Staff from all grades were invited to attend a series of fatigue and well-being workshops (classroom sessions) to identify individual development needs and preferred learning styles. As such, our training content specifically addressed the factors that influenced fatigue and wellness for our staff (Figure 5.1.3).

We took a blended learning approach and used an electronic training platform to provide core fatigue and wellness information—**for example, information on sleep, diet, exercise, and lifestyle management techniques;** this was supplemented by trainer-led classroom sessions that encouraged open discussion and checked understanding of the subject matter covered.

TABLE 5.1.3
The Two Stages of Fatigue Training

Stage 1: Definition and Causes	Stage 2: Effects of Fatigue
• Encouraged open conversations with staff about fatigue, its causes and effects • Provided staff with information to recognise fatigue onset and techniques to effectively manage it • Used the CIRAS DVD to help build awareness of key messages and promoting a reporting culture.	• Developed awareness of our Fatigue Management process • Carried out an interview to determine whether any lifestyle factors were causing fatigue at work, for example, a new baby at home or childcare/ school arrangements • A medical assessment by a qualified occupational health provider was performed for each member of staff that had triggered a fatigue event on our fatigue monitoring device (Guardian). The need for a medical review is identified after the interview. • A fatigue management plan was developed for any driver who had a fatigue event. The plan allowed for monitoring changes to the driver's performance.

Core training was provided to all staff members; safety critical staff groups and those that had direct control on how fatigue is managed, drivers, our controllers, schedulers, and managers received supplementary training that was tailored to their roles and responsibilities.

We recognised that fatigue and wellness management does not apply solely to the workplace; therefore, in addition to our blended learning programme we hosted a family open day in September 2019. The purpose of the day was to extend our learning with our employees' families so that the impact of fatigue and wellness on family life could be discussed. This was expected to enable families to learn and identify the symptoms of fatigue in themselves and in other family members, so that they could identify and support potential mitigations, including any coping strategies each family had that could be shared with other families attending the day.

5.1.5.2 NEW DRIVER ROSTERS

Following the internal audit of our FRMS during **May 2017**, we revised our rules:

- Reduced the number of consecutive days someone in a safety critical role was allowed to work from 12 days to 8.
- New rules applied to our four types of staff rosters: Main, Early, Late and Spare.
- No one was rostered to work more than 7 consecutive days.

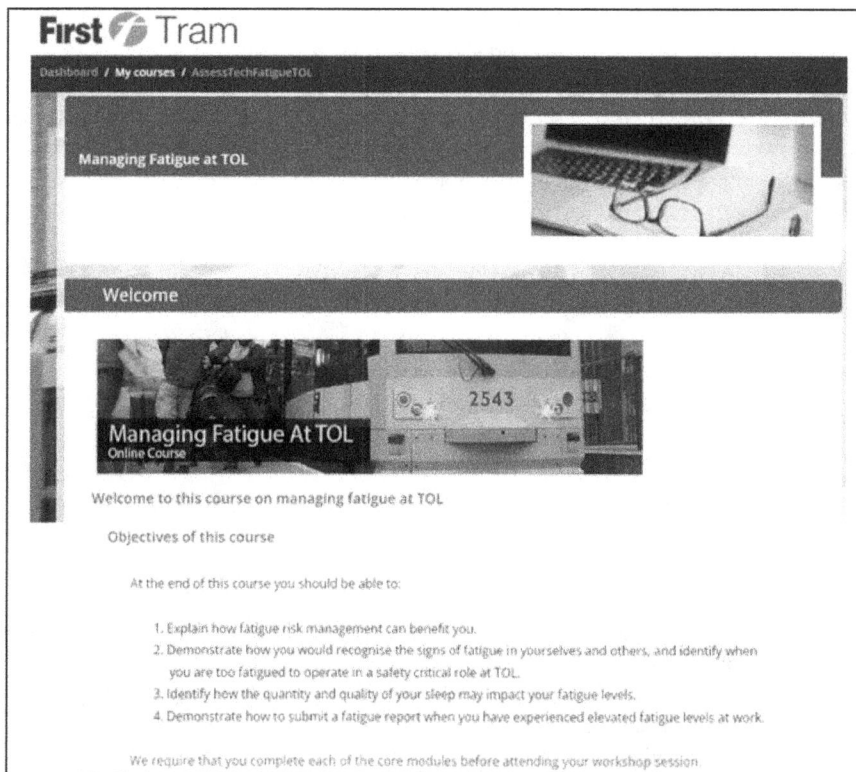

FIGURE 5.1.3   A screenshot from our online fatigue training page.

These new rules meant that the safety critical roles could be rostered to work 7 days, with the ability to work an additional day. The new rule was applied in two ways:

- Staff member can volunteer to work their day off, known as a working rest day. A list of volunteers was maintained; or
- Staff submitted a request to change their rostered rest day.

Most rest day changes were at the request of staff. We rarely asked staff to change a rest day unless there was an operational need to do so. On those occasions we referred to our volunteer list and applied the 8-day rule to identify the most suitable staff member.

Our rule stated you must have one rest day in each pay week, which began on a Sunday. Staff could change a rest day whereby it is swapped to another day. The outcome of working a rest day meant they worked an "additional" day.

Our procedures ensured that working an additional day or changing a rest day does not break our 8 consecutive day rule.

A second roster update was implemented during **July 2019**; the principles were based on drivers working a 5-day, rather than a 7-day week. These new rosters considered feedback from our drivers, fatigue self-reports, and 13 periods of data collected from our in-cab fatigue and alertness monitoring system.

Subtle changes were made to the Sunday roster to address work patterns that were understood to bring on the onset of fatigue; examples of the changes made included reducing excessively long driving periods on areas of our route where low cognitive load exists and re-allocated the distribution and length of meal breaks to allow drivers to take on food, water, and rest at optimum times:

- Reduced from working 7 consecutive days to 6.
- Shorter first half of duty.
- Content of duties varied to take account of low workload areas.
- Long breaks on Sundays reduced from 2 hours to 1 hour.
- Break timings used to address known fatigue spikes within shift-halves.
- Increased rest time when transitioning between shifts.

A third review of the rosters was carried out in **September 2019** that saw further reductions in the HSE Fatigue and Risk indices, which we used to measure our rosters.

During 2020 driving rosters were reviewed and modified for a fourth time:

- The average driving hours per week were reduced to just over 35 hours, resulting in an additional rest day.
- The roster pattern was changed to extend the time-off between finishing with an early shift and returning on to a late shift.
- A reduced number of split rest days.
- No 4-hour blocks of driving in the first half of any early duties.
- On long weekends where duties finished on a late and returned on an early duty, this was reversed to maximise the total rest period.

These latest rosters came into effect on **31 October 2021**. To deliver the new duties, we needed to recruit an additional ten drivers.

5.1.5.3 Driver Self-Reporting

Increased awareness of fatigue amongst our staff following the fatigue training led to a positive behaviour of drivers self-reporting when they felt that they were too fatigued to drive. We updated our fatigue procedure so that it described clear and specific actions to be carried out with any instance of fatigue being reported.

A combination of the fatigue training coupled with the knowledge that there are no disciplinary consequences for reporting fatigue has resulted in a sustained increase in drivers' self-reporting instances of being fatigued.

We were proactive and took immediate action when staff became too fatigued to work safely. Table 5.1.4 shows the guidance we have developed for the managers of drivers who self-report fatigue either before or whilst on duty.

The number of drivers self-reporting fatigue has increased with the introduction of a positive environment to report before or whilst on duty with no fear of retribution. Following our refresher training in 2021 we can see the number of drivers positively self-reporting fatigue has risen, which is a good outcome (see Figure 5.1.4).

TABLE 5.1.4
Guidance for Managers of Drivers Who Self-report Fatigue

Before Duty Commences
- Record the reason the individual is unfit for duty in the Control Duty Log
- Arrange for a fatigue report to be completed
- Advise the individual to attend a fatigue interview after a suitable period of rest.
- This will be carried out on the same day as the fatigue event, and is not considered to be a day off
- The driver will be removed from any safety-critical work for that day
- Develop a personal fatigue management plan that supports the individual affected.

Whilst on Duty
- Prevent the individual from carrying out further safety critical work
- Make arrangements for the individual to return to the depot and complete a fatigue report
- Conduct a fatigue interview, on the same day, after a period of rest for the driver
- Develop a personal fatigue management plan that supports the individual affected
- Prevent the individual from driving any other company or personal vehicle.

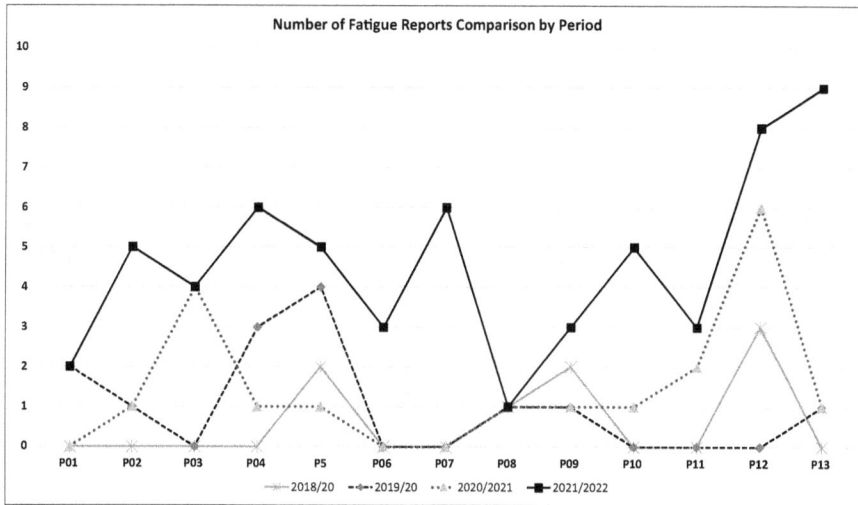

FIGURE 5.1.4 Comparison over 4 years for drivers self-reporting fatigue. Fatigue incidents occurring prior to Period 4* 2018/2019 were treated as sickness or absence. 2021/2022 covers up to Period 8 (November 2021).

*NB: A period is four weeks in length, P1 starts on 1 April and P13 is the last four weeks in March each year.

5.1.5.4 Fatigue Detection Technology

The Seeing Machines Guardian system was fitted in all tram cabs during December 2017. This fatigue detection technology uses an in-cab face three-point sensor camera to track eye closure or eye distraction and head position. The device sits on the dashboard of each tram cab. If fatigue is detected, the driver is alerted through an alarm consisting of a vibration on the bottom of the driver's seat and an audible warning. The alarm will last for approximately 5 seconds. The event along with the previous 3 seconds is recorded and shared as an immediate Executive alert for the Management Team. It is subsequently stored on a Cloud server for company use and post-event discussions with the driver. The initial classification of a fatigue event is carried out by Seeing Machines. Upon receipt TOL will amend if needed to meet our Significant Events categorisation which is for microsleep and drowsiness only.

These Significant events are captured and reported. If a driver does not trigger the device, there will not be any associated footage.

Using the fatigue detection technology, we had the ability to track any driver who triggered the Guardian more than six times within a four-week period.

Figure 5.1.5 shows the first year of monitoring the data from the fatigue monitoring device which was installed in December 2017. We took 3 months to baseline the alerts. Following this first year and over time the number of detected fatigue events by drivers has reduced.

Eighteen drivers triggered the device more than six times in a four-week period. Each of those drivers had a post-event interview and a fatigue support plan was put in place.

In Figure 5.1.6, we can see a significant decrease in the number of drivers who have triggered the device six or more times in a period—a reduction of 16 drivers to only 2, circa 10% of our drivers. We believe that these are excellent results.

Another component we analysed was the spread of events across different times of the operating day, and where within the timeframe of a driving duty a significant event happened.

Analysis over the same period shows that the spread of events across different times of our 22-hour operating day has also reduced. In Figure 5.1.7 the dotted line

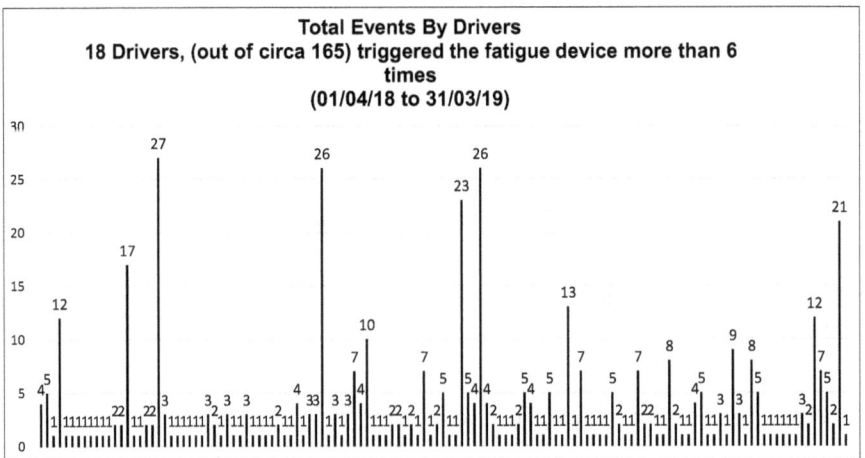

FIGURE 5.1.5 Analysis of all 165 drivers' fatigue events (as detected by the Guardian) over the period from 1 April 2018 to 31 March 2019.

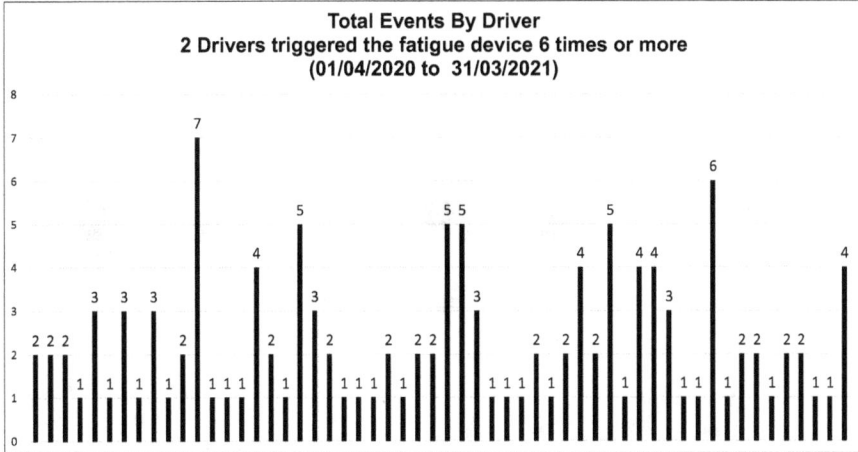

FIGURE 5.1.6   Analysis of all 165 drivers over the period from 1 April 2020 to 31 March 2021.

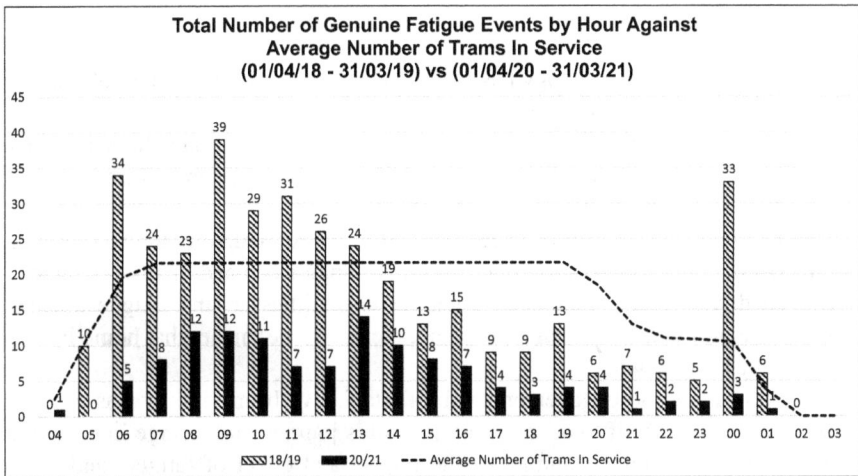

FIGURE 5.1.7   Comparison of fatigue events by hour against average number of trams in service.

shows the average number of trams in service across the day. In this comparison there is a significant reduction in the number of fatigue events per hour from 2018–2019 to 2020–2021.

We looked at how many hours into a driver's shift a fatigue event happened. The numbers have reduced significantly since we introduced fatigue detection technology. The comparison is presented in Figure 5.1.8.

We analysed the duty in two halves, to determine the impact of the break times within a duty. The outcome of changing our roster and associated timing of breaks can be seen from the reduction shown in this comparison.

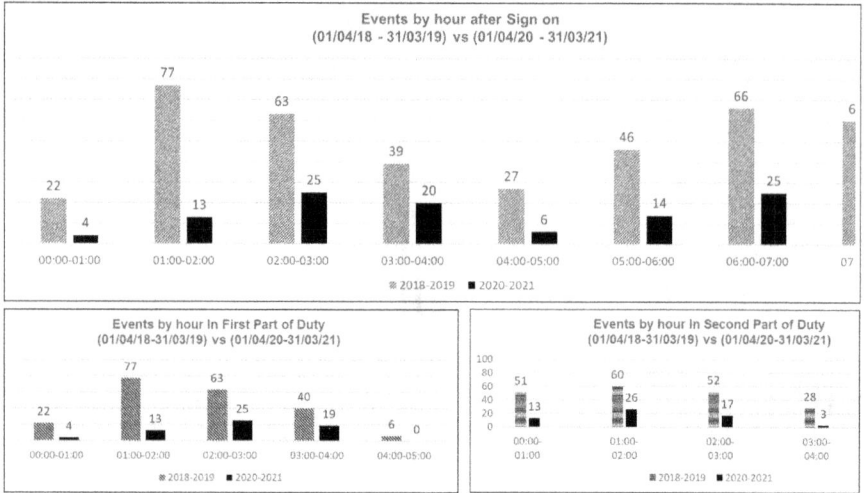

FIGURE 5.1.8   Comparison of fatigue events by number of hours after signing on for duty.

Fatigue monitoring technology has undoubtedly improved the welfare of our staff and resulted in a safer environment for our customers.

The main outcome has been more successful than we could have hoped for. The fatigue risk management training has increased staff knowledge and awareness about fatigue, its causes and effect.

Another significant benefit has been the ability for some drivers to get diagnosed for previously unknown medical conditions that impair sleep and increase fatigue.

Trained drivers better understand their responsibilities around fatigue management and the importance of their well-being, including the impact that home life and lifestyle may have on work.

Communication and engagement with all staff have been vital; it was essential for all safety critical staff to accompany us on this journey and change in behaviour to build a collective understanding of the impact and effect of fatigue, and of the measures to mitigate it.

Our blended fatigue training was important due to its nature and the combination of using visuals, hands-on insights and sharing insights to build awareness of fatigue has played an important role with staff, as has the refresher training.

One analogy we use within the Executive Team at TOL is to imagine being on a racetrack. If we see one or several colleagues on the track, don't assume they have absorbed all of the key information the first time around. Rather than lap them, slow down, and take them with us on the journey, driving forward together.

Figures 5.1.9 and 5.1.10 show the summary analysis for three years: 2018 to 2019, 2019 to 2020, and 2020 to 2021.

The results show an overall 43% reduction in all events for 2020/21 in comparison to 2019/20, and 69% when 2020/21 is compared to 2018/19.

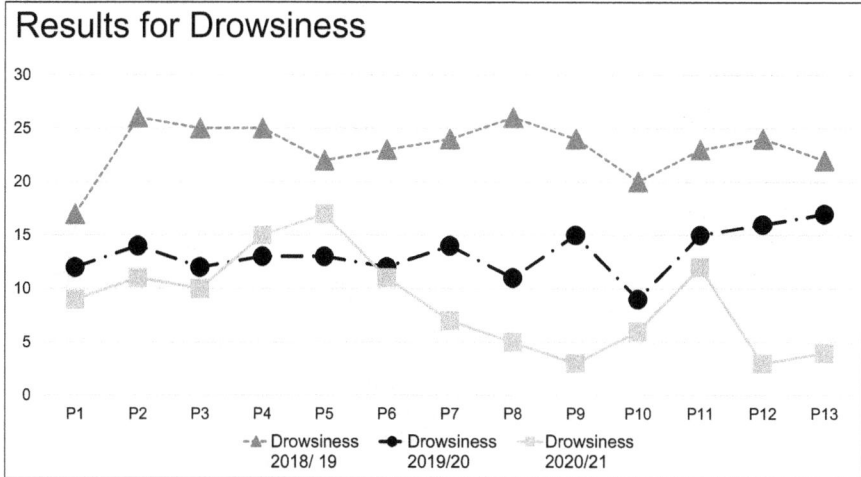

FIGURE 5.1.9 Three-year comparison of drowsiness events each period. Each year runs from April to March.

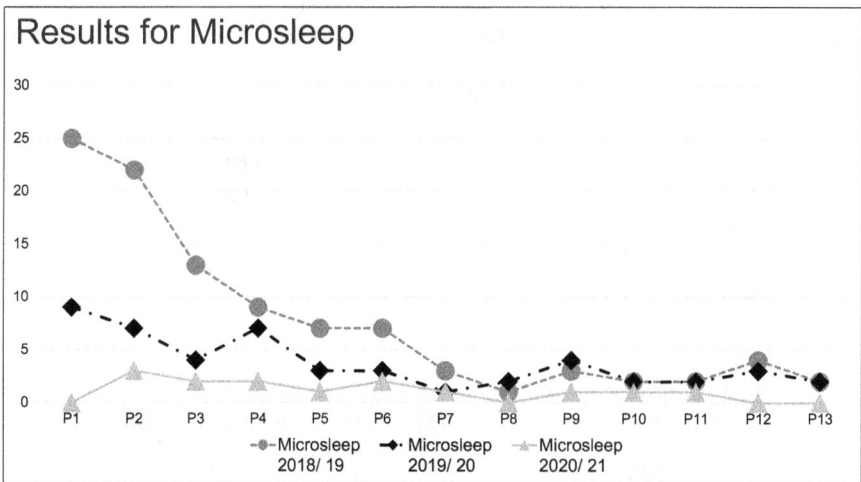

FIGURE 5.1.10 Three-year comparison of microsleep events each period.

5.1.6 OTHER BENEFITS: TANGIBLE IMPACT ON HEALTH MEASURES

Since the introduction of the fatigue monitoring device and its data, we have supported a small number of staff who, through our fatigue and welfare management arrangements, have identified underlying health conditions that they were previously unaware of. They all followed up with their family doctor and

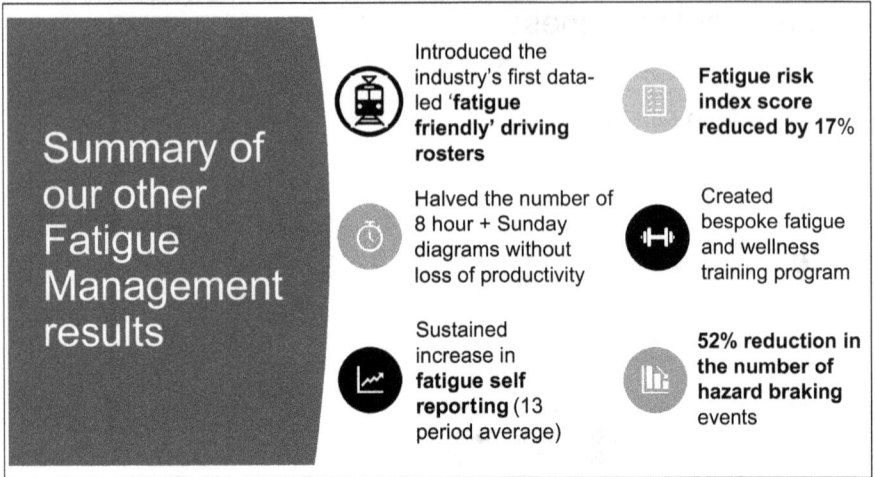

FIGURE 5.1.11 Summary of other fatigue management results of the project.

received a diagnosis and the proper medical treatment. We can now monitor more closely any known health condition of our staff members that may have an impact on fatigue or sleep.

The conditions that affect fatigue that were identified by the fatigue monitoring device included **diabetes, underactive thyroid function,** and **obstructive sleep apnoea**—all of which if untreated have potential to cause serious health issues.

We believe that well-being has been built around a relationship of trust between staff and managers:

- Results can be seen from our experience of a sustained year-on-year **increase in the number of staff fatigue self-reports**.
- Showed a clear demonstration of a **shift in culture** from one of uncertainty to one of trust—indicated that staff members were confident in the quality of management support provided in the event of a fatigue episode occurring.

A summary of other fatigue management results of this project is presented in Figure 5.1.11.

5.1.7 REFLECTIONS

If we were to start the programme again, we would revisit the speed of implementation of the fatigue detection technology. The quick implementation met with some initial pushback from staff who did not fully understand the essence of urgency or the potential benefits. Staff expressed feeling that we were "doing this to them". This in turn put an element of strain on our historically good staff management and relationship with our trade unions.

Our wider communication with staff could have achieved more, to bring more staff with us from the beginning, which could have reduced some of the resistance from staff and embraced the fatigue detection technology quicker.

As part of our continuous improvement, and the recent implementation of our new rosters in October 2021, we continue to monitor for fatigue using the fatigue monitoring device, which is active the whole time any tram is in operation.

We will continue periodically with our refresher fatigue training to ensure it remains top of mind for our drivers, and any new drivers continue to receive fatigue training as part of their induction. We believe that we still have a way to go to fully embed the fatigue programme into the company culture, and recognise that this will take time, but we are getting there. Keeping staff engaged is an important element of the programme that cannot be underestimated. We will continue to provide staff with regular updates as part of our ongoing safety training days and key awareness messages.

5.1.7.1 EXTERNAL INTEREST

News of our success has travelled fast. In 2019 we hosted visitors from many different business sectors to discuss and share learnings. These included companies that operate light rapid transit systems across Europe, America, Australia, Asia, and Africa; UKTram, UK bus operators, Transport for London, Tideway (operator of the Thames Barrier System); the ORR, the Rail Safety and Standards Board (RSSB), the Rail Delivery Group, Loughborough University, and the Royal Air Force Safety Centre.

5.1.8 CONCLUSIONS: SUMMARY OF THE SUCCESS

As an employer, TOL has a duty of care for their safety critical staff. This can be seen in our responsibility for developing "fatigue-friendly" rosters and scheduling duties for the drivers.

Before and throughout all changes, engagement with trade unions was a vital component when the new rosters and duties were developed. This engagement continues.

We wanted to ensure that our changes were making a difference, and so, using a new process that focuses on just safety culture principles, we gathered feedback and found tangible benefits. Staff absence rates have improved.

Our monitoring of fatigue has helped identify underlying health conditions that some members of staff had but were unaware of them, and we reduced the overall number of significant events identified using the fatigue detection device. Events of microsleep/drowsiness reduced by over 50% each year since it was first monitored in 2018.

Further benefits of investing in our Total Fatigue Management Programme can be seen first-hand in the reduced number of safety incidents resulting from fatigue and distraction.

We have seen a 52% reduction in drivers applying their hazard brake in the first 13 periods since the programme began to date. This type of event is one of the greatest contributors to passenger injuries on board our trams.

By reducing the number of hazard brake applications, we have directly made the on-tram environment safer for our customers and other system users.

Our Fatigue and Wellness Management Programme addresses individual, workplace, and organisational issues that affect fatigue. The programme included:

- cutting-edge staff fatigue and wellness training processes;
- a data-led fatigue friendly roster;
- increased staff engagement in fatigue management;
- used technology to monitor driver alertness.

We are very pleased with the results to date!

5.1.8.1 INDUSTRY RECOGNITION

We have been delighted to receive recognition from both inside and outside of our light rail sector and have captured some of them below:

- TOL won with London Trams–**Highly Commended–for Safety and Security Excellence** in 2018—for the introduction of the Guardian device.
- TOL won with London Trams–Rail Business Awards 2019–**Highly Commended–for Safety and Security Excellence—**for the introduction of the Guardian device.
- 2019 TfL Supplier awards—**Best Safety Initiative** for Total Fatigue Management.
- TOL won **the Significant Safety Initiative** in 2019.
- 2020—Shortlisted for (heavy rail) Safety Health Excellence (SHE) Awards for **Best Safety Project** for Total Fatigue Management.

SUMMARY POINTS FOR PRACTITIONERS

The following points summarise the key takeaways from Tram Operations Ltd.'s journey to improve their fatigue risk management capability:

- Engagement with unions and staff is important to have a clear fatigue management process, which is based on a Just/Open Culture, to enable staff to report when they are fatigued, using a supportive rather than disciplinary approach.
- Using real live staff data helps build insight and trends on your network. Develop and apply fatigue-based rules to your rosters and duties using your own staff data.
- Using insights from hours of work and hours of rest when developing rosters helps to build suitably timed rest periods, reduce impacts from moving between early starts/late finishes, or when returning after days off. Consider any on-call arrangements. Review rosters against a recognised Fatigue Index.
- Establish clear responsibilities for employer, employees, and employees' families.

- Use fatigue and welfare management arrangements to help identify unknown health conditions such as diabetes, sleep apnoea, and thyroid irregularities and to strengthen employee trust through discussions focussing on health, well-being, eating well, exercise and mental well-being.

REFERENCES

European Union (2003). Directive 2003/88/EC of the European Parliament and of the Council. Directives originating from the EU, *88*, 4 November. Accessed December 3, 2022 at: www.legislation.gov.uk/eudr/2003/88/contents/adopted.

HSE (Health and Safety Executive) (2006). Managing shift work: Health and safety guidance. Report no. HSG256. Accessed December 3, 2022 at: www.hse.gov.uk/pubns/priced/hsg256.pdf.

(ORR) Office of Rail and Road (2021). Good practice guidelines–Fatigue Factors. December. Accessed December 3, 2022 at: www.orr.gov.uk/sites/default/files/2021-12/good-practice-guidelines-fatigue-factors.pdf.

(ORR) Office of Rail and Road (2022). ROGS–The regulatory requirements for managing safety on the railways, tramways and other guided transport systems. Accessed December 8, 2022 at: www.orr.gov.uk/guidance-compliance/rail/health-safety/laws/rogs.

(ORR) Office of Rail Regulation (2013). Revised ORR guidance on managing rail staff fatigue. December 17. Accessed December 8, 2022 at: www.orr.gov.uk/media/18545.

SAFTE-FAST (2022). SAFTE-FAST–The Science of Performance at Work. www.saftefast.com.

UK (1998). The Working Time Regulations. UK Statutory Instruments, *1833*. Accessed December 3, 2022 at: www.legislation.gov.uk/uksi/1998/1833/contents/made.

5.2 Assessing Railway Traffic Controller Safety with an Hourly Risk Index

Bart Roets[1,2] and Simon Folkard[3]

[1]Faculty of Economics and Business Administration, Ghent University, Ghent, Belgium
[2]On Track Lab Research Centre and Performance Data Division, Infrabel Belgian Railways, Brussels, Belgium
[3]Department of Psychology, Swansea University, Swansea, UK

CONTENTS

DOI: 10.1201/9781003213154-36

5.2.1 INTRODUCTION: FATIGUE PREVALENCE AND RESEARCH IN RAILWAY TRAFFIC CONTROL

This chapter presents a real-world case study based on Belgium's railway traffic control centres. Building on an intense and continuous collaboration between researchers and practitioners, we not only produced a risk-based model for assessing work schedules, but also validated it with large-scale traffic control data. The model is now implemented through a custom-built business intelligence tool called "EDISON". Our research and implementation efforts were performed in close cooperation with operational and data experts from Infrabel, the public company managing Belgium's railway infrastructure. Infrabel owns and operates the entire Belgian railway infrastructure and is one of the key players in Belgian mobility. Its core activities are asset management (building, maintaining, and renewing the infrastructure) and real-time traffic control.

"Railway traffic controllers" or "train dispatchers" are shiftworkers that work around the clock, in "traffic control centres", "signal boxes", or "dispatching centres". We define railway traffic control as the combination of (1) signalling activities (i.e., the authorisation of train movements), (2) real-time traffic management (i.e., decisions such as re-routing trains to ensure a fluid traffic flow and mitigate train delays), and (3) safety actions. Examples of safety actions are the protection of track maintenance workers through safety locks in the signalling system or launching safety procedures at level crossings. Belgian railway traffic controllers are aligned 24/7 in non-overlapping 8-hour shifts, starting at 06:00, 14:00, and 22:00, and with a maximum of seven consecutive days of shift work.

In Europe, railway traffic control is characterised by a large-scale technological migration towards computerised control centres (Wilson & Norris, 2005; Roets & Christiaens, 2015), which increasingly opens opportunities for in-depth and data-driven research. More generally, the European Union is pursuing the development of a competitive single European railway area that encourages railway infrastructure companies to reduce their costs (see the European Directive 2012/34/EU, 2012). At the same time, railways should maintain and even improve safety levels where practicable (see the European Directive 2016/798/EU on railway safety, 2016). This "Safety Directive" explicitly demands a consideration of human factors, and specifically mentions fatigue as one of the contributing circumstances to be examined in safety investigations.

Despite railway traffic controllers' safety-critical role and the recognised importance of fatigue, fatigue research in the railways has mainly focused on train drivers, and there have been only a limited number of studies involving them (Dorrian et al., 2011). Regardless, research on railway traffic controller fatigue and sleep is growing and has been undertaken world-wide: In Europe (e.g., Sallinen et al., 2005; Fan & Smith, 2018), the US (e.g., Popkin et al., 2001; Raslear et al., 2013), and Australia (Dorrian et al., 2011).

The current paucity of research stands in contrast with the prevalence of traffic controller fatigue in US railways, where traffic controllers and train staff (train and engine workers) have been found to exhibit the highest exposure to fatigue (Gertler et al., 2013). In the United Kingdom, an official investigation (UK Rail Safety and

Standards Board [RSSB], 2015) revealed that fatigue-related incidents were mainly attributable to train drivers, followed however by traffic controllers.

This chapter (1) presents the "Hourly Risk Index" (Roets & Folkard, 2022), a recently developed risk-based model for the evaluation of staff rosters; (2) examines its validity with a large-scale and real-world data set; (3) presents EDISON, a custom-developed business intelligence tool; and (4) concludes with suggestions for future research efforts, for both academics and practitioners.

5.2.2   ESTIMATING WORK SCHEDULE RISK WITH THE HOURLY RISK INDEX

5.2.2.1   Fatigue as a Contributing Factor in Railway Incidents

Patterns of risk can be less predictable in complex and highly protected systems such as railways, aviation, or the nuclear power industry (Gander et al., 2011). In these systems, human performance deficits (due to fatigue or other causes) interact with several safety barriers such as teamwork, automation, or procedures, and as such the link between human performance and safety events is not always clear (Gander et al., 2011; Cabon et al., 2012). Fatigue is typically one of many contributing factors to safety events, whereas in less complex systems, safety events can more easily be linked to a single identifiable cause (such as an individual car driver being fatigued).

The UK RSSB report (RSSB, 2015) identified fatigue as a contributing factor in 21% of 246 "high risk railway incidents" (when considering the entire railway system, and not only traffic control). Within these 51 incidents, work-related fatigue factors were found in 38% of the cases, and home-life-related fatigue factors in 40%. This shows that the employer has some leverage in avoiding fatigue-related incidents, for example, by improving its staff schedules using fatigue risk models. It also makes clear that there is an equally important responsibility of the employee for fatigue management, who must be aware of the possible consequences of being fatigued and should show up to work adequately rested and ready.

5.2.2.2   Why Consider Fatigue-Related Risk and Not Fatigue as Such?

Shiftworkers (such as railway traffic controllers) are particularly prone to safety-related fatigue problems. Improved scheduling of shift work has been recognized as a main countermeasure against fatigue risk (e.g., Anund et al., 2015; Xu & Hall, 2021). In addition to the scientific research on modelling and predicting fatigue levels, another strand of research has focused on the link between fatigue and safety. In other words, this strand of research is concerned with whether increasing fatigue is necessarily accompanied by an increase in safety events.

There is some evidence that this is not always the case. It appears that during a night shift the peak in risk occurs long before that in fatigue. The peak in risk normally occurs around midnight, while that in fatigue occurs in the early hours of the morning (Williamson et al., 2011). In addition, when fatigue levels do reach their maximum, and sleep onset is likely, risk levels have been known to go down again. One explanation for this divergence is the concept of "fatigue awareness", introduced by Cabon et al. (2012). When aware of their own fatigue, tired staff may adopt risk mitigating strategies, such as an intentional increased use of automation (e.g., a higher reliance on autopilot by aircrew) or a greater reliance on team cooperation. The level of awareness is expected to be lower at moderate levels of fatigue, which leads to less protective measures, which in turn leads to a higher safety risk.

For this reason, Infrabel decided to adopt the concept of the "Risk Index" (Folkard et al., 2007). The Risk Index approach can be used to assess the fatigue-related risk associated with an organisation's work schedules. It has the specific advantage that it is directly based on the risk of a safety event, instead of relying on intermediate variables such as fatigue or alertness. This not only takes account of the above-mentioned divergence in fatigue and (fatigue-related) risk patterns, but also makes it more understandable and meaningful for non-academic practitioners (Folkard & Lombardi, 2004).

5.2.2.3   A Brief Historic Overview of the Risk Index and Its Use in Railways

A first prototypic version of the Risk Index was presented by Folkard and Lombardi (2004). The model was innovative in the sense that, in contrast with the prevailing approaches for fatigue assessment, it was directly based on data and trends in safety events in real-world working environments instead of laboratory-based estimations of fatigue and alertness. Evidence-based on several work schedule parameters such as shift sequence and shift length, it provides a risk score for the entire work shift that can easily be interpreted by practitioners. This 2004 Risk Index was further refined by Folkard et al. (2006, 2007). In 2006, the UK Health and Safety Executive (HSE) integrated the Risk Index into their freely available "Fatigue and Risk Index Calculator" tool which organisations could use to assess work schedules. A more complete description of the HSE Risk Index can be found in Folkard et al. (2007).

According to a report from the UK Rail Safety and Standards Board (RSSB) (2015), the HSE Risk Index and its counterpart the Fatigue Index were thought to be the most widely used fatigue risk models in the UK rail industry. A fatigue management survey from 2021 undertaken by the International Union of Railways showed that, among the participating European railway companies that applied a work schedule assessment tool, the HSE Fatigue and Risk Index Calculator was the most commonly used (Macgregor-Curtin et al., 2021). Nevertheless, in June 2021 the HSE removed the old, Excel format calculator from its website arguing that it was "being misused in order to justify work patterns that clearly require further action to reduce fatigue-related risk" (see also Chapter 2.2, Basacik et al.).

In 2017, 10 years after the Folkard et al. (2007) publication on the HSE Risk Index, the Risk Index was updated after an extensive review of the existing literature (Fischer et al., 2017). This led to a revised version of the Risk Index, in which the Risk Index model was re-quantified, based on the most recent research data.

5.2.2.4   Adding Hourly Detail: Creating the "Hourly Risk Index"

Although the Risk Index has the advantage of directly estimating risk through work schedule characteristics, a major shortcoming is its lack of hourly detail. The original

Risk Index was designed to compare overall shift systems/schedules, not as a tool for safety event analysis, and it consequently lacked hourly or within-shift risk estimates.

Therefore, for the purpose of introducing the Risk Index as a tool for Infrabel safety investigators, we developed an hourly version: the "Hourly Risk Index" (Roets & Folkard, 2022). By lifting the temporal resolution of the Risk Index to the hourly level (instead of the current work shift average), we raised the practical applicability of this risk-based model to the same level as the fatigue-based models (which generally make hourly predictions). This is particularly warranted given the fundamental and empirically evidenced discrepancies between time-of-day variations in fatigue and risk (see above). Furthermore, the hourly detail not only substantially improved the accuracy for the current use of the Risk Index as an ex-ante work schedule risk evaluation tool, but also opens the possibility of its use for ex-post enquiries by safety investigators.

5.2.2.5   STRUCTURE AND INTERPRETATION OF THE HOURLY RISK INDEX

For introductory purposes, we provide a brief overview of the concept behind the Hourly Risk Index. The development of the hourly version is based on the most recent scientific insights (provided by Fischer et al., 2017). More details about the Hourly Risk Index model and the underlying empirical studies can be obtained by contacting the authors.

The Hourly Risk Index is based on three components:

1.   The Cumulative risk: shift sequence, recovery afterwards, quick returns between shifts.
2.   The Time-of-Day risk: hour of the day.
3.   The Hours-on-Duty risk: successive hours on duty.

The overall risk score is calculated, in a simple but very transparent way, by multiplying these three individual components:

$$\text{Hourly Risk Index} = \text{Cumulative} * \text{Time-of-Day} * \text{Hours-on-Duty}$$

It is important to note that this approach of considering all risk-contributing factors at the same time (by multiplying them) leads to an evaluation of fatigue risk in its totality: The multiplication simultaneously considers all relevant characteristics of the staff schedule. This stands in contrast with more traditional Hours of Service regulations, whereby violations are only detected for separate, individual aspects of the staff schedule (such as exceeding allowed shift length). In addition, the within-shift detail provided by the enhanced temporal resolution of the Hourly Risk Index delivers insights that go beyond the shift-level protocols and rules imposed by Hours of Service regulations.

It is also important to note that the risk calculation produces a relative risk. This risk is generally expressed as being relative to a chosen "standard" schedule, which means that a score of 1.25, for example, should be interpreted as a "25% higher risk" than the risk of the standard schedule it is compared against. For its application at Infrabel, we took a slightly different approach: After calculating the Hourly Risk Index, we normalised the risk scores by dividing them by the yearly average over the period 2013 to 2018. As such, all Risk Indexes are relative to this 6-year average, which provides an interesting additional characteristic of our risk estimates: Scores higher than 1 are associated with a higher risk than the average of 2013 to 2018, while scores lower than 1 indicate a lower risk than the 6-year average. In addition, and to further increase its transparency for the railway practitioners, we multiplied the risk scores by 100. As such, an Hourly Risk Index value of, for example, 120, can then immediately be interpreted as "a risk level that is 20% above the 6-yearly average", and a score of 80 as being "20% lower than the 6-yearly average".

5.2.3   VALIDATING THE MODEL

5.2.3.1   THE IMPORTANCE OF REAL-WORLD VALIDATION

The HSE Risk Index has been the subject of several validation studies (Greubel & Nachreiner, 2013; Roets & Christiaens, 2019). Validation not only helps in evaluating the power of the Hourly Risk Index, but is also, and most importantly in a real-world context, a crucial instrument for facilitating practitioner buy-in. Validation means, in short, that the developed model is tested to ensure that it does what it is supposed to do. In the case of our risk model, this can be interpreted as "does the Hourly Risk Index adequately reflect an increase in fatigue risk?".

It is important to note that validation of fatigue models in a real-world environment is not a trivial exercise. It can be considerably more challenging than in a well-controlled laboratory environment, where rostering or fatigue effects can be studied "in isolation" and most other extraneous influences or "confounding variables" can be carefully monitored or kept constant (see Fletcher & Dawson, 2001, and Philip et al., 1999 for some good real-world validation examples). We have approached the validation process from two complementary angles: (1) a subjective validation ("face-validation") and (2) an objective validation ("statistical validation").

5.2.3.2   FACE VALIDATION

Face validity means that, when comparing the output of a model with what we would expect using common sense, they seem similar, that is, the model seems to measure what it is supposed to measure. At its core, the concept behind the Risk Index (calculating fatigue risk directly from data from incidents) is much easier to explain than traditional fatigue modelling approaches (which are based not only on laboratory studies but also on more abstract notions such as alertness). As such, the Risk Index is easily understood and has a high face validity. In addition, and because of this high face validity, it should prove easy to verify or dispute (Folkard & Lombardi, 2004). This was clearly confirmed in expert meetings with Infrabel practitioners. The Hourly Risk Index concept, modelling, and interpretation were discussed in detail and, in addition to face validation, the expert feedback was also used subsequently to improve on model interpretation and visualisation (such as normalising against the 6-yearly risk average, see sub-section 5.2.2.5; or displaying relevant operational details such as the duty number, see sub-section 5.2.4.2).

5.2.3.3 GENERATING A LARGE-SCALE DATA SET FOR A STATISTICAL VALIDATION

To statistically validate the Hourly Risk Index, and in close cooperation with Infrabel data engineers, we constructed a unique, purpose-built data set (Roets & Folkard, 2022). The real-world data set contains shift schedule and human error data for approximately 2000 controllers (fully anonymised), for the period 2013 to 2018 (some 8 million working hours). Although the controllers work non-overlapping 8-hour shifts, starting at 06:00, 14:00, and 22:00, and with a maximum of seven consecutive workdays, local management has the flexibility to freely adapt the work schedules (e.g., change the number of consecutive shifts). We considered the actual rosters, and as such captured modifications such as shift swapping or unscheduled absences. To investigate the potential performance improvement of the Hourly Risk Index over the original HSE index, the data set also contains the latter's values, which were calculated at work shift level (and not at the hourly level).

Generated through a custom-built business intelligence tool, our large-scale data set not only contains the risk scores but is also linked with the safety-critical human errors made by the controllers. As all operator actions are supported by a safety system, the probability of a safety event is drastically reduced. However, and although very rare (with less than one safety event per million events: Railways in Europe are labelled as "ultra-safe systems", Amalberti, 2001), safety-critical human errors cannot be totally excluded. All occurring safety events are registered in a specifically designed database that contains the safety-critical errors made by the controllers. All errors are subjected to a thorough examination by safety investigators, who make a distinction between errors without consequences (severity level 1) and those with consequences (severity level 2). Examples of errors with consequences (4.6% of all safety-critical errors) are damages to track switches, damages to rolling stock and overhead wires, or other material damage. During the 6-year period considered in the data (2013 to 2018), there were no safety events that resulted in injuries or fatalities.

5.2.3.4 STATISTICAL VALIDATION

Using the large-scale data set created in the previous step, we evaluated the validity of the Hourly Risk Index and benchmarked it against the HSE Risk Index. We discuss only the main results here; a more detailed analysis can be found in Roets and Folkard (2022).

Figure 5.2.1 displays the average Risk Index values, both for the HSE version and the new hourly version, for the three categories of working hours: hours where no safety event occurred ("no error"), hours where a safety-critical event of level 1 happened ("errors without consequences"), and hours where the more severe errors occurred ("errors with consequences").

The average Hourly Risk Indexes are depicted with the dark bars. The average for the severity level 1 errors (108.9) was clearly higher than the average without error (which is equal to 100). Severity level 2 had an average risk of 149.9, which was

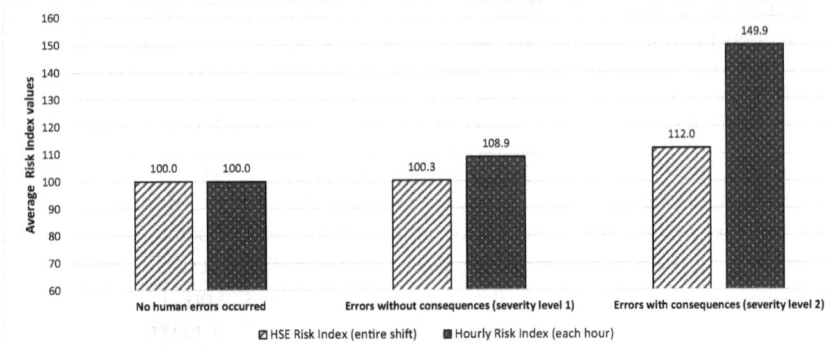

FIGURE 5.2.1 Comparison of risk estimates produced by the HSE Risk Index with the new Hourly Risk Index, for three error categories (no safety-critical errors, errors without consequences, and errors with consequences).

about 50% higher than the risk level in the errorless category. The observed difference in risk for severity level 1 and level 2 was 41. All these differences were statistically significant using a one-tailed t-test, which means that the observed differences are not coincidental, but most likely due to an actual difference in average Hourly Risk Index values.

When we repeated this analysis with the HSE version of the Risk Index (see the pale coloured bars) we observed that the more severe errors were also characterised by a clear, but less pronounced, higher average Risk Index (112.0). However, contrary to the Hourly Risk Index, this shift-level Risk Index did not distinguish significantly between the less severe safety-critical errors (average of 100.3) and the errorless shifts.

We also analysed the impact of each separate component of the Hourly Risk Index (Cumulative risk, Time-of-Day risk, and Hours-on-Duty risk) on error occurrence. The results corroborate the above conclusions, and show that the individual Risk Index components exhibit some predictive power. Importantly, the predictive power of the overall Hourly Risk Index—which multiplies all the individual components and therefore simultaneously considers all relevant work schedule characteristics—is clearly higher.

Taken together, and in addition to the face validity discussed above, these empirical results provide some real-world evidence that the newly constructed Hourly Risk Index has potential in assessing work schedules for safety-relevant fatigue risk, while improving and outperforming its previous version, the Folkard et al. (2007) HSE Risk Index.

5.2.4   PRACTICAL IMPLEMENTATION

5.2.4.1   A "Risk Index Engine" Calculating Hourly Risk

A "risk index engine" implements the Hourly Risk Index functions defined above. Taking work schedules as an input, the engine's algorithms calculate the hourly risk and its components. In the spirit of Open Science, the engine is freely available (along with other biomathematical models, without any warranty and licenced under the GNU Affero General Public License v3.0) in the open source "FIPS" R package (Wilson et al., 2020).

5.2.4.2 A Business Intelligence Tool for Daily Use

Given the high face validity of the Hourly Risk Index, and the evidence provided by the statistical validation, a business intelligence tool called "EDISON" is currently being tested at Infrabel. The application that generated the necessary data sets for the validation study was transformed into a practical tool for safety investigators, with the intention to gradually evolve its systematic use in the context of the company's safety management.

The custom-developed EDISON software tool is designed for daily use by Infrabel safety investigators. The core of the server-based IT system is the risk index engine. The engine is directly connected to the Infrabel's staff rostering application and is seamlessly integrated in a QlikView (Qlik Software Company) business intelligence application. Automatically updated every hour, by querying the staff roster database, the engine calculates the Hourly Risk Index for the past 6 months (for an ex-post safety investigation analysis) and for the next 4 months (for an ex-ante view). Results are immediately displayed in EDISON. Access to this application is strictly limited, and all staff data are anonymised. Only authorised safety investigators can look up the identity of an actual controller, and only on a case-by-case basis.

5.2.4.3 Visualising Fatigue Risk

Simplicity and intuitiveness were the keywords for our visualisation strategy when designing EDISON. Figures 5.2.2 (daily variations) and 5.2.3 (hourly detail) show some screenshots of the EDISON tool. As demonstrated in Figure 5.2.3, users can

Date	Begin	End	Type	Sequence	Duty	Task	Fatigue risk (average)	Fatigue risk (average)	Fatigue risk (maximum)	Cumulative score	Cumulative score
1/12/2020	06:00	14:00	Early	1	4112	B7 SCR CLM		58	69	1,21	
2/12/2020	06:00	14:00	Early	2	4112	B7 SCR CLM		61	73	1,27	
3/12/2020	06:00	14:00	Early	3	4112	B7 SCR CLM		64	76	1,34	
4/12/2020	06:00	14:00	Early	4	4112	B7 SCR CLM		68	80	1,40	
5/12/2020		off			CX	zCX-Compensatie Onr Cyclu				1,18	
6/12/2020		off			RX	zRX-Rust Onreg Cyclus				1,04	
7/12/2020	06:00	14:00	Early	1	4112	B7 SCR CLM		53	62	1,09	
8/12/2020	06:00	14:00	Early	2	4112	B7 SCR CLM		55	65	1,14	
9/12/2020		off			CX	zCX-Compensatie Onr Cyclu				1,07	
10/12/2020	22:00	06:00	Night	1	4312	B7 SCR CLM		125	140	1,20	
11/12/2020	22:00	06:00	Night	2	4312	B7 SCR CLM		142	158	1,36	
12/12/2020	22:00	06:00	Night	3	4612	B7 SCR CLM		160	178	1,54	
13/12/2020	22:00	06:00	Night	4	4912	B7 SCR CLM		180	201	1,73	
14/12/2020		off			RX	zRX-Rust Onreg Cyclus				1,57	
15/12/2020		off			RX	zRX-Rust Onreg Cyclus				1,20	
16/12/2020		off			CX	zCX-Compensatie Onr Cyclu				1,03	

FIGURE 5.2.2 Screenshot of the EDISON tool showing *daily* variations, and presenting, for each shift, the average and maximum Hourly Risk Indexes. For the days off, the cumulative component C is also shown (recovery curve, on the far right).

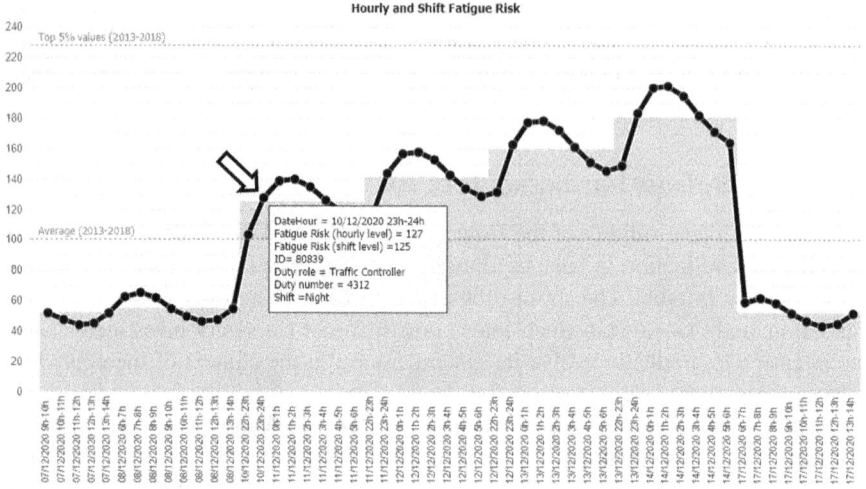

FIGURE 5.2.3   Screenshot of the EDISON tool displaying the *hourly* detail, with the black line showing the Hourly Risk Index, and the grey bars the work shift average (only for the working days).

hover over each individual hour to display more detailed information, such as hourly risk scores or staff roster details (operator role, duty number, anonymous ID, etc.).

5.2.5   CONCLUSIONS AND SOME SUGGESTIONS FOR FUTURE ACADEMIC-PRACTITIONER RESEARCH

In this chapter, we presented a case study rooted in the real-world environment of railway traffic control. We put forward a risk-based model (Roets & Folkard, 2022) that allows the prediction of risk at the hourly level and evaluated its performance by analysing a large-scale data set from Belgium's railway traffic control centres (containing close to 8 million round-the-clock working hours). The validation efforts provided some expert-based and statistical evidence that the development of the Hourly Risk Index is headed in the right direction. Given the results, the model is currently being deployed at Belgian national railways through the "EDISON" tool. It is also currently being tested by Infrabel safety investigators. The tool allows the addition of a fatigue component to safety investigations, and the examination of whether roster-induced fatigue is a contributing factor. Based on the NASA Technology Readiness Level (TRL) scale, EDISON is currently at level 7 out of the nine implementation levels ("prototype demonstration in the operational environment").

The current version of the Hourly Risk Index could be improved in several ways. For example, the existing model does not take into account workload, rest breaks, or the age of the traffic controller. To keep improving the Hourly Risk Index and to address issues like this, the development of the Hourly Risk Index is done iteratively, where (1) scientific literature and research, (2) increasingly more and better real-world data, and (3) feedback from operational experts support the continuous improvement of our fatigue risk estimations. This iterative modelling approach (see Civil Aviation Safety Authority, 2014) will allow us not only to refine the risk model, but also to improve visualisations, increase user acceptance, and gradually move towards its systematic use. Figure 5.2.4, which visualises this approach, was consistently presented to each Infrabel expert, as a basic principle underpinning the intense researcher-practitioner collaboration. In addition to this within-company feedback, we also hope that the free availability of the risk engine in the open source R-package "FIPS" (Wilson et al., 2020) will further support the interaction between fatigue scientists and operations managers (of all kinds of industries), and as such lead to further improvements of the Hourly Risk Index model.

Looking further ahead, research on fatigue-related human error in complex systems (such as railway traffic control) should also consider aspects such as operational complexity and organisational factors (Gander et al., 2011). We are therefore gathering highly disaggregated traffic control data on features such as task complexity, traffic complexity, train delays, coordination tasks, and the use of automation by the operators. Building on this premise, and focusing on railway traffic control operators, we have established strategic partnerships with several European and US universities. Our most recent research has already (1) revealed that traffic control tasks with a highly variable workload are more prone to human error (Roets et al., 2018), (2) identified "operational clusters" (or working conditions) of similar fatigue risk and task complexity (Topcu et al., 2019), (3) empirically examined the impact of workload, fatigue, and operator experience on the use of automation (Dillon et al., 2020), and (4) performed System Dynamics computer simulations to explore the

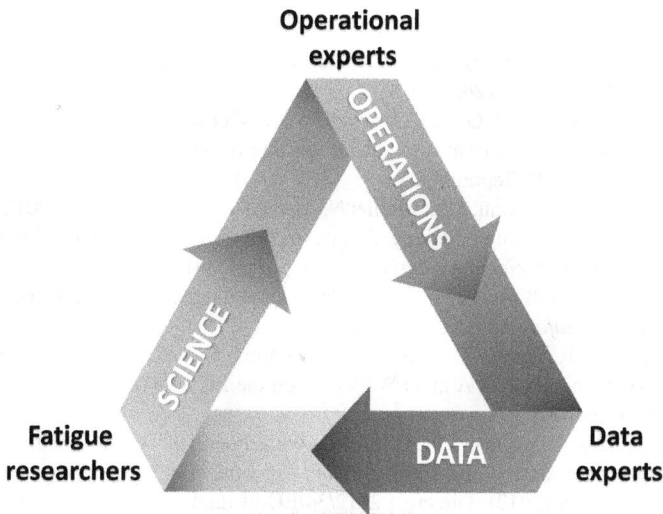

FIGURE 5.2.4 Iterative development approach based on data, science, and operational insight.

non-linear interactions among fatigue, the use of automation, operator workload, and human error (Mahmoudi et al., 2020).

To conclude, there is a need and the potential for work schedule risk assessment in railway traffic control. Since many railway organisations in Europe still seem to focus primarily on Hours of Service regulations (Macgregor-Curtin et al., 2021), it is high time that they also consider managing fatigue risk. Further, railway traffic controller fatigue remains a severely under-researched area, and intense and continuous researcher-practitioner collaborations, such as the one presented in this chapter, are one of the ways to address this shared challenge.

SUMMARY POINTS FOR PRACTITIONERS

- We discuss a real-world case study based on Belgium's railway traffic control centres.
- We present the Hourly Risk Index, a risk-based model for the evaluation of staff rosters.
- The Hourly Risk Index outperforms its predecessor, the Risk Index.
- The model is now being deployed and tested at Belgian national railways.
- A continuous researcher-practitioner collaboration will allow further refinement.

NOTE

The views expressed in this chapter are those of the authors and do not necessarily reflect the opinions of Infrabel.

REFERENCES

Amalberti, R. (2001). The paradoxes of almost totally safe transportation systems. *Safety Science*, 37(2–3), 109–126.

Anund, A., Fors, C., Kecklund, G., van Leeuwen, W., & Åkerstedt, T. (2015). Countermeasures for fatigue in transportation: A review of existing methods for drivers on road, rail, sea and in aviation. VTI Report 852A.

Cabon, P., Deharvengt, S., Grau, J. Y., Maille, N., Berechet, I., & Mollard, R. (2012). Research and guidelines for implementing fatigue risk management systems for the French regional airlines. *Accident Analysis & Prevention*, 45, 41–44.

Civil Aviation Safety Authority (2014). Biomathematical fatigue models, guidance document. *Civil Aviation Safety Authority Australia*.

Dillon, R., Madsen, P., Roets, B., Topcu, T., & Triantis, K. (2020). The autonomous decision system choice. 20th Annual Workshop on the Economics of Information Security (WEIS), Brussels.

Dorrian, J., Baulk, S. D., & Dawson, D. (2011). Work hours, workload, sleep and fatigue in Australian rail industry employees. *Applied Ergonomics*, 42(2), 202–209.

European Commission (2012). Directive 2012/34/EU of the European Parliament and of the Council 21 November 2012 establishing a single European railway area. *Official Journal of the European Union*.

European Commission (2016). Directive 2016/798/EU of the European Parliament and of the Council of 11 May 2016 on railway safety. *Official Journal of the European Union*.

Fan, J., & Smith, A. P. (2018). A preliminary review of fatigue among rail staff. *Frontiers in Psychology*, 9, 634.

Fischer, D., Lombardi, D. A., Folkard, S., Willetts, J., & Christiani, D. C. (2017). Updating the "Risk Index": A systematic review and meta-analysis of occupational injuries and work schedule characteristics. *Chronobiology International*, 34(10), 1423–1438.

Fletcher, A., & Dawson, D. (2001). Field-based validations of a work-related fatigue model based on hours of work. *Transportation Research Part F: Traffic Psychology and Behaviour*, 4(1), 75–88.

Folkard, S. & Lombardi, D. A. (2004). Toward a "risk index" to assess work schedules. *Chronobiology International*, 21(6), 1063–1072.

Folkard, S., Lombardi, D. A., & Spencer, M. B. (2006). Estimating the circadian rhythm in the risk of occupational injuries and accidents. *Chronobiology International*, 23(6), 1181–1192.

Folkard, S., Robertson, K. A., & Spencer, M. B. (2007). A fatigue/risk index to assess work schedules. *Somnologie-Schlafforschung und Schlafmedizin*, 11(3), 177–185.

Gander, P., Hartley, L., Powell, D., Cabon, P., Hitchcock, E., Mills, A., & Popkin, S. (2011). Fatigue risk management: Organizational factors at the regulatory and industry/company level. *Accident Analysis & Prevention*, 43(2), 573–590.

Gertler, J., Di Fiore, A., & Raslear, T. (2013). Fatigue status of the US railroad industry (DOT/FRA/ORD-13/06). Washington, DC: US Department of Transportation, Federal Railroad Administration.

Greubel, J. & Nachreiner, F. (2013). The validity of the risk index for comparing the accident risk associated with different work schedules. *Accident Analysis & Prevention*, 50, 1090–1095.

Macgregor-Curtin I., Nora Balfe, & M. Chiara Leva (2021). Managing and measuring fatigue: a survey of rail industry practices. *Proceedings, Seventh International Rail Human Factors conference*, London.

Mahmoudi, H., Liu, N.Y., Triantis, K., & Roets, B. (2020). A dynamic model of workload and fatigue as predictors of errors in safety critical monitoring roles: Railway traffic controllers. Institute for Operations Research and the Management Sciences (INFORMS), INFORMS 2020 Annual Meeting.

Philip, P., Taillard, J., Guilleminault, C., Quera, S., Bioulac, B., & Ohayon, M. (1999). Long distance driving and self–induced sleep deprivation among automobile drivers. *Sleep*, 22(4), 475–480.

Popkin, S., Gertler, J., & Reinach, S. (2001). A preliminary examination of railroad dispatcher workload, stress, and fatigue (DOT/FRA/ORD-01/08). Washington, DC: U.S. Department of Transportation, Federal Railroad Administration.

[RSSB] Rail Safety and Standards Board (2015). Fatigue and Its Contribution to railway incidents. London, England.

Raslear, T. G., Gertler, J., & DiFiore, A. (2013). Work schedules, sleep, fatigue, and accidents in the US railroad industry. *Fatigue: Biomedicine, Health & Behavior*, 1(1/2), 99–115.

Roets, B., & Christiaens, J. (2015). Evaluation of railway traffic control efficiency and its determinants. *European Journal of Transport and Infrastructure Research*, 15(4).

Roets, B., & Christiaens, J. (2019). Shift work, fatigue, and human error: An empirical analysis of railway traffic control. *Journal of Transportation Safety & Security*, 11(2), 207–224.

Roets, B., & Folkard, S. (2022). Estimating hourly work schedule risk in railway traffic controllers. *Safety Science,* 151, 105757.

Roets, B., Verschelde, M., & Christiaens, J. (2018). Multi-output efficiency and operational safety: An analysis of railway traffic control centre performance. *European Journal of Operational Research*, 271(1), 224–237.

Sallinen, M., Härmä, M., Mutanen, P., Ranta, R., Virkkala, J., & Müller, K. (2005). Sleepiness in various shift combinations of irregular shift systems. *Industrial Health*, 43(1), 114–122.

Topcu, T. G., Triantis, K., & Roets, B. (2019). Estimation of the workload boundary in socio-technical infrastructure management systems: The case of Belgian railroads. *European Journal of Operational Research*, 278(1), 314–329.

Williamson, A., Lombardi, D. A., Folkard, S., Stutts, J., Courtney, T. K., & Connor, J. L. (2011). The link between fatigue and safety. *Accident Analysis & Prevention*, 43(2), 498–515.

Wilson, M. D., Strickland, L., & Ballard, T. (2020). FIPS: An R Package for Biomathematical Modelling of Human Fatigue Related Impairment. *Journal of Open Source Software*, 5(51), 2340.

Xu, S., & Hall, N. G. (2021). Fatigue, personnel scheduling and operations: Review and research opportunities. *European Journal of Operational Research*, 295(3), 807–822.

5.3 Rail Transport

Lessons Learnt in Implementing a Sleep Apnoea Assessment Programme in the Transportation Industry

Daria Luisi[1], Tamara Dumanovsky[2], Laura Bienenfeld[1], Muataz Jaber[1], Nelson Gonzalez[1], and Patrick Warren[1]

[1]Metropolitan Transportation Authority, Brooklyn, NY, USA
[2]Joslyn Levy & Associates, New York, NY, USA

CONTENTS

Disclaimer: This chapter summarises and discusses observations by the authors, who are involved in the Metropolitan Transportation Authority's (MTA) Sleep Apnoea programme. The views and recommendations contained in this chapter represent the personal views of the authors and are not official statements on behalf of the MTA or any other organisation.

DOI: 10.1201/9781003213154-37

5.3.1　OVERVIEW AND INTRODUCTION

Obstructive sleep apnoea (OSA) is a significant medical condition associated with excessive daytime fatigue and a major risk factor for motor vehicle accidents (Patil et al., 2019; Colvin et al., 2016; Karimi et al., 2015; Parks et al., 2009; Tregear et al., 2009). The prevalence of mild, moderate, and severe OSA in the US adult population 30 to 70 years of age is estimated to be 26%, and 10% for moderate and severe OSA (Peppard et al., 2013).

Untreated OSA has been identified as a contributing factor in several major train incidents in the past decade. During this time, the US National Transportation Safety Board (NTSB) recorded three major incidents in the New York City area, which are likely attributable to undiagnosed severe OSA and resultant fatigue. In 2013, a passenger train derailment resulted in four fatalities and 61 injuries. In 2016, injuries associated with a passenger train over-running a bumper post resulted in one fatality and more than 100 injuries. In 2017, a passenger train crash resulted in 108 injuries. Incidents where undiagnosed and/or untreated OSA is a contributing factor can be extremely costly and often tragic for the employees, employers, and the public.

The most commonly recommended treatment for moderate to severe OSA is continuous positive airway pressure (CPAP) which delivers air pressure during sleep, reducing the number of respiratory events during sleep, which improves daytime sleepiness and quality of life. CPAP is recommended because it has been well studied and had demonstrated effectiveness in treating OSA. Other positive airway pressure treatments include bilevel positive airway pressure (BPAP) and autotitrating positive airway pressure (APAP). Oral mouth pieces might also be used in cases of mild or moderate OSA where CPAP is not tolerated, but not recommended for severe OSA. Surgery is recommended only in cases where other treatments have been tried and have not been effective (Mayo Clinic). Research has found that with CPAP treatment and normal amounts of sleep, OSA is no longer a risk for fatigue among older males with OSA (Filtness et al., 2011).

Despite the known risks of untreated OSA to personal and public safety, no federal standards for the transportation industry have been accepted and implemented for the screening, diagnosis, and treatment of sleep disorders. The Railroad Safety Administration Committee (RSAC) of the US Federal Railroad Administration (FRA) recognised this need for federal standards in September 2006 and established a Medical Standards Working Group to develop standards for identifying conditions that could lead to sudden incapacitation or impairment of safety critical personnel (RSAC, 2006). The group convened a Physicians Task Force that developed draft medical standards and protocols. However, the FRA put the working group on hiatus due to the requirement for the FRA to focus on activities mandated in the Rail Safety Improvement Act of 2008, and the critical safety and health issues associated with OSA among safety-sensitive transportation workers were left unaddressed by the FRA.

In November 2016, the Motor Carrier Safety Advisory Committee (MCSAC) and Medical Review Board (MRB) of the US Federal Motor Carrier Safety Administration (FMCSA), the lead federal agency responsible for regulating and providing safety oversite of commercial motor vehicles, submitted a joint recommendation in response to a request for comments on the FRA's Advanced Notice of Proposed Rulemaking (ANPRM) on OSA (MCSAC and MRB, 2016). In 2017, the advanced notice was withdrawn, with the determination that existing safety programmes and the FRA's rulemaking addressing fatigue risk management are the appropriate avenues to address OSA (FMCSA, 2017). Instead, FMCSA continues to recommend drivers and employers use the North American Fatigue Management Program. FRA continues to monitor railroads' OSA programmes and fatigue management plans as part of its Risk Reduction Program, a voluntary, non-regulatory approach to risk management, and its System Safety programme.

A recent position statement by the American Academy of Sleep Medicine on the need to diagnose and treat OSA in the transportation industry recognises the serious health, safety, and financial implications—including fatigue-related crashes and incidents—that can be attributed to transportation workers who perform safety-sensitive functions (Das et al., 2021). In the absence of regulatory requirements, the authors recommend that the transportation industry follow, at a minimum, the 2016 guidelines issued by the FMCSA's MSCAC and MRB in their submission to the FRA, alone or in combination with 2006 guidance by the joint task force of the American College of Chest Physicians, the American College of Occupational and Environmental Medicine, and the National Sleep Foundation (Hartenbaum et al., 2006).

Currently, FMCSA and the US Federal Aviation Administration (FAA) require periodic comprehensive medical evaluations for safety-sensitive employees, while the FRA and US Federal Transit Administration (FTA) regulations do not. For example, transit organisations under FTA oversight have no medical evaluation requirements for passenger vehicle drivers or dispatch and control, which potentially introduces unnecessary risk for organisations regulated by federal entities and their clientele. It is left to states or individual organisations to implement these requirements. Those that choose to do so generally follow the FMCSA's medical evaluation requirements for commercial motor vehicle (CMV) drivers.

As part of its medical evaluation protocols, FMSCA outlines regulatory requirements and guidance for certifying Medical Examiners. This includes standards for medical examination, diagnosis, treatment, and disease management for numerous medical conditions that may severely impair a driver, such as epilepsy, schizophrenia, hypertension, and diabetes mellitus on insulin, with specific determinations for work status requirements. In contrast, OSA is mentioned in the regulations, but without specific medical guidance. While physicians are instructed to evaluate for OSA, the recommendations cover only screening and diagnosis criteria, but do not provide specific guidance on treatment or determinations of work status (FMCSA, 2020).

A national unified framework for OSA evaluation and follow-up would benefit the transportation industry. While the industry currently relies on FMCSA 2016 recommendations, these do not include enough specificity in relation to OSA screening, diagnosis, follow-up treatment, compliance monitoring, and work status determination, and are not consistently implemented across the industry. Federal regulations and standards under a national unified framework would eliminate the variability in implementing OSA programmes and provide clear direction for transportation industry employers to protect their employees and the public from risks associated with untreated OSA.

5.3.2   INCORPORATING OSA SCREENING AS PART OF A BROADER SYSTEM SAFETY PROGRAMME

The MTA has close to 70,000 employees, of which 62,300 across five agencies are in safety-sensitive positions, providing safe and reliable passenger services to 8 million customers daily (before the coronavirus disease 2019 [COVID-19] pandemic). MTA's OSA screening programme is one element in an overall system safety effort to ensure operational safety and improve health and wellness among employees. MTA's Occupational Health Services (MTA OHS) began implementing its OSA screening programme in 2015 and had it fully operational in March 2017. The programme initially focused on screening locomotive engineers and railroad conductors, an approach recommended by the NTSB and the FRA. The programme was later expanded to include other safety-sensitive titles related to passenger services, including train operators, subway conductors, bus operators, tower operators, and employees who operate a company vehicle and have a commercial driver license (CDL). Taken together, these seven titles represent approximately one-third of the unionised workforce and 50% of safety-sensitive titles of the MTA.

MTA OHS incorporates OSA screening, diagnosis, and treatment in all work-related regulatory exams for safety-sensitive workers to determine if the employee has an unacceptable risk for moderate to severe OSA, and has established uniform medical screening criteria across all agencies, which include railroad, subway, and bus systems. Initial screening to identify those at risk of OSA is performed by MTA OHS licenced physicians at MTA medical facilities. As part of the MTA's risk reduction action plan, OSA screenings are conducted at the time of pre-employment physicals, regularly scheduled periodic medical examinations, revisits for diabetes and hypertension, fitness for duty as part of a return-to-work physical, and post-accident evaluation. Specified intervals for OSA compliance are dependent upon periodic regulatory exams. Depending on the exam, these may be annual, or may occur on a 2- to 3-year cycle and may vary across the MTA agencies; these periodic exams are mandated under other federal, state, or company programmes.

Upon arrival at an MTA medical facility, employees complete a screening questionnaire before their medical examination. The initial screening questionnaire includes items that can identify risk for moderate and severe OSA based on the current medical guidelines for fatigue management. The questionnaire includes items from the Snoring, daytime Tiredness, Observed apnoea, and high blood Pressure (STOP) questionnaire (Chung et al., 2008), the Epworth Sleepiness Scale (epworthsleepinessscale.com), additional questions on inappropriate sleepiness during the day (or work shift), and history of motor vehicle crashes or near misses due to fatigue. In addition to the self-reported screening questionnaire, MTA OHS assesses employees against physical criteria that were established as a guideline for physicians based on 2016 FMCSA MCSAC and MRB joint recommendations (MCSAC and MRB, 2016). The physical criteria for OSA risk include:

- BMI>35 AND neck circumference >17″ for men or >16" for women OR
- BMI>35 OR neck circumference >17″ for men (>16" for women) PLUS any of the following: loud snoring, observed apnoeas, diagnosed hypertension requiring medication, and diagnosed diabetes or glucose intolerance.

MTA has an OHS physician review the questionnaire responses with the employee or applicant. The physician conducts a physical assessment when warranted and refers possible cases of OSA to a board-certified sleep specialist for further assessment, including a diagnostic sleep study. MTA OHS then instructs employees and applicants to bring the results of the sleep specialist evaluation, sleep study report, and any treatment recommendations to their designated MTA medical facility for evaluation and documentation. If treatment is recommended by the sleep specialist, MTA permits employees to work during the evaluation process and are given approximately 90 days from screening to achieve treatment compliance. When treatment requires continuous positive airway pressure (CPAP), MTA defines satisfactory compliance as at least 21 out of 30 consecutive days (70%) usage for 4 hours or more (Kribbs et al, 1993). For employees who require CPAP treatment but do not achieve satisfactory compliance, MTA restricts their performance of safety-sensitive duties until they demonstrate satisfactory compliance with treatment. OHS will schedule employee revisits to an MTA medical facility to monitor continued compliance; revisit scheduling varies by MTA agency due to challenges obtaining compliance reports for ongoing post-treatment surveillance, union involvement, and staff resources.

The MTA OHS tracks employee OSA screenings and referrals on a monthly basis. Program data indicate that, at the time of screening, 17% of employees are referred for testing. Among those referred for testing, 90% are diagnosed with moderate to severe OSA. This represents 15% of all employees screened. It is important to note that screening is dependent, in part, on self-reported information. Because of this, the OSA prevalence rate of 15% for MTA safety-sensitive employees is likely a low estimate of the true prevalence in the employee population.

5.3.3 CHALLENGES TO IMPLEMENTING A SCREENING PROGRAMME WITHOUT FEDERAL REGULATORY REQUIREMENTS

In 1989, the MTA developed medical standards to evaluate safety-sensitive employees, and continues to monitor, maintain, and update these standards as needed. These medical standards are designed to ensure that applicants and employees in jobs directly affecting safety of passengers and the broader public are medically and physically fit to perform their job duties without risk to themselves or the public. Over the years, the MTA OHS expanded the medical standards to include additional medical conditions and added standards for OSA in 2015.

To develop its OSA medical standards, the MTA engaged an expert panel from New York University's Occupational and Industrial Orthopedic Center to work with MTA OHS physicians, nurses, and technicians to design an OSA medical assessment process for MTA applicants and employees. After reviewing the relevant research studies and professional organisation guidelines, the MTA medical standards panel outlined criteria for OSA treatment compliance for employees with diagnosed moderate to severe OSA. These compliance criteria closely align with the FMCSA's MSAC and MRB 2016 recommendations. The medical standards establish procedures to guide MTA OHS professional and technical employees in OSA assessment, including tracking forms and protocols for use in documenting medical assessments and obtaining necessary information from the applicants' and employees' health care providers. MTA OHS updated its medical standards at the end of 2016 to include an enhanced screening questionnaire and specific physical screening criteria for OSA.

Implementing a successful screening programme requires key stakeholders to acknowledge the problem, the risks it poses to employees and public safety, and the potential costs and consequences for the organisation and public, and agree that screening, diagnosis, and treatment of employees are needed. The stakeholders include the employer, employees, labour unions, insurance plans, and the public.

The MTA is a unionised workforce with different labour organisations representing workers in each of its five subordinate agencies. Engagement with the MTA workforce and their respective unions is key to implementing and maintaining an effective medical screening programme. As part of the process of developing medical standards for sleep apnoea, beginning in 2015, the MTA held a series of planning meetings with the unions to encourage participation and provide information on the importance and seriousness of OSA to their union members.

MTA's OSA programme is designed so that safety-sensitive employees, who provide passenger service, are appropriately screened for OSA, are referred for further diagnostic testing when needed, and that referral and treatment guidance are followed. The MTA's construction of its OSA programme has highlighted organisational and operational challenges associated with implementing a medical screening programme in the absence of federal regulatory requirements and guidance.

5.3.3.1 IDENTIFYING SAFETY-SENSITIVE TITLES

In creating an OSA screening programme, the MTA first needed to identify which employees should be included in the programme. To this end, the MTA initially focused on passenger services titles that involved the movement of customers on the system, relying on other regulated programmes (including asbestos and silica surveillances, hearing conservation, and respirator testing) and recent incidents to assist with identifying the high-risk safety-sensitive titles. As the programme evolved, and with the support of labour unions, additional safety-sensitive titles were added.

5.3.3.2 IDENTIFICATION OF DIAGNOSTIC TESTING PROTOCOLS

MTA's next challenge was to determine which of the various OSA diagnostic testing protocols would best suit a surface transportation organisation. In 2007, the American Academy of Sleep Medicine recommended that applicants and employees suspected of or diagnosed with OSA undergo an evaluation with a sleep medicine certified pulmonary specialist or other sleep medicine certified specialist to confirm the diagnosis (Collop et al., 2007). When the MTA began its OSA screening programme in

2015, MTA OHS physicians often recommended that employees found to be at risk for moderate or severe OSA follow up with their primary care physicians. However, at that time, the primary care physicians often did not recognise sleep apnoea in the employee as a worker safety risk and so did not refer the employee to a sleep specialist—a practice that inhibited appropriate diagnosis of the condition. As the programme progressed, it became apparent that a sleep specialist was necessary for appropriate diagnosis and treatment.

Consequently, in 2016 the MTA added the requirement for assessment by a sleep specialist to its medical standards. In cases where an MTA OHS physician determines that an employee or applicant requires further assessment based on responses to the screening questionnaire or on the physical criteria, they will be informed that they must be evaluated by a certified sleep specialist before they will be permitted to perform safety-sensitive duties. If employees do not comply, they may be placed on work restrictions; continued non-compliance could lead to termination. The MTA OHS outsourced the screening and diagnosis to three large vendors to cover the service area. To facilitate screening and diagnosis, the MTA recommended a portable monitoring home sleep test (PM HST) for all employees who were referred by the MTA OHS physician, as this was the most efficient and cost-effective way to operationalise the programme. The MTA further determined that the PM HST was the optimal addition to the OSA diagnostic test because it was the quickest process for screening and came at a lower cost, as well as greater availability, and convenience. As part of this process, the sleep specialist would review the PM HST results and determine if an in-lab overnight sleep test (polysomnography, or PSG) was clinically warranted and, if needed, could pre-scribe any additional treatment.

5.3.3.3 MONITORING TREATMENT

Another challenge for the MTA was monitoring OSA treatment compliance and effect-iveness once an employee began treatment. In cases where an MTA OHS screening finds a need for further diagnostic testing, an employee is given 90 days to see a sleep specialist complete a sleep study, begin treatment (if required), and provide a 30-day treatment compliance report. Employees continue in their regular duties during these 90 days. If an employee who is being monitored for treatment compliance presents at one of the MTA medical facilities and has not achieved proper compliance, the employee will be restricted to work they can safely perform for a specified time. For prospective employees, applications will be held for 90 days to allow for compliance.

To monitor continued compliance, employees must routinely provide CPAP usage data. CPAP is the most common treatment recommended by sleep specialists, and this is the case among MTA employees that are assessed for moderate to severe OSA. In the rare cases where the sleep specialist recommends an alternative treatment, OSH will monitor compliance under that treatment. However, differences in programme implementation and union negotiations across the MTA agencies prevented con-sistency in the frequency of continued monitoring. For example, while most agency workforces must provide a 90-day compliance report only once a year, one of the agencies tracks compliance quarterly. To streamline reporting, the MTA encouraged employees to authorise the MTA OHS physicians to directly download compliance data from the CPAC electronic device or the sleep specialist. When an employee fails to provide timely documentation of treatment, the MTA removes the employee from service. An employee's failure to provide timely documentation and subsequent removal from safety-sensitive service are costly to the MTA and can potentially adversely impact operations and maintenance of full service because of the reduction in the active workforce on any given day.

5.3.3.4 INSURANCE COVERAGE

When the MTA committed to implementing an OSA screening and intervention programme there were questions related to insurance coverage for sleep specialists and treatment options. Ultimately, because the MTA is a self-insured organisation, it extended its company health plan to cover OSA screening, diagnosis, and treatment. However, other organisations with limited health plans may have a greater challenge.

Of significance, both self-insured and non-self-insured organisations need to negotiate with management and union health plans for coverage for OSA services. For example, health plans could cover the PSG in an accredited sleep centre, but employees would be responsible for the deductible and/or co-insurance payment. Other insurance plans cover the PM HST or PSG only for those meeting the plan's internal criteria for OSA risk factors.

When adding coverage for OSA to insurance plans, organisations must establish criteria for testing based on whether it is medically necessary for the diagnosis of suspected OSA and outline specific criteria that need to be met to determine whether an in-lab PSG or PM HST is indicated. Each organisation must consider cost-benefit and productivity analyses as they make decisions on how frequently safety-sensitive workers should be screened/rescreened and what type of screenings are acceptable (PM HST and/or PSG). Organisations must then negotiate with their own insurance providers for the costs and procedures covered.

5.3.3.5 UNEXPECTED SUPPLY CHAIN CONSTRAINTS

Each time medical equipment or medications are introduced into a medical protocol, availability of these products can become problematic. Such was the case for the MTA with the June 2021 recall by the US Food and Drug Administration of CPAP and BPAP machines produced by a major manufacturer. This recall caused an unexpected external challenge to the programme. Specifically, it affected employees' ability to comply with the programme and the availability of crews to operate the transportation system. To overcome this challenge, the MTA proactively secured as many machines on the market as possible to give employees new equipment in cases where their CPAP equipment had been recalled. In addition, MTA negotiated with one of the health plans to assist with appropriate messaging and established a dedicated hotline for employees to call and receive information on the recalled machine. MTA's procurement department covered all costs related to providing new machines and instructed payment to go directly to the durable medical equipment company. The MTA considered access to this medical equipment to be a high priority for its OSA-affected employees. The identification and follow-up with employees placed an increased burden on OHS staff in the middle of the COVID-19 pandemic. When supply chain issues occur, significant work is required to ensure employee access to equipment, or the agency must be prepared to pull the employees from service for safety reasons.

5.3.4 DISCUSSION

The MTA's experience with its OSA screening programme over the last 6 years has highlighted several challenges that are not directly addressed in the current FMCSA recommendations and would benefit from more specific guidance from the federal government to support the surface transportation industry.

As part of its programme, the MTA identified specific job titles related to the movement of passengers and to customer safety. The MTA evaluated which titles to include by considering the level of risk for occupational sleep loss or fatigue, and the likelihood of an existing yet untreated sleep disorder contributing to an accident or incident. During the development of the programme, the MTA identified a list of risk factors that may affect performance of shift workers and workers in passenger service. The MTA continues to review these and other risk factors related to OSA and the potential impacts on safety to identify additional titles for inclusion in the screening programme. The establishment of federal standards, consistent with existing medical standards for other medical conditions, could provide clear definitions of titles and work responsibilities for inclusion in the OSA screening programme.

Decisions about the appropriate testing protocols were influenced, in large part, by the challenges of screening many employees in the shortest amount of time, establishing contracts that could meet the demand across multiple agencies with many locations, the need to keep some containment on budgetary considerations, and by the need to maintain a consistent and steady workforce. The MTA and similar agencies would benefit from having government or industry standards or recommendations that would ensure coverage of appropriate employees.

The MTA found establishing protocols to monitor long-term treatment adherence and imposing work restrictions for non-adherence to be especially challenging. Specifically, there was limited research and guidance as to how often compliance should be checked, when an employee should be removed from service for non-compliance, or when it is safe to return them to duty after restarting treatment. For example, the accepted CPAP compliance rate of at least 70% (Kribbs et al., 1993) does not address non-compliance and the ability to perform work safely, and questions remain as to whether compliance rate is the best criterion to measure treatment effectiveness. For example, significant improvements in reaction time and attention may be demonstrable within one week of continuous nightly use of effective pressure; however, maximum improvement in these functions may require several months, and improvement in overall cognitive and executive functions may require longer compliance (Sutherland at al., 2015).

Monitoring continuing, long-term compliance with CPAP treatment varies by MTA agency due to a variety of factors. These include differences in employee populations at each of the agencies, work tasks that require sustained attention, shift work, employees who work alone, safety critical positions, employees who operate equipment, likelihood of loss of life and damage to property as a result of a hazard, and negotiations with union agreements for restrictions. Consequently, organisations must include their labour partners early in the programme development process.

Another concern is that there are no standardised criteria for determining work status, which is often established in negotiations with key stakeholders and not based on medical research. The MTA was left to decide through internal policy development the duration of any work restrictions by adapting work restriction policies developed with key stakeholders to include physical and medical limitations due to OSA. In addition, it is critical that unions and employees understand that discontinuation of CPAP or other recommended therapy for even one night may result in significant impairment even if the employee is not aware (Filtness et al., 2012). At the MTA, the OHS physician considers the possibility of other medical conditions that could cause an acute serious reaction. Some medical conditions will not be known to the employee or their operating department and often a decision made by the OHS physician to place restrictions on an employee is questioned by both the union and the employee as to its validity. The MTA OHS physician, using their professional judgement, may recommend work restrictions that create challenges with union leadership and operations and result in a shortage of employees and the inability to meet desired service levels.

5.3.5 CONCLUSIONS

The MTA continues to be responsive to the safety concerns of its employees, customers, and the public, while at the same time providing reliable service. The addition of the OSA screening and compliance monitoring to its safety management or programme further ensures this commitment to safety. Given the experiences described above and illustrated by MTA's OSA programme, it would be useful for the FRA Railroad Safety Administration Committee to revisit OSA recommendations to further protect the railroad workforce and their customers. Current federal OSA recommendations for annual medical examinations for transportation employees do not explicitly require transportation organisations to enforce sleep apnoea guidelines (American Academy of Sleep Medicine, 2016).

Many of the challenges outlined above could be clarified and addressed in the FMCSA recommendations, or with additional FRA guidance for the transportation industry, providing companies with clear direction on programme implementation and ongoing operations. Regardless of whether there are any mandated requirements, below are some key steps to consider before implementing an OSA programme that are based on the MTA's experiences to date.

SUMMARY POINTS FOR PRACTITIONERS

- Establish a fatigue management committee as part of the organisation's system safety programme. This should include internal and external stakeholders.
- Develop and enforce medical standards for transportation employees in safety-sensitive positions. Include:
  a. Identification criteria for who to screen, by title or work responsibilities.
  b. Criteria for screening: when, how, and frequency.
  c. Interpretation of the treatment protocols in relation to fitness for duty and restrictions.
  d. Definitions of specific treatment methods as part of the overall benefits for improvement.
- Define acceptable risk for an individual with comorbidities such as diabetes or hypertension.
- Develop a post-OSA surveillance programme.
- Establish a tracking and monitoring system which interfaces with the organisation's safety system(s).

REFERENCES

American Academy of Sleep Medicine. (2016). *Hidden health crisis costing America billions: underdiagnosing and undertreating obstructive sleep apnea draining healthcare system.* https://aasm.org/advocacy/initiatives/economic-impact-obstruct ive-sleep-apnea/

Chung, F., Yegneswaran, B., Liao, P., Chung, S. A., Vairavanathan, S., Islam, S., Khajehdehi, A., & Shapiro, C. M. (2008). STOP questionnaire: A tool to screen patients for obstructive sleep apnea. *Anesthesiology,108*(5):812–821.

Collop, N. A., Anderson, W. M., Boehlecke, B., Claman, D., Goldberg, R., Gottlieb, D.J., Hudgel, D., Sateia, M., & Schwab, R. (2007). Clinical guidelines for the use of unattended portable monitors in the diagnosis of obstructive sleep apnea in adult patients. *JCSM: Official Publication of the American Academy of Sleep Medicine, 3*(7):737–747.

Colvin, L. J., & Collop, N. A. (2016). Commercial motor vehicle driver obstructive sleep apnea screening and treatment in the United States: An update and recommendation over-view. *Journal of Clinical Sleep Medicine: JCSM: Official Publication of the American Academy of Sleep Medicine, 12*(1):113–125. https://doi.org/10.5664/jcsm.5408

Das, A. M., Chang, J. L., Berneking, M., Hartenbaum, N. P., Rosekind, M., Ramar, K., Malhotra, R. K., Carden, K. A., Martin, J. L., Abbasi-Feinberg, F., Aurora, R. N., Kapur, V. K., Olson, E. J., Rosen, C. L., Rowley, J. A., Shelgikar, A. V., Trotti, L. M., & Gurubhagavatula, I. (2021). Enhancing public health and safety by diagnosing and treating obstructive sleep apnea in the transportation industry: An American Academy of Sleep Medicine position statement. *Journal of Clinical Sleep Medicine: JCSM: Official Publication of the American Academy of Sleep Medicine.* Advance online publication. https://doi.org/10.5664/jcsm.9670

Federal Motor Carrier Safety Administration. (2017, August). *FMCSA and FRA Withdraw Advance Notice of Proposed Rulemaking on Obstructive Sleep Apnea among Commercial Motor Vehicle Drivers and Rail Workers.* U.S. Department of Transportation. www. fmcsa.dot.gov/newsroom/fmcsa-and-fra-withdraw-advance-notice-proposed-rulemak ing-obstructive-sleep-apnea-among.

Federal Motor Carrier Safety Administration. (2020, April). *National Registry of Certified Medical Examiners Program: Medical Examiner Handbook 2020 Edition.* U.S. Department of Transportation. www.fmcsa.dot.gov/advisory-committees/mrb/draft-fmcsa-medical-examiner-handbook-4-23-2020.

Filtness, A. J., Reyner, L. A., & Horne, J. A. (2011). Moderate sleep restriction in treated older male OSA participants: Greater impairment during monotonous driving compared with controls. *Sleep Medicine, 12*(9):838–843.

Filtness, A. J., Reyner, L. A., & Horne, J. A. (2012). One night's CPAP withdrawal in otherwise compliant OSA patients: Marked driving impairment but good awareness of increased sleepiness. *Sleep and Breathing, 16*(3):865–871.

Hartenbaum, N., Collop, N., Rosen, I. M., Phillips, B., George, C. F., Rowley, J. A., Freedman, N., Weaver, T. E., Gurubhagavatula, I., Strohl, K., Leaman, H. M., Moffitt, G. L., American College of Chest Physicians, American College of Occupational and Environmental Medicine, & National Sleep Foundation (2006). Sleep apnea and commercial motor vehicle operators: Statement from the joint task force of the American College of Chest Physicians, the American College of Occupational and Environmental Medicine, and the National Sleep Foundation. *Chest, 130*(3):902–905. https://doi.org/10.1378/chest.130.3.902

Karimi, M., Hedner, J., Häbel, H., Nerman, O., & Grote, L. (2015). Sleep apnea-related risk of motor vehicle accidents is reduced by continuous positive airway pressure: Swedish Traffic Accident Registry data. *Sleep, 38*(3):341–349. https://doi.org/10.5665/sleep.4486

Kribbs, N. B., Pack, A. I., Kline, L. R., Smith, P. L., Schwartz, A. R., Schubert, N. M., Redline, S., Henry, J. N., Getsy, J. E., & Dinges, D. F. (1993). Objective measurement of patterns of nasal CPAP use by patients with obstructive sleep apnea. *The American Review of Respiratory Disease, 147*(4):887–895. https://doi.org/10.1164/ajrccm/147.4.887

Mayo Clinic. Patient Care and Health Information, Diseases and Conditions, Obstructive Sleep Apnea (July 27, 2021). www.mayoclinic.org/diseases-conditions/obstructive-sleep-apnea/diagnosis-treatment/drc-20352095.

Motor Carrier Safety Advisory Committee and Medical Review Board. (2016, November). *MRB Task 16-01 Report.* Federal Motor Carrier Safety Administration, U.S. Department of Transportation. www.fmcsa.dot.gov/advisory-committees/mrb/final-mrb-task-16-01-letter-report-mcsac-and-mrb

Parks, P., Durand, G., Tsismenakis, A. J., Vela-Bueno, A., & Kales, S. (2009). Screening for obstructive sleep apnea during commercial driver medical examinations. *Journal of Occupational and Environmental Medicine, 51*(3): 275–282. https://doi.org/10.1097/jom.0b013e31819eaaa4

Patil, S. P., Ayappa, I. A., Caples, S. M., Kimoff, R. J., Patel, S. R., Harrod, C. G. (2019). Treatment of adult obstructive sleep apnea with positive airway pressure: An American Academy of Sleep Medicine systematic review, meta-analysis, and GRADE assessment. *Journal of Clinical Sleep Medicine, 15*(2):301–334.

Peppard, P. E., Young, T., Barnet, J. H., Palta, M., Hagen, E. W., & Hla, K. M. (2013). Increased prevalence of sleep-disordered breathing in adults. *American Journal of Epidemiology, 177*(9), 1006–1014. https://doi.org/10.1093/aje/kws342

Railroad Safety Advisory Committee. (2006, September). *Railroad Safety Advisory Committee Task Statement: Medical Standards for Safety-Critical Personnel, Task No.: 06-03.* Federal Railroad Administration, U.S. Department of Transportation. https://rsac.fra.dot.gov/tasks

Sutherland, K., Phillips, C. L., & Cistulli, P. A. (2015). Efficacy versus effectiveness in the treatment of obstructive sleep apnea: CPAP and oral appliances. *Journal of Dental Sleep Medicine, 2*(4):175–181.

Tregear, S., Reston, J., Schoelles, K., & Phillips, B. (2009). Obstructive sleep apnea and risk of motor vehicle crash: Systematic review and meta-analysis. *Journal of Clinical Sleep Medicine: JCSM: Official Publication of the American Academy of Sleep Medicine, 5*(6):573–581.

U.S. Food and Drug Administration. (2021, November). *Philips Respironics CPAP, BiPAP, and Ventilator Recall: Frequently Asked Questions.* www.fda.gov/medical-devices/saf ety-communications/philips-respironics-cpap-bipap-and-ventilator-recall-frequently-asked-questions

5.4 Marine Transport
Using Technologies for Managing the Risk of Fatigue at Sea

Michelle Grech

The University of Queensland, Brisbane, Australia

CONTENTS

5.4.1 FATIGUE IN MARITIME TRANSPORT

For decades, seafarer fatigue has been and continues to be a major concern in shipping and for the international maritime safety regulators. Maritime groundings and collisions at sea continue to highlight the issue of fatigue and the limited recognition still evident on the need to apply effective fatigue risk management approaches (Grech, 2016). This is still an ongoing issue with more recent marine accident investigation reports continuing to point to limited or lack of effective fatigue risk management approaches at sea.

As an example, on 17 October 2020, in the early hours of the morning (04:46 hours) the oil tanker *Atina* with a crew of 21 onboard struck a stationary oil and gas production platform while attempting to anchor in the Gulf of Mexico, off the coast of Louisiana (NTSB, 2021). According to the report, the master had not slept in the 24-hour period prior to the collision. The master[1] indicated that he had wanted to anchor the ship as soon as possible because he was tired. The location he chose to anchor did not match the planned anchoring location, a situation which resulted in the *Atina* getting too close to the oil and gas production platform, subsequently making heavy contact. The platform's four crew members and one technician had to evacuate by helicopter to another nearby platform after

DOI: 10.1201/9781003213154-38

activating the emergency shutdown. No one was injured; however, damages to the platform and vessel were estimated to be around $73.5 million. The US National Transportation Safety Board (NTSB) determined that the ship operating company did not allow sufficient time for a proper handover[2] to the master prior to him joining the ship, which resulted in the master being fatigued during an attempted night-time anchoring operation. The incoming master, without having any hand-over period, was required to take command of a vessel that he had never served on before, under pilotage (pilotage is required for the passage due to the complexities associated with navigating the ship through the Mississippi River and into the Gulf of Mexico) on the Mississippi River, at night, after having travelled by air and other means for a journey of about 54 hours from his home in Turkey. The use of fatigue monitoring wearable technologies in this case would have likely detected the level of fatigue that the master was experiencing at the time. This would have alerted and/or provided an early indication to both the master and the company that performance and safety were potentially compromised and with proper training and procedures early control measures would have been put in place to mitigate such a situation.

Similar to the above example, accident investigation reports and research continue to identify several shortfalls, such as long working hours without break, shortened sleep, poor scheduling practices, high work demands, and others with limited application of science-based fatigue management practises at sea (Grech, 2016; Dohrmann & Leppin, 2016). Operational challenges posed by shipping create conditions conducive to fatigue. Apart from being a 24 hours per day operation, seafarers spend long periods of time working on a ship, with some working up to 11 continuous months at sea, which is the maximum period allowed by international regulations. As well, seafarers may need to work under harsh environmental conditions, such as extreme temperatures, humidity, and ship motion. There is also evidence to suggest that some operators may limit the size of the crew to the minimum complement allowed by the regulations (World Maritime University, 2020). Such conditions can have their toll, with sleep loss identified as a common issue at sea (Jepsen, Zhao, Pekcan, Barnett & Van Leeuwen, 2017). Continuous exposure to sleep loss leads to situations in which individuals lose their ability to recognise their diminished performance and can lead to a mismatch in how they feel and how they perform, which increases the potential of operational errors with negative safety outcomes. Thus, the need to manage the risk of fatigue appropriately is crucial to make maritime transport safer.

The use of fatigue monitoring technologies supplemented by training and procedures at sea can provide an important layer of defence to manage the risk of fatigue, with wearable technology now able to track the level of fatigue. Such systems can allow the master and/or the shipping company to manage and schedule working hours based on the actual fatigue level among the crew rather than just relying on fixed schedules. The rest of this chapter will focus on the current state of fatigue risk management at sea and illustrate how various technologies could be used to manage the risk of fatigue at sea.

5.4.2   CURRENT STATE OF FATIGUE RISK MANAGEMENT AT SEA

The International Maritime Organisation (IMO) is the global standard-setting authority for safety, security, and environmental protection of international shipping. Its main objective is to create a regulatory framework for the shipping industry that is fair and effective, universally adopted, and universally implemented. The International Labour Organisation (ILO) sets out global labour standards on ships through the Maritime Labour Convention (2006). Its main aim is to ensure that seafarers are afforded the same protection and rights as shore-based workers ensuring decent working and living conditions for all seafarers on ships.

Presently, strategies to mitigate the effects of fatigue in maritime transport are primarily centred on regulatory approaches, including limits to "hours of work and rest" and to some extent safe crewing determination levels. These regulations are set out by the IMO and the ILO, and are in turn applied by Flag States that are required to regulate ships registered under their Flag. Port States provide a level of oversight through Port State control inspections ensuring ships registered in any country coming into their port are meeting their obligations and are complying with the various conventions that apply to them, as set out by the IMO and the ILO. Ensuring that they operate with a safe crewing level as per IMO requirements, which is approved by the Flag State, is one of these requirements. The safe crewing determination incorporates an evaluation of the appropriate number of qualified crew required to ensure safe shipboard operations. Consideration of fatigue is critical in evaluating the number of crew required to operate a ship safety and effectively. However, the global industry mainly relies on hours of work and rest requirements to manage the risk of fatigue at sea with these minimum standards put in place to create a level playing field for all ship operations across the industry. So, although they can be considered as sensible and generally positively affect shipboard safety, there are limitations in these approaches. The main issue here is that the hours of work and rest requirements are not enough to guarantee that the appropriate quality and quantity of sleep has been obtained. In effect, the combination of utilising the minimum regulatory requirements for hours of rest or work (i.e., ten hours rest in any 24-hour period and 77 hours rest in any seven-day period, or 14 hours work in any 24-hour period and 72 hours work in any seven-day period) and the maximum time onboard allowed prior to repatriation (11 months) for seafarers guarantees that fatigue will be present, with more work needed to manage the risk of fatigue at sea. Importantly, several independent recent studies (Sampson, Ellis, Acejo & Turgo, 2017; Baumler, Singh Bhatia & Kitada, 2021) have identified systemic hours of work and rest recording malpractices across the industry, with some companies even ignoring the minimum safe crewing levels making the situation more dire.

It is common for seafarers to end up working longer schedules than originally planned with the continued pressure to complete tasks and deliver cargo with minimum delays. Unfortunately, fatigue impacts their ability to accurately assess their fitness for duty and make decisions that put themselves and/or others at increased risk. This also brings into question the effectiveness of current company managed recording practices limiting accurate feedback related to seafarers' workload and rest.

These issues were recognised internationally in 2015, with the IMO embarking on a review of the guidelines on fatigue, aiming to ensure the reviewed guidelines meet contemporary approaches and science to fatigue management. This brought to attention the fact that the existing legislation and regulations are not singularly able to address some of the systemic risks that cause fatigue. For example, even if crewmembers work within time limits set by regulations, they may still be unable to sleep if their rest periods are at times when they are used to being awake. So, although the prescriptive approach to fatigue management provides a good starting point, it does not properly address all the factors that can lead to fatigue, such as quality of sleep obtained, work duties, personal situation, general health, time of day, etc. In addition, seafarers have limited and, in some cases, no ability to take action to manage fatigue because of the minimal support in understanding its emergence and its potential dire consequences. Most importantly, there is limited support in what to do if it does manifest. The tendency among many seafarers is to continue working and ignore the warning signs and, in combination with the pressures to complete tasks, ensure the ship continues to deliver on time as per schedule (Andrei, Grech, Ho, McIlroy, Crous, Griffin & Neal, 2018).

The aspect of managing the risk of fatigue using goal-based approaches has become best practise in industries such as aviation (Hobbs, Bedell Aver & Hiles, 2011), with maritime attempting to follow a similar approach through the IMO. The use of a fatigue risk management approach is also based on the premise that fatigue is an inevitable part of work and, in some contexts such as the maritime domain, this cannot be avoided and hence needs to be appropriately managed. For example, a person working during night-time, irrespective of how well-rested, is still battling their circadian rhythms and will experience some level of fatigue. Prescriptive approaches that specify limits to hours of work and rest alone do not consider these circadian aspects and hence the implementation of fatigue risk-based approaches is crucial to ensure safety in the maritime domain.

5.4.3 CURRENT APPROACHES TO FATIGUE RISK MANAGEMENT

The IMO revised their *Guidelines on Fatigue* (MSC 1598), which were published in 2019 (International Maritime Organisation, 2019). Central to these guidelines is the concept of a risk-based approach to fatigue management. This means applying a scientifically based, data-driven approach to continuously monitor and manage fatigue-related safety risks. Since fatigue affects the safe operation of a ship, fatigue management should logically be an integral part of safety management systems. In all circumstances, the guideline encourages that fatigue risk management approaches should ensure that seafarers are provided with the recovery, rest and sleep periods necessary to enable them to perform their work effectively and safely irrespective of the type of work schedules in place. The revised guidelines on fatigue management are intended to be used as part of a ship's safety management system (SMS), as it follows the same principles of risk identification, assessment, and mitigation. Figure 5.4.1 depicts a fatigue risk management framework that is based on Dawson and McCulloch's (2005) conceptual basis of managing fatigue model and has been adopted by the IMO to manage the risk of fatigue at sea (Grech, 2016).

Risk Based Approach

Hazard Assessment Listed in order of effectiveness with risk mitigations for the top rows providing for more robust fatigue control measures.	Risk Mitigation
A. Is company providing effective **support** for managing the risks of fatigue?	• Training and Awareness • Adequate Resources • Healthy shipboard environment
B. Are seafarers provided with adequate **sleep opportunity**? (Quantity and Quality)	• Hours of work and rest requirements • Duty Scheduling and Planning • Workload Management • Work and Living Environment
C. Is the **sleep obtained** adequate? (Quantity and Quality)	• Company and seafarer responsibility
D. Are seafarers able to **maintain adequate alertness** and performance while on duty?	• Self and Peer Fatigue Monitoring • Ensuring 'Fit for Duty'
E. Are fatigue related events (near miss and accidents) **reported and analysed**?	• Fatigue Reporting and Analysis

FIGURE 5.4.1 Fatigue risk management framework adopted in the IMO guidelines on fatigue (Grech, 2016).

The IMO's guideline on fatigue includes some information on self-assessment tools that can be utilised by companies and seafarers alike to monitor sleep, levels of fatigue and sleepiness. These are mainly presented in the form of manual checklists for conducting risk assessments. Although self-assessment tools are useful and valid methods to assess and monitor sleep and fatigue, they require manual input which can be cumbersome, and subject to error and information gaps. Using technology to supplement fatigue risk management approaches has gained some traction in recent years as advanced science-based technological developments have emerged in this area.

5.4.4 TECHNOLOGY TO SUPPORT FATIGUE RISK MANAGEMENT AT SEA

Technologies that objectively predict or detect seafarer fatigue can be used to effectively complement or even replace current prescriptive hours of work and rest regulatory approaches. Such technologies can be used to support fatigue risk management to holistically manage the risk of fatigue. Aspects such as planning and monitoring work and sleep are associated with reducing the risk of fatigue as they can support work scheduling and workload management, and ensure that work and living environments support sleep, alertness, and performance. Most of these planning and monitoring aspects of fatigue risk management can now be supported through the use of technology. Some of these are described next.

5.4.4.1 Technology to support Fatigue Planning

As highlighted in Section 3, fatigue is affected by many factors. Many of the key aspects that impact fatigue are captured by biomathematical models—which are used to predict the risk of fatigue (e.g., through reduced alertness and/or perform-ance), sleepiness, and sleep opportunity based on sleep/wake histories and/or work schedules (Mallis, Mejdal, Nguyen & Dinges, 2004; Dawson, Darwent, & Roach, 2017; Chapter 4.3 of this book). Biomathematical models have been used to some degree in the maritime industry mainly in research settings to quantify the degree of sleep opportunity afforded by a watch schedule and, by inference, the *relative likelihood* of a fatigue-related error occurring (Dawson, Noy, Harma, Åkerstedt & Belenky, 2011; Riedya, Fekedulegn, Andrew, Vila, Dawson & Violanti, 2020). Biomathematical modelling tools assist in planning and designing work schedules which reduce the risk of fatigue and allow for science-based approaches to be used in predicting the most conducive work schedules to apply and identify "hot spots" for consideration.

Most of these biomathematical models are based on Borbély's (1982) two-process model of sleep regulation, which includes the interaction of (1) homeo-static need for sleep and (2) circadian rhythm, reflecting the underlying mechanism of fatigue. A three-process model which has recently become more pervasive in the scientific literature adds a sleep inertia process that captures the decrease in alertness that occurs immediately after waking (Ingre et al., 2014). Both the two- and three-process models are commonly applied as fatigue forecasting tools in aviation (Civil Aviation Safety Authority, 2014), but are not yet widely used in a maritime setting. A recent study applying biomathematical models in a submarine context identified that such models are useful for general scheduling purposes such as comparing prospective shift schedules (Wilson, Ballard, Strickland, Boeing, Cham, Griffin & Jorritsma, 2021). Biomathematical models are typically used by those responsible for shift scheduling to identify schedules that place individuals at high risk of fatigue during vulnerable periods at work, such as when sleep loss and circadian misalignment may combine to increase the risk for performance degradation. It is conceivable that such models could be used in a maritime context and would allow better scheduling that is, for example, more conducive to circadian rhythms and sleep need.

There are many biomathematical models in use, with some available commercially [e.g., FAID (Roach, Fletcher & Dawson, 2004), SAFE (Belyavin & Spencer, 2004), SAFTE (Hursh, Redmond, Johnson, et al., 2004)] or publicly (Ingre et al., 2014)]. It is important that biomathematical tools selected for use in a maritime operational setting include the key criteria of being valid, reliable, sensitive, specific, and gener-alisable. In addition, validation of these criteria should be done in the actual maritime operational environment. Notwithstanding, compared to compliance with prescrip-tive hours of work and rest requirements, there is little doubt that biomathematical fatigue modelling tools significantly improve the capacity to predict the likelihood of fatigue across different watch schedules and should be part and parcel of any fatigue risk management approach.

Although such technologies are useful for planning purposes, they do not con-sider the reality of individual differences and are limited in terms of how well they model medical conditions, including sleep disorders. Due to these limitations of biomathematical models, monitoring each person onboard a ship can provide that added layer of information to monitor what is actually happening in "reality" and whether tweaking the prediction and planning in place is necessary. There have been recent advances in fatigue science making monitoring more accessible and affordable by measuring fatigue through wearable devices and video-based technologies, which can be done in "real time" and/or retrospectively. Fatigue monitoring can support shift scheduling and countermeasures put in place for planning purposes by allowing issues to be identified early on and rectified as necessary.

5.4.4.2 TECHNOLOGY TO SUPPORT FATIGUE MONITORING

Technologies that objectively detect or predict worker fatigue may be used effectively to complement or even replace prescriptive regulatory approaches. Over the last decade, there have been substantial advances in these technologies, which have been validated in operational settings. Devices mainly include wearable (i.e., devices that measures actigraphy or electroencephalography (EEG)) and video-based (i.e., those that measure ocular movement) devices that are able to support fatigue management approaches through real-time monitoring.

Wrist actigraphy devices, also referred to as activity monitor watches, have been used in research for decades to study fatigue and sleep. These devices provide the advantages of being portable, easy to use and able to collect sleep data over a long period of time. However, the cost associated with these devices limits their use to research applications. Recent advancements in a new generation of wearable devices such as wrist activity watches that measure actigraphy and smart caps that measure EEG (which measure changes in brainwaves which have been shown to be valid biomarkers of fatigue) have made them more accessible and provide for a larger array of measures (Dawson, Searle & Peterson, 2014). Wrist actigraphy provides an objective and accurate measure of sleep/wake timing and duration (Sadeh, Hauri, Kripke & Lavie, 1995). Some of these technologies can now be harnessed to a smartphone, which makes fatigue and performance monitoring less invasive and widely available. A study conducted onboard 13 ships using a combination of actigraphy data through wearable devices, reaction time tests, and subjective performance measures examined the effects of shift schedules on fatigue in 30 participating seafarers. Although the study was limited in size and focused on Swedish ships, the results identified dangerously high levels of sleepiness among some of the crew, showing the usefulness of such technology in identifying seafarer fatigue risks on certain shifts (Lutzhoft, Dahlgren, Kircher, Thorslund & Gillberg, 2010). More recently, maritime protection and indemnity (P&I) insurance clubs, recognising the impact of fatigue and its potential serious consequences, started working with shipping companies, investigating the use of wearable technology to monitor fatigue and enable the identification of fatigue "hot spots" within ship operations as a risk mitigation strategy. Another wearable technology which is being trialed in a maritime setting is the SmartCap, validated and widely used in mining in Australia. SmartCap technology uses EEG sensors embedded under a baseball cap with a sweatband, or a headband, with an electronic processor card attached. Data is wirelessly transmitted and allows for remote monitoring through an App (Universidad de Chile, 2015). It provides threshold scores of sleepiness and alerts the wearer if they start showing signs of fatigue. P&O maritime logistics have teamed up with SmartCap technology to trial this wearable technology to test its effectiveness in monitoring fatigue across their crew (P&O News, 2021).

Advances in the area of wearable technology now allow for biomathematical model predictions to be "individualised" through the use of individual "actual" sleep data (such as actigraphy), which takes into account individual differences and provides for more accurate predictions. These predictions can be used in combination with fitness for duty testing (performance measures), which can be, for example, applied prior to a watch schedule, to individuals conducting safety critical tasks (i.e., navigating). In combination with historical actigraphy data, such information could be used to validate the biomathematical model and, in turn, to estimate changes in an individual's alertness or performance over the ensuing watch schedule.

Performance-based monitoring systems can use embedded measures of performance (i.e., vessel track keeping; closest point of approach (CPA) and the frequency and magnitude of engine and rudder orders as a measure of performance) which are generally non-intrusive.

Today, fatigue monitoring technology allows for real-time monitoring of alertness or performance during work, with such measures able to show a trend in alertness or performance prior to reaching a set threshold at which operational performance is negatively impacted. These approaches may not necessarily detect fatigue; rather they detect behaviours and performance that can lead to unsafe conditions (i.e., performance is used as a proxy for fatigue).

This provides the ability to monitor operational readiness and assess the situation facilitating informed decision-making to ensure that appropriate control measures are put in place, if and when required.

Other monitoring technologies which are currently primarily applied for car driver fatigue monitoring use video-based analysis utilising modulated infra-red light that capture eyelid behaviour or indirect measures. PERCLOS (percent eye closure) is one example and has been reliably associated with attentional lapses and driving performance (Ayoob, Grace & Steinfeld, 2005; Balkin, Horrey, Graeber, Czeisler & Dinges, 2011). There now exist technologies supported by research that permit automated analysis in real-time, making this technology a viable option for monitoring in a variety of operational environments (Fredriksson, Lenné, van Montfort & Grover, 2021). This has also informed the development of European Commission regulations which have now mandated this type of technology in European Union cars from 2023 onwards (Hynd, McCarthy, Carroll, Seidl, Edwards, Visvikis, et al., 2015; Euro NCAP, 2017). To ensure reliability, these types of monitoring systems are designed to collate multiple measures of drowsiness including blink duration, amplitude-velocity ratio, and frequency which are more likely to capture more patterns of drowsiness behaviour (Ingre, Åkerstedt, Peters, Anund, & Kecklund, 2006). Currently being extensively applied for driver monitoring, the system uses strategically placed cameras to capture driver attention and level of alertness. New systems are being integrated into cars and being programmed to escalate actions through alerts or warnings to progressively slow or stop the car if the driver is no longer able to drive the car safely. These types of technologies offer new opportunities to manage individual distraction and drowsiness in real time and could present real opportunities for similar technologies to be installed on the bridge of a ship.

5.4.5   CONCLUSIONS

Fatigue risk management systems supported by technology provide the ability to predict and plan for fatigue to minimise risk while ensuring minimal disruption and operational safety. Biomathematical models and tools that are widely available provide the ability to assess the risks associated with various watch schedules that may be under consideration. Technology can now measure and monitor fatigue and performance both retrospectively and in real time. Doing so can also provide the feedback loop and check required to evaluate the biomathematical models' predictions and planned schedules and provides the ability to intervene when potential "hot spots" or issues are identified.

Technologies available today are sensitive enough to detect early indications of fatigue and are capable of accurately and proactively predicting fatigue in individual operators, making tools like actigraphy and other monitoring devises especially suitable for fatigue management in operational environments. With the use of such technologies, rules and regulations on hours of work and rest could be supported or redesigned to require that shipboard operations maintain adequate levels of objectively monitored alertness/performance of seafarers. This would reflect a more goal-based approach and is a change in emphasis that would more directly address the issues of ultimate concern. This could potentially provide for a more effective approach to limiting fatigue. However, of equal importance is the organisational safety culture within which such technology is being used. Therefore, for such technological approaches to work effectively they must occur within a positive safety culture of learning (awareness training), non-disciplinary, no blame reporting of fatigue/not being fit for duty, and other elements of good fatigue management practices.

SUMMARY POINTS FOR PRACTITIONERS

- Fatigue impairment is recognised as a hazard and continues to be a major risk in maritime operations
- Accident investigations and research continue to highlight work-related shortfalls and limited application of fatigue risk management approaches at sea.
- Maritime operations rely on traditional prescriptive approaches to managing fatigue at sea, through limiting hours of work and rest.
- Commercially available fatigue detection and monitoring technologies can be used as a way to mitigate fatigue risk and support fatigue management systems. These technologies allow for real-time monitoring of sleep, alertness and/or performance during work allowing the identification of "hot spots" during operations.
- Technologies available today are sensitive enough to provide early indications of fatigue and are capable of accurately and proactively predicting fatigue in individual operators.
- This technology shows promise as useful elements of a broader fatigue risk management system at sea.

NOTES

1 The Master is the highest seafarer rank on a ship with overall responsibility for everything that happens onboard his or her ship, including the security of the ship, as well as the safety of the crew and cargo, both when in port and when at sea.
2 Handover is an important function that is carried out when an incoming master relieves the current master with several formalities and procedures involved as part of the process. This process is critical to taking command of a ship especially if the incoming master is new to the ship and its crew, as it provides for a smooth and safe transition. In this case, the investigation identified that the company's safety management system required an overlapping period of at least one day for senior officers, and at least seven days for new senior officers. This would have enabled the incoming master to get some rest and receive a proper handover.

REFERENCES

Andrei, D., Grech, M., Ho, J., McIlroy, T., Crous, R., Griffin, M., & Neal, A. (2018). *Assessing the determinants and consequences of safety culture in the maritime industry.* A report based on the findings of research grant LP130100215. Accessed 28 February 2022 assessing-the-determinants-consequences-of-safety-culture-in-maritime-ind.pdf (amsa.gov.au)

Ayoob, M.A., Grace, R., & Steinfeld, A. (2005). *Driver-Vehicle-Interface (DVI) Development of a Drowsy Driver Detection and Warning System for Commercial Vehicles* (Report CMU-RI-TR-05-46). Carnegie Mellon University, Pittsburgh, Pennsylvania.

Balkin, T. J., Horrey, W. J., Graeber, R. C., Czeisler, C. A. & Dinges, D. F. (2011). The challenges and opportunities of technological approaches to fatigue management. *Accident Analysis and Prevention, 43* (2011), 565–572.

Baumler, R., Singh Bhatia, B., & Kitada, M. (2021). Ship first: Seafarers' adjustment of records on work and rest hours. *Marine Policy,* 130, August 2021, 104186.

Belyavin, A. J., & Spencer, M. B. (2004). Modeling performance and alertness: The QinetiQ approach. *Aviat. Space Environ. Med., 75* (Suppl. 3), A93–A103.

Borbély, A. A. (1982). A two-process model of sleep regulation. *Human Neurobiology, 1* (3), 195–204.

Civil Aviation Safety Authority (2014). *Biomathematical Fatigue Models Guidance Document. Australian Government*, Civil Aviation Safety Authority. Accessed 27 February 2022, http://refhub.elsevier.com/S0003-6870(21)00059-4/sref21.

Dawson, D., Darwent, D., & Roach, G. D. (2017). How should a bio-mathematical model be used within a fatigue risk management system to determine whether or not a working time arrangement is safe? *Accident Analysis and Prevention, 99*, 469–473. https://doi.org/ 10.1016/j.aap.2015.11.032.

Dawson, D., & McCulloch, K. (2005). Managing fatigue: It's about sleep. *Sleep Medicine Reviews, 9*(5), 365–380.

Dawson, D., Noy, Y. I., Härmä, M., Åkerstedt, T., & Belenky, G. (2011). Modelling fatigue and the use of fatigue models in work setting. *Accident Analysis and Prevention, 43*(2), 549–564.

Dawson, D., Searle, A. K., & Paterson, J. L. (2014). Look before you (s)leep: Evaluating the use of fatigue detection technologies within a fatigue risk management system for the road transport industry. *Sleep Medicine Reviews, 18*(2), 141–152.

Dohrmann, S. B. & Leppin, A. (2017). Determinants of seafarers' fatigue: A systematic review and quality assessment. *International Archives of Occupational and Environmental Health, 90*, 13–17.

Euro NCAP (2017). *Euro NCAP 2025 Roadmap—In pursuit of Vision Zero.* Available online at: https://cdn.euroncap.com/media/30700/euroncaproadmap-2025-v4.pdf.

Flynn-Evans, E. E., Kirkley, C., Young, M., Bathurst, N., Gregory, K., Vogelpohl, V., End, A., Hillenius, S., Pecena, Y., & Marquez, J. J. (2020). Changes in performance and bio-mathematical model performance predictions during 45 days of sleep restriction in a simulated space mission. *Science Reports, 10* (1), 15594. https://doi.org/10.1038/s41598-020-71929-4.

Fredriksson, R., Lenné, M. G., van Montfort, S., & Grover, C. (2021). European NCAP program developments to address driver distraction, drowsiness and sudden sickness. *Frontiers in Neuroergonomics, 2*, 786674. doi: 10.3389/fnrgo.2021.786674

Grech, M. R. (2016). Fatigue risk management: A maritime framework. *International Journal of Environmental Research and Public Health, 13*, 175. doi:10.3390/ijerph 13020175.

Hobbs, A., Bedell Avers, K., & Hiles, J. J. (2011). *Risk management approaches in aviation maintenance: Current best practise and potential future countermeasures.* Report No: DOT/FAA/AM-11/10. Assessed 13 July 2022, http://rosap.ntl.bts.gov/view/dot/20808.

Hursh, S. R., Redmond, D. P., Johnson, M. L., Thorne, D. R., Belenky, G., Balkin, T. J., Storm, W. F., Miller, J. C. & Eddy, D. R. (2004). Fatigue models for applied research in warfighting. *Aviation, Space and Environmental Medicine, 75* (Suppl. 3), A44-A60.

Hynd, D., McCarthy, M., Carroll, J., Seidl, M., Edwards, M., Visvikis, C., et al. (2015). *Benefit and Feasibility of a Range of New Technologies and Unregulated Measures in the Field of Vehicle Occupant Safety and Protection of Vulnerable Road Users.* Transport Research Laboratory for the European Commission.

Ingre, M., Åkerstedt, T., Peters, B., Anund, A., & Kecklund, G. (2006). Subjective sleepiness, simulated driving performance and blink duration: Examining individual differences. *Journal of Sleep Research, 15*, 47–53. doi: 10.1111/j.1365-2869.2006.00504.x

Ingre, M., Van Leeuwen, W., Klemets, T., Ullvetter, C., Hough, S., Kecklund, G., Karlsson, D., & Åkerstedt, T. (2014). Validating and extending the three process model of alertness in airline operations. *PloS One, 9* (10), e108679. https://doi.org/ 10.1371/journal.pone.0108679.

International Maritime Organisation (2019). *Guidelines on Fatigue.* MSC.1/Circ.1598. 24 January 2019.

Jepsen, J., Zhao, Z., Pekcan, C., Barnett, M., & Van Leeuwen, W. (2017). Risk factors for fatigue in shipping, the consequences for seafarers' health and options for preventive intervention. In: MachLachlan, M. (Ed.) *Maritime Psychology,* Springer, Cham, pp. 127–150.

Lutzhoft, M., Dahlgren, A., Kircher, A., Thorslund, B., & Gillberg, M. (2010). Fatigue at sea in Swedish shipping-A field study. *American Journal of Industrial Medicine, 53*, 733–740.

Mallis, M. M., Mejdal, S., Nguyen, T. T., & Dinges, D. F. (2004). Summary of the key features of seven biomathematical models of human fatigue and performance. *Aviation Space and Environmental Medicine, 75* (Suppl. 1), A4–A14.

[NTSB] National Transportation Safety Board (2021). *Contact of Tanker Atina with Oil and Gas Production Platform SP-57B.* Issued November 10, 2021. MAB-21/24.

P&O News (2021). P&O *Maritime Logistics launches industry-first deployment of SmartCap fatigue management system.* Accessed 17 July 2022. https://pomaritime.com/news/po-maritime-logistics-launches-industry-first-deployment-of-smartcap-management-system/.

Riedya, S. M., Fekedulegn, D., Andrew, M., Vilaa, B., Dawsone, D., & Violanti, J. (2020). Generalizability of a biomathematical model of fatigue's sleep predictions. *Chronobiology International, 37*(4), 564–572. doi:10.1080/07420528.2020.1746798.

Roach, G. D., Fletcher, A. & Dawson, D. (2004). A model to predict work-related fatigue based on hours of work. *Aviation, Space and Environmental Medicine, 75* (Suppl. 3), A61–A69.

Sadeh, A., Hauri, P. J., Kripke, D. F., & Lavie, P. (1995). The role of actigraphy in the evaluation of sleep disorders. *Sleep, 18*(4), 288–302.

Sampson, H., Ellis, N., Acejo, I., & Turgo, N. (2017). *Changes in Seafarers' Health 2011-16: A Summary Report. Cardiff.* Retrieved 13 February 2019 from http://orca.cf.ac.uk/116526/1/Changes%20to%20seafarers%27%20health%202011-2016.pdf.

Universidad De Chile (2015). *Evaluation of "SmartCap" technology designed to monitor on-line the fatigue level of workers.* Sleep and Chronobiology Laboratory, Department of Physiology and Biophysics, School of Medicine. University of Chile. Accessed 17 June 2022, at SmartCap-Field-Validation-UdC-Full-Report.pdf (ukconstructionmedia.co.uk).

Van Dongen, H. P., Maislin, G., Mullington, J. M. & Dinges, D. F. (2003). The cumulative cost of additional wakefulness: dose-response effects on neurobehavioral functions and sleep physiology from chronic sleep restriction and total sleep deprivation. *Sleep, 26*, 117–126.

Wilson, M. D., Ballard, T., Strickland, L., Boeing, A. A., Cham, B., Griffin, M. A., & Jorritsma, K. (2021). Understanding fatigue in a naval submarine: Applying biomathematical models and workload measurement in an intensive longitudinal design. *Applied Ergonomics, 94*, 103412.

World Maritime University (2020). *A culture of adjustment, evaluating the implementation of the current maritime regulatory framework on rest and work hours (EVREST).* World Maritime University. (Attributed authors: Baumler, R., De Klerk, Y., Manuel, M.E., and Carballo Piñeiro, L.). Accessed 27 February 2022. https://commons.wmu.se/lib_reports?utm_source=commons.wmu.se%2Flib_reports%2F66&utm_medium=PDF&utm_campaign=PDFCoverPages.

5.5 Fatigue and Sleepiness in UK Policing

Yvonne Taylor

National Police Wellbeing Service, College of Policing, Ryton-on-Dunsmore, Warwickshire, UK

CONTENTS

5.5.1 INTRODUCTION: ORGANISATION AND PRIMARY DUTIES

The Metropolitan Police, established in September 1829 with the introduction of the Metropolitan Police Act, was the first organised police force within England and Wales. Today, there are 43 territorial police forces within England and Wales with similar boundaries to local government geographical areas (Emsley, 2012). These are shown in Figure 5.5.1.

The primary duties of police officers have not altered greatly over the years. The Statement of Common Purpose and Values for the Police Service in England & Wales, adopted in 1990, stated that

> The purpose of the police service is to uphold the law fairly and firmly; to prevent crime; to pursue and bring to justice those who break the law; and to keep the Queen's Peace; to protect, help and reassure the community; and to be seen to do all this with integrity, common sense and sound judgement.

> *Association of Chief Police officers, 1990*

In order to fulfil these duties, policing operates on a 24-hour basis, incorporating variable shift patterns, to service incoming demand, operate efficiently, and conduct the pro-active prevention, reduction, and detection of crime and disorder (Taylor, 2020).

The number of police officers in the 43 territorial police forces is approximately 123,171, with 103,347 of those in frontline policing roles (Home Office, 2019). Although exact numbers of those working shifts (as opposed to those consistently

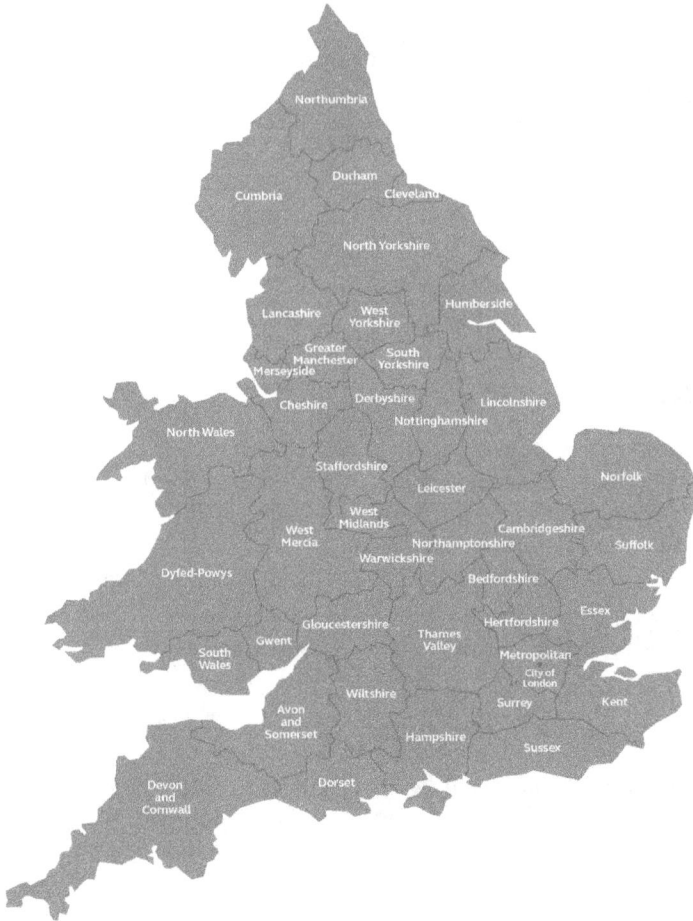

FIGURE 5.5.1 Police forces in England and Wales. © College of Policing Ltd—Reproduced and adapted by Yvonne Taylor with permission under licence number SF00266.

working regular daytime hours) are not available, it is presumed that those in the frontline roles would be the officers providing that 24-hour response service—there to respond to emergencies, whatever the time of day or night. There are also civilian staff members, such as control room staff, who work shift patterns. All of these personnel are working long hours, around the clock, often at times when it is not customary to be awake (Horrocks & Pounder, 2006). These staff and officers often have to make rapid decisions under time pressure, or are required to drive under stressful conditions, for example, having to respond to emergency calls in a timely fashion (Vila, 1996).

Vila (2006) suggests that police officers are a group of workers that are of concern with regard to their risk of fatigue. However, their experiences could also be similar to those in other occupational groups who work long hours or extended shifts (Caruso,

2014), such as those in the transportation industry, medical staff, and others. Shift work, extended hours, and fatigue are all thought to increase the risk of impaired performance, workplace accidents, and road traffic collisions (Dorrian et al., 2017). Fatigue is thought to contribute to up to 20% of serious collisions in the UK (Jackson et al., 2011). However, as a causation factor, it is believed to be under-represented in road traffic collision statistics, often attributed to other causes, such as driver distraction (Jackson et al., 2011).

Those individuals having to drive for work purposes are potentially at higher risk of being involved in a fatigue-related collision than those who do not drive for work purposes (Clarke et al., 2009). In addition, shift workers suffer from more fatigue whilst travelling to and from work, than those who work daytime hours (Rogers et al., 2001). The reasons for this difference are not fully understood; however, sleep restriction and circadian disruption are believed to be a contributory factor to fatigue amongst shift workers (Clarke et al., 2009).

Fatigue, along with irregular and disrupted sleep, is often seen as a "normal" aspect of policing, with police shift workers often sleep deprived and in a chronic state of "shift lag" (Vila, 1996). However, these topics have traditionally been given little attention within policing in England and Wales, possibly because managers typically have little knowledge or awareness of the effects of shift work on fatigue (Oexman et al., 2002), or what to do to alleviate the related problems. Often, joining the policing family will be the first time that officers or staff have worked shifts or irregular hours. Due to this, they may be unaware of many of the risks associated with lack of sleep and the disruption of the circadian rhythm, particularly whilst working night shifts (Horrocks & Pounder, 2006). This lack of knowledge and inability to address the consequences of fatigue have implications for the health and well-being of police officers and staff and also affects the wider organisation, as it often results in increased instances of stress-related illness and work absences (Scholarios et al., 2017).

5.5.2 PECULIARITIES IN POLICING AND HOW SHIFT PATTERNS HAVE EVOLVED

Shift work, particularly night shift or rotating shift work, is known to cause sleep disturbances and reduction (Scholarios et al., 2017). Currently, there is no universally agreed, ideal shift system that will suit all shift workers and eliminate the associated problems. However, there are suggested recommendations that will minimise the adverse effects of these working patterns. For example, a rapid forward rotating system, which begins with day shifts, followed by afternoon shifts, then night shifts, with sufficient time for rest between shifts, and the avoidance of extended shifts, may be preferable to other systems such as weekly, backward rotation, for example (Knauth & Hornberger, 2003). This is because delaying the rhythm is more compatible with the human body clock, and is associated with improved sleep quality and reduced fatigue, along with fewer social and psychological problems (Tucker, Smith, Macdonald, & Folkard, 2000). Despite this recommendation (which will not work for all organisations), fatigue associated with shift work can still be problematic, causing safety concerns, including those related to driver fatigue (James & Vila, 2015).

TABLE 5.5.1
Traditional Regulation Police Shift System

Week	Monday	Tuesday	Wednesday	Thursday	Friday	Saturday	Sunday
1	Night	Night	Night	Night	Night	Night	Night
2	Rest Day	Rest Day	Afternoon	Afternoon	Afternoon	Afternoon	Afternoon
3	Afternoon	Afternoon	Rest Day	Rest Day	Day	Day	Day
4	Day	Day	Day	Day	Rest Day	Rest Day	Rest Day

Shift systems have changed and developed in policing over the years, as they have in other industries. However, shift patterns are still many and varied and involve a difficult balance of managing public demand, organisational need, and officer and staff welfare (Mason, 1999). Traditional, regulation police shift systems in England and Wales provided a continuous, 24-hour cover by officers and staff working a "traditional regulation shift pattern" of 8-hour shifts, covering nights (22:00 to 06:00 hours), then afternoons (14:00 to 22:00 hours) and then days (06:00 to 14:00 hours). This was originally believed to be the most effective method of covering the 24-hour period (Stone et al., 1993). This backward rotating pattern is shown in Table 5.5.1.

The effectiveness of the traditional regulation shift pattern, such as performance indicators, along with officer welfare and morale, was challenged over the years, and shift systems in policing have evolved. This was, in the main, to try to match police resources to crime patterns and demands for service in order to deploy resources where and when they were required (Richbell et al., 1998), rather than just covering the 24-hour period with equal numbers of officers and staff on three 8-hour teams. For example, by providing longer shift length, it allowed a shift overlap at times of greatest demand (Totterdell & Smith, 1992). This has also resulted in individual police forces choosing their own shift patterns, rather than all forces following the same pattern.

Trials of alternative shift patterns began in 1989, with various forms of 8-hour shifts and compressed working week systems. One of these systems, known as the "Ottawa shift system" (believed to have first been used by Canadian police, hence the adopted name), was most favoured by UK officers and staff (Richbell et al., 1998; Stone et al., 1993; Totterdell & Smith, 1992). The Ottawa system is shown in Table 5.5.2. The idea of this system was to retain 8-hour night shifts, but to extend the day and afternoon shifts to 10-hour duration, in order to provide additional time for the 6-day rest period following the series of night shifts (Totterdell & Smith, 1992). This system also allowed for a 07:00 hours day shift start time, as opposed to the 06:00 hours start time on the regulation shift pattern (Stone et al., 1993). As such, the shift times for the Ottawa system were generally 07:00 to 17:00 day shifts, 14:00 to 00:00 or 17:00 to 03:00 (Thursday, Friday, and Saturday) afternoon shifts, and 22:30 to 07:00 (Saturday to Thursday) or 23:00 to 07:00 (Friday) night shifts.

When compared with the regulation shift pattern, it was found that those officers working the Ottawa system reported a significant improvement in well-being, reduced disruption of personal life and an increase in average sleep duration (Stone et al.,

TABLE 5.5.2
Ottawa Shift System

Week	Monday	Tuesday	Wednesday	Thursday	Friday	Saturday	Sunday
1	Rest Day	Rest Day	Day	Day	Day	Rest Day	Rest Day
2	Afternoon	Afternoon	Afternoon	Rest Day	Rest Day	Day	Day
3	Day	Day	Rest Day	Rest Day	Night	Night	Night
4	Night	Night	Night	Night	Rest Day	Rest Day	Rest Day
5	Rest Day	Rest Day	Rest Day	Afternoon	Afternoon	Afternoon	Afternoon

1993). However, Totterdell and Smith (1992) also suggested that, due to officers only attaining an average of 6.4 hours daily sleep duration when working the seven consecutive night shifts, a review of the block of night shifts may be required.

In 2004, a study of police resource management revealed that very little research had been done on a national basis in relation to shift patterns. The Home Office (2004) report, later reiterated by the Home Office (2010) circular regarding police officer shift arrangements, put forward a number of observations and recommendations, which included the following:

- Shifts should be forward rotating (days, then afternoons, then nights). This assists in minimising circadian sleep disruption and extending opportunity for sleep.
- Shift length should ideally be between 8 and 10 hours.
- There should be no more than six consecutive shifts before rest days, and no more than four consecutive night shifts in any shift pattern.
- Day shifts should start as late in the morning as possible, for example, 07:00 hours is better than 06:00 hours.
- Rest days should be in blocks of no less than two consecutive days.
- The most effective and efficient shift systems are either a Variable Shift Arrangement (VSA) or a 2×2×2 pattern. VSA allows variation in shift lengths and start and finish times. This provides overlap and additional staff at times of peak demand. This is presented in Table 5.5.3. The 2×2×2 pattern repeatedly rotates two day shifts, two afternoon shifts, and two night shifts, followed by four rest days.
- 12-hour shifts are not recommended, as significant concern exists around health and safety implications of these shifts.

Little additional research has taken place since that described in the 2010 Home Office circular regarding police shift patterns in England and Wales. However, favourable shift patterns are likely to improve safety, welfare, and officer morale and therefore lead to more efficient use of resources and a better quality of service being delivered to the public (Home Office, 2004). Shift changes similar to those recommended by the Home Office and exploration of alternative shift patterns have taken place internationally. In a study of American police officers (Amendola et al., 2011), it was found that

TABLE 5.5.3
Example of a Variable Shift Arrangement (VSA) Shift System

Week	Monday	Tuesday	Wednesday	Thursday	Friday	Saturday	Sunday
1	Day	Day	Day	Day	Rest Day	Rest Day	Afternoon
2	Afternoon	Afternoon	Rest Day	Rest Day	Night	Night	Night
3	Night	Rest Day	Rest Day	Rest Day	Day	Day	Day
4	Rest Day	Rest Day	Afternoon	Afternoon	Afternoon	Afternoon	Rest Day
5	Rest Day	Night	Night	Night	Rest Day	Rest Day	Rest Day

those working 10-hour shifts reported having more sleep and a better quality of life than their colleagues who were working 8-hour shifts. However, when shift length was extended to 12-hours, those officers reported greater levels of fatigue, and lower levels of alertness, when compared with those working 8-hour shifts. As such, it seems that a compressed working week, with 10-hour shifts, provides some compromise and well-being advantages over the shorter or longer alternatives.

All shift systems have some advantages and disadvantages and there is no system that suits all industries and all those who work in them. However, organisations still have much to learn about shift systems in general, including the negative effects that working shifts may have on health, psychological well-being, errors, and performance (Caruso, 2014).

In recent years, austerity has been a driver for police forces seeking to improve efficiency and effectiveness across all areas of policing, and this has resulted in further changes in shift patterns (Barton, 2013). These changes have not always been positive in terms of the effect on fatigue. There is no "one-size-fits-all" approach to policing, including shift patterns (House of Commons Home Affairs Committee, 2008). However, as individual police forces specify their own shift systems, some shift patterns currently in existence, such as multiple consecutive 12-hour shifts, do not appear to take into account the best practice recommendations of the Home Office (2004) and Home Office (2010) reports or the findings from academic research that have shown them to be less favourable.

Ultimately, today's 24/7 policing places a lot of forces and officers under increased pressure to work extended hours (Houdmont & Elliot-Davies, 2016) and shift patterns need to be reviewed regularly to ensure that the best possible balance of health and welfare can be achieved, whilst also meeting the demands of providing a 24-hour service (Taylor, 2020).

Whilst there are many differences in legislation and policing practice around the world, it is suggested that there are also many similarities. Findings in terms of shift patterns, safety, alertness, and well-being are therefore likely to be transferable in many cases.

5.5.3 STAFF HEALTH, SAFETY, AND WELFARE

The Health and Safety at Work etc. Act (1974) and the Police (Health and Safety) Act (1997) impose a duty of care on employers in respect of employee physical and mental health, safety, and welfare, including working practices and working hours. In addition, there are duties on employees to co-operate with their employer, and to take reasonable care of themselves and others. One element of the relevant legislation is the requirement for safe working systems, including working times and practices, staffing levels, supervision and training. Legislation also specifies the need for employers to consult with employees regarding the introduction of measures likely to affect their health and safety, such as, for example, a change in shift patterns (Health and Safety at Work etc. Act, 1974).

In 1998, The Working Time Regulations (1998) were introduced and incorporated into British law as a result of European Working Time Directives. As a result, there were restrictions placed on the maximum average number of hours worked per week (currently 48 hours), a minimum between-shift time period of 11 hours, and a stipulation that a night worker's normal hours of work should not exceed an average of 8 hours in each 24-hour period (The Working Time Regulations, 1998). There are partial exemptions from the directives when it comes to policing, for instance, where there are peculiarities in relation to some operations, such as spontaneous public order incidents, where it cannot be determined how long these may last, and therefore how long officers may be on duty (Wardman & Mason, 1999). However, despite the regulations, most shift patterns currently followed in policing require night shift durations of more than 8 hours, with some forces operating consecutive 12-hour night shifts.

Until recently, fatigue has largely been ignored in police settings. However, excessive fatigue could put other members of the public at risk, if officers make ill-informed decisions when, for example, handling firearms, or driving at high speed, and under pressurised conditions (Vila et al., 2000). In their study of 379 officers in four local police agencies in the USA, Vila and colleagues (Vila et al., 2000) measured the extent of fatigue in police patrol officers, in a bid to identify relationships between fatigue, health, safety, and performance. They found that 59% of officers reported regularly having less than 7 hours sleep per day, and that there was concern amongst the group regarding fatigued colleagues. The authors concluded that police officers should receive training in relation to managing their fatigue, relevant policies should be put in place regarding working hours, and employees should be involved in any fatigue-related policy implementation. The National Police Wellbeing Service surveys conducted in England and Wales in 2019, 2020 and 2021 (Graham et al., 2019; Graham et al., 2020; Graham et al., 2021) concurred with these findings, highlighting high levels of self-reported sleep disturbance and reduced sleep duration amongst officers and staff.

Police officers often perform emotionally and physically demanding roles in a high-pressure environment, and have been found to experience psychological distress and be at high risk of developing post-traumatic stress disorder (PTSD) (Green, 2004). This can come about due to repeated exposure to physically or emotionally distressing and difficult scenes, or from work demands such as extended shifts leading to reduced sleep quality and quantity (Kinman et al., 2012). In this respect, it is perhaps all the more important, then, that work–life balance and officer welfare need to be considered by employers when designing and implementing any changes to shift patterns.

The agenda to improve well-being and welfare is relatively new to policing in England and Wales and has been introduced as a result of research into specific well-being issues in policing and the prevalence of PTSD (Graham et al., 2019, 2020). In addition to health and safety legislation, the onus for welfare and well-being lies on the organisation, and Chief Constables hold a statutory responsibility to manage the welfare of officers and staff (Home Office, 2018). The Home Office is now striving to ensure that every member of policing feels that their welfare and well-being is actively supported by their police force, and that all individuals have access to appropriate support whenever it is needed. The plan to assist in achieving this goal includes promoting a culture focused on support, early intervention, and prevention, with evidence-based standards throughout policing, including through occupational health departments, effective line management, and relevant signposting to external experts, for example, for counselling when required (Home Office, 2018). This clearly must include considerations around working practices, shift patterns, and fatigue management (Taylor, 2020).

5.5.4 STANDARDS OF PROFESSIONAL BEHAVIOUR

Policing has responsibility for many prevention services, different from those of other emergency services, such as fire and rescue. This dictates the need for officers to be alert, available, and on patrol during night shifts in order to prevent and detect crime, or respond to other calls for service (Charman, 2018). This need largely inhibits police officers and staff from sleeping during their night shifts, and indeed, sleeping on duty could be construed as being in conflict with the standards of professional behaviour (Taylor, 2020).

The standards of professional behaviour are a framework outlining the expectations that the police and the public have regarding police behaviour. They are designed to enable everyone to understand what is acceptable versus unacceptable conduct. In particular, sleeping on duty could come into conflict with the following sections of the Code of Ethics (College of Policing, 2014):

- Duties and Responsibilities—*"I will be diligent in the exercise of my duties and responsibilities"*.
- Fitness for work—*"I will ensure, when on duty or at work, that I am fit to carry out my responsibilities"*
- Discreditable Conduct—*"I will behave in a manner, whether on or off duty, which does not bring discredit on the police service or undermine public confidence in policing."*

Police officers are required to behave in a manner which does not discredit the police service or undermine public confidence in it, whether on or off duty (College of Policing, 2014). Arguably, police officers may not be diligent in the exercise of their duties and responsibilities if they are found to be asleep whilst on duty. It could also undermine public confidence in the police service.

On the other hand, if officers comply with these expected standards of professional behaviour and do not nap on duty, they may be awake for many hours, sometimes more than 24 hours and at times when their natural circadian rhythm dictates that they should be asleep. This is then likely to put them at risk of excessive fatigue, experiencing poor physical and mental performance, along with the possibility of impairment levels more than those associated with the current drink drive limit in England and Wales (Dawson & Reid, 1997; Gov.UK, n.d.; Rajaratnam et al., 2013).

As the public service that upholds and enforces the law in relation to road safety, and being open to public scrutiny and accountability, policing organisations need to manage working hours with suitable rest breaks and in consideration of staff well-being (Bullock & Garland, 2019), whilst educating their employees about the dangers of driver fatigue (James et al., 2022).

5.5.5 DRIVER TRAINING, DRIVER SAFETY AND FATIGUE MANAGEMENT IN POLICING

More than a quarter of all recordable road traffic incidents in the UK are thought to be work related (Department for Transport, 2019). In view of that, it may be prudent that those drivers who do drive for work receive some form of additional driver training and fatigue management education relevant to their particular role.

Police drivers have different levels of driver training, depending on their role and requirement to drive within the organisation; however, all generally undergo some form of police-led driver training prior to driving police vehicles. This usually includes both classroom-based and on-road training. The training is in line with the current recommendations in *Roadcraft: The Police Driver's Handbook*, which includes input on driver vulnerabilities and human factors, amongst other topics (Mares, Coyne, & MacDonald, 2013). The College of Policing also specifies national learning standards for police driving through Authorised Professional Practice (APP), which includes various goals for driver education. The APP points out that poor driver attitude and behaviours may undermine the reputation of the police and specify factors that may be influential, including both driving at night and fatigue (College of Policing, 2019). The APP also specifies that police drivers are expected to continually, dynamically self-assess actions and performance and should notify a supervisor if any of the factors, such as fatigue, affects them (College of Policing, 2019). However, nothing is provided by the APP in terms of maximum recommended drivers' hours, or what actions are available to drivers or supervisors should an officer come to them. It remains, then, that there is very little guidance on driver fatigue, whether an officer is on duty, or whilst commuting to and from the workplace. Incorporating further fatigue management training into this syllabus is one way in which to educate staff and improve overall safety (Taylor, 2020).

To better understand whether fatigue management training can improve fatigue amongst police officers, a pilot study (James et al., 2022) trialled a fatigue-management training intervention programme in selected forces within England. The study utilised wrist actigraphy along with validated questionnaires to evaluate the fatigue management training intervention. The results showed that positive behaviour change was evident, leading to significant improvements in both sleep quantity and quality. In addition, there were improvements in overall sleep satisfaction, elimination of dozing at the wheel incidents, along with a reduction in nightmares, daytime sleepiness, constant tiredness, trouble sleeping and hypervigilance symptoms. This is an encouraging step for policing in England and Wales, where effective fatigue management strategies are in their infancy.

5.5.6 CONCLUSIONS

There remains a lack of understanding in relation to fatigue and the effects of shift work in policing in England and Wales, and therefore a lack of guidance on how to manage and mitigate workplace fatigue. In particular, understanding how fatigue and shift work impact safety-critical areas, such as road safety, is needed. Methods to document related information is currently inconsistent, and there is a particular lack of consistency in policies, procedures, and training. Fatigue risk management in policing is in its infancy, but fatigue remains a critical problem that warrants further attention (James et al., 2022; Taylor, 2020).

SUMMARY POINTS FOR PRACTITIONERS

- Policing in England and Wales needs to acknowledge that long working hours and shift work can cause or contribute to fatigue, increasing the likelihood of general ill-health, accidents, injury, and road traffic collisions.
- It may be timely for a national review of shift patterns, with a refresh of guidance on the patterns thought most suitable in terms of balancing well-being with organisational need. This would be beneficial not only for policing, but also for other emergency services and large shift working organisations.
- The Common Goal for Police Wellbeing (Home Office, 2018) stipulates a clear focus on standards related to welfare and well-being. Strategies to deliver these standards need to be developed and fatigue risk management systems should be considered as a necessary part of ensuring statutory responsibilities are met.

REFERENCES

Amendola, K. L., Weisburd, D., Hamilton, E., Jones, G., Slipka, M., Heitmann, A., … Tarkghen, E. (2011). The impact of shift length in policing on performance, health, quality of life, sleep, fatigue, and extra-duty employment. Washington, DC: Police Foundation.

Association of Chief Police officers. (1990). *Statement of Common Purpose and Values.*

Barton, H. (2013). 'Lean' policing? New approaches to business process improvement across the UK police service. *Public Money & Management, 33*(3), 221–224.

Bullock, K., & Garland, J. (2019). 'The organisation doesn't particularly consider itself responsible for you': Organisational support for officers injured in the line of duty and organisational (in) justice. *Policing and Society*, 1–17.

Caruso, C. C. (2014). Negative impacts of shiftwork and long work hours. *Rehabilitation Nursing, 39*(1), 16–25. https://doi.org/10.1002/rnj.107

Charman, S. (2018). From crime fighting to public protection: The shaping of police officers' sense of role. *Perspectives on Policing: Paper, 3.*

Clarke, D. D., Ward, P., Bartle, C., & Truman, W. (2009). Work-related road traffic collisions in the UK. *Accident Analysis & Prevention, 41*(2), 345–351.

College of Policing. (2014). *Code of Ethics: A Code of Practice for the Principles and Standards of Professional Behaviour for the Polising Profession of England and Wales.*

College of Policing. (2019). Police driving. Retrieved December 4, 2021, from www.app.coll ege.police.uk/app-content/road-policing-2/police-driving/.

Dawson, D., & Reid, K. (1997). Fatigue, alcohol and performance impairment. *Nature, 388*(6639), 235. https://doi.org/10.1038/40775

Department for Transport. (2019). Casualties involved in reported road accidents. Retrieved December 4, 2021, from www.gov.uk/government/statistical-data-sets/ras30-repor ted-casualties-in-road-accidents#casualties-involved-in-reported-road-accidents-excel-data-tables.

Dorrian, J., Mclean, B., Banks, S., & Loetscher, T. (2017). Morningness/eveningness and the synchrony effect for spatial attention. *Accident Analysis and Prevention, 99*, 401–405. https://doi.org/10.1016/j.aap.2015.11.012

Emsley, C. (2012). The birth and development of the police. In *Handbook of Policing* (pp. 100–117). Willan.

Gov.UK. (n.d.). The drink drive limit. Retrieved June 17, 2022, from www.gov.uk/drink-drive-limit.

Graham, L., Brown, N., Plater, M., Gracey, S., Legate, N., & Weinstein, N. (2019). *National Police Wellbeing Survey.* Retrieved from https://oscarkilo.org.uk/app/uploads/2020/06/ISSUED-2019-National-Police-Wellbeing-Survey-1.pdf.

Graham, L., Plater, M., & Brown, N. (2021). *National Police Wellbeing Survey.* Retrieved from www.oscarkilo.org.uk/media/2826/download?inline.

Graham, L., Plater, M., Brown, N., & Gracey, S. (2020). *National Police Wellbeing Survey.* Retrieved from https://oscarkilo.org.uk/national-wellbeing-survey-results-published/.

Green, B. (2004). Post-traumatic stress disorder in UK police officers. *Current Medical Research and Opinion, 20*(1), 101–105. https://doi.org/10.1185/030079903125002748

Haslam, C., & Mallon, K. (2003). A preliminary investigation of post-traumatic stress symptoms among firefighters. *Work & Stress, 17*(3), 277–285.

Health and Safety at Work etc. Act. Health and Safety at Work etc. Act 1974, Pub. L. No. 37, Legislation (1974). Retrieved from www.legislation.gov.uk/ukpga/1974/37/contents.

Home Office. (2004). *Study of Police Resource Management and Rostering Arrangements.* London. Retrieved from www.intellicate.com/whitepapers/HO_police_rostering.pdf.

Home Office. (2010). *Guidance on designing variable shift arrangements (VSA) for police officers. 016-2010.* London.

Home Office. (2018). *A common goal for police wellbeing.* London. Retrieved from https://assets.publishing.service.gov.uk/government/uploads/system/uploads/attachment_data/file/721646/common-goal-for-wellbeing-version-3.pdf.

Home Office. (2019). Police workforce open data tables. Retrieved December 4, 2021, from www.gov.uk/government/statistics/police-workforce-open-data-tables.

Horrocks, N., & Pounder, R. (2006). Working the night shift: Preparation, survival and recovery–A guide for junior doctors. *Clinical Medicine, Journal of the Royal College of Physicians of London.* https://doi.org/10.7861/clinmedicine.6-1-61

Houdmont, J., & Elliot-Davies, M. (2016). Police Federation of England and Wales 2016 Officer Demand, Capacity, and Welfare Survey. *Initial Report–Descriptive Results.* London: Police Federation of England and Wales.

House of Commons Home Affairs Committee. (2008). *Policing in the 21st Century: Report, Together with Formal Minutes* (Vol. 2). The Stationery Office.

Jackson, P., Hilditch, C., Holmes, A., Reed, N., Merat, N., & Smith, L. (2011 Fatigue and road safety: A critical analysis of recent evidence. Road safety web publication no . 21, 1–85.

James, L., James, S., & Hesketh, I. (2022). Evaluating the effectiveness of the fatigue and shift working risk management strategy for UK Home Office police forces: Pilot study. *International Journal of Emergency Services, 11*(2), 292–299.

James, S. M., & Vila, B. (2015). Police drowsy driving: Predicting fatigue-related performance decay. *Policing, 38*(3), 517–538. https://doi.org/10.1108/PIJPSM-03-2015-0033

Kinman, G., McDowall, A., & Cropley, M. (2012). Work-family conflict and job-related well-being in UK police officers: The role of recovery strategies.

Knauth, P., & Hornberger, S. (2003). In-depth review: Shift work preventive and compensatory measures for shift workers, 109–116. https://doi.org/10.1093/occmed/kqg049

Mares, P., Coyne, P., & MacDonald, B. (2013). *Roadcraft: The Police Driver's Handbook.* London: The Stationery Office.

Mason, C. (1999). *Healthy Nights?* Home Office, Policing and Reducing Crime Unit.

Morris-Stiff, G. J., Sarasin, S., Edwards, P., Lewis, W. G., & Lewis, M. H. (2005). The European Working Time Directive: One for all and all for one? *Surgery, 137*(3), 293–297.

Oexman, R. D., Knotts, T. L., & Koch, J. (2002). Working while the world sleeps: A consideration of sleep and shift work design. *Employee Responsibilities and Rights Journal, 14*(4), 145–157.

Police (Health and Safety) Act. Police (Health and Safety) Act 1997, Pub. L. No. 42 (1997). Retrieved from www.legislation.gov.uk/ukpga/1997/42/contents.

Rajaratnam, S. M. W., Howard, M. E., & Grunstein, R. R. (2013). Sleep loss and circadian disruption in shift work: Health burden and management. *Medical Journal of Australia, 199*(8), S11–S15. https://doi.org/10.5694/mja13.10561

Richbell, S., Simpson, M., Sykes, G. M. H., & Meegan, S. (1998). Policing with the Ottawa shift system: A British experience. *Policing, 21*(3), 384–396. https://doi.org/10.1108/13639519810228714

Rogers, A., Holmes, S., & Spencer, M. (2001). The effect of shiftwork on driving to and from work. *Journal of Human Ergology, 30*(1–2), 131–136.

Scholarios, D., Hesselgreaves, H., & Pratt, R. (2017). Unpredictable working time, well-being and health in the police service. *The International Journal of Human Resource Management, 28*(16), 2275–2298.

Stone, R., Kemp, T., Rix, B., & Weldon, G. (1993). *Effective Shift System for the Police Service.* Great Britain, Home Office, Police Research Group.

Taylor, Y. L. H. (2020). Shift workers, fatigued driving and the impact on road safety-An investigation involving police service employees. University of Leeds.

The Working Time Regulations. The Working Time Regulations, Pub. L. No. 1833 (1998). UK. Retrieved from www.legislation.gov.uk/uksi/1998/1833/contents/made.

Totterdell, P., & Smith, L. (1992). Ten-hour days and eight-hour nights: Can the Ottawa shift system reduce the problems of shiftwork? *Work & Stress, 6*(2), 139–152.

Tucker, P., Smith, L., Macdonald, I., & Folkard, S. (2000). Effects of direction of rotation in continuous and discontinuous 8 hour shift systems. *Occupational and Environmental Medicine, 57*(10), 678–684. https://doi.org/10.1136/oem.57.10.678

Vila, B. (1996). Tired cops: Probable connections between fatigue and the performance, health and safety of patrol officers. *American Journal of Police, 15*(2), 51–92.

Vila, B. (2006). Impact of long work hours on police officers and the communities they serve. *American Journal of Industrial Medicine, 49*(11), 972–980. https://doi.org/10.1002/ajim.20333

Vila, B., Kenney, D. J., Gregory, B., & Reuland, M. (2000). Evaluating the Effects of Fatigue on Police Patrol Officers: Final Report. National Institute of Justice Research Report No. 184188, February 1 (122 p.). Retrieved from https://nij.ojp.gov/library/publications/eva luating-effects-fatigue-police-patrol-officers-final-report.

Wardman, K., & Mason, C. (1999). The working time directive: Officer health and safety and police efficiency. *The Police Journal*, *72*(1), 2–13.

5.6 Managing Commercial Vehicle Driver Fatigue in Canada

A Government Perspective

Pierre Thiffault

Transport Canada, Ottawa, Canada

CONTENTS

5.6.1 INTRODUCTION AND BACKGROUND

Picture it: early July 1990, and I am driving from Montreal to Hunting Island, South-Carolina—a 2,200 km, two-day trip. Quite a long journey for a 25-year-old with no professional driving experience. Adding to the length of the trip was the stress accumulated throughout the previous week at work, the late-night packing, and the very early morning start. The first day, from Montreal to Richmond, VA, was quite long with a 12-hour drive. However, it is during the second day that insight struck that would later inspire the main experiment for my doctoral thesis, later reported in Thiffault and Bergeron (2003).

I was driving south on Interstate 95, going across Virginia, North Carolina, and, eventually, South Carolina. This is a long, low-demand, monotonous drive. The highway was made of concrete sections separated by repetitive perpendicular fissures in the pavement. Driving at constant speed created an all-encompassing, rhythmic sensory experience. Not only did I see the lines on the pavement, but I could also feel the movement of the car and hear the clicking of the tires as I passed over them.

After a while, I felt that this empty monotonous road coupled with this repetitive sensory experience was having a sort of hypnotic effect, bringing me into a lower state of alertness. Slumped forward in my seat with heavy eyes—although I had slept a full night and it was now only 11:00 am—I started worrying that this monotonous driving context and the increasing heat were going to put me to sleep. I began to struggle against a progressively growing internal sleep pressure.

Then came the opposite phenomenon. In the vast uninterrupted roadside, I saw in the distance a massive billboard advertising a well-known shopping centre situated on the border between North and South Carolina. The sign indicated that the centre was still 150 miles away, and the message was very salient, colourful, and even slightly amusing. Another one came soon, again with a joke, more colours, and even mechanical movement in the scene. The billboards became more and more frequent. I ended up expecting them, looking for them, calculating distances and time, etc. Finding the signs became front and centre to my driving experience. I then realised that the painful struggle with fatigue had now faded away. When I eventually passed the shopping centre, I was alert, awake, and felt safe and comfortable as I continued driving.

This anecdotal experience repeated itself the following year. I found that I would experience lowered alertness and increasing fatigue when driving on monotonous highways, but that it would fade away when I exited highways to join winding rural roads or urban settings. Given my training in psychophysiology and familiarity with concepts such as the habituation response, which explains the inhibition of an orientation response after repeated stimulation, I started formulating a hypothesis: by itself, task (road) monotony has an impact on driver alertness and vigilance, and this task-induced effect can become critical and precipitate more acute drowsiness when coupled with endogenous sleep-related or circadian fatigue contributors. Consequently, I decided to conduct a review of the research literature in this area and to test this hypothesis using the driving simulator at University of Montreal.

The literature related to the impact of fatigue in operational settings, looking all the way back to the original work of Norman and Jane Mackworth in the 1950s (Mackworth, 1948; Mackworth, 1950) to more recent publications in the mid 1990s, mainly focused on vigilance. Vigilance—defined as the ability to detect critical signals in a low demanding task environment—is central to performance and safety in all modes of transportation. From prior research, it was understood that the *vigilance decrement*, or reduction in the ability to detect those critical signals over time, was the main mechanism by which fatigue impacts performance in operational settings and transportation safety. The aim of this research was, not surprisingly, to develop a better understanding of the factors that impact vigilance and how to best mitigate them.

During this *vigilance paradigm* period, the causes of fatigue were classified as endogenous or exogenous. Endogenous factors are those that stem from within the organism, such as sleep deficit, time awake, and time-of-day. These factors create the base level of alertness and represent the strongest influence on vigilance. Exogenous factors describe external task characteristics such as monotony and underload, which produce milder phasic decreases of arousal that also have the potential to induce hypovigilance, even in well-rested operators. At the centre of vigilance research is the notion that there is a systemic interaction between endogenous and exogenous factors, and that it is their joint influence, at all times, that determines the level of operator vigilance and associated levels of performance and safety.

To explore the possibility that roadside monotony by itself decreases driver alertness and vigilance, I developed a driving simulator task where the monotony of visual stimulation was controlled and manipulated. Then, in 1995, my studies were sidelined for 18 months while I recuperated from serious injuries sustained in a collision. When I resumed my research in 1997, the latest research literature had shifted focus from a vigilance to a sleep research paradigm, with significant involvement of the sleep research community. I realised then that the outcome variable of driver fatigue research had shifted towards drowsiness, microsleeps, and falling asleep and that it was no longer focused on the vigilance decrement, which is likely to happen before drowsiness is even felt. Instead of representing a critical outcome of endogenous and exogenous factors, performance decrements on vigilance tasks became a dependent variable to assess basic endogenous alertness. The milder contributions of exogenous factors, such as task underload and monotony, on vigilance and safety fell off the radar. This state of driver fatigue research lasted for a decade or so.

Today, further to this transition from a vigilance to a sleep research paradigm, we are seeing a new surge in studies looking at task monotony and underload and how it impacts alertness and vigilance. The issue, now labelled as passive (task-related) fatigue (see Chapter 3.4 of this book), is mainly focused on the impacts of driving automation and the issue of partial automation of the driving task (where only some elements, such as lane-keeping and maintaining headway to a lead vehicle, are managed by the automation). The requirement in these situations for drivers to remain vigilant while task monotony is increased goes against some of the basic scientific principles related to alertness and sustained attention (Körber et al., 2015; Jarosch et al., 2017; May and Baldwin, 2009; Thiffault and Bergeron, 2003; Saxby et al., 2013; Zeller et al., 2020).

5.6.2 COMMERCIAL VEHICLE[1] DRIVER FATIGUE

This chapter focuses on commercial vehicle driver fatigue and how it is being addressed by the Federal Government in Canada. The fatigue risk factors are described, as are the difficulties in quantifying the effects of fatigue on crashes and the prescriptive and non-prescriptive components of current efforts to address the problem.

Due to its impacts on performance in tasks that require vigilance, fatigue has been recognised as a significant safety problem in all modes of transportation. Among those, the road transportation sector has received a substantial amount of attention from scientists and regulators over the past three decades or so (see National Academies of Sciences, Engineering, and Medicine, 2016, for a review). The significant fatigue risk factors associated with long-haul trucking and motorcoach operations, as well as the fact that heavy vehicles operate on public roads while constantly interacting with light duty vehicles with a significant weight and mass differential, create a risk that needs to be mitigated. This chapter focuses on how this is being addressed by Transport Canada and our stakeholders.

5.6.2.1 FATIGUE RISK FACTORS IN COMMERCIAL VEHICLE OPERATIONS

In 2011, I assessed the research literature relative to fatigue risk factors present in the motor carrier industry (Thiffault, 2011). A fresh look at more recent literature indicates that the conclusions from 2011 remain accurate (Dawson et al., 2021; National Academies of Sciences, Engineering, and Medicine, 2016; Davidovic et al., 2018; Hege et al., 2015). To better understand why commercial motor vehicle (CMV) drivers continue to be at risk of fatigue, and why regulatory and complementary non-regulatory fatigue management initiatives are necessary, it is important to first identify the main fatigue causes. These are:

- acute and chronic sleep loss (getting less than 8 hours of sleep over one night, or over a number of consecutive nights);
- time-of-day (driving during the circadian low point, mainly between 02:00 and 06:00 and, to a lesser extent, in the afternoon);
- time-on-task (driving for prolonged periods of time);
- time awake (driving after one has been awake for more than 16 hours);
- irregular and unpredictable sleep patterns (potential for circadian phase shifting, sleep loss, and poor sleep quality);
- obstructive sleep apnoea (OSA—impairs sleep quality and quantity, relates to obesity);
- task underload and monotony (performing a task that relies on vigilance in low-demand, monotonous conditions);
- the macroergonomic structure of the industry (being paid by the mile, operating in a just-in-time delivery context, not being paid for waiting time, etc.).

In light of these fatigue causes, it is straightforward to understand that CMV drivers are at higher risk: They tend to have short, irregular, and often-interrupted sleep patterns; many obtain their core sleep period in a sleeping berth in the truck; they operate for extended periods of time each day; they tend to be overweight with high rates of OSA; they often operate in low-demanding, unstimulating highway driving conditions; and they tend to be paid by the mile, which creates a motivation to drive as many miles as possible (i.e., longer time-on-task), producing a fertile ground for fatigue as well as health and wellness issues (Belzer, 2020). As a result, driver fatigue has been identified as a pervasive phenomenon in the life of CMV drivers. It is related to health and wellness (National Academies of Sciences, Engineering, and Medicine, 2016; Crizzle et al., 2020) and is identified as a key contributing factor for heavy vehicle crashes in numerous studies, using various methodologies, whether they are based on comprehensive crash causation assessments (FMCSA, 2006), naturalistic observations conducted in field operational tests (Hanowski et al., 2007), subjective measures of CMV drivers' experience with regard to fatigue and safety incidents (Sieber et al., 2014) or national crash databases (Thiffault, 2011; Transport Canada, 2021).

5.6.3 DATA LIMITATIONS

It is difficult to assess the presence of fatigue in safety incidents. As a result, estimates of the contribution of fatigue to crashes tend to vary consistently, ranging from as low as 5% to as high as 50% of all crashes, with a median of about 15 to 25% (see Dawson et al., 2018 and Chapter 2.1 of this book for comprehensive reviews). In an important consensus statement published in 2000, a group of leading fatigue experts stated:

> ...fatigue is the largest identifiable and preventable cause of accidents in transport operations (between 15 and 20% of all accidents), surpassing that of alcohol or drug related incidents in all modes of transportation. Official statistics often underestimate this contribution. Underestimation of the impact of fatigue can lead to the underutilization of important countermeasure.

Åkerstedt, 2000

Two key factors can explain the difficulties in assessing the extent to which fatigue contributes to crashes: Enduring conceptual complexities in the field and challenges with fatigue assessment. Under a sleep research paradigm, one would identify fatigue as a crash contributor when it can be demonstrated, or if it is deemed possible, that an operator was either seriously drowsy or fell asleep, which represents the extreme end of the alertness or sleep-wake continuum. Under a vigilance paradigm, although more difficult to assess and demonstrate, one would also include the more central portion of that continuum which defines the earlier signs of fatigue; when the operator first becomes hypovigilant (inattentive), even before experiencing physical drowsiness. As Dinges (1995) emphasised, *the vigilance decrement is the most robust effect of fatigue and sleepiness*. This statement implies that the vigilance decrement is *always* present when fatigue takes place, and that it has a *critical impact* on operator performance, especially in the transportation sector where performance relies heavily on sustained attention/vigilance.

When we consider the effect of hypovigilance on critical aspects of driving performance (increased reaction time, poor tracking and speed management, missed signals, decreased defensive driving and proactive scanning behaviour, lower situational awareness, etc.), it becomes apparent that a significant portion of fatigue-related crashes are related to this early fatigue phase. Fatigue-related hypovigilance is both critical to performance and highly prevalent, especially in low-demanding monotonous driving conditions such as highways. It is therefore highly prevalent among long-haul CMV drivers, who are affected by numerous endogenous fatigue risk factors and tend to operate on monotonous roads for extended periods of time.

There is currently in the culture of road safety practitioners a tendency to attribute all inattention-based safety incidents to driver distraction, which is problematic. Distraction and hypovigilance (fatigue-related inattention) are two different problems involving different causal mechanisms, which necessitate different mitigation strategies. While distraction is based on a dual-task paradigm and is mitigated by modulating attentional demands and attentional resource allocation, hypovigilance relates to lowering brain alertness (explained by both endogenous and exogenous—or task-induced—factors) and is mitigated by strategies aimed at improving operators' alertness, such as providing better sleep opportunities, treating sleep disorders, decreasing time-on-task, avoiding circadian low points, and decreasing or interrupting task monotony.

What I call the "flashlight beam" analogy provides a good example of this dual reality of inattention. The beam of a flashlight can be compared to attention and, given that attention is a single channel process, there is only one flashlight beam. Distraction happens when primary task signals are missed because the beam of attention was oriented towards a secondary task. On the other hand, hypovigilance happens when task signals are missed because the intensity of the beam is weak (or too low), even if it is oriented towards signals in the primary task.

The tendency to associate all inattention incidents to driver distraction and the dual-task paradigm creates a situation where reality is not well represented. It contributes to the underestimation of the role of fatigue in crashes and it channels resources away from the field of research on driver fatigue. It also reinforces a societal perception that the risks of fatigue in transportation are only related to acute drowsiness and falling asleep. This, in turn, has the potential to negatively impact how road safety practitioners and, consequently, road users understand and try to mitigate the risks associated with driver fatigue.

A second reason for the difficulty in assessing the contribution of fatigue to crashes is that it is impossible to measure fatigue directly. Fatigue does not leave physiological or metabolic traces that can be detected after a crash has occurred. Identifying the contribution of fatigue therefore mainly relies on observing and analysing crash parameters in light of specific sets of criteria (operational definitions of fatigue) or referring to subjective accounts (Dawson et al., 2018). And subjective accounts tend to be unreliable since professional drivers may not be willing to disclose the information and incriminate themselves or because they might not be aware that they were fatigued prior to a crash (mainly because being involved in a crash will jolt the driver wide awake). Note that this is even more true in cases where milder hypovigilance caused a crash, given that there is no salient physical experience associated with it that can be remembered. Lastly, subjective accounts of fatigue are not available in the case of fatal crashes.

In Canada, the main source of data on crashes and crash contributing factors comes from Transport Canada's National Collision Database (NCDB[2]), which is an aggregate of data stemming from police reports related to all reportable crashes in the country. While this comprehensive data set is a highly valuable source of information to depict and better understand the reality of road crashes in the country, it is a well-documented fact, in light of the above assessment difficulties, that data sets based on police reports have limitations with regard to fatigue-related crashes. Police reports tend to seriously underestimate the prevalence of fatigue as a crash contributor, with identified rates as low as 1% to 4% of crashes (Li et al., 2018). Mining the entirety of the NCDB database from its inception in 1992 to 2019, we see that fatigue is identified as a contributing factor in only 2% of fatal crashes involving light duty vehicles and in 1.2% of commercial vehicle crashes.

Today, it is understood and accepted that these fatigue assessment difficulties limit the utility of official crash databases to examine fatigue-related crashes. When trying to represent this reality, road safety practitioners tend to rely on wider assessments that triangulate various methodologies (e.g., lab studies, large-scale surveys, and naturalistic studies) and on consensus statements from experts which unite these data sources and assess them in light of the continuously expanding body of scientific knowledge about fatigue in transportation. It is widely agreed that, although precise estimates will vary, fatigue is a key transportation safety hazard that needs to be mitigated (National Academy of Sciences, Engineering, and Medicine 2016). According to the Infrastructure Health & Safety Association, driver fatigue is a top-ranked risk for the Ontario trucking industry[3].

As described in the main deliverable from the Canadian Council of Motor Transport Administrators (CCMTA's) Human Factors and Motor Carrier Safety Task Force (Thiffault, 2011), there is no silver bullet for driver fatigue and the problem should ideally be addressed using a multifaceted, systemic approach. In that report we identified a series of interventions, including:

- improving motor carriers' safety culture and fatigue management practices;
- improving drivers' ability to manage their own level of alertness and their willingness to do so via improved training;
- screening for and treating OSA;
- using biomathematical software to improve scheduling practices;
- improving driver remuneration schemes;
- implementing fatigue monitoring technologies and Advance Driver Assistance Systems (ADAS);
- improving rest area infrastructure;
- implementing central and lateral rumble strips; and
- implementing evidence-based health and wellness programmes for CMV drivers.

As a whole, these interventions are in line with the precepts of the Safe System Approach, which is the foundational component of the Global Decade of Action for Road Safety, central to current international efforts to curb road fatalities. Many of these elements are also at the core of fatigue management programmes (FMPs), and our approach to this is described in sub-section 5.6.4 of this chapter.

However, given the reality of the motor carrier industry, including economic pressures, inherent market competitive processes, and the deep-rooted fatigue risk factors associated with the profession, there is also a need for government to use the regulatory tools at its disposal to implement legal limits to duty and driving time as well as imposing minimal rest periods, in order to ensure that a sufficient level of safety is met. Hours of service regulations provide the means to achieve this. They are instrumental for protecting the safety of both general road users and CMV drivers; they help in promoting CMV drivers' health and wellness, and they ensure a level-playing field for the industry. It is however fundamental that the regulations be evidence-based, respecting basic principles of fatigue science, and that the development process includes genuine and documented consultations with government and industry stakeholders as well as representatives from public interest groups. These consultations will help to ensure that the operational realities of the industry are factored in, they will increase industry and social acceptance and they will make the regulations more agile while maximising compliance.

5.6.4   THE COMMERCIAL VEHICLE DRIVERS HOURS OF SERVICE (HOS) REGULATIONS

The responsibility for managing the safety of trucks and buses in Canada is shared between the federal and provincial governments. As part of the *Motor Vehicle Transport Act* (MVTA), the federal government has jurisdiction over certain aspects of the safety of extra-provincial motor carriers and bus undertakings. The MVTA outlines the federal role in regulating the safe operation of motor carriers. One of these regulations, first enacted is 1994 and updated in 2007, is the *Commercial Vehicle Drivers Hours of Service Regulations*[4].

There are two general approaches that a governing body can use to address operator fatigue in transport operations: The prescriptive and the performance-based, or non-prescriptive, approach. The HOS regulations represent the prescriptive component of how the Canadian federal government aims at mitigating commercial vehicle driver fatigue. As will be described later, in Canada and the US, it is also completed by a non-prescriptive voluntary approach.

At the time when the first Canadian HOS regulations were enacted in 1994, the Canadian and US federal governments jointly launched a major field study entitled the *Driver Fatigue and Alertness Study* (Wylie et al., 1997). The study, conducted on a sample of 80 drivers in Canada and the US, was the first North American field trial on driver fatigue. The goal was to observe the evolution of driver fatigue and alertness in order to make recommendations for countermeasures. Drivers were observed in the naturalistic driving environment while operating on revenue-generating trips. Key findings were that time-of-day was the most determining factor influencing fatigue and alertness, and that there was evidence of cumulative fatigue across days of driving. The results of this foundational research effort created a momentum among government and industry stakeholders, as well as within academia, which eventually led to the reformulation of the Canadian HOS regulations in 2007. The 2007 Regulations, which represent a significant update to the 1994 edition, were further amended in 2019 and 2021 to introduce the mandatory use of Electronic Logging Devices (ELD) to automatically record information related to drivers' hours of driving and rest. This is expected to improve accuracy and prevent falsification, as was the case with the self-reported paper logbooks they replaced, and therefore help to enforce the regulations and better mitigate driver fatigue.

The 1994 Regulations were based on a 23-hour rotational shift principle (15 on duty/8 off-duty), allowing for up to 16 hours on-duty in a day and 108 hours in 7 days. This many hours represents very long workdays, few sleep/rest opportunities and creates the potential for circadian phase shifting within a cycle. The 2007 Regulations provided solutions for these problems and brought further improvements. They were developed over a 10-year period on the basis of intense consultations between government and industry representatives. They also relied on an iterative development process that included fatigue expert panels that were consulted on numerous occasions to answer specific questions related to fatigue science and scheduling practices. A comprehensive presentation of the current Canadian HOS regulations is out of scope for this chapter; however, below are the key requirements:

- The HOS regulations are based on a 24-hour day principle, with the log start time fixed at the beginning of the cycle, promoting scheduling stability and preventing phase shifting.
- There is a minimum of 10 hours off-duty in a day, 8 of which are consecutive, representing a 25% increase in off-duty time compared to the 1994 Regulations.
- The maximum on-duty time in a day is 14 hours, and the maximum driving time is 13 hours, which is 19% less than that stipulated in the former regulations.
- On-duty time must be completed within a 16-hour window, in an effort to mitigate the time-awake factor.
- Drivers can choose to operate according to either cycle 1 (70 hours on-duty in 7 days, 36-hour restart) or cycle 2 (120 hours on-duty in 14 days, with 24 consecutive hours off-duty after 70 hours on-duty and a 72-hour restart). For clarity, the restart period defines an extended period of continuous off-duty time that is needed to mitigate chronic fatigue accumulated during the cycle.

It needs to be emphasised that HOS regulations have clear objectives and limitations. They are designed to set maximum legal limits to on-duty time and minimum legal limits to off-duty time and to stabilise scheduling within a cycle, but they do not represent a comprehensive fatigue management approach and are not intended as such. HOS regulations provide a regulatory framework that sets boundaries to ensure that CMV drivers do not operate in contradiction of some of the essential sleep science principles and that they are provided with enough time, on a daily basis and between cycles, to get sufficient consolidated sleep as well as napping opportunities. In terms of key limitations, HOS regulations:

- do not address time-of-day effects;
- set legal limits but these maximum/minimal limits should not be understood as optimal scheduling practices;
- cannot account for individual differences in fatigue susceptibility;
- do not provide the fatigue knowledge, motivation, and safety culture elements that are important to facilitate the self-management of alertness; and
- do not provide fatigue management tools, such as scheduling software, biomathematical models, fatigue monitoring technologies or screening and treatment options for sleep problems, which should all be part of a comprehensive fatigue management approach (Thiffault, 2011).

There are therefore solid arguments to support the notion that HOS regulations should ideally be complemented by a comprehensive fatigue management programme which provides means to address most of the above-mentioned limitations. And it was these arguments that drove the development of the North American Fatigue Management Program (NAFMP).

5.6.5 THE NORTH AMERICAN FATIGUE MANAGEMENT PROGRAM

The NAFMP (https://nafmp.org) is a voluntary, non-regulatory tool that supports fatigue management in the motor carrier industry. It is widely used by industry professionals in Canada and the US. The programme is presented as a voluntary, no-fee website and learning management system (LMS) that provides motor carriers, managers, dispatchers, commercial drivers and their families with information and tools to enhance fatigue knowledge and management practices. It is designed to be a comprehensive complement to the Canadian and US HOS regulations by providing a framework for training and education on:

- improving organisational safety culture;
- fatigue and fatigue management;
- work, rest, and scheduling practices;
- sleep disorders screening and treatment;
- fatigue monitoring technologies; and
- bio-mathematical scheduling tools.

The programme includes 10 training modules (approximately 15 hours of training) available in French and English and can be downloaded or completed online via the interactive LMS, with or without audio narration. The programme also includes a comprehensive implementation manual with detailed instructions explaining how it can be implemented following some of the key principles of the fatigue risk management system (FRMS) approach, an organisational risk mitigation model used to address fatigue in transport operations in various modes (see Sprajcer et al., 2021). Finally, the programme includes a return-on-investment calculator, where motor carriers can estimate the financial benefits of using the programme, either as a whole or by selecting specific components, and considering the unique configuration of their organisation. Next is a brief overview of how the NAFMP was developed and deployed in Canada and the US.

In 2000, a report was commissioned by Transport Canada to assess the efficiency of various fatigue countermeasures in transport operations. The report recommended the development of an education-based fatigue management programme as a complement to HOS regulations. This recommendation fostered the interest of government officials in the Canadian province of Alberta. Together with industry representatives, they created a joint committee, which generated the initial R&D effort into what would eventually become the NAFMP. The committee contracted a research team to carry out conceptual work aimed at exploring various fatigue countermeasures and refining the notion of an organisational FMP. The Alberta team soon expanded to include Transport Canada, the province of Quebec and the US Federal Motor Carrier Safety Administration (FMCSA).

This expanded team conducted an initial field study to assess the applicability of FMP in operational settings and to explore its effectiveness. This first iteration of the programme, comprised of educational modules, operational tools, and stepwise clinical sleep disorder screening and treatment, was applied to motor carriers in Alberta, Quebec, and Texas (US). As part of the FMP, drivers suffering from OSA were identified and treated. A follow-up revealed that, compared to when untreated, their daily average sleep time increased by 73 per cent (from an average of 3.9 hours of sleep per day to an average of 6.8 hours). Furthermore, these drivers experienced 44% fewer lapses ("misses" in target detection) on a psychomotor detection task used to assess vigilance following the FMP intervention. These results highlighted the important role of the diagnosis and treatment of commercial drivers' sleep disorders in reducing fatigue in the motor carrier industry (Moscovitch et al., 2006).

A second study was commissioned to another research team to develop further the elements of the programme and to observe their efficacy in an operational environment (Smiley et al., 2011). The project involved a field operational test with 77 commercial vehicle drivers in Alberta, Quebec, and California (US). The study revealed positive trends in average daily sleep duration and sleep efficiency post-FMP as well as reduced safety-critical events on the road. Key findings include improved reported sleep quality on duty days; 20 minutes longer main sleep on duty days; duty day main period sleep duration and sleep efficiency improved compared to rest days; a trend showing less subjective fatigue reported by drivers and a reduction in the proportion of drivers reporting critical events (from 46% to 29%), as well as a 40% reduction in the number of critical events per km driven (Smiley et al., 2011).

In the next and final phase of R&D, a team from Virginia Tech Transportation Institute (VTTI) developed the final educational modules and implementation manual, while another team from the American Transportation Research Institute (ATRI) created the first website of the NAFMP, which was launched in July 2013.

In 2021, after eight years in operation, the website and the courses, used by thousands of commercial drivers and motor carriers, were updated to reflect the latest technologies for online courses. The Commercial Vehicle Safety Alliance (CVSA) became the host of the programme with a key objective to continue its promotion and increase its visibility and use within the North American motor carrier industry. Finally, following recommendations from a US National Academy of Science panel in 2016, a new field operational trial is taking place in 2022–2023 to assess the efficacy of the latest iteration of the NAFMP and to make recommendations for potential improvements. The study, funded by NIOSH and the US FMCSA, will implement the NAFMP in an operational environment, with an objective of enrolling 180 drivers. The aim is to assess the effects of the programme from an organisational standpoint, as well as through a comprehensive and cutting-edge fatigue assessment approach that will include real-time fatigue detection technologies.

5.6.6 CONCLUSIONS

After 25 years working in this field, I am always surprised to see how conceptual difficulties remain an issue and how decades of research have not sufficiently percolated into the common understanding of fatigue, what it encompasses, how it impacts performance, and how to mitigate these effects. As discussed in the anecdote presented in the foreword, my early work was dedicated to bringing back some emphasis to the notions of monotony, task-induced fatigue and vigilance as genuine, fatigue-related, safety concerns. It is interesting to note that those issues are now central to the current discussion on the human factors' implications of driving automation. In terms of motor carrier safety, we are using these same notions to improve CMV driver training, to widen the scope of fatigue-related crash data to include inattention errors, and to highlight the importance of mitigating potential task-induced fatigue risks associated with automation.

The main scope of this chapter highlighted how the Federal government in Canada has dealt with the issue of CMV driver fatigue since the mid-1990s. This was done through benchmarking field research underlying the development of a hybrid approach based on prescriptive rules yet complemented with a comprehensive voluntary programme inspired by the key principles of the non-prescriptive FRMS approach.

The central position is that, given the reality of the motor carrier industry, HOS regulations are necessary but they have limitations and are not intended to represent a comprehensive all-encompassing fatigue management strategy. The NAFMP was developed to complement these regulations and to address these limitations. Together with our partners in the US and the CVSA, we are now working actively to increase industry penetration of this programme and to improve it on the basis of sound empirical evidence.

SUMMARY POINTS FOR PRACTITIONERS

- Fatigue is not only caused by time-of-day, time-awake, task duration, or sleep-related factors, and fatigue-related crashes include more than acute drowsiness and falling asleep incidents. Although these are the strongest causal factors, task monotony and underload also contribute to fluctuations in alertness that can generate a vigilance decrement (inattention) which also significantly contributes to fatigue-related crashes. As such, the management of fatigue needs to focus on the usual endogenous factors, but also on making sure that drivers are kept alert by the task itself. From a fatigue perspective, if vigilance is still necessary, increasing task monotony by removing drivers from the loop and decreasing their input may be counterproductive.
- It is difficult to quantify the contribution of fatigue to crashes in official crash databases. On the basis of a large body of research using various methodologies, the consensus is that fatigue contributes to 15 to 25% of crashes, and potentially more for commercial vehicle drivers, who are more exposed to fatigue risk factors than the general driving population.
- There are two general means by which governments can mitigate the risk of commercial vehicle driver fatigue: A prescriptive and a non-prescriptive approach. Hours-of-service regulations represent the prescriptive component used in Canada. They mainly set maximum limits to duty time and minimal limits to off-duty time. However, on their own, the regulations are not intended as a comprehensive fatigue management strategy.
- The North American Fatigue Management Program (https://nafmp.org), a non-prescriptive approach that was developed to complement HOS regulations, is intended as a comprehensive fatigue management strategy. It is a voluntary, no-fee programme that provides motor carriers, managers, dispatchers, commercial drivers, and their families with information and tools to enhance current fatigue knowledge and management practices.
- Finally, in light of the Safe System Approach, which is the foundational component of the Global Decade of Action for Road Safety, addressing commercial

vehicle driver fatigue necessitates a systemic multifaceted approach that should also include countermeasures at the enforcement (ELD), infrastructure (rumble strips, frequent and acceptable rest areas), and vehicle safety levels (advanced driver assistance systems and crash avoidance technologies). Transport Canada and its stakeholders are constantly working to develop new approaches at all three levels.

NOTES

1 In this chapter, the term *commercial vehicle* refers to a truck with a Registered Gross Vehicle Weight (RGVW) of more than 4,500 kg or a bus with a designated seating capacity of more than 10 persons, including the driver.
2 /wwwapps2.tc.gc.ca/Saf-Sec-Sur/7/NCDB-BNDC/p.aspx?l=en.
3 www.ihsa.ca/Road-Safety-Solutions/Driver-fatigue-is-a-top-ranked-risk-in-Ontario.aspx.
4 https://laws-lois.justice.gc.ca/eng/regulations/SOR-2005-313/.

REFERENCES

Åkerstedt, T. (2000). Consensus Statement: Fatigue and accidents in transport operations. *Journal of Sleep Research, 9,* 395.

Belzer, M. (2020). The economics of long work hours: How economic incentives influence workplace practice. *Industrial Health, 58,* 399–402.

Crizzle, A.M., Mirsosseini, N., Bigelow, P., Shubair, M., Zello, G., & Thiffault, P. (2020). *A neglected sector: Improving the health and working conditions of long-haul truck drivers in Alberta.* Report prepared for the Government of Alberta Occupational Health and Safety Branch, Project #095237350.

Davidovic, J., Pesic, D., & Antic, B. (2018). Professional drivers' fatigue as a problem of the modern era. *Transportation Research Part F, 55,* 199–209.

Dawson, D., Reynolds., A.C., Van Dongen, H.P.A., & Thomas, M.J.W. (2018). Determining the likelihood that fatigue was present in a road accident: A theoretical review and suggested accident taxonomy. *Sleep Medicine Review, 42,* 202–210.

Dawson, D., Sprajcer, M., & Thomas, M. (2021). How much sleep do you need? A comprehensive review of fatigue related impairment and the capacity to work or drive safely. *Accident Analysis and Prevention, 151,* 1–13.

Dinges, D.F. (1995). An overview of sleepiness and accidents. *Journal of Sleep Research, 4,* 4–14.

Federal Motor Carrier Safety Administration. (2006). *Report to Congress on the Large Truck Crash Causation Study.*

Hanowski., R.J., Hickman., J., Fumero, M.C., Olson, R.L., & Dingus, T.A. (2007). The sleep of commercial vehicle drivers under the 2003 hours-of-service regulations. *Accident Analysis and Prevention, 39,* 1140–1145.

Hege., A., Perko, M., Johnson, A., Yu., C.H., Sönmez., S., & Apostopoulos, Y. (2015). Surveying the impact of work hours and schedules on commercial motor vehicle driver sleep. *Safety and Health at Work, 6,* 104–113.

Jarosch, O., Kuhnt, M., Paradies, S., & Bengler, K. (2017). *It's out of our hands now! Effects of non-driving tasks during highly automated driving on drivers' fatigue.* In: Proceedings of the Ninth International Driving Symposium on Human Factors in Driver Assessment, Training and Vehicle Design. Manchester, Vermont.

Körber, M., Zimmerman, M., & Bengler, K. (2015). Vigilance and passive fatigue caused by monotony in automated driving. *Procedia Manufacturing, 3*, 2403–2409.

Li, Y., Yamamoto, T., & Zhang, G. (2018). Understanding factors associated with misclassification of fatigue-related accidents in police record. *Journal of Safety Research, 64*, 155–162.

Mackworth, N.H. (1948). The breakdown of vigilance during prolonged visual search. *Quarterly Journal of Experimental Psychology, 1*, 6–21.

Mackworth, N.H. (1950). Researches on the measurement of human performance (*Medical Research Council Special Report Series No. 268*). London, England: Her Majesty's Stationery Office.

May, J.F., & Baldwin, C.L. (2009). Driver fatigue: The importance of identifying causal factors of fatigue when considering detection and countermeasures technologies. *Transportation Research Part F, 12*, 218–224.

Moscovitch, A., Reimer, M., Heslegrave, R., Boivin, D., Hirshkowitz, M., Rhodes, W., & Kealey, M. (2006). *Development of educational material and testing of tools and Procedures to be used in phase 3 fatigue management program.* Report submitted to Transport Canada.

National Academies of Sciences, Engineering, and Medicine. (2016). *Commercial Motor Vehicle Driver Fatigue, Long-Term Health, and Highway Safety: Research Needs.* Washington, DC: The National Academies Press. https://doi.org/10.17226/21921.

Saxby, D.J., Matthews, G., Warm, J.S., Hitchcock, E.M., & Neubauer, C. (2013). Active and passive fatigue in simulated driving: Discriminating styles of workload regulation and their safety impacts. *Journal of Experimental Psychology Applied, 19(4)*, 287–300.

Sieber, W.K., Robinson, C.F., Birdsey, J., Chen, G-X., Hitchcock, E.M., Lincoln, J.E., Nakata, A, & Sweeney, M.H. (2014). Obesity and other risk factors: The national survey of long-haul truck driver health and injury. *American Journal of Industrial Medicine, 57(6)*, 615–626.

Smiley, A., Smahel, T., Boivin, D.B., Boudreau, P., Remmers, J., Turner, M., Rosekind, M.R., & Gregory, K.B. (2011). *Effects of a fatigue management program on fatigue in the commercial motor carrier industry.* Research report prepared for Transport Canada.

Sprajcer, M., Thomas, M.T.W., Sargent, C., Crowther, M.E., Boivin, D.B., Wong., I.S., Smiley, A., & Dawson., D. (2021). How effective are fatigue risk management systems (FRMS)? A review. *Accident Analysis and Prevention.* https://doi.org/10.1016/j.aap.2021.106398.

Thiffault, P. (2011). *Addressing human factors in the motor carrier industry in Canada.* Report prepared for the Canadian Council of Motor Transport Administrators (CCMTA). www.bv.transports.gouv.qc.ca/mono/1081534.pdf.

Thiffault, P., & Bergeron, J. (2003). Monotony of road environment and driver fatigue: A simulator study. *Accident Analysis and Prevention, 35*, 381–391.

Transport Canada. (2021). *Commercial Vehicle Safety in Canada: 2012–2018 Seven-Year Review.* Report tabled to Parliament.

Wylie, C.D., Shultz, T., Miller, J. C., Mitler, M.M., & Mackie, R.R. (1997). *Commercial Motor Vehicle Driver Fatigue and Alertness Study: Technical Summary.* Report # FHWA-MC-97-001 for the United States and TP1287E for Canada.

Zeller, R., Williamson. A., & Friswell, R. (2020). The effect of sleep-need and time-on-task on driver fatigue. *Transportation Research Part F, 74*, 15–29.

5.7 Friend or Foe?

The Use of Digital Devices in the Fight Against Monotony and Boredom in Air Traffic Management

Lea Sophie Vink

Head of Human Performance, Austro Control, Vienna, Austria

CONTENTS

5.7.1 INTRODUCTION

Air Traffic Management (ATM) is a complex system that is designed to be sustainable at full capacity. What this means in practical human performance terms is to move as many aircraft as possible across the sky safely with as few human operators as required. It is well established that too little workload can result in fatigue creeping in from monotony and boredom (Straussberger & Schaefer, 2007) just as having workload that is too high can result in overloading and acute fatigue as the body runs out of energy. One of the main goals of the supervisors of operations rooms and towers is to keep human performance output optimised, meaning that the operators are kept at optimum workload.

Prior to 2020, as Air Traffic continued to increase after the 2009 financial crisis, there were warnings that ATM was running out of Air Traffic Controllers (ATCOs) to handle the increased traffic. There was growing evidence that the rate of overloads, for example, during the summer months was increasing beyond acceptable hazard

DOI: 10.1201/9781003213154-41

levels (Vink, 2021). This meant that the focus for safety management in ATM was to avoid the overload condition—where workload is too high, because this posed the most immediate safety risk.

One of the solutions to combat reduced numbers of ATCOs (and pilots) to meet future demand has been to focus on how automation in ATM can and should be used. One scenario would involve controllers becoming less and less interventionist and hands-on and therefore switching to more passive and monitoring roles. This would make the role more like that of operators of power stations, pilots, or ship operators. A key question for this scenario is to what extent can a human be expected to intervene when something rarely goes wrong with an automated system? And a subsequent question would be how can you combat monotony and boredom in operators monitoring safety systems (Metzger & Parasuraman, 2005).

So far, the ATM system is optimised to run at full capacity and so there has been little opportunity to research the effect on ATM operators of prolonged significantly reduced workload. The Covid-19 pandemic has provided this opportunity. When the pandemic began, there was a rapid loss of air traffic and many of the larger operations centres found themselves with the unusual situation of having too many staff on shifts (Vink, 2021). In Europe, the EU authorities issued requests to individual Air Navigation Service Providers (ANSPs) to provide safety analysis on the most immediate risks. One of the key risks identified for human operators was monotony, boredom, and fatigue. After taking immediate action to prevent increased safety risk such as by offering extra human factors training, awareness campaigns about increased risk, added simulator training days to maintain sharp skills, and modifications to duty rosters, focus then shifted in many ANSPs towards capturing the lessons learnt for human performance. Aside from the safety risk of the underloading condition, the Covid-19 pandemic also provided a very useful opportunity for research into future automation scenarios because it represented an ultra-low air traffic situation.

Since the arrival of the cell phone in the 1990s, there has been a strong rejection of the use of digital devices during the operation of safety systems. For example, the early 2000s saw a wave of anti-cell phone legislation particularly aimed at drivers. The consensus is that digital devices such as cell phones or e-readers are a major distraction and should not be used (Castro et al., 2019). But the reality in ATM is quite different. Although many people will not admit it, the use of digital devices has crept into the operations room in the last ten years, especially with smart phones. Although many operations have outright banned the use of devices, this can unfortunately push their use into hiding which could be more dangerous (Rudin-Brown et al., 2009). An open and honest discussion of the use of digital devices by ATCOs needs to happen because there has been promising research showing potential benefits of keeping the mind stimulated during quiet periods of operation.

This chapter presents the case for a nuanced and mature approach to safely allowing the use of digital personal devices in ATM to off-set monotonous periods of work and ultimately argues that future ATM systems must create a way to keep operators stimulated as systems become more automated and the job becomes more "monitoring" focused. Digital devices such as cell phones may provide this necessary stimulus.

5.7.2 "WE ALL TRAIN FOR THE OUT OF THE ORDINARY, BUT WHAT ABOUT THE ORDINARY?"

On 10 June 1990, a British Airways Flight 5390 between Birmingham, UK and Málaga, Spain suffered an extremely unusual problem. The aircraft departed on schedule at 07:20 UTC and climbed normally, without any cause for concern. The co-pilot had been handling the aircraft during the take-off and, as the plane was transferred to the Bristol Sector flying southwest, both pilots loosened their harnesses to settle into the flight (Department of Transport (U.K.), 1992).

However, at approximately 13 minutes after take-off as the aircraft passed through 17,300 feet, there was a loud bang, and the cabin began to fill with condensation. The cabin crew knew immediately that an explosive decompression had occurred. Air Steward Nigel Ogden immediately rushed into the cockpit where he saw the unimaginable. The left windscreen of the cockpit had been sucked outside and, due to the decompression, the captain had been partially dragged out with it. His legs and knees pinned him against the flight controls and Ogden immediately rushed forward and held on to him. Meanwhile, the co-pilot took control of the aircraft and began an immediate emergency descent as the aircraft was not equipped with oxygen for all the passengers. At a safe altitude, he re-engaged the autopilot and issued a mayday.

Eventually, after holding on desperately to the captain, Ogden was assisted by another flight attendant who managed to tie himself onto the left jump seat. The two continued their courageous efforts, trying to pull the captain back inside. The co-pilot finally received vectors to the nearest airport—Southampton—where he managed to land the aircraft safely at 07:55. After landing, the captain was discovered to still be alive and was rushed to hospital, where he was treated for bone fractures, frostbite, and shock. Eventually, it was concluded that a maintenance engineer had used the wrong thread of screws to replace the windscreen, which led to the loosely secured windscreen being ejected (Department of Transport (UK), 1992).

In civil aviation operations all around the world, pilots and ATCOs are trained to be prepared for many unusual and unexpected situations. What is most remarkable in the case of Flight 5390 is that everyone involved eventually went back to work and continued with their jobs. Captain Lancaster returned to the air only 5 months later and continued flying with British Airways until 2003 (New Zealand Herald, 2020)!

Some of the ATCOs who had been involved in this incident have been interviewed subsequently and they have continued to stress the rareness of such an event. One controller stated, "we all train for the out of the ordinary. But almost none of us train for the 99% of our careers which are spent in blissful quiet."

This example highlights the reality of being an operator within safety systems or high reliability organisations. Advances in training, human factors, and lesson learning from incidents have meant that operators today are prepared for almost anything. Human Performance has become a key commodity in these systems as organisations try to get the most out of their people. But as systems become more and more advanced, the role of humans is shifting from operations towards a more passive role. How can we keep our operators engaged and alert on an everyday basis while being ready for that one unusual incident in a 40-year career?

5.7.3 WHAT ARE WE FIGHTING? —WHAT IS THE DANGER?

Endsley defined situational awareness (SA) as "the perception of the elements in the environment within a volume of time and space, the comprehension of their meaning and the projection of their status in the near future" (Endsley, 1995). A loss of SA therefore means that an operator does not sub-consciously understand all the information presented to them to be able to fully appreciate the context and what is happening. When there is reduced SA, the mind therefore cannot make optimal conscious decisions. This exchange between sub-conscious and conscious decision-making is where most of the human error happens (Kahneman, 2011).

For example, on a quiet night shift at an airport there are sometimes no ground movements, no departures or arrivals for several hours and the tower controller simply has to monitor radio frequencies in case there is an emergency. A controller may keep themselves occupied with other tasks such as weather reports, approving and monitoring ground maintenance work or keeping an eye on radars, but generally the battle is within themselves to stay awake and alert in case something goes wrong.

But what does this mean in terms of cognitive processes? Normally, we would assume that the crucial capability of "thinking" with logic and rationality was the most critical function needed to solve a problem (Kahneman, 2011). However, as suggested by Wickens (2008) with his multiple-resource theory, as individuals become more tired, the brain actively tries to divert energy away from these higher functions to maintain sub-conscious abilities. The brain prefers to take sub-conscious shortcuts to make decisions rather than expend energy on the slower thinking brain (Kahneman, 2011). Higher thought is reserved for critical functions and costs more energy to the operator (Wickens, 2008) and, therefore, when we become fatigued, bored, or have low workload, our minds cannot focus.

During the night-time hours, or in periods of low air traffic activity, controllers face an additional cognitive challenge as the brain tries to conserve energy. The reduction of light at night triggers the release of melatonin and this actively prepares the body for sleep (Walker, 2017). Especially overnight, the body is focused on preparing to shut down and repair itself. Walker (2017) contends that sleep is the most essential bodily function for maintaining all our systems—including the logging of memories and for calibrating higher thought. In fact, it has been confirmed that up to 25% of ATCOs are affected by momentary shift-sleepiness, which is normally caused by low workload and monotonous situations (Teixeira de Freitas et al., 2017). Excessive sleepiness is especially prominent between the later evening hours of 21:30 and 23:30 and again between 02:00 and 04:00 (Chang et al., 2019). Even regular sleep cannot avert the phenomenon of sleepiness triggered by night hours and reduced activity. For example, a 2016 study found that despite 90% of controllers indicating they sleep quite well, they can still suffer from momentary sleepiness at work (Yuan et al., 2016). Essentially, controllers are battling the normal circadian rhythms that are trying to shut their brains down to sleep and this in turn leads to reduced higher cortical function. As discussed above, when higher cortical function is reduced, this makes intervention and decision-making slower and less effective.

Fatigue in ATCOs is managed actively by global and regional regulators. For example, in Europe, the latest rules pertaining to fatigue management were issued in 2017 and came into effect in 2019/2020 (European Union, 2017). The European rules cite specific rostering guidelines found in ICAO Document 9966 which are globally adopted (ICAO, 2016). These regulations provide a scientific-based envelope that in theory should protect controllers while maximising the allocation of staffing resources against demand. Detailed fatigue countermeasure implementation is left up to the individual operators and countries to enforce and manage (ICAO, 2016). There are several traditional fatigue countermeasures that can be taken during shifts. For example, ATCOs should not sit at a workstation longer than 2 hours maximum. On average, a controller will spend about 1 to 1.5 hours before taking a break, when they are usually relieved by a teammate. Regular breaks and support from teams, as well as regular training and fatigue monitoring systems, can (and do) go a long way to off-set monotony, boredom, and fatigue.

But the Covid-19 pandemic has revealed several issues with current practices. For instance, some operations maintaining two controllers in a sector to provide additional safety protection, but this can potentially increase the danger of monotony and boredom if the shared workload becomes too low. It is also expensive and often difficult to have fully staffed operations rooms during extremely quiet periods because the overnight hours are unattractive for many staff members. During the pandemic, most airports suffered almost 95% losses in commercial air traffic movements. However, many smaller regional airports experienced increases in general aviation (GA) traffic (i.e., smaller pleasure aircraft) at unexpected times outside of normal commercial traffic patterns (Vink, 2021). This situation proved that the traditional ATM watch structure was ineffective to both off-set the higher spikes in workload from the GA traffic and the now extended periods of monotony. Even before Covid-19, ANSPs and operators were downsizing the number of controllers per shift and implementing single-person operations (Chang et al., 2019). This, coupled with increasing remote airport operations and even multiple remote airport operations maintained by one controller, has revealed that more active management of in-watch fatigue and human performance is needed.

5.7.4 THE COVID-19 PANDEMIC AS OPPORTUNITY

When the global Covid-19 pandemic confronted the aviation industry in March 2020, the European Air Traffic Network experienced the sharpest contraction in traffic numbers it has ever seen (ICAO, 2021). The outcome of the disruption to "normal" operating routines because of the pandemic was a new focus on the risk of the pandemic to rapidly changing human factors issues in ATM. The conclusion at Austro Control was that the biggest threat to ATCOs was a loss of situational awareness caused by underloading and exacerbated by skill fade and monotony (Vink, 2021).

Aviation has previously focused on the opposite phenomenon—"overloading" which is where an ATCO or pilot reports that they have more cognitive workload than they consider safe to manage (Edwards et al., 2017). In cognitive terms this means that the number of synaptic signals that must be detected and processed exceeds what the brain can cope with, leading to significant performance consequences, even inability to continue working (Smolensky, 1990). This is a very dangerous situation of course but a large body of research exists that is focused on protecting the system from this scenario (e.g., Pinska et. al., 2006). Significantly less research has been focused on what happens to ATCOs when nothing (or very little) is going on. This may seem surprising given that the probability of catastrophic accidents such as mid-air collision is so low that it is guaranteed most operators will never come across an unusual situation in their careers (Ostroumov et al., 2020).

The Covid-19 pandemic provided an opportunity to study human performance in ATCOs under these ultra-low traffic circumstances. Several European ANSPs conducted studies looking into these phenomena including at Austro Control where studies were conducted looking specifically at the impact to human performance (Vink, 2021).

After immediate measures to combat monotony, fatigue, and boredom such as increased breaks, re-planning of traffic, and reduced opening hours were taken, a prediction of the types of skills that would fade fastest was made using literature analysis from other industries, such as the medical, education, and military sectors (e.g., Fischer et al., 2018). Particularly, it was concluded that recently learnt skills such as new procedures and technologies would be forgotten faster while more ingrained motor skills such as specific keyboard and mouse inputs required for specialised systems and tasks would take over 9 months to fade. Findings from the research at Austro Control confirmed these skill fade criteria, but a more interesting finding was the impact of monotony and boredom, specifically how controllers were coping with these issues.

A European study conducted just before the Covid-19 period found that, although most controllers would be unlikely to admit it, electronic devices were already being used by ATCOs in most ANSPs across Europe (FABCE Airspace Alliance, 2019). Because it was known that many operational ATM units already had some rules around the use (and non-use) of devices, and in an attempt to be honest about the use of these devices, some of the ANSPs, with a focus on combating the reduction of skills and off-setting monotony, relaxed their rules banning cell phones and other devices (e.g., reading tablets). This was done under controlled rules. For example, in one unit, a controller could only use a device if there were no more than two aircraft on the radio frequencies. In another unit—an airport—the rules stated that a controller could use a digital device if no aircraft were on the ground frequencies or man-oeuvring and there were no more than two aircraft on the approach frequencies. These rules were issued internally after human factors experts conducted an updated review of the use of digital devices (see proposed model below) and implemented them as an experiment to investigate whether these devices could be safely used at all in ATM operations rooms and towers. The initial results suggest that, in certain conditions, digital devices can be a positive stimulus.

5.7.5 CELL PHONE "DISTRACTION" VS. "STIMULUS"

The conclusion of 20 years of research on "cell phone-induced distraction" is that, in almost all cases, human beings are not as good at multi-tasking as they think they are. Regularly, drivers in driving simulators will miss key visual and audible signals when focusing on cell phones (Parnell et al., 2017) as do drivers of real vehicles (Hansma et al., 2020). They are reduced in their abilities to form memories of situations and therefore less likely to retain situational awareness. Interestingly, Strayer et al. (2004) concluded that drivers using cell phones exhibited greater impairment than intoxicated drivers, when controlling for driving difficulty and time on task.

There is a consistent finding of the effect of age on cell phone-induced driver distraction, with younger drivers (under 30) and older drivers (over 65) suffering most (Guo et al., 2016). This makes some sense when factoring driving inexperience (in younger drivers) and slowing of reaction time for older drivers. This could probably be extrapolated to ATM in the case of younger controllers for two reasons. Firstly, less experienced controllers can be more distracted because they are not as "tuned in" as well as more experienced controllers who know what to look and listen for and secondly, when things do happen, they have less problem-solving options because they have not necessarily developed as many yet. However, it is questionable whether the same effect would be seen in older ATCOs since significant reductions in temporal lobe functions tend to be seen in people over 65 and very few ATCOs are still practising above this age (Berron et al., 2018). However, given that more incidents and occurrences happen with controllers over the age of 50 (van de Merwe et al., 2012), it is important to continue being cautious with management techniques for older controllers.

However, despite the overwhelming evidence of the cell phone distraction phenomenon in motor vehicle drivers, the earlier research (i.e., between 2001 and 2015 and see, e.g., Strayer & Drews, 2007 or Overton et al., 2014) focused on traditional approaches to human factors whereby a cause–effect relationship was suggested (implicating cell phones as being causal and blaming the end user). Instead, Parnell et al. (2017) stress that a systems approach to interpreting this research is needed. They also point to the ineffectiveness of total bans on cell phones on efforts to reduce crashes. For example, in the UK, it has been illegal to use a phone while driving since 2003; however 1.6% of drivers across the UK were observed to be on their phones in 2014 (Parnell et al., 2017). Out of 45.5 million drivers, that is a large proportion. The UK's response has been simply to increase the penalty, but drivers continue to break the law at the same rate. The number of incidents where cell phone use was a factor has remained consistent however, suggesting that cell phones are not the only causes.

Although cell phone usage does indeed reduce concentration, distracts from the driving task and plays a role in accidents and occurrences, cell phone usage is not necessarily the only, or even primary, causal factor. Distraction is a concern, but it may not necessarily be a major threat to safety, at least not in some circumstances.

To extrapolate this argument to ATM, more research is needed to establish conclusions but, the number of potential safety gains from the use of cell phones / devices in ATM is likely far greater than those for driving, meaning that distraction is perhaps not the biggest threat—when factoring in many other things such as culture, Human Machine Interface (HMI) design, tower ergonomic layout, and ATCO fatigue (which is still overwhelmingly the major cause of distraction and under-stimulation (Tomic & Liu, 2017)). The systems approach suggests that we need to be careful not to equate the use of digital devices with **causality of occurrences** (Parnell et al., 2017).

In the wider context of aviation operations there are also Just Culture and Safety Culture issues at play. A Just Culture is one in which operators are not punished for actions, omissions or decisions taken by them that are commensurate with their experience and training but where gross negligence, violations and destructive acts are not tolerated (Eurocontrol, 2022). Safety Culture refers to the collected shared beliefs regarding safety and predicts shared safety behaviours (Kirwan et al., 2021). Often, behaviours such as using cell phones to off-set monotony or fatigue are collectively conducted but not reported or discussed due to cultures that are more likely to blame or punish. But many ATCOs would admit—albeit anonymously—that they already use cell phones when on watch in different settings. If we are honest with ourselves, cell phones and devices have crept into every facet of our lives. Denying that personnel are using digital devices to keep themselves awake and alert may be more dangerous than actively managing their usage. A safer approach is to have an open and honest discussion about the potentially constructive use of digital devices and to find a safer means to have oversight on their usage (Schwarz et al., 2016).

5.7.6   THE ATM CONUNDRUM AND POSSIBLE WAYS FORWARD

Although it would be dangerous to allow digital devices into high intensity ATM operations, what about cases where under-load combined with fatigue or drowsiness is the bigger concern? This is increasingly the ATM conundrum. In towers where single-person operations are common, or in operations rooms overnight where traffic levels are quite low, and given the known risk of fatigue on concentration, digital devices might provide a welcome stimulus.

To test this possibility, an increasing number of research studies are looking at drivers in automated vehicles who must intervene in emergency situations. The hypothesis was that, over time, a distraction such as reading, watching a show or playing on one's cell phone would lead to a reduced ability to intervene. However, two studies in 2017 and 2020 have shown that, **while increasing time-on-task** leads to decreased ability to intervene, there is **no significant** reduction in ability to intervene because of a driver's engagement in secondary tasks (Feldhütter et al., 2016). This suggests that engaging in a secondary task in less-stimulating environments does not inhibit one's ability to refocus as and when required. In fact, a 2020 study by Lassmann et al. found that the secondary task produced a positive effect on drivers' ability to intervene—participants reported feeling better and more alert in potentially monotonous situations (Lassmann et al., 2020).

This is a radical new way of thinking about the use of devices while driving. It indicates that, in periods of significant underloading, or under reduced operations such as single-person operational towers, or in overnight watches in larger operations rooms, secondary tasks (not necessarily devices, but games, books, etc.) might be beneficial for operators by keeping them alert.

Crucially, a finding of no significant reduction in ability to intervene when interacting with a cell phone suggests that operators' **cognitive pathways are primed** to react in the normal ways that they have been trained to do, just by virtue of being present in the responsible position. In other words, someone conducting other secondary tasks, but remaining present on watch, can intervene and resume their primary task(s) without a loss of ability (Naujoks et al., 2018). There are parallels here with other industries such as the maritime industry, where bridge watchkeepers are regularly engaged in other tasks—such as plotting fixes or having their attention away from looking out—but can resume the primary task of keeping the ship safe when an alarm is raised (Straussberger, 2006).

Therefore, it is possible that, with the rise of underloading and automation resulting in controller tasks moving to monitoring rather than tactical handling of traffic, a secondary task such as digital device usage may provide beneficial stimulation without loss of ability to intervene.

5.7.6.1 A WAY OF DEPLOYING DEVICES SAFELY

Like many challenges in safety management, the probability of an event must be weighed against the severity of an outcome. It is possible therefore to predict, using several criteria, the risk probabilities and likelihoods involved in allowing the usage of digital devices into operations. However, a responsible and valid amount of data needs to be collected. Some of the criteria for consideration are presented here in a **potential model** for risk modelling the use of digital devices in ATM operations rooms. Austro Control utilised such an approach during the Covid-19 pandemic to provide guidance to units as to when it might be safe and beneficial to use digital devices.

5.7.6.2 METHODOLOGY

To create the model, a selection of 12 ATCOs from different domains held workshops facilitated by human factors specialists. Based on literature reviews such as Parnell et al. (2017) it was decided that the best way to allow safe and controlled use of stimulants would be to map the units/domains of ATM by risk. The choice of "distraction" and "decreased time to respond" (representing two established hazards) were placed on the y-axis against "positive stimulant" and "increased time to respond" (two positive countermeasures) on the x-axis.

Next, the workshops created a list of criteria for consideration during risk assessment. Table 5.7.1 outlines the most imporant criteria identified that could be used.

After establishing the risk assessment criteria, the workshops identified all the possible domains that existed (within Austria) in which to test the mapping. These domains are listed in Table 5.7.2. Using the number label for each domain, this was transferred to the operational risk matrix shown in Figure 5.7.1.

Finally, the workshop evaluated the domains using the two sets of axes. The amount of distraction that a device/stimulant might present was weighted against the assessed positive outcome. The second was "decreased time to respond" vs "increased time to respond" (e.g., to a urgent task such as an aircraft calling in via radio) that refers to the danger present in an operation if time is a crucial factor. For example, usually, approach sectors over large airports are extremely time critical (see number 3) whereas a tower controller operating overnight when there is no traffic is not as time critical.

TABLE 5.7.1
Criteria for Risk Assessment of Units by Use of Stimulants

1	Probability of under-stimulation vs normal human performance capacity
2	Frequency of traffic (e.g., ACC sectors are combined to provide controllers with enough to do vs. Single-person Tower who has one movement every 2 hours)
3	Number of sectors and the associated Monitor Values (maximum traffic capacity of sectors)
4	Environmental conditions (e.g., Weather phenomenon)
5	Amount of available support staff
6	Severity of failing to intervene in time
7	Probability that intervention would be needed
8	Comfort or social interaction factor (e.g., Enjoyment, Meaning, team-work, and social company)
9	Probability of boredom, monotony, or fatigue (e.g., single-person operations vs. multi-team operations)
10	Amount of additional safety nets (e.g., communication frequencies connected, multiple people monitoring same info in other countries/areas, alarms etc.)

TABLE 5.7.2
Types of ATM and Engineering Support Domains

1	En-Route Controllers with normal traffic
2	En-Route Controllers with 5–10% of normal traffic levels ("Covid" conditions)
3	Approach Controllers with normal traffic
4	Approach Controllers with 20–25% of normal traffic ("Covid" conditions)
5	En-Route/Approach Supervisors with Normal Traffic
6	En-Route/Approach Supervisors with Covid-19 levels of Traffic
7	Tower Controllers at a Large Airport with normal traffic
8	Tower Controllers at a Large Airport overnight with 10% traffic
9	Tower Controllers at a Regional Airport with normal traffic
10	Tower Controllers at a Regional Airport with 10% traffic (e.g., overnight traffic levels)
11	Tower Controllers in Single-person operations during the day
12	Tower Controllers in Single-person operations overnight
13	Operational Engineers during the day
14	Operational Engineers during the night with no maintenance

Note. The numbers in the left column correlate with the numbers in Figure 5.7.1.

The use of the operational risk matrix allowed for controlled, risk managed introduction of digital devices and stimulants into some operations during the Covid-19 pandemic period which helped to mitigate some of the monotony and boredom experienced by low traffic levels.

Over the 24-month Covid-19 period, occurrence data was regularly reviewed but no evidence of distraction from personal device use was found as a contributing factor to occurrences. These data suggested that, when digital devices were allowed into operations rooms to off-set monotony, they may have helped and were safely used. This also provides

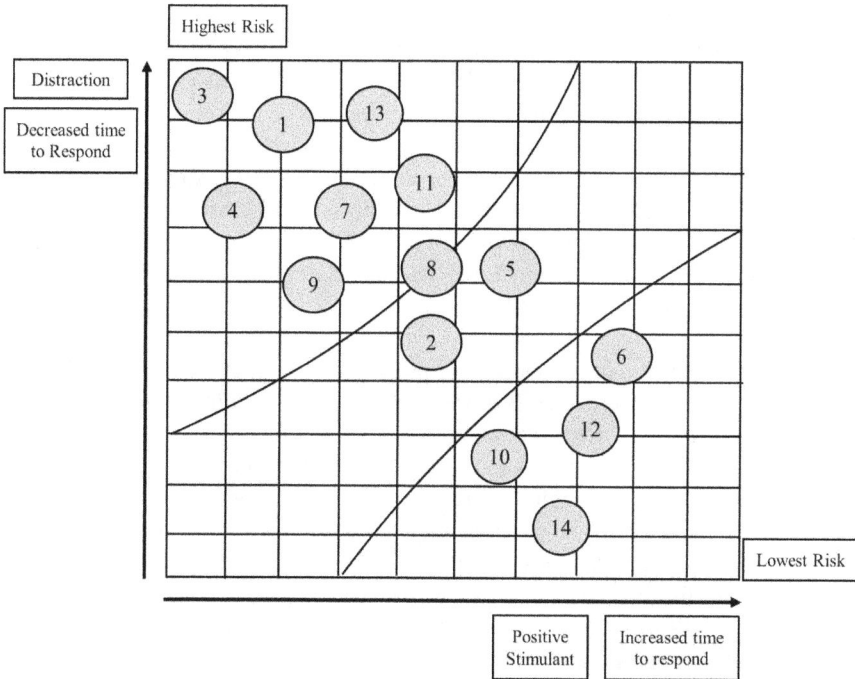

FIGURE 5.7.1 Proposed operational risk matrix for the safe use of digital devices in ATM operations.

some early evidence of the usefulness of such an approach. However, more research is required. For example, shifts or domains where devices or stimulants are not used should be compared to domains where devices are used. Simulated traffic levels and other methods of controlling distractions and task-drivers should also be used to test this approach.

Additionally, to safely use the above model, human performance metrics are needed. A possibility would be to combine objective measures from the criteria above such as the maximum and average amounts of aircraft that can be managed by a sector (known as Monitor Values), traffic frequencies, scheduled frequencies, etc., with other HMI data such as mouse clicks or keyboard inputs. This would give an indication of the aggregate amount of integration required per flight. From there, simulations could assess the ability of controllers to intervene or respond whilst using cell phones. Importantly, ratings of situational awareness and workload should also be collected to model this most accurately (Arico et al., 2017). Metrics such as these could provide a very accurate picture of the true risks associated with using digital devices.

5.7.7 CONCLUSIONS

The use of digital devices as a means of off-setting monotony, boredom, and fatigue is promising. However, the full impact to ATCOs—where tasks can be complex and where there are periods of peak mental activity and performance—is not yet conclusively known. The majority of evidence still supports the common-sense view: That digital devices are distracting in complex, busy operations where attention and focus is needed (e.g., Hansma et al., 2020). However, in periods of significantly lower workload, such as single manned towers, overnight periods, remote tower monitoring or as watches become less hands-on, digital devices may provide a positive effect keeping controllers awake and alert without having an impact on their ability to refocus when required. During the Covid-19 pandemic, this approach was observed and there was no statistically significant effect in terms of occurrences.

A common theme throughout the research is that fatigue and drowsiness have a larger impact on safety regardless of the usage of digital devices, and in ATM we should defend against these effects more strongly. While eliminating digital devices **may seem like a quick win**, the larger systematic view suggests **that we should focus on policies and procedures to reduce fatigue,** which could include the use of stimulation devices such as digital devices or other secondary tasks. Further research is needed that could capitalise on already existing research programmes such as the SESAR Joint Undertaking (a European private-public research collaboration to accelerate delivery of the Single-European Sky policy (SESAR) Joint Undertaking, 2022) as well as on exploratory research projects both internal and external to ANSPs. The model could be further developed and introduced as an operational risk matrix tool. Ultimately, as our systems become more automated and more digital, capable of real-time analysis and adoption of safety features, the possibility for a more nuanced and mature approach to fatigue management and the use of digital devices is becoming a reality.

SUMMARY POINTS FOR PRACTITIONERS

- The role of humans in Air Traffic Management is changing. Covid-19 has shown us that many traditional watch structures and measures to off-set fatigue, monotony, and boredom are not agile enough.
- Human operators are gradually moving towards a more passive role with the rise of automation and technology. This has potential to reduce their ability to intervene in critical situations.
- Traditionally there has been hesitancy at allowing digital personal devices into the ATM operations rooms because of the possibility of distraction. But ATM has a higher number of safety nets and distraction alone might not be the biggest risk.
- Monotony, boredom, and fatigue decrease the brain's ability to intervene. New research from driverless cars and cockpits shows that keeping brains stimulated increases the ability to intervene correctly.
- A careful and controlled use of digital personal devices such as cell phones or e-readers may therefore provide more benefits and stimulus to ATCOs in order to maintain alertness. More research is needed into the effects for ATM.

REFERENCES

Arico, P., Borghini, G., di Flumeri, G., Bonelli, S., Golfetti, A., Graziani, I., Pozzi, S., Imbert, J. P., Granger, G., Benhacene, R., Schaefer, D., & Babiloni, F. (2017). Human factors and neurophysiological metrics in air traffic control: A critical review. *IEEE Reviews in Biomedical Engineering*, *10*, 250–263. https://doi.org/10.1109/rbme.2017.2694142

Berron, D., Neumann, K., Maass, A., Schütze, H., Fliessbach, K., Kiven, V., Jessen, F., Sauvage, M., Kumaran, D., & Düzel, E. (2018). Age-related functional changes in domain-specific medial temporal lobe pathways. *Neurobiology of Aging*, *65*, 86–97. https://doi.org/10.1016/j.neurobiolaging.2017.12.030

Castro, S. C., Strayer, D. L., Matzke, D., & Heathcote, A. (2019). Cognitive workload measurement and modeling under divided attention. *Journal of Experimental Psychology: Human Perception and Performance*, *45*(6), 826–839. https://doi.org/10.1037/xhp0000638

Chang, Y. H., Yang, H. H., & Hsu, W. J. (2019). Effects of work shifts on fatigue levels of air traffic controllers. *Journal of Air Transport Management*, *76*, 1–9. https://doi.org/10.1016/j.jairtraman.2019.01.013

Commision Implementing Regulation 2017/373. Laying down common requirements for providers of air traffic management/air navigation services and other air traffic management network functions and their oversight.

Department of Transport. (1992, April). *Report on the accident to BAC One-Eleven, G-BJRT, over Didcot, Oxfordshire on 10 June 1990* (No. 1/1992). https://assets.publishing.service.gov.uk/media/5422faa7e5274a131400078d/1-1992_G-BJRT.pdf

Edwards, T., Gabets, C., Mercer, J., & Bienert, N. (2017). Task demand variation in air traffic control: Implications for workload, fatigue, and performance. In *Advances in human aspects of transportation* (pp. 91–102). Springer, Cham.

Endsley, M. R. (1995). Toward a theory of situation awareness in dynamic systems. *Human Factors: The Journal of the Human Factors and Ergonomics Society*, *37*(1), 32–64. https://doi.org/10.1518/001872095779049543

Eurocontrol. (2022). *Just culture*. SKYbrary. Retrieved 8 August 2022, from https://skybrary.aero/articles/just-culture.

FABCE Airspace Alliance. (2019, April). *FABCE safety survey electronic devices*. FABCE.

Feldhütter, A., Gold, C., Schneider, S., & Bengler, K. (2016). How the duration of automated driving influences take-over performance and gaze behavior. *Advances in Ergonomic Design of Systems, Products and Processes*, 309–318. https://doi.org/10.1007/978-3-662-53305-5_22

Guo, F., Klauer, S. G., Fang, Y., Hankey, J. M., Antin, J. F., Perez, M. A., Lee, S. E., & Dingus, T. A. (2016). The effects of age on crash risk associated with driver distraction. *International Journal of Epidemiology*, *46*(1), 258–265. https://doi.org/10.1093/ije/dyw234

Hansma, B. J., Marulanda, S., Chen, H. Y. W., & Donmez, B. (2020). Role of habits in cell phone-related driver distractions. *Transportation Research Record: Journal of the Transportation Research Board*, *2674*(12), 254–262. https://doi.org/10.1177/0361198120953157

ICAO. (2016). *Manual for the oversight of fatigue management approaches* (No. 9966). International Civil Aviation Organization. www.icao.int/safety/fatiguemanagement/FRMS%20Tools/Doc%209966.FRMS.2016%20Edition.en.pdf.

ICAO. (2021, December 14). *Effects of novel coronavirus (COVID-19) on civil aviation: Economic impact analysis* [Slides]. PowerPoint.

Image of pilot hanging out window captures heroic story 30 years on. (2020, November 18). *NZ Herald*. Retrieved 2 December 2021, from www.nzherald.co.nz/travel/image-of-pilot-hanging-out-window-captures-heroic-story-30-years-on/GR2HBBCBUGMOTA7MEYPI7UR54A/.

Kahneman, D. (2011). *Thinking, fast and slow* (1st ed.). Farrar, Straus and Giroux.

Kirwan, B., Shorrock, S., & Reader, T. (2021, February). *The future of safety culture in European air traffic management*. Eurocontrol. https://skybrary.aero/sites/default/files/bookshelf/5993.pdf

Lassmann, P., Fischer, M. S., Bieg, H.-J., Jenke, M., Reichelt, F., Tuezuen, G.-J., & Maier, T. (2019). Keeping the balance between overload and underload during partly automated driving: Relevant secondary tasks. In T. Bertram (Ed.), *Automatisiertes Fahren 2019. Proceedings*. (pp. 233–250). Springer Publishing. https://doi.org/10.1007/978-3-658-27990-5_19

Metzger, U., & Parasuraman, R. (2005). Automation in future air traffic management: Effects of decision aid reliability on controller performance and mental workload. *Human Factors: The Journal of the Human Factors and Ergonomics Society*, *47*(1), 35–49. https://doi.org/10.1518/0018720053653802

Naujoks, F., Höfling, S., Purucker, C., & Zeeb, K. (2018). From partial and high automation to manual driving: Relationship between non-driving related tasks, drowsiness and take-over performance. *Accident Analysis and Prevention*, *121*, 28–42. https://doi.org/10.1016/j.aap.2018.08.018

Ostroumov, I., Ivashchuk, O., Shmelova, T., & Babichev, S. (2020). Risk of mid-air collision in a lateral plane. *CITRisk*, 297–307.

Overton, T. L., Rives, T. E., Hecht, C., Shafi, S., & Gandhi, R. R. (2014). Distracted driving: Prevalence, problems, and prevention. *International Journal of Injury Control and Safety Promotion*, *22*(3), 187–192. https://doi.org/10.1080/17457300.2013.879482

Parnell, K. J., Stanton, N. A., & Plant, K. (2017). Where are we on driver distraction? Methods, approaches and recommendations. *Theoretical Issues in Ergonomics Science*, *19*(5), 578–605. https://doi.org/10.1080/1463922x.2017.1414333

Pinska, E., Tijus, C., Jouen, F., Poitrenaud, S., & Zibetti, E. (2006). Reducing cognitive load of air traffic controllers through the modeling of the hierarchical segmentation of inputs. In *Fifth Eurocontrol Innovative Research Workshop & Exhibition* (pp. 137–144).

Rudin-Brown, C. M., Young, K. L., & Lenné, M. G. (2009). Behavioural adaptation to mobile phone legislation: Could there be unintended consequences of partial bans? *Proceedings of the First International Conference on Driver Distraction and Inattention*.

Schwarz, M., Kallus, K. W., & Gaisbachgrabner, K. (2016). Safety culture, resilient behavior, and stress in air traffic management. *Aviation Psychology and Applied Human Factors*, *6*(1), 12–23. https://doi.org/10.1027/2192-0923/a000091

SESAR Joint Undertaking. (2022). *Discover SESAR*. Retrieved 5 August 2022, from www.sesarju.eu/discover-sesar.

Smolensky, M. W. (1990, December). *The effect of work load history on operational errors in air traffic control simulation: The hysteresis effect—expectancy perseverance or short-term memory overload?* (Dissertation, Psychology). Texas Tech University. https://ttu-ir.tdl.org/ttu-ir/bitstream/handle/2346/18923/31295005967517.pdf?sequence=1.

Straussberger, S. (2006, November). *Montony in air traffic control–contributing factors and mitigation strategies* (No. 15/06). EEC. https://citeseerx.ist.psu.edu/viewdoc/download?doi=10.1.1.75.9999&rep=rep1&type=pdf

Straussberger, S., & Schaefer, D. (2007). Monotony in air traffic control. *Air Traffic Control Quarterly*, *15*(3), 183–207. https://doi.org/10.2514/atcq.15.3.183

Strayer, D. L., Crouch, D. J., & Drews, F. A. (2004). A comparison of the cell phone driver and the drunk driver. *SSRN Electronic Journal*. https://doi.org/10.2139/ssrn.570222

Strayer, D. L., & Drews, F. A. (2007). Cell-Phone–Induced driver distraction. *Current Directions in Psychological Science*, *16*(3), 128–131. https://doi.org/10.1111/j.1467-8721.2007.00489.x

Teixeira De Freitas, S., Kolstein, H., & Bijlaard, F. (2017). Fatigue assessment of full-scale retrofitted orthotropic bridge decks. *Journal of Bridge Engineering*, *22*(11). https://doi.org/10.1061/(asce)be.1943-5592.0001115

Tomic, I., & Liu, J. (2017). Strategies to overcome fatigue in air traffic control based on stress management. *The International Journal of Engineering and Science*, *06*(04), 48–57. https://doi.org/10.9790/1813-0604014857

van de Merwe, K., Oprins, E., Eriksson, F., & van der Plaat, A. (2012). The influence of automation support on performance, workload, and situation awareness of air traffic controllers. *The International Journal of Aviation Psychology*, *22*(2), 120–143. https://doi.org/10.1080/10508414.2012.663241

Vink, N. (2021). The effect to human performance and wellbeing of air traffic management operational staff through the COVID-19 pandemic. In *91st International Symposium on Aviation Psychology* (pp. 370–375). International Symposium on Aviation Psychology.

Walker, M. (2017). *Why we sleep: Unlocking the power of sleep and dreams*. Scribner.

Wickens, C. D. (2008a). Multiple resources and mental workload. *Human Factors: The Journal of the Human Factors and Ergonomics Society*, *50*(3), 449–455. https://doi.org/10.1518/001872008x288394

Yuan, L., Ma, G., & Sun, R. (2016). An analysis of fatigue and its characteristics: A survey on Chinese air traffic controllers. In D. Harris (Ed.), *Engineering Psychology and Cognitive Ergonomics. EPCE 2016. Lecture Notes in Computer Science, vol 9736* (pp. 38–47). Springer, Cham. https://doi.org/10.1007/978-3-319-40030-3_5

Section 6

Fatigue Risk Management of the Future

6.1 Road Vehicle Automation and Its Effects on Fatigue, Sleep, Rest, and Recuperation

Christer Ahlström,[1] Johanna Wörle,[2] Mikael Ljung Aust,[3] and Frederik Diederichs[4]

[1]Swedish National Road and Transport Research Institute (VTI), and Department of Biomedical Engineering, Linköping University, Linköping, Sweden
[2]Würzburg Institute for Traffic Sciences (WIVW) Veitshöchheim, Germany
[3]Volvo Cars Safety Centre, Volvo Car Corporation, Gothenburg, Sweden
[4]Fraunhofer Institute of Optronics, System Technologies and Image Exploitation (IOSB), Karlsruhe, Germany

CONTENTS

6.1.1 INTRODUCTION

As more driving assistance functions are introduced, our vehicles gradually become more capable of both driving and handling risky situations by themselves. Today, for example, anti-lock braking systems help us preserve tyre traction when we do emergency steering and braking manoeuvres. Lane keeping assistance systems gently steer us back

DOI: 10.1201/9781003213154-43

if we drift out of the lane. Adaptive cruise control adapts a set cruise speed and headway time to slower-moving vehicles ahead. Automatic emergency braking systems detect slow or stopped traffic and urgently apply the brakes, if needed. Even highly automated vehicles, such as robot taxis that can drive from A to B with no human intervention, have started to appear on public roads. However, these highly automated systems have not yet reached the level of technical sophistication where they can be widely deployed and used everywhere on all types of roads. Until this happens, a responsible driver should therefore always be present when automated functions are active. In case an assistance function malfunctions, or if the automated system leaves the specific domain in which it is designed to operate properly, the driver must be ready to take over control and manage any part of the driving task that a function has assumed control over.

There are different ways to define the capabilities and responsibilities of an automated vehicle system. The commonly referred to Society of Automotive Engineers (SAE) standard J3016 suggests six levels of driving automation (SAE, 2021). To understand the SAE structure, it is important to know that future automated driving systems often are assumed to operate only in a pre-defined situation/environment, called the systems' Operational Design Domain (ODD). Level 0 equals unassisted manual driving in any ODD. Levels 1 to 2 are *assisted* driving where the human driver still is responsible for maintaining vehicle control. Levels 3 to 4 represent *piloted* driving where the automated system is responsible within a specific ODD and a human driver is responsible for all driving outside the ODD. Level 5 is also *piloted driving*, but can also be referred to as "robot taxi"; no driver involvement in controlling the vehicle is needed at any point.

These six automation levels can be summarised as follows (see Table 6.1.1):

Level 0: Manual driving, the driver performs all driving tasks.

Level 1: An advanced driver assistance system (ADAS) on the vehicle can assist the human driver with either steering or braking/accelerating, but not both simultaneously. The driver must constantly supervise the support features when they are engaged.

Level 2: Partial Automation ("hands off")—An ADAS can itself control both steering and braking/accelerating simultaneously within the systems' ODD. The human driver must monitor the driving environment and be ready to take control at all times, even without a notification.

Level 3: Conditional Automation ("eyes off")—An automated driving system (ADS) can perform all aspects of the driving task within the systems' ODD. When the system is available and active, the human driver can engage in non-driving-related activities (NDRA), but must always be ready to take control with short notice (a few seconds). Outside of the system's ODD, the human driver performs the driving task.

Level 4: High Automation ("mind off")—An ADS can do all of the driving within the system's ODD. The human need not pay attention within the ODD and will be notified well in advance (several minutes) before having to resume control. Outside of the system's ODD, the human driver performs the driving task.

Level 5: Full Automation ("body off")—An ADS can do all of the driving in all situations. The human occupants are just passengers and need never be involved in the driving task.

TABLE 6.1.1
Levels of Automation Set Forth in SAE J3016 Standard, Complemented with Fatigue-Related Issues in the Last Column

Level	Name	Control	Monitoring	Fallback	Operational Design Domain	Fatigue-related issues and opportunities
Manual 0	No automation				Limited	Task-related fatigue, sleepiness
Assisted 1	Driver assistance				Limited	Task-related fatigue, sleepiness
2	Partial automation				Limited	Task-related fatigue, sleepiness
Piloted 3	Conditional automation				Limited	Underload, sleepiness
4	High automation				Limited	Sleep inertia, sleepiness, recovery by nap and sleep
5	Full automation				Unlimited	Recovery by nap and sleep

Note: Levels of Automation Set Forth in SAE J3016 Standard, complemented with fatigue-related issues in the last column.

These six levels have different implications for fatigue. For instance, in manual driving (level 0), fatigue commonly arises during the night or in the early morning hours. It can also appear after too many uninterrupted hours of wakefulness spent behind the wheel or after extended periods of high or low workload (Williamson et al., 2011). Assisted driving (levels 1 to 2) has the potential to reduce fatigue caused by high workload, at least to the extent the driving task itself is causing the overload. However, since the driver's role in that case shifts from driving to monitoring, levels of fatigue may then instead increase due to boredom, monotony and/or exhaustive attentive monitoring without an active task. With more sophisticated and reliable forms of driving automation, it thus becomes more difficult for a human driver to maintain the level of vigilance needed to monitor both the automation and the roadway (Bainbridge, 1983; Carsten & Martens, 2019; Noy et al., 2018).

An effective countermeasure for fatigue due to underload is to stop driving and take a short break, or to activate oneself by, for example, engaging in an NDRA while driving. Engaging in NDRAs while driving becomes feasible during piloted driving (SAE levels 3 to 5). However, in level 3, the human must remain alert enough to be able to resume manual driving with short notice. The real game changer from a fatigue point of view is therefore when level 4 and level 5 systems are introduced. These will allow a travelling human to sleep, recover, and recuperate from fatigue while on the move. As such, these ADS will facilitate a truly effective countermeasure for fatigue (given that sleep inertia issues can be managed, see below).

The remainder of this chapter summarises the current state of the art on how assisted and piloted automated driving can affect driver fatigue. Fatigue is here defined as the biological drive for recuperative rest. The type of rest that is needed depends on what type of fatigue the driver experiences (May & Baldwin, 2009). If the driver is suffering from high levels of task-related fatigue due to overload, which often occurs in parallel to stress, adequate rest refers to cease driving and temporarily shut off demands of sustained attention. In comparison, if fatigue is due to under-stimulation or boredom, then activation rather than rest is required to reduce the level of fatigue. In contrast, if fatigue is due to sleep deprivation or driving at night-time, actual sleep is needed.

6.1.2 DEVELOPMENT OF FATIGUE IN ASSISTED DRIVING

Many new vehicles are equipped with level 1 technologies designed to actively prevent crashes. Examples include lane departure warnings and lane keeping assistance systems. Such systems considerably reduce single-vehicle, sideswipe, and head-on injury crash rates, that is, crashes that are often associated with driver fatigue and/ or inattention (Cicchino, 2018; Sternlund et al., 2017; Wang et al., 2020). The extent to which more advanced automated functions, such as level 2 systems, have safety benefits above and beyond level 1 functions has yet to be determined (Mueller et al., 2021). For example, there are concerns that problems with driver fatigue may become worse when using level 2 systems as compared to manual driving (Ahlström, Zemblys, et al., 2021; Dunn et al., 2021; Flynn-Evans et al., 2021; Kundinger et al., 2020). One hypothesis is that fatigue increases due to boredom and underload when the vehicle takes over both the lateral and longitudinal continuous control tasks. Another hypothesis is that attentive monitoring without active task engagement is very demanding (Warm et al., 2008) and leads to fatigue due to overload (Greenlee et al., 2019; Solís-Marcos et al., 2018; Stapel et al., 2019).

6.1.3 DEVELOPMENT OF FATIGUE IN PILOTED DRIVING

Piloted automated systems have not yet reached the market. Most research on piloted driving is therefore based on driving simulator experiments with participants who have no previous experience of such systems. This can be problematic for several reasons. Firstly, compared to manual driving on real roads, fatigue develops faster and to higher levels in driving simulators (Fors et al., 2018; Hallvig et al., 2013). It is possible that automated simulated driving could lead to even faster development of fatigue, especially if the drivers are not allowed to engage in NDRAs. Secondly, it is not known how experience and familiarity with ADS affect drivers' trust of and reliance on the systems, and how this in turn might affect fatigue. The results described here and in the next sub-section should therefore be interpreted with these limitations in mind.

In contrast to SAE level 2 systems, levels 3 to 4 systems are designed to work without human intervention when the system is within its ODD. Importantly, piloted systems are not allowed to disengage before a human driver resumes manual control in a verified manner. This means that the driver does not have to continuously monitor the roadway and the automation; rather, they need to only remain alert enough to be able to start driving manually within a given time frame. An interesting research question on level 3 systems is thus if drivers can remain alert enough to safely resume control when requested to do so. Available research shows that driver performance after a takeover request is affected both by fatigue level (Kreuzmair et al., 2017) and by type of fatigue (Vogelpohl et al., 2019), where sleep-related fatigue leads to slower resumption of manual control compared to task-related fatigue. Also, reduced performance prevails after the takeover when driving manually again, especially during the night (Kaduk et al., 2021a, 2021b).

Not surprisingly, drivers seem to have a difficult time staying alert during extended periods of piloted driving. Feldhütter et al. (2019) found that 25% of their participants temporarily showed strong evidence of fatigue or fell asleep when driving with a level 3 system in a simulator. Similarly, Vogelpohl et al. (2019) reported that drivers showed signs of fatigue already after only 15 to 35 minutes of piloted driving. This is in contrast to a condition with manual driving where fatigue only arose in sleep-deprived drivers and then only after a longer period of driving (about 40 minutes). Furthermore, testing in 2012 and 2013 in the Google Self-Driving Car Project showed that employees, when asked to supervise during piloted driving in freeway environments, frequently engaged in behaviours such a prolonged use of personal devices (Favaro et al., 2022). They were also subject to signs of fatigue including microsleep events and some participants were even seen asleep at the wheel for extended periods of time.

To avoid fatigue due to underload and boredom in piloted driving, it is important that drivers are allowed to "activate" themselves (Jarosch, Paradies, et al., 2019). Examples of activities include working, watching movies, playing games, and interacting with social media. By engaging in various NDRAs, drivers can limit the development of task-related fatigue, which in turn improves takeover performance (Jarosch, Bellem, et al., 2019; Jarosch, Paradies, et al., 2019; Naujoks et al., 2018; Neubauer et al., 2014; Schömig et al., 2015). Similarly, a richer and more engaging driving environment reduces fatigue in piloted driving (Jamson et al., 2013; Zhang et al., 2021). The actual "amount" of driver fatigue that can be countered by engagement in NDRAs is however limited and eventually the NDRA itself will start to contribute to fatigue, which may be a reason why long-duration piloted drives show poorer driver takeover performance compared to shorter duration piloted drives (Bourrelly et al., 2019).

6.1.4 SLEEP AND SLEEP INERTIA IN PILOTED DRIVING

A game changer in fighting driver fatigue could be the introduction of piloted driving systems at SAE levels 4 and 5. Since these systems do not require the driver to resume manual control on short notice, drivers may then choose to rest or sleep and only resume control in planned takeovers if/when the ODD ends. In modern society with long working and commuting hours, shift work, and social duties, this could have major benefits for users. For example, one-fourth of employed people in Europe spend 30 to 60 minutes on their daily commute to work (eurostat, 2020). Also, an increasing number of Americans—about one-third of the US adult population in 2019—claim to not to get enough sleep (Sheehan et al., 2019). Using the daily commute to catch up on sleep could therefore be highly beneficial, since even a short 10-minute nap can improve alertness and performance (Milner & Cote, 2009). Indeed, potential users of ADS state that sleeping in the vehicle would be one of their preferred activities (Becker et al., 2018; Schoettle & Sivak, 2014). For commercial drivers, particularly long-haul truck drivers with long working hours, planned sleep periods on a journey could even become part of Fatigue Risk Management Systems (Gander et al., 2016) to restore alertness, performance, and well-being (Ahlström, van Leeuwen, et al., 2021).

At SAE level 4, the automation is only available during part(s) of a trip, e.g., only on certain highway sections. When the automated system's ODD ends, the driver still needs to resume manual driving. If drivers use some or all of the ODD time to sleep, they will need to be awakened in time to resume driving safely. One therefore must ask whether drivers can resume high quality driving after sleeping, given that sleep inertia (the transitional state of lowered arousal occurring after awakening from sleep—see also Chapter 3.2) has been identified as a safety issue in other modes of transport like aviation (Hartzler, 2014).

Only a few studies have investigated the effects of sleep inertia on driver takeover behaviour when transitioning from piloted driving to manual control. One driving simulator study found that, when sleeping drivers were awakened by a request to intervene, their takeover reactions were delayed, and they showed visual disorientation compared to when they were not sleeping (Wörle et al., 2020). Under the influence of sleep inertia, participants' overall takeover performance yielded "errors", such as strong oscillations in the lane and missing safety glances when changing lanes, compared to only "imprecisions" when they operated the vehicle when awake. Drivers in that study experienced the situation of taking back control after sleep as "stressful" and "unpleasant" as compared to when taking over vehicle control at normal alertness (Wörle et al., 2021; Wörle et al., 2020). On the other hand, a similar study in a driving simulator yielded no differences in driving performance or mental workload ratings between a nap-condition and a no-nap condition (Hirsch et al., 2020). In the Wörle et al. studies, participants were always awakened in stable sleep (sleep stage N2) which was verified with EEG, while in the Hirsch et al., study, the sleep stage was not controlled, suggesting that the sleep stage before awakening influenced performance in the takeover situation.

The extent to which sleep results in sleep inertia can depend on a number of factors including sleep history, circadian timing, duration of the sleep episode, the sleep stage from which the driver is awakened from, if one eats before sleeping and also situational variables such as the difficulty of the takeover scenario or the wake-up modality (Hilditch & McHill, 2019; Tassi & Muzet, 2000). Furthermore, the intensity and duration of sleep inertia can vary, and no empirical data is available on the impacts of strong versus light sleep inertia. It is however clear that sleep inertia is common after sleep and that it impairs physical and cognitive performance, including driving performance (Wörle et al., 2020). The effects of sleep inertia on driver behaviour during and after transition of control therefore needs to be investigated further before sleep can become a use case in automated driving. System designers need to consider that a driver's physical and cognitive performance might be impaired for up to 30 minutes after waking up (Tassi & Muzet, 2000).

While SAE level 4 systems may at some point allow drivers to sleep while the system is in the ODD, the quality of sleep obtained during automated driving will likely not be as recuperative as sleeping in one's bed at home. This issue challenges the expectation that automated driving could extend driving hours to any larger extent in the haulage industry (Ahlström, van Leeuwen, et al., 2021). To overcome that difference, automated driving systems and vehicle interiors need to be designed to maximise the benefits of sleeping while still maintaining adequate vehicle crash-worthiness. In other words, for drivers of levels 4 and 5 systems, achieving high-quality sleep should not increase the risk of personal injury should the vehicle be involved in a crash. This presents a considerable additional challenge for automotive manufacturers.

6.1.5   DRIVER MONITORING SYSTEMS IN AUTOMATED VEHICLES

Current driver monitoring and fatigue detection systems are based on:

i. vehicle-based information such as lane keeping performance;
ii. behavioural information such as inactivity, yawning, and eye movements; and
iii. driver physiological data such as heart rate and brain activity.

The most common driver fatigue detection systems in today's production vehicles are based on drivers' lane keeping performance. This kind of measure does not work when an ADS is doing the lane keeping, and so more direct physiological–and/or behavioural-based ways to determine drivers' fatigue levels are needed (Halin et al., 2021; Mueller et al., 2021).

Note that at SAE levels 1 to 2, a fatigue detection system should monitor the driver's fatigue level continuously, just as it would do in manual driving. This aspect of driver monitoring is covered in Chapter 4.6. At levels 3 to 5 the driver does not need to supervise the system when it is engaged. However, in levels 3 and 4, the driver must resume manual driving at some point, when the system alerts them that driver takeover is necessary. A fatigue detection system suitable for levels 3 and 4 systems must therefore (i) continuously assess whether the driver is fit to drive, and (ii) verify that the driver is attentive and physically positioned to drive safely before the actual transfer of control takes place. The second requirements arise as the driver may have been out of the loop for a considerable amount of time when requested to resume manual control. Verifying that the driver is attentive and positioned to drive is therefore a necessary precaution.

An important practical issue for fatigue detection in automated systems is that behaviour-based fatigue detection systems which work for manual driving may not be entirely applicable in automated driving. When a driver disengages from driving, she/ he may lay down, move around, or engage in other tasks in ways that block the sensors and/or mislead the algorithms analysing the sensor data. This issue was highlighted in a study by Feldhütter et al. (2019) where the percentage of eyelid closure (PERCLOS) was used to monitor fatigue. During automated driving, participant drivers engaged in an NDRA on a handheld device in their lap, which thus required them to look down. The camera-based driver monitoring system used in the study incorrectly interpreted this behaviour as long periods of driving with eyes closed. This resulted in very high PERCLOS values, even though the drivers had their eyes open and were alert.

For automated features at SAE level 5, no fatigue detection is needed since the driver is never in control, and becomes, in effect, a passenger of the vehicle.

6.1.6 FATIGUE COUNTERMEASURES IN AUTOMATED VEHICLES

For automated systems at SAE levels 1 and 2, the types of fatigue countermeasures needed are roughly the same as for manual driving. This includes escalated warning strategies that gradually make use, and increases the saliency, of multimodal alerts. For example, warnings could ramp up from visual only to later include tactile and auditory alerts and eventually also pulse braking (Mueller et al., 2021). Proactive countermeasures are also plausible, especially those warning systems that simultaneously promote situational awareness. One example is a lane-keeping assistance system in which a motor acts on the steering wheel by adding torques (Mulder et al., 2012). Proactive and corrective countermeasures on the strategic, tactical, and operational level for manual driving can be found in Section 4 of this book.

In piloted driving, automated functions can, in and of themselves, act as fatigue countermeasures. At levels 3 to 4, the vehicle system must be capable of initiating minimal-risk manoeuvres such as parking the car in a safe location. Thus, if the driver is non-responsive to a takeover request, the vehicle should still be able to stop safely even if the driver does not intervene. Also, if the driver is detected to be asleep while the vehicle is still in its ODD, the system can try to wake the driver. Such wake-up measures should escalate in message urgency and increase the number of modalities used for alerts when the vehicle approaches the end of its ODD. In addition to previously mentioned multimodal alerts, it would also be possible to use olfactory (smell) cues to prepare a fatigued or sleeping driver before the takeover (Tang et al., 2021).

One must remember that task-related fatigue will primarily be affected by these types of alerts, while sleepiness-related fatigue will not. A sleepy driver may momentarily become less fatigued, but typically will return to pre-alert fatigue levels after about 5 to 10 minutes (Anund et al., 2008). Still, these 5 to 10 minutes may be enough if the goal is to manually bring the vehicle to a complete stop or to manually manoeuvre the vehicle through, for example, a roadwork section.

6.1.7 CONCLUSIONS

Piloted automated driving brings new challenges and opportunities both for detecting and counteracting fatigue in driving. In terms of counteracting, on vehicles equipped with automated systems at SAE level 3 and up, the driver is allowed and even encouraged to engage in NDRAs, which is one way to counter task-related fatigue. With systems at levels 4 to 5, it may even be possible for a driver to sleep while on the move. Aside from making it possible for private car owners to take strategic naps during a drive, this also opens up the possibility for more flexible, risk management-based, hour of service regulations for professional drivers who are able to sleep while the automated features are active. It may eventually be possible to extend the maximum daily driving period without causing less safe working conditions or increased crash risk. Of course, this would require that an automated system's ODD has sufficient time extension so that the driver could disengage for a sufficiently long period.

Regarding fatigue detection, piloted driving requires robust and continuous assessment of the driver's fitness to drive level, and this assessment must be made through direct observation of the driver. The assessment of driver fatigue with automated systems will be made more difficult in the future due to the expected increase in body position variability and NDRA types which come with piloted driving. In addition to developing the ADS itself, vehicle manufacturers must therefore resolve additional challenges regarding vehicle crashworthiness and interior comfort and sensing capabilities to realise the full potential of safe, piloted driving.

SUMMARY POINTS FOR PRACTITIONERS

- In terms of vehicle support, driving can be seen as either assisted or piloted, depending on if the human driver is responsible (assisted) or if the vehicle is responsible (piloted) for vehicle control.
- During assisted driving, the demand that comes from having to monitor the road and the vehicle in combination with boredom may lead to driver fatigue, especially at night when the sleep pressure is high.
- Task-related fatigue during piloted driving can be mitigated if drivers are allowed (and encouraged) to engage in non-driving-related activities (NDRA).
- Future piloted driving may allow drivers to take rest breaks and strategic naps while on the move, thus facilitating more flexible hour of service regulations.
- Piloted driving brings new challenges for fatigue detection. Vehicle behaviour no longer provides a viable source of information, and increased variability in drivers' body positioning and non-driving-related activity repertoire challenge interior sensing capabilities.

REFERENCES

Ahlström, C., van Leeuwen, W., Krupenia, S., Jansson, H., Finér, S., Anund, A., & Kecklund, G. (2021). Real-time adaptation of driving time and rest periods in automated long-haul trucking: Development of a system based on biomathematical modelling, fatigue and relaxation monitoring. *IEEE Transactions on Intelligent Transportation Systems, 23*(5), 4758–4766.

Ahlström, C., Zemblys, R., Jansson, H., Forsberg, C., Karlsson, J. G., & Anund, A. (2021). Effects of partially automated driving on the development of driver sleepiness.

Accident Analysis & Prevention, *153*, 106058. https://doi.org/https://doi.org/10.1016/j.aap.2021.106058

Anund, A., Kecklund, G., Vadeby, A., Hjälmdahl, M., & Åkerstedt, T. (2008). The alerting effect of hitting a rumble strip—A simulator study with sleepy drivers. *Accident Analysis and Prevention*, *40*(6), 1970–1976. https://doi.org/10.1016/j.aap.2008.08.017

Bainbridge, L. (1983). Ironies of automation. In *Analysis, design and evaluation of man–machine systems* (pp. 129–135). Elsevier.

Becker, T., Hermann, F., Duwe, D., Stegmüller, S., Röckle, F., & Unger, N. (2018). Enabling the value of time. Implications for the interior design of autonomous vehicles. In: Fraunhofer IAO. www.muse.iao.fraunhofer.de/content/dam/iao/muse/de/documents/projekte/180611_EVoT_study_report_EN_final.pdf

Bourrelly, A., de Naurois, C. J., Zran, A., Rampillon, F., Vercher, J., & Bourdin, C. (2019). Long automated driving phase affects take-over performance. *IET Intelligent Transport Systems*, *13*(8), 1249–1255. https://digital-library.theiet.org/content/journals/10.1049/iet-its.2019.0018

Carsten, O., & Martens, M. H. (2019). How can humans understand their automated cars? HMI principles, problems and solutions. *Cognition, Technology & Work*, *21*(1), 3–20.

Cicchino, J. B. (2018). Effects of lane departure warning on police-reported crash rates. *Journal of Safety Research*, *66*, 61–70.

Dunn, N. J., Dingus, T. A., Soccolich, S., & Horrey, W. J. (2021). Investigating the impact of driving automation systems on distracted driving behaviors. *Accident Analysis & Prevention*, *156*, 106152.

eurostat. (2020). *Majority commuted less than 30 minutes in 2019*. Retrieved 2022-08-10 from https://ec.europa.eu/eurostat/web/products-eurostat-news/-/ddn-20201021-2

Favaro, F., Hutchings, K., Nemec, P., Cavalcante, L., & Victor, T. (2022). Waymo's Fatigue Risk Management Framework: Prevention, monitoring, and mitigation of fatigue-induced risks while testing automated driving systems. *arXiv preprint arXiv:2208.12833*.

Feldhütter, A., Hecht, T., Kalb, L., & Bengler, K. (2019). Effect of prolonged periods of conditionally automated driving on the development of fatigue: With and without non-driving-related activities. *Cognition, Technology & Work*, *21*(1), 33–40.

Flynn-Evans, E. E., Wong, L. R., Kuriyagawa, Y., Gowda, N., Cravalho, P. F., Pradhan, S.,..... Wilaiprasitporn, T. (2021). Supervision of a self-driving vehicle unmasks latent sleepiness relative to manually controlled driving. *Scientific Reports*, *11*(1), 1–13.

Fors, C., Ahlström, C., & Anund, A. (2018). A comparison of driver sleepiness in the simulator and on the real road. *Journal of Transportation, Safety and Security*, *10*(2), 72–87.

Gander, P. H., Wu, L. J., van den Berg, M., Lamp, A., Hoeg, L., & Belenky, G. (2016). Fatigue risk management systems. In M. Kryger, T. Roth, & W. C. Dement (Eds.), *Principles and Practice of Sleep Medicine. 6th ed.* (pp. 697–707). Elsevier.

Greenlee, E. T., DeLucia, P. R., & Newton, D. C. (2019). Driver vigilance in automated vehicles: Effects of demands on hazard detection performance. *Human Factors*, *61*(3), 474–487.

Halin, A., Verly, J. G., & Van Droogenbroeck, M. (2021). Survey and synthesis of state of the art in driver monitoring. *Sensors*, *21*(16), 5558.

Hallvig, D., Anund, A., Fors, C., Kecklund, G., Karlsson, J. G., Wahde, M., & Åkerstedt, T. (2013). Sleepy driving on the real road and in the simulator—A comparison. *Accident Analysis and Prevention*, *50*, 44–50. https://doi.org/10.1016/j.aap.2012.09.033

Hartzler, B. M. (2014). Fatigue on the flight deck: The consequences of sleep loss and the benefits of napping. *Accident Analysis & Prevention*, *62*, 309–318.

Hilditch, C. J., & McHill, A. W. (2019). Sleep inertia: Current insights. *Nature and Science of Sleep*, *11*, 155.

Hirsch, M., Diederichs, F., Widlroither, H., Graf, R., & Bischoff, S. (2020). Sleep and take-over in automated driving. *International Journal of Transportation Science and Technology*, *9*(1), 42–51.

Jamson, A. H., Merat, N., Carsten, O. M. J., & Lai, F. C. H. (2013). Behavioural changes in drivers experiencing highly-automated vehicle control in varying traffic conditions. *Transportation Research Part C: Emerging Technologies*, *30*, 116–125. https://doi.org/ https://doi.org/10.1016/j.trc.2013.02.008

Jarosch, O., Bellem, H., & Bengler, K. (2019). Effects of task-induced fatigue in prolonged conditional automated driving. *Human Factors*, *61*(7), 1186–1199.

Jarosch, O., Paradies, S., Feiner, D., & Bengler, K. (2019). Effects of non-driving related tasks in prolonged conditional automated driving–A Wizard of Oz on-road approach in real traffic environment. *Transportation Research Part F: Traffic Psychology and Behaviour*, *65*, 292–305.

Kaduk, S. I., Roberts, A. P. J., & Stanton, N. A. (2021a). Driving performance, sleepiness, fatigue, and mental workload throughout the time course of semi-automated driving— Experimental data from the driving simulator. *Human Factors and Ergonomics in Manufacturing & Service Industries*, *31*(1), 143–154. https://doi.org/https://doi.org/ 10.1002/hfm.20875

Kaduk, S. I., Roberts, A. P. J., & Stanton, N. A. (2021b). The manual shift in phase: The impact of circadian phase on semi-autonomous driving. What can we learn from current understanding in manual driving? *Theoretical Issues in Ergonomics Science*, *22*(1), 103–123. https://doi.org/10.1080/1463922X.2020.1758829

Kreuzmair, C., Gold, C., & Meyer, M.-L. (2017). The influence of driver fatigue on take-over performance in highly automated vehicles. *25th International Technical Conference on the Enhanced Safety of Vehicles (ESV) National Highway Traffic Safety Administration*.

Kundinger, T., Riener, A., Sofra, N., & Weigl, K. (2020). Driver drowsiness in automated and manual driving: insights from a test track study. *Proceedings of the 25th International Conference on Intelligent User Interfaces, Cagliari, Italy*. https://doi.org/10.1145/3377 325.3377506

May, J. F., & Baldwin, C. L. (2009). Driver fatigue: The importance of identifying causal factors of fatigue when considering detection and countermeasure technologies. *Transportation Research Part F: Psychology and Behaviour*, *12*(3), 218–224. https://doi.org/10.1016/ j.trf.2008.11.005

Milner, C. E., & Cote, K. A. (2009). Benefits of napping in healthy adults: Impact of nap length, time of day, age, and experience with napping. *Journal of Sleep Research*, *18*(2), 272–281.

Mueller, A. S., Reagan, I. J., & Cicchino, J. B. (2021). Addressing driver disengagement and proper system use: Human factors recommendations for level 2 driving automation design. *Journal of Cognitive Engineering and Decision Making*, *15*(1), 3–27.

Mulder, M., Abbink, D. A., & Boer, E. R. (2012). Sharing Control with Haptics: Seamless Driver Support from Manual to Automatic Control. *Human Factors*, *54*(5), 786–798. https://doi.org/10.1177/0018720812443984

Naujoks, F., Höfling, S., Purucker, C., & Zeeb, K. (2018). From partial and high automation to manual driving: Relationship between non-driving related tasks, drowsiness and take-over performance. *Accident Analysis & Prevention*, *121*, 28–42.

Neubauer, C., Matthews, G., & Saxby, D. (2014). Fatigue in the automated vehicle: Do games and conversation distract or energize the driver? *Proceedings of the Human Factors and Ergonomics Society Annual Meeting*.

Noy, I. Y., Shinar, D., & Horrey, W. J. (2018). Automated driving: Safety blind spots. *Safety Science*, *102*, 68–78.

SAE. (2021). Taxonomy and definitions for terms related to driving automation systems for on-road motor vehicles (Standard J3016_202104). In: SAE International.

Schoettle, B., & Sivak, M. (2014). *Public opinion about self-driving vehicles in China, India, Japan, the US, the UK, and Australia.*

Schömig, N., Hargutt, V., Neukum, A., Petermann-Stock, I., & Othersen, I. (2015). The interaction between highly automated driving and the development of drowsiness. *Procedia Manufacturing*, *3*, 6652–6659. https://doi.org/https://doi.org/10.1016/j.promfg.2015.11.005

Sheehan, C. M., Frochen, S. E., Walsemann, K. M., & Ailshire, J. A. (2019). Are US adults reporting less sleep?: Findings from sleep duration trends in the National Health Interview Survey, 2004–2017. *SLEEP*, *42*(2).

Solís-Marcos, I., Ahlström, C., & Kircher, K. (2018). Performance of an additional task during Level 2 automated driving: An on-road study comparing drivers with and without experience with partial automation. *Human Factors*, 0018720818773636.

Stapel, J., Mullakkal-Babu, F. A., & Happee, R. (2019). Automated driving reduces perceived workload, but monitoring causes higher cognitive load than manual driving. *Transportation Research Part F: Traffic Psychology and Behaviour*, *60*, 590–605. https://doi.org/https://doi.org/10.1016/j.trf.2018.11.006

Sternlund, S., Strandroth, J., Rizzi, M., Lie, A., & Tingvall, C. (2017). The effectiveness of lane departure warning systems—A reduction in real-world passenger car injury crashes. *Traffic Injury Prevention*, *18*(2), 225–229.

Tang, Q., Guo, G., Zhang, Z., Zhang, B., & Wu, Y. (2021). Olfactory facilitation of takeover performance in highly automated driving. *Human Factors*, *63*(4), 553–564.

Tassi, P., & Muzet, A. (2000). Sleep inertia. *Sleep Medicine Reviews*, *4*(4), 341–353.

Vogelpohl, T., Kühn, M., Hummel, T., & Vollrath, M. (2019). Asleep at the automated wheel—Sleepiness and fatigue during highly automated driving. *Accident Analysis & Prevention*, *126*, 70–84. https://doi.org/https://doi.org/10.1016/j.aap.2018.03.013

Wang, L., Zhong, H., Ma, W., Abdel-Aty, M., & Park, J. (2020). How many crashes can connected vehicle and automated vehicle technologies prevent: A meta-analysis. *Accident Analysis & Prevention*, *136*, 105299. https://doi.org/https://doi.org/10.1016/j.aap.2019.105299

Warm, J. S., Parasuraman, R., & Matthews, G. (2008). Vigilance requires hard mental work and is stressful. *Human Factors*, *50*(3), 433–441.

Williamson, A., Lombardi, D. A., Folkard, S., Stutts, J., Courtney, T. K., & Connor, J. (2011). The link between fatigue and safety. *Accident Analysis & Prevention*, *43*(2), 498–515. https://doi.org/https://doi.org/10.1016/j.aap.2009.11.011

Wörle, J., Metz, B., & Baumann, M. (2021). Sleep inertia in automated driving: Post-sleep take-over and driving performance. *Accident Analysis & Prevention*, *150*, 105918. https://doi.org/https://doi.org/10.1016/j.aap.2020.105918

Wörle, J., Metz, B., Othersen, I., & Baumann, M. (2020). Sleep in highly automated driving: Takeover performance after waking up. *Accident Analysis & Prevention*, *144*, 105617. https://doi.org/https://doi.org/10.1016/j.aap.2020.105617

Zhang, Y., Ma, J., Zhang, C., & Chang, R. (2021). Electrophysiological frequency domain analysis of driver passive fatigue under automated driving conditions. *Scientific Reports*, *11*(1), 1–9.

6.2 Through the Darkness of Future Past
A Cautionary Tale

Anjum Naweed[1], Verna Blewett[1],
Lily Hirsch[1], and Ashleigh J. Filtness[2]

[1]Central Queensland University, Appleton Institute for
Behavioural Science, Adelaide, Australia
[2]Loughborough University, Loughborough, UK

CONTENTS

6.2.1   INTRODUCTION

In 2013, a specific fatigue-related safety concern in rail transport was explored in a series of workshops. Each workshop considered the concern by presenting its past, helping participants map its present, and then envision their "ideal" future 10 years from the day—in this case, the year 2023. Ten years on, we explore these futures, the ways organisations believed they would be achieved, and the extent to which their vision corresponded with a future now all but realised. These previously unpublished findings stem from broader research (e.g., Filtness & Naweed, 2017; Naweed, 2013; Naweed & Rainbird, 2015; Naweed, Rainbird & Chapman, 2015; Naweed, Rainbird

DOI: 10.1201/9781003213154-44

& Dance, 2015; Rainbird & Naweed, 2017). While we refrain from jargon, there is an abbreviated term we cannot avoid: SPAD, or "signal passed at danger", representing the safety issue in workshops. By "workshop", we refer to a group of diverse individuals (in this case, the rail industry) working together to determine agreed outcomes on a particular subject (i.e., SPADs) using a facilitated process.

6.2.2   THE LINK BETWEEN SAFETY AND FATIGUE IN RAIL TRANSPORTATION

Rail operations is a broad and distributed system driven by service delivery and safety targets, but it relies on the actions of just one or two individuals (Naweed, 2014). The size, speed, and limited manoeuvrability of trains require the driver to act early, and traditional rail systems use multiple signals so that instructions to proceed or drive cautiously can be shown ahead of the danger point (i.e., a stop signal). Driver action is thus supported by existing route knowledge.

As tracks can vary in length and frequency of driver inputs, the role can be monotonous and demanding, requiring drivers to maintain concentration and vigilance. Monotonous routes create high risk for fatigue (Dunn & Williamson, 2012), and as rail is typically a 24/7 operation, there are safety implications for fatigue resulting from sleep loss and disruption (Åkerstedt, 1991). A fatigued state can easily impact driving performance, for example, by increasing propensity to become distracted, reducing situation awareness, delaying reaction times; this increases SPAD risk—which increases collision/derailment risk (Naweed, 2020).

6.2.3   THE CONTEXT OF THE RESEARCH AND THE FUTURE INQUIRY WORKSHOP

SPADs are a measure of safety performance and any occurrences are notified to agencies charged with rail regulation (Naweed, Trigg, et al., 2018). Rail operators are required to have a fatigue risk management system (FRMS) in place, with fatigue modelling a common (though not required) approach for developing rosters.

In 2013, the authors (AN, VB, and LH) ran five "Future Inquiry Workshops" (FIW) across Australia and New Zealand (i.e., Australasia) to explore SPAD management, with the goal to extract insights and inform enhanced mitigation practice. The FIW (Blewett & Shaw, 2008; 2017) is a large group process that enables diverse participants representing "the whole system in the room", to seek and identify common ground and determine strategies for action that lead to a commonly desired future. FIW is underpinned by appreciative inquiry (Cooperrider et al., 2003) and Future Search (Weisbord & Janoff, 2000)—grounded in the work of early theorists on leadership, socio-technical systems, and group dynamics. The process is highly participative throughout with actors embracing self-management and responsibility for action at the outset.

For each workshop, participants were identified through two questions: *"who influences SPADs?"* and *"who is influenced by SPADs?"* Throughout the day, the Past, Present, and Future are considered (see Figure 6.2.1) and facilitators "direct traffic" rather than attempting to impose pre-determined outcomes or influence thinking.

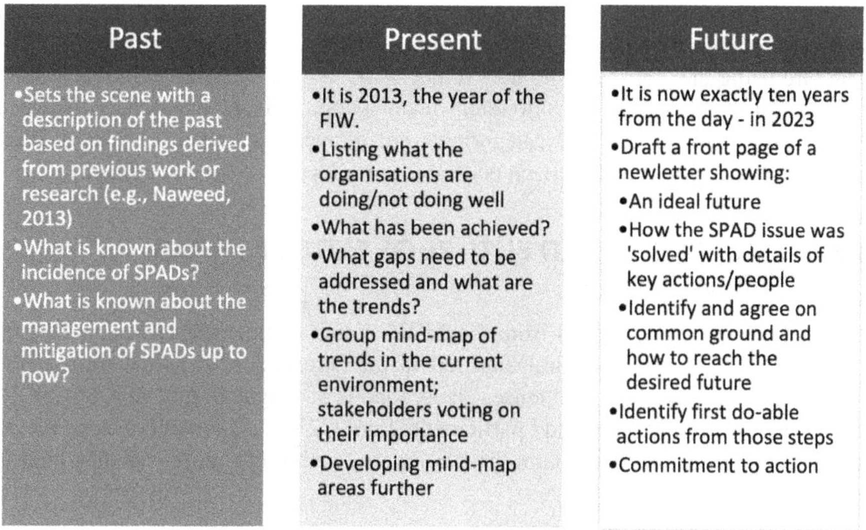

Past	Present	Future
•Sets the scene with a description of the past based on findings derived from previous work or research (e.g., Naweed, 2013) •What is known about the incidence of SPADs? •What is known about the management and mitigation of SPADs up to now?	•It is 2013, the year of the FIW. •Listing what the organisations are doing/not doing well •What has been achieved? •What gaps need to be addressed and what are the trends? •Group mind-map of trends in the current environment; stakeholders voting on their importance •Developing mind-map areas further	•It is now exactly ten years from the day - in 2023 •Draft a front page of a newletter showing: •An ideal future •How the SPAD issue was 'solved' with details of key actions/people •Identify and agree on common ground and how to reach the desired future •Identify first do-able actions from those steps •Commitment to action

FIGURE 6.2.1 Activities associated with the past, present, and future phases of the FIW.

The principles of seeking common ground, focusing on the future (not presenting problems and conflicts), and taking responsibility for action were foundational. Participant involvement is constant and vocal, and the workshop is tightly directed within a one-day timeframe. It is designed to use the conflict in the room, rather than ignore it, and to achieve future-focused outcomes embedded in common ground. These foundations were key as Australasian rail is characterised by conflict and differentials in positional power among system actors.

6.2.4　THE FUTURE INQUIRY WORKSHOP: METHODOLOGY

A total of 220 participants took part across five workshops at local (Auckland-NZ: $n = 48$; South Australia: $n = 41$; Queensland[1]: $n = 38$; Western Australia: $n = 39$) and industry (Victoria: $n = 54$) levels, with the latter including Australasian representation. Stakeholder groups included users and maintainers of signals; employee representatives; controllers of signals; builders and designers of signals, infrastructure, and rail safety; policy developers and designers; policy influencers; frontline supervisors; and broader industry representatives. There were slight differences between the names and composition of the stakeholder groups in each workshop, but they were broadly comparable.

All workshop data linked with fatigue were isolated and extracted. For the "present" phase, FIW data were taken from four aspects of that phase: listing what organisations are/are not doing well; creating nodes on the mind-map (a visual form of a group brainstorm, see Figure 6.2.2); voting on the mind-map; and taking mind-map nodes away for further development. For the "future" phase, all statements relevant to fatigue were taken from the newsletters created by participants.

Together, two researchers (AN and AF) coded data using conventional content analysis (Hsieh & Shannon, 2005). High-level categories were drawn from the FIW structure using the "present" and the "future",[2] and a generic socio-technical system categorisation (i.e., job/task, individual, team/social, and organisational) (Naweed et al., 2019). All subordinate categories were derived inductively, and high-level industry grouping was added. Each code was considered in relation to fatigue.

6.2.5   THE PRESENT AND FUTURE OF FATIGUE IN RAIL OPERATIONS

This section presents findings from the FIWs as two distinct narratives on fatigue. The first is of fatigue in Australasian rail in the "present" (2013—the time of the workshops), told in the present tense. The second is of fatigue in the "future" (2023), and as the process "transported" participants into 2023, it is also told in the present tense. Both narratives reflect participant perspectives through consensus on common ground.

6.2.5.1   FATIGUE IN (THE YEAR 2013 AND) A CHAOTIC PRESENT

Table 6.2.1 presents an overview of fatigue in the present ("2013") and Figure 6.2.2 reflects this "chaotic" present in the mind-maps. At an industry level, changes to health standards have provoked reactivity in risk management, but general regulation of fatigue is improved.

At the job/task level, fatigue has been causally linked to SPADs, but biomathematical modelling is flawed, inaccurate, and lacks validation. The inaccuracies are essentially *"garbage in, garbage out"*.[3]

At the organisational level, fatigue is not being managed well. There is also increasing pressure to use biomathematical modelling. Issues around staffing/resourcing and rostering are present, the former through poaching (of drivers/controllers) by mining companies, and the latter through insufficient resourcing to enable the awareness creation needed for fatigue management. Rostering issues are occurring through late notice of rostering changes and inadequate time off between shifts, leading to short staffing.

Insufficient time is impeding timetabling analysis, leading to timetables that are poorly designed and increase driver workload. An increased focus and reliance on technical analysis of SPADs is creating an inability to capture the *"truth about fatigue"* because non-technical factors (e.g., culture, norms, and pressures) are being overlooked.

At a team/social level, presenteeism is concerning. Train drivers are being pressured to work overtime, on their days off, and feel bullied into doing long hours. There is a push to *"keep going"* even when a driver is fatigued. People are not being honest about fatigue, influencing the accuracy of information about fatigue and fitness to drive. Trust among management and drivers is lacking and family and friends do not understand the pressures of the drivers' job.

Individually, drivers are self-managing fatigue through sick leave and swapping shifts, which when not officially recorded means that biomathematical modelling is

TABLE 6.2.1
Fatigue in the Year 2013 as Expressed in the Present Phase across the Future Inquiry Workshops

Factors	Major Category	Minor Category
Industry	Changes to health standards	Including body mass index (BMI) and sleep apnoea in health standards, provoking reactivity
	Improved regulation	Fatigue regulations have been improved
Organisational	Barriers to analysis	Increasingly detailed and technical analysis of SPADs is obfuscating the role of fatigue
		Lack of time and resourcing available for timetable analysis
	Staffing/resourcing issues	Drivers and controllers are being poached by other rail operators
		Fatigue management awareness is hindered by limited time and resourcing availability
	Rostering is not being done effectively	Notice of changes to the roster are late
		Time off between shifts is inadequate
	Fatigue management is not being done well, or at all	Management of workload is not being done well
		Fatigue is not being managed
		There is increasing pressure on railways to use FAID [a biomathematical modelling system]
Team/Social	A "presenteeism" problem	There is a push to keep going even when drivers are fatigued
		Drivers feel pressured and bullied to do long hours and work on days off
	No broader awareness of pressures	Family and friends do not realise the drivers' job pressures
	Trust, or lack thereof	A lack of trust in management and in drivers around managing fatigue
		People are generally not honest about fatigue
Job/Task	The fatigue-SPAD link	Fatigue is causally linked with SPADs
	Issues with biomathematical modelling	Fatigue models need additional data
		FAID is inaccurate and flawed—garbage in garbage out
Individual (Driver)	Self-management of fatigue	Maladaptive use of sick leave to manage fatigue
		Swapping shifts to manage fatigue
	Individual pressure(s) for productivity	Money motivates drivers to work on days off
		Feeling obliged to take a job when fatigued and to avoid disappointing others
	To report, or not to report	Scared to report fatigue as it results in job loss
		Not reporting overtime pressures
	Individual responsibility	Not taking responsibility for one's own actions
		Fatigue is important for some but not others

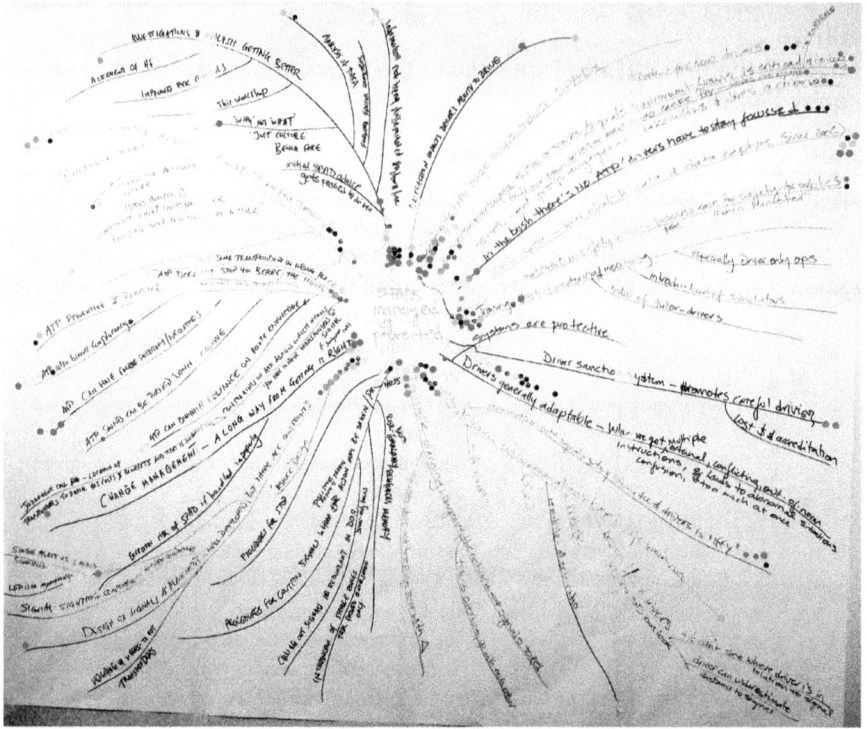

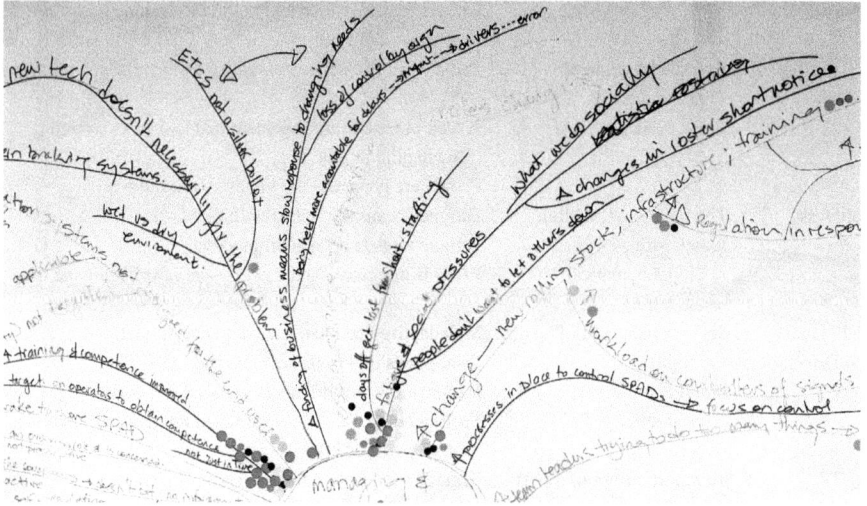

FIGURE 6.2.2 Full (top) and cropped (bottom) photos of mind-maps created during Future Inquiry Workshops. Notes: For illustrative purposes; full mind-map size = approx. 3300 x 3500 mm; clustered dots reflect stakeholder voting and density of voting for each node; cropped map displays a fatigue node. Each stakeholder group has a different colour dot.

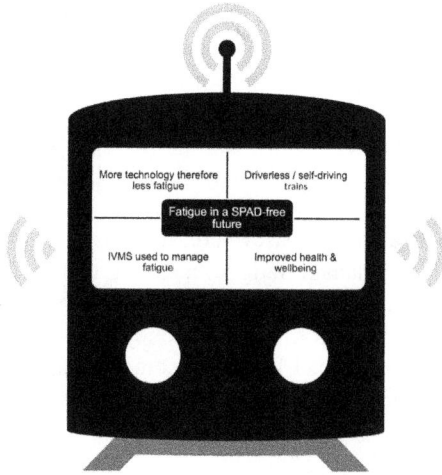

FIGURE 6.2.3 Factors associated with fatigue in a SPAD-free future (as expressed in the 2013 FIW newsletters for the year 2023). IVMS = in-vehicle monitoring systems.

inaccurate for the actual shifts worked. Drivers feel obliged to work fatigued and are being financially motivated to work on their days off. Individuals are not reporting fatigue or overtime pressures to management for fear of job loss, so management is not aware of the size of the issue. Some are not taking responsibility for their own actions around fatigue, and while fatigue is important for some stakeholders (e.g., users of signals, policy influencers, and developers), it is unimportant to others (e.g., controllers, maintainers of signallers).

6.2.5.2   FATIGUE IN A POSSIBLE SPAD-FREE FUTURE (THE YEAR 2023)

Figure 6.2.3 presents an overview of fatigue in a future ("2023")—as imagined during the 2013 FIWs—where SPADs are now extinct. A positive change in worker well-being is palpable: *"There is less fatigue"*, *"the health of drivers has improved"*; moreover, *"people sleep better"* and *"are happier"*, and managers *"can sleep at night"*. In some parts of Australasia, passenger trains are now driverless, which equates to *"less fatigue, and faster, safer, more efficient"* operations. Elsewhere, trains are not driverless, but in-vehicle monitoring systems (IVMS) are being used to manage fatigue effectively. *"Driver fatigue attentiveness technology"*, *"eye-tracking cameras for fatigue management"*, and *"driver fatigue vigilance systems"* are everywhere. There is more technology, therefore less fatigue.

6.2.6   ALTERNATE FUTURES, REPEATING HISTORIES

Across workshops, participants documented a present and possible future. The present was characterised by challenges in systemic issues with impacts at organisational and team/social levels, including resourcing, rostering and fatigue management, barriers around analysis of SPADs and timetabling, presenteeism, and trust. At job/task level, major concerns were identified in the systems being used to drive rostering processes. Consequently, much of the burden was placed on individual drivers' self-management and job control.

While a plethora of ideas contributed to SPAD extinction, many risk factors in the chaotic present were addressed in the imagined future by one mechanism: Removing the human from the train. No longer was there a need to roster driving, manage fatigue, or worry about reporting. Elsewhere, humans were still driving trains, but IVMS were being used to manage fatigue, meaning that in the 10 years since the workshops, numerous technical (i.e., technology reliability, systems integration) and non-technical (matured culture, formation of policy, union non-acceptance) barriers to safely implementing IVMS had been overcome. What an achievement! In this future, there was a sense of optimised work–life balance, of happiness at work/home, and reduced stresses.

6.2.6.1 What Predictions Came True?

The first fully "driverless" heavy haul train arrived in Western Australia in 2018 (five years after the FIWs), delivering 28,000 tonnes of iron ore autonomously over 280 km (RioTinto, 2022). The first fully "driverless" Australian passenger train arrived in Sydney in 2019 (six years after the FIWs), and currently runs on a 36 km section of track (Zasiadko, 2019).

While IVMS designed for road vehicles were prevalent in 2013, today their number is greater than a hundred. To date, IVMS have not found their way into Australasian rail. Barriers to their implementation (e.g., false positives, trust, and acceptance issues) are well documented (Balkin et al., 2011), and a recent national open consultation for consideration of IVMS use in trains (Office of the National Rail Safety Regulator, 2020a) was labelled *"draconian and dangerous"* by rail unions (Zhang, 2021), and *"fervently opposed"* (Rail Tram and Bus Union, 2021).

Since the FIWs, issues in work–life balance, stress, physical and mental health, well-being, job satisfaction, and rostering remain prevalent in the workforce (see Chapter 4.9 in this volume).

SPADs have not gone extinct. Aside from the introduction of driverless trains in Australia, which represent a fraction of train services in the country, none of the future predictions made during the 2013 FIWs have come true.

6.2.6.2 What Was the Contribution of the Workshops to Realising the Desired Future?

SPADs are a complex problem, and a 10-year "future" was invariably too short a period in which to expect significant change. Stepping into the future in an FIW is a guided physical and psychological relocation. The future the participants emerge in has the problem solved and looking back allows them to focus on solutions instead of being stymied by the problems in the (real) present. In terms of being able to be imagined, our planning groups selected 10 years as the better option, and the FIWs contributed to SPAD discourse by identifying the commonly agreed "first do-able steps" towards achieving the desired future.

Given the gulf between the predictions and reality that came to pass, what contribution did the FIWs make to moving to a SPAD-free world? There was no "mandate" for change in the lead up to the FIWs in that the industry recognised a problem and supported a research-driven forum to explore the issues around it. As per the FIW process, a handful of individuals volunteered to lead the work on the first do-able steps, which provided an opportunity for commitment and consistency in the execution of a collective agenda. This involved publicly announcing their commitment to the group and gaining its approval (Blewett & Shaw, 2017). Thus, the FIW outcomes rely on champions, agreement, discovery, and transdisciplinarity in participative processes to flourish (having the whole system in the room), and engender new values and philosophies (Naweed, Ward, et al., 2018).

In 2013, the FIWs had system-wide involvement with key stakeholders so quantifying or apportioning the contribution of the FIWs to change within the industry is difficult. Issues remain in SPAD-risk management (Naweed, Trigg, et al., 2018), and driver rostering and fatigue risk management problems persist. The impact of the FIWs may be questioned on the basis of the process relying on non-mandated effort from individuals for whom this effort was vulnerable to the very issues the FIWs identified (e.g., paucity of time and resourcing). These individuals also worked within an industry prone to restructure and high turnover, meaning the champions across the FIWs were vulnerable to job loss and unexpected change. The FIWs staged a complex issue at an industry level in a country where rail remains under state control. As a wicked problem (Rittel & Webber, 1973), the barriers for the ongoing participation to tackle SPADs were many.

Apportioning the contribution of the FIWs to change is difficult, but was that the point of the exercise? In the decade since the FIWs, the area of SPADs and fatigue has seen development in open discussion. A dedicated SPAD symposium has taken place four times (2015, 2016, 2018, and 2023) in Australia, with ~100 delegates in each. In 2019, a "Good Practice in the Management of Rail Driver Health and Wellbeing" guideline (Rail Industry Safety & Standards Board, 2019) was published, emphasising the role of the "organisational" parts of the system for ameliorating performance pressures and managing resourcing. Likewise, the role of "job design" when building rosters, managing sleep, fatigue, and the intersection between work and family life, was emphasised. In 2020, the first fatigue risk management guideline for Australian rail (industry) was published (Office of the National Rail Safety Regulator, 2020b), aiming to provide practical guidance on how to manage fatigue-related risks and meet legislative requirements. The change has been incremental and somewhat incidental, but conversation has continued, and the FIWs likely played a role as the starting blocks to change and inspiring the unfolding story.

6.2.6.3 A DESIRE FOR CHANGE

Whether technology is viewed as a silver bullet, panacea, or pipedream, tales of its lure echo throughout rail history (Dawson et al., 2017; Naweed & Rose, 2018) as well as in many other transport and non-transport sectors. How technology was viewed in the "present" (year 2013) and the "future" (year 2023) did not reflect its role in "fixing" fatigue as much as a desire for change, with technology as the driving force (Naweed & Golightly, 2022). But what of fatigue management for those with the responsibility for managing, controlling, and maintaining the trains? What of the policies, and the infrastructure for capturing and handling big data now possible with the use of IVMS? Driverless trains and IVMS may seem an "easy" fix, but a great deal of work, engagement, innovation, and strategy would be needed to realise the technology-driven future envisioned for 2023—and there would still be no escaping the need to effectively manage fatigue.

6.2.7 MANAGING FATIGUE IN TRANSPORTATION IN THE FUTURE YET TO COME: SIX PRINCIPLES FOR CHANGE

As yet, fatigue management of the future is unwritten. Retrospectively analysing how one future was envisioned after a different future came to pass provides a rare opportunity of getting a forward viewpoint from across an industry sector, and extracting lessons that can contribute to writing the future yet to come. What can we learn from the FIW process as well as the outcomes and their impact on progress towards a SPAD-free world? Change has thus far been characterised by small, incremental steps; what opportunities exist for larger change and how might this be enabled? We offer six principles for change.

1–Commitment to Change

The FIWs were a researcher initiative, not industry-led. Industry and organisations accepted them and participated, seeing value without making any commitment to change. This lack of commitment to implementing FIW outcomes limited the capacity of the FIWs to lead to lasting change. As a research tool, the FIWs were successful: They provided valuable data; the industry agreed on their conclusions; and researchers could make data-driven recommendations, safe in the knowledge that they were backed by the whole rail system. However, this is not the same as FIWs generated by the industry, which would demonstrate industry-level buy-in and be driven by a commitment to change. Commitment to change by the industry is the first principle that we have learnt from this work.

2–Ongoing Reflection and Review

In any future, changes can be expected, but what is unknown and unpredictable is the nature and importance of those changes. Since the FIWs, new issues have emerged that highlight the burden of fatigue in rail. Workforce development and retention continue to pose a problem (Australasian Railway Association, 2018), and the COVID-19 pandemic introduced pressures that altered priorities (Naweed et al., 2021). What is critical, then, is that systems be developed that provide reliability, flexibility, and resilience in the face of unexpected events. The second principle from this work is the need for ongoing reflection and review of progress towards the desired change. This was outside the remit of the research, but could have been taken up by the industry.

One may argue that this valuable opportunity, provided by the research, was lost by the industry. Such review would allow goals and strategy to be shifted in response to unexpected events. Alternatively, the whole question could be revisited with additional FIWs if the changed (internal or external) environment demands it.

3–Provide Resources

In a transport service industry, a paucity of time and resourcing to develop initiatives for managing fatigue risk are workplace norms, for those in the frontline and in management. It is important to find a way of promoting fatigue management in a way that can overpower these barriers. This could be read as a sub-plot to the principle of commitment to change on the part of not only the leaders of industry, but also other system actors who have power (e.g., union leaders, regulators, and governments). Our third principle to inspire change is to provide resources.

4–Provoke a Paradigm Shift

Whether fatigue is managed through IVMS or eliminated by removing the human from the train, fatigue is regarded as little more than a hazard across the industry. In a service transport sector, fatigue tends to be examined through a safety lens, but, and paradoxically, it creates competing tensions with productivity. Our fourth principle asserts the need for a paradigm shift on big issues. There is a reliance on human behaviours and people doing the right thing and not making errors, but we know that errors will never be eliminated because humans are error-prone beings. A paradigm shift would help us reframe fatigue as something more than a hazard.

5–Mind the Technology

In terms of their benefits to any government, the narrative about driverless trains is obvious: There would be no driver rosters, no calling in sick, and no driver error. On the other hand, such technological change is a fundamental threat to driver employment. Despite this, there was general agreement in the FIWs that technological change was inevitable and although it was a potential threat to employment, it could be a solution to mitigate fatigue and poor safety outcomes. However, technology that leads to increased driver monotony could exacerbate fatigue problems. So, in determining the best use of technology, the whole system needs to be heard so that threats at all levels are minimised and new hazards are not introduced. Our fifth principle is therefore the importance of being mindful of different narratives about technology.

6–Infiltrate Corporate Memory

Common ground identified in the FIWs included that fatigue was an issue that needed to be managed within each organisation and by the industry. Do-able first steps were identified; however, the nature of the one-day workshops, the lack of commitment by the rail industry to own the outcomes, the lack of consistent follow-up of change actions, and the passage of time have meant that, regrettably, the sands of change may have passed through the sieve of corporate memory.

Without a mandate implemented in policy documents and woven into the fabric of an organisation, we see that any change promised through agreement will be lost with the next restructure, or the next takeover, or the next wave of employees—from management to signal operators, to drivers. Corporate memory resides across each organisation; it is not confined to management but sits with all actors who contribute to participatory processes that govern the life of an organisation. To maintain momentum for change, the drive for change needs to be distributed, and not confined to individuals. This is particularly critical in an industry where there is considerable career mobility.

6.2.8 CONCLUSIONS

The process of the FIW is by its nature aspirational. It is a way of determining the collective good; that is, what is best for everyone in the system given there may be many differing needs and desires. It identifies the first do-able steps towards achieving those goals. However, the only way to make a workplace or industry healthy and safe is to *make* it healthy and safe—that is, committing to and then taking the necessary action to change the environment. This might include improved training, but change cannot be reliant on people "doing the right thing"; it requires feedback loops reflecting changes in management approach, systems of work, policy, and organisational politics. To be effective, change in these areas requires broad commitment across the organisation/industry. Thus, bringing diverse system actors together in one place to work together to determine what the future should look like is an efficient starting point for change. Everyone involved brings their own perspective and must listen and respond to the views of the others. And everyone has the right to change their minds and forge new and unexpected alliances. However, those who have the power to implement change (e.g., management, union leaders, industry leaders, and government officials) need to make the commitment to implement the identified changes before the workshop even takes place, and to commit time and resources to follow up progress regularly with a "whole system" team. Regular and consistent follow-up allows the strategy for change to adapt to unexpected or unanticipated changes in the social, physical, technological, and regulatory environments. Without commitment to change and follow-up, a foray into the future will likely remain "interesting" and "aspirational", rather than the first firm step towards lasting change.

SUMMARY POINTS FOR PRACTITIONERS

- Fatigue is linked with safety concerns such as SPADs in rail industries.
- Technology is envisioned as a way of "fixing" fatigue.
- The Future Inquiry Workshop identifies the first do-able steps towards achieving future goals and starting blocks to change.
- Commitment to change across industry and systems actors increases the chances of realising the commonly desired future.
- The six principles for enabling large and lasting change on effective management of fatigue-related risk in transport are commitment to change, ongoing reflection and review, provide resources, provoke a paradigm shift, mind the technology, and infiltrate corporate memory.

NOTES

1 The workshop in Queensland included representation of rail organisations in New South Wales.
2 The "past" was used to set the scene for the FIW.
3 A colloquialism for poor-quality data entry leading to unreliable data output.

REFERENCES

Åkerstedt, T. (1991). Shift work and sleep disturbances. In: Peter, J.H., Penzel, T., Podszus, T., von Wichert, P. (eds) *Sleep and Health Risk* (pp. 265–278). Springer, Berlin, Heidelberg.

Australasian Railway Association. (2018). Skills crisis: A call to action. Retrieved, Jan 15, 2022, from https://ara.net.au/wp-content/uploads/ARA-Skills-Capability-Study.pdf.

Balkin, T. J., Horrey, W. J., Graeber, R. C., Czeisler, C. A., & Dinges, D. F. (2011). The challenges and opportunities of technological approaches to fatigue management. *Accident Analysis & Prevention, 43*(2), 565–572.

Blewett, V., & Shaw, A. (2008, 11–13 August). *Future Inquiry: Participatory Ergonomics at Work*. Paper presented at the Nordic Ergonomics Society Conference, Reykjavik, Iceland.

Blewett, V., & Shaw, A. (2017). Future inquiry: A participatory ergonomics approach to evaluating new technology. In C. Bearman, A. Naweed, J. Dorrian, J. Rose & D. Dawson (Eds.), *Evaluation of Rail Technology* (pp. 111–124). Surrey, UK: CRC Press.

Cooperrider, D. L., Whitney, D. K., & Stavros, J. M. (2003). *Appreciative Inquiry Handbook*. Bedford Heights, OH: Lakeshore Publishers.

Dawson, D., Bearman, C., Naweed, A., & Hughes, G. (2017). Introduction: The promise and perils of new technology. In C. Bearman, A. Naweed, J. Dorrian, J. Rose & D. Dawson (Eds.), *Evaluation of Rail Technology* (pp. 1–8). Surrey, UK: CRC Press.

Dunn, N., & Williamson, A. (2012). Driving monotonous routes in a train simulator: The effect of task demand on driving performance and subjective experience. *Ergonomics, 55*(9), 997–1008.

Filtness, A. J., & Naweed, A. (2017). Causes, consequences and countermeasures to driver fatigue in the rail industry: The train driver perspective. *Applied Ergonomics, 60*, 12–21.

Hsieh, H.-F., & Shannon, S. E. (2005). Three approaches to qualitative content analysis. *Qualitative Health Research, 15*(9), 1277–1288.

Naweed, A. (2013). Psychological factors for driver distraction and inattention in the Australian and New Zealand rail industry. *Accident Analysis & Prevention, 60*, 193–204.

Naweed, A. (2014). Investigations into the skills of modern and traditional train driving. *Applied Ergonomics, 45*(3), 462–470.

Naweed, A. (2020). Getting mixed signals: Connotations of teamwork as performance shaping factors in network controller and rail driver relationship dynamics. *Applied Ergonomics, 82*, 102976.

Naweed, A., & Golightly, A. (2022). Advancement in rail transportation and safety: Key themes for human factors and systems thinking. In N. Bugalia, S. Misra, A. Mahalingam & K. E. Seetha Ram (Eds.), *Policy Messages for Planning and Implementing High-Speed Rail in Asia* (pp. 89–97). Japan: Asian Development Bank Institute. 10.56506/PWXS1277.

Naweed, A., Jackson, J. E., & Read, G. J. M. (2021). Ghost trains: Australian rail in the early stages of the global COVID-19 pandemic. *Human Factors and Ergonomics in Manufacturing & Service Industries, 31*(4), 438–444.

Naweed, A., & Rainbird, S. (2015). Recovering time or chasing rainbows? Exploring time perception, conceptualization of time recovery, and time pressure mitigation in train driving. *IIE Transactions on Occupational Ergonomics and Human Factors, 3*(2), 91–104.

Naweed, A., Rainbird, S., & Chapman, J. (2015). Investigating the formal countermeasures and informal strategies used to mitigate SPAD risk in train driving. *Ergonomics, 58*(6), 883–896.

Naweed, A., Rainbird, S., & Dance, C. (2015). Are you fit to continue? Approaching rail systems thinking at the cusp of safety and the apex of performance. *Safety Science, 76*, 101–110.

Naweed, A., & Rose, J. (2018). Assessing technology acceptance for skills development and real-world decision-making in the context of train driving. *Transportation Research Part F: Traffic Psychology and Behaviour, 52*, 86–100.

Naweed, A., Trigg, J., Cloete, S., Allan, P., & Bentley, T. (2018). Throwing good money after SPAD? Exploring the cost of signal passed at danger (SPAD) incidents to Australasian rail organisations. *Safety Science, 109*, 157–164.

Naweed, A., Ward, D., Gourlay, C., & Dawson, D. (2018). Can participatory ergonomics process tactics improve simulator fidelity and give rise to transdisciplinarity in stakeholders? A before–after case study. *International Journal of Industrial Ergonomics, 65*, 139–152.

Naweed, A., Young, M. S., & Aitken, J. (2019). Caught between a rail and a hard place: a two-country meta-analysis of factors that impact track worker safety in lookout-related rail incidents. *Theoretical Issues in Ergonomics Science, 20*(6), 731–762.

Office of the National Rail Safety Regulator. (2020a). In-cab audio and video safety recordings: Consultation Regulatory Impact Statement. Retrieved, Jan 15, 2022, from www.onrsr.com.au/industry-information/latest-news/in-cab-audio-and-video-safety-recordings-consultation-regulatory-impact-statement.

Office of the National Rail Safety Regulator. (2020b). ONRSR Guideline: Fatigue Risk Management. Retrieved, Jan 15, 2022, from www.onrsr.com.au/publications/fact-sheets-guidelines-and-policies/guidelines.

Rail Industry Safety & Standards Board. (2019). Good Practice in the Management of Rail Driver Health and Wellbeing. Retrieved, Jan 13, 2022, from www.rissb.com.au/products/good-practice-in-the-management-of-rail-driver-health-and-wellbeing/.

Rail Tram and Bus Union. (2021). RTBU members force safety regulator back to the drawing board. *Transport NOW*. www.rtbu.org.au/rtbu_members_force_safety_regulator_back_to_the_drawing_board

Rainbird, S., & Naweed, A. (2017). Signs of respect: embodying the train driver–signal relationship to avoid rail disasters. *Applied Mobilities, 2*(1), 50–66.

RioTinto. (2022). How did one of the world's largest robots end up here? Retrieved Jan 15, 2022, from www.riotinto.com/en/news/stories/how-did-worlds-biggest-robot.

Rittel, H. W., & Webber, M. M. (1973). Dilemmas in a general theory of planning. *Policy Sciences, 4*(2), 155–169.

Weisbord, M. R., & Janoff, S. (2000). *Future Search: An Action Guide to Finding Common Ground in Organizations and Communities* (2nd ed.). San Francisco: Berrett-Koehler.

Zasiadko, M. (2019). First driverless metro launched in Australia. *RailTech.com*. www.railtech.com/infrastructure/2019/05/27/first-driverless-metro-launched-in-australia/.

Zhang, J. (2021). Public Transport Union concerned CCTV on trains will lead to 'big brother style' surveillance. *The Epoch Times*. www.theepochtimes.com/public-transport-union-concerned-cctv-on-trains-will-lead-to-big-brother-style-surveillance_3815252.html.

6.3 Space Transport and Fatigue

Crystal L. Kirkley[1], Zachary L. Glaros[1], Nicholas G. Bathurst[1], Cassie J. Hilditch[2], and Erin E. Flynn-Evans[1]

[1]Fatigue Countermeasures Laboratory, Human Systems Integration Division, NASA Ames Research Center, Moffett Field, CA, USA
[2]Fatigue Countermeasures Laboratory, Department of Psychology, San José State University, San José, CA, USA

CONTENTS

6.3.1 INTRODUCTION

To date, over 600 individuals, representing almost 40 countries, have travelled into space (Roberts, 2021; Roulette, 2021). Space missions can range in duration from several hours to more than a year. In the past, crews have been comprised of exceptionally healthy individuals, but recent advances in the commercial space sector have led to a more diverse population of individuals travelling to space as tourists (Cohen and Spector, 2019). Space travel presents numerous challenges to fatigue management for astronaut crews (Brainard et al., 2016; Mallis & DeRoshia, 2005). In this chapter, the term "crew" refers to the group of individuals ("crewmembers") who are

DOI: 10.1201/9781003213154-45

onboard a space vehicle to complete a dedicated mission. Fatigue in space results from many of the same challenges that shift workers face on Earth, including inadequate sleep, circadian misalignment, and elevated workload. However, spaceflight also presents unique challenges including non-24-hour light-dark cycles, erratic work schedules, a microgravity sleep environment, constraints to habitat design, and an isolated and confined living environment. This chapter outlines the current challenges facing space travel and then discusses fatigue management strategies and countermeasures aimed at addressing these challenges. The chapter concludes with a future-facing approach to what challenges may arise as advancements in space travel continue to develop at a rapid pace.

6.3.2 WHAT ARE THE CHALLENGES TO SLEEP IN SPACE?

As on Earth, fatigue in space largely arises from sleep deficiency and circadian misalignment. Numerous studies have demonstrated that crews sleep an average of six hours a night while in space, compared to longer durations when on Earth, irrespective of the mission directives or duration (Barger et al., 2014a; Dijk et al., 2001; Frost et al., 1976; Gundel et al., 1993; Gundel et al., 1997; Monk et al., 1998; Santy et al., 1988; Stoilova et al., 2000). Although microgravity itself may influence an individual's ability to sleep in space, other causes of sleep loss have been identified, including circadian disruption, irregular schedules, sub-optimal sleep environments, and living and working in an isolated and confined environment (Figure 6.3.1).

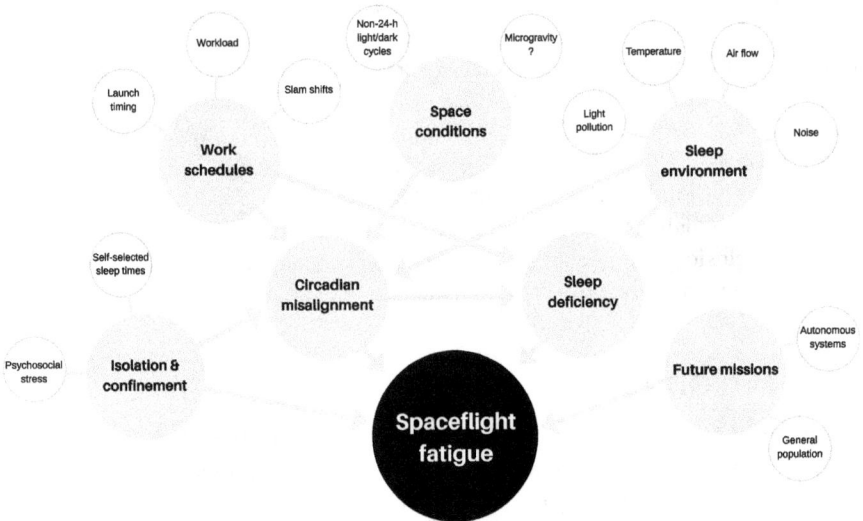

FIGURE 6.3.1 A schematic of the multiple factors contributing to fatigue in spaceflight. Dashed lines represent unexplored impacts on spaceflight fatigue. "Slam shifts" refer to changes in sleep timing of up to 12 hours, as discussed in sub-section 6.3.2.2 (work schedules). The impact of microgravity is as yet undefined, hence is displayed with a question mark.

6.3.2.1 Circadian Entrainment/Misalignment

Human sleep and circadian rhythms have evolved to adapt to the 24-hour light-dark cycle on Earth. However, crewmembers in space are no longer exposed to the light-dark cycle generated by the rotation of the Earth, which can contribute to sleep and circadian disruption (Guo et al., 2014; Mallis & DeRoshia, 2005). Such sleep loss and circadian misalignment have been associated with decrements in performance that have impacted the success and safety of a mission (Ellis, 2000).

Circadian misalignment among crewmembers can arise from both an inappropriate light-dark cycle and an irregular scheduling. Astronauts in low-Earth orbit, such as when aboard the International Space Station (ISS), experience approximately 16 orbits per day, resulting in a 90-minute light-dark cycle with ~45 minutes of light and darkness per orbit. Humans are unable to entrain their circadian clock to a 90-minute photoperiod (Buysse et al., 2005) and this can result in misalignment between a crewmember's circadian drive for sleep and the scheduled sleep opportunity. This circadian misalignment can occur even when crewmembers follow a nominal 24-hour sleep-wake schedule (Gundel et al., 1997; Monk et al., 2001). In contrast, schedule-induced circadian misalignment, as described in the next section, occurs during as much as 20% of nights during long-duration missions, resulting in increased use of medication and an hour less sleep compared to nights of circadian alignment (Flynn-Evans et al., 2016a).

As humans venture further into space, such as future missions to Mars, new issues arise that will impact the human circadian system. Mars rotates with a period of 24.65 hours, roughly 39 minutes longer than on Earth. This longer day length will require crewmembers to shift to a schedule that is similar to travelling two time zones westward every three days (Barger et al., 2012). Studies of individuals working on a Mars day length while on Earth have demonstrated that most people can adapt to the 39-minute daily shift if provided with appropriate lighting countermeasures (Barger et al., 2012). However, one report found that personnel working on Mars time in support of the Mars Exploration Rover mission experienced increases in fatigue and sleepiness, and decreases in energy and alertness compared to the crew's baseline performance under normal (24-hour) working conditions (DeRoshia et al., 2008). Collectively, these findings support the need for more research in this area to ensure that future Mars astronauts are provided with resources to facilitate their adaptation to a non-24-hour day length.

6.3.2.2 Work Schedules

Designing work schedules that allow for adequate and appropriately timed opportunities for sleep and personal activities is central to proactive fatigue risk management. Spaceflight scheduling involves many considerations and trade-offs that are not often encountered among other shift workers on Earth. In addition, every type of spaceflight mission, including low-Earth orbit missions, lunar orbit and landings, and long-duration missions such as missions to Mars, each present unique scheduling challenges (Barger et al., 2014a; Flynn-Evans et al., 2016a; Monk et al., 2004).

Unlike many Earth-based shiftwork operations, where schedules are driven by a need to staff blocks of time, limited crew size and time-sensitive mission events often determine when sleep can occur, both before and during spaceflight. For example, there is often a limited window of time available for a launch, which could occur at any time of day or night. Crewmembers are required to wake approximately five hours before launch (Czeisler et al., 1991; Flynn-Evans et al., 2016a), which means that they may need to shift their pre-flight sleep in order to accommodate all of the activities required for launch. Crewmembers use numerous countermeasures to help them adjust their circadian rhythms to minimise sleep loss and to enhance alertness during pre-flight shifting of sleep, including the use of specialised lighting (Czeisler et al., 1991) and optimised schedule shifting protocols (Monk et al., 2004; Whitson et al., 1995) (discussed further in sub-section 6.3.3 of this chapter).

In-flight work–rest schedules are also shaped by the nature of the mission. For example, Apollo missions in the late 1960s and early 1970s permitted only limited time for sleep due to task demands that required action by the small crews (Nicholson, 1972). Many short-duration missions aboard the Space Shuttle required crews to shift sleep progressively earlier or later, following non-24-hour schedules that allowed them to be awake during launch and landing activities (Dijk et al., 2001; Monk et al., 1998). Although most long-duration space station spaceflight operations have prescribed a nominal 24-hour schedule, mission operations often necessitate frequent schedule changes (Barger et al., 2012; Flynn-Evans et al., 2016a; Nicholson, 1972), including "slam shifts" (i.e., changes in sleep timing of up to 12 hours), whereby crewmembers must shift their sleep in order to be awake for time-sensitive mission activities.

All spaceflight missions have typically involved a high tempo workflow, with minute-by-minute scheduling of tasks that the crewmembers must strictly follow. Due to the challenges associated with working in space, crewmembers can fall behind on their schedule, which can encroach into their scheduled sleep opportunity and further curtail sleep (Beard, 2020).

6.3.2.3 SLEEP ENVIRONMENT

An adequate sleep environment is a foundational element of fatigue risk management. The primary factors that challenge sleep during spaceflight include environmental issues that are common to individuals on Earth, such as inadequate lighting, noise, and thermal management, as well as factors unique to spaceflight, such as inadequate airflow leading to carbon dioxide (CO_2) build-up. There are numerous challenges to ensuring that space vehicles or habitats are equipped with the proper sleep environment for crew. Since the beginning of multi-day human spaceflight, crews have slept during their missions. In some early missions, the spacecraft was not designed for quality sleep (Flynn-Evans et al., 2016b). Upon return to Earth, the crews provided feedback about the lack of adequate sleep and sleeping accommodations. From this feedback, engineers, designers, operations teams, and human performance specialists have endeavoured to identify and mitigate the factors that negatively impact sleep by improving sleep environment design. Short-duration missions, such as those on the

Space Shuttle, typically involved a small habitable volume, where all crews slept in a shared space (Flynn-Evans et al., 2016b). In contrast, long-duration missions, such as on Skylab, Mir, and the ISS, typically provided crews with private sleep quarters. However, sleep environment issues have persisted in both short- and long-duration missions.

The challenge of designing an appropriate sleep environment for spaceflight is apparent when considering the interactions between acoustic emissions, airflow, and temperature. Sleep disruption due to acoustic emissions, or noise, affects crewmembers' sleep just as it affects the sleep of individuals on Earth (Basner et al., 2011). Crews report that, during short-duration missions, noise from other crewmembers is disruptive to sleep (Barger et al., 2014a). Fatigue arising from noise disturbances to sleep among crew has resulted in impairment of cognitive abilities, declines in psychological well-being, increased sleepiness, and mood changes, including increased irritability-nervousness (Begault, 2018). During long-duration missions in which crews have had access to private sleep quarters, the fan used to provide airflow and CO_2 clearance can be an "annoyance" and disruptive to sleep (Maryatt et al., 2018). However, turning the fan off leads to the development of potentially dangerous increases in CO_2 as well as increased temperature within the sleep quarters, where temperatures can reach close to 27°C (80°F) (Maryatt, 2019). These environmental sleep disruptions all contribute to fatigue and can impact the cognitive capabilities of the crew (Maryatt et al., 2018).

As described in sub-section 6.3.2.1, circadian misalignment occurs during spaceflight due, in part, to non-24-hour patterns of light exposure. The lighting and window coverings within a space vehicle have the potential to counteract inappropriate light exposure, but the majority of space vehicles to date have used fluorescent lamps, with little regard for their brightness, spectral composition, and mounting location (Maryatt et al., 2018). Similarly, window coverings have often been insufficient to block light during the 90-minute light-dark cycle in low-Earth orbit (Dijk et al., 2001). Inadequate and mistimed light exposure makes it difficult to entrain to a 24-hour rhythm and likely contributes to the reduced sleep duration observed during spaceflight and subsequent fatigue.

6.3.2.4 Isolation and Confinement

Isolation and confinement are issues that are somewhat unique to spaceflight and can contribute to circadian misalignment and fatigue. Space station missions, including those on Mir and ISS, involve crewmembers living and working in space for 4 to 6 months or more, with 4 to 6 crewmembers (Morphew, 2001). Future missions to Mars will involve crews that will live and work in an isolated and confined space vehicle for up to three consecutive years (Cranford and Turner, 2021). Long-duration missions have negative impacts on crewmembers' psychological and physical health (in spaceflight and on Earth-based stations), including increased fatigue, decreased motivation, and other physical complaints (e.g., headaches and digestive issues) (Kanas, 1990), as well as negative psychosocial consequences (e.g., symptoms of depression, insomnia, irritability, and anxiety) (Christensen and Talbot, 1986; Kanas,

1985). Earth-based analogue studies designed to mimic the isolation and confinement experienced during spaceflight have elucidated the mechanisms by which these conditions lead to fatigue. Isolated and confined environments can contribute to increased social tension between crewmembers over time, which, in turn, can lead crewmembers to withdraw from social interactions and adopt a self-selected sleep and work schedule (Basner et al., 2014). In an isolated and confined environment absent of daily 24-hour photoperiodic cues, this can increase the potential for an individual to experience a circadian rhythm "free run" (i.e., when the circadian rhythm is not entrained to an external cue, like light, sleep-wake patterns cycle according to the length of the individual's biological clock, which is often not exactly 24 hours (Czeisler et al., 1999)). Such a phenomenon has occurred among some crewmembers during Mars analogue missions (Barger et al., 2014b; Basner et al., 2013) and during isolated and confined Antarctic winter-over missions (Kawasaki et al., 2018; Najjar et al., 2014). This type of circadian misalignment has not only been associated with fatigue-related performance impairment (Barger et al., 2014b; Basner et al., 2014; Mairesse et al., 2019), but has also exacerbated interpersonal conflict (e.g., decreased group cohesion and social interaction (Palinkas, 1992; Sandal et al., 1995)), which can cause further sleep disruption and fatigue (Palinkas & Suedfeld, 2008). In addition, one analysis of a 520-day Mars mission simulation found that over time the crew began to experience more extreme fatigue, known as torpor, suggesting that longer missions in isolation and confinement may have an even more severe impact on fatigue (Basner et al., 2013).

6.3.3 HOW CAN WE PROTECT SLEEP AND MANAGE FATIGUE DURING SPACE TRAVEL?

6.3.3.1 LIGHT INTERVENTIONS

Light interventions in other transport and occupational settings are discussed in Chapter 4.8 of this book. This chapter discusses the application of light to manage fatigue in spaceflight. The lack of appropriate 24-hour photoperiodic cues (discussed in sub-section 6.3.2.1), combined with a need for frequent schedule shifts (discussed in sub-section 6.3.2.2), has led to a high prevalence of circadian misalignment and subsequent fatigue and performance impairment during spaceflight. Indeed, the need to promote and maintain optimal crewmember alertness and performance drove many of the foundational studies in this area (Mallis and DeRoshia, 2005). Light interventions to manage fatigue in spaceflight include protocols to help crews either maintain stable entrainment with a 24-hour schedule, adapt to a non-24-hour schedule, or phase shift to meet operational demands pre-flight and during flight.

As mentioned in sub-section 6.3.2.2, preparing for missions often requires shifting sleep-wake patterns to align crew sleep-wake schedules with launch timing. Just like preparing for a night shift on Earth, strategic exposure to, and avoidance of, light pre-flight can help to phase-shift circadian rhythms to meet the operational demands of the mission (Czeisler et al., 1991). The use of light as an intervention pre-flight has been shown to accelerate adaptation to new schedules, regardless of whether the changes are abrupt (within three days) or more gradual (more than three days)

(Santy et al., 1994). For example, bright light exposure in the evening for seven days, combined with delayed sleep patterns, shifted the melatonin and cortisol rhythms of nearly all crewmembers to within two hours of a 12-hour shifted schedule before a flight (Whitson et al., 1995).

During spaceflight, light interventions may be able to be used to maintain alignment of circadian rhythms to stable 24-hour schedules, or to non-24-hour light-dark exposures or schedules, such as those that will be experienced during Mars missions. The use of standard interior lighting and light shades alone has not been successful based on the observation of circadian drift in crewmembers (Gundel et al., 1997). However, ground-based spaceflight analogues have demonstrated the potential of specialised dynamic lighting, which manipulates light levels during crew wake episodes, to accelerate in-flight phase shifting. For example, 450 lux of light administered during the first half of a wake episode is sufficient to entrain individuals to shorter than 24-hour schedules similar to those used during short-duration spaceflight (Scheer et al., 2007). Conversely, 450 lux of light during the second half of the wake episode appears sufficient to entrain individuals to a Mars Sol (24.65 hours) (Scheer et al., 2007). Similarly, two 45-minute bright 9500 lux light pulses timed in the biological evening appear to be sufficient to facilitate phase delays of one hour per day, which have been useful during both short- and long-duration missions (Gronfier et al., 2007). Such exposure to bright light pulses in the evening should also be sufficient to facilitate human circadian entrainment to the Mars Sol. A field study examining individuals living and working on a Mars Sol during the Phoenix Mars Lander mission found that blue light boxes aided circadian adaptation, thereby improving sleep and reducing fatigue when the individuals were aligned with the Mars Sol relative to phases when they were misaligned (Barger et al., 2012). Moreover, lighting delivered across a 24-hour period to mimic the intensity and spectral composition of the Earth's light-dark cycle (i.e., bright, blue-enriched light during the working day; dim, blue-depleted light before bedtime; and darkness during the primary sleep opportunity (Brainard et al., 2013)) is currently being tested on the ISS to determine if this lighting schedule can improve sleep, circadian alignment, fatigue, and performance (Brainard et al., 2016).

Together, these studies highlight the potential benefits of light to manage fatigue during spaceflight by promoting alertness during night shifts, shifting the circadian rhythm to a new phase, stabilising 24-hour rhythms, or adapting to a non-24-hour cycle. Appropriate lighting (e.g., timing, intensity, and spectral composition) is, therefore, an important consideration when designing spacecraft and for managing the fatigue of all crewmembers involved in spaceflight transport.

6.3.3.2 SCHEDULING TOOLS

Numerous biomathematical models have been developed to predict levels of fatigue and performance, as well as to estimate optimal work timing and circadian phase shifts (described in Chapter 4.3). Some of these models have been used to determine the appropriate timing for light interventions (Gronfier et al., 2007; Scheer et al., 2007), and to assess the consequences of sleep loss during spaceflight analogue missions (Flynn-Evans et al., 2020). Such models are used by ground support scheduling teams to help plan crew schedules that minimise sleep loss, circadian misalignment, and fatigue.

As scheduling becomes more autonomous in long-duration missions, crew will need more intuitive scheduling tools that are easy to use without ground support (Marquez et al., 2021). As a result, models that help crewmembers self-schedule the optimal timing of work tasks, sleep, and countermeasures could be integrated within existing scheduling tools. For example, studies are underway to determine whether providing crews with performance model predictions in a system where they can freely move tasks around on their schedule could be beneficial for future long-duration missions (Shelat et al., 2022).

6.3.3.3 HABITAT DESIGN

Although there are few data describing how changes in spaceflight habitat design impact sleep and fatigue, numerous studies suggest that sleeping in an appropriate sleep environment is a key element of good sleep hygiene and associated daytime functioning on Earth (Caddick et al., 2018). Features of the sleep environments that crew experienced during long-duration missions on Skylab, Mir, and ISS have informed improvements to the spaceflight sleep environment over time. In particular, the crew quarters (CQ) used on ISS have incorporated many of the best practices from Earth and lessons learnt from space to provide an adequate sleep environment, providing a model for the design of future spaceflight sleep environments. Specifically, the CQ provide a private sleep space that minimises sleep disruption due to environmental factors. For example, the location of the CQ within the space station is away from sources of noise, such as the galley and waste management system (Broyan et al., 2010). In addition, the ambient noise level in the CQ is targeted to be below a noise criterion (NC) rating of 40 for continuous noise and ± 10 dB for intermittent and impulsive noise to minimise sleep disruption (Broyan et al., 2010; NASA, 1995). The CQ include a solid-state lighting assembly which is a dimmable light source with three different spectral modes to reduce pre-sleep light disruption (Brainard et al., 2013). The CQ also have an intake duct diffuser with a fan speed control switch located within the reach of the crewmember that maintains appropriate ventilation and helps to regulate temperature (Broyan et al., 2010).

Even though improvements have been made to the sleep environment on the space station, it is unclear whether the CQ environment improves sleep and reduces fatigue, and not every space mission will be able to integrate similar CQ. For example, lunar expeditions will likely involve crewmembers living and working in a small vehicle without volume for private sleep accommodations (NASA, 1995). Moreover, lunar and Mars surface expeditions will require a horizontal sleep positioning, to account for different forces of gravity (Caddick et al., 2018). Hence, more research is needed to understand the benefits and consequences of different designs for providing the optimal sleep environment under varying conditions.

6.3.3.4 PHARMACOLOGICAL COUNTERMEASURES

In situations where the use of proactive countermeasures such as those described above is insufficient to mitigate fatigue, crews may use reactive countermeasures such as wake- and sleep-promoting medications (Barger et al., 2014a; Putcha et al., 1999; Santy et al., 1988; Wotring, 2015; Wotring & Smith, 2020). There are few data on the use of wake-promoting medications in space, although crews typically have access to caffeine and other wake-promoting medications (Barger et al., 2014a). Up to 50% of crewmembers have used hypnotics during spaceflight, but it is unclear whether these medications were beneficial. In fact, in ground tests, the use of hypnotics by crew has been associated with worsened sleep inertia (Dinges et al., 2019), raising concerns that hypnotic use in spaceflight could compromise a crewmember's ability to respond to an emergency. During flight, hypnotics appear to reduce sleep onset latency but do not lengthen sleep duration (Barger et al., 2014a), and are used more often when crews are circadian misaligned (Flynn-Evans et al., 2016a). These findings suggest that hypnotic use may be driven by crewmembers feeling unable to fall asleep. Studies examining the efficacy of medication use and their impact on subsequent fatigue are needed.

6.3.4 FUTURE CHALLENGES TO MANAGING FATIGUE IN SPACE

The nature of spaceflight is changing at a rapid pace. While space travel has previously been limited to candidates who meet stringent health and fitness screening requirements, the race towards commercial space travel is opening this opportunity up to a broader population. As space travel becomes more accessible, it is unlikely that the current rigorous selection processes will be applied, which increases the potential for travellers with health problems, including sleep disorders. Furthermore, the acceleration of commercial space operations may require pilots and ground crews to support short frequent missions, much like commercial aviation. It is unknown whether the current controls and strategies used to reduce fatigue for highly selected astronauts and cosmonauts will be sufficient to manage fatigue in a more diverse population.

Another potential change to spaceflight travel is the shift from crewmembers who are all actively involved in operating the space vehicle, to passive passengers. This may reduce the need to manage fatigue in this passenger group, with screening requirements and mitigation strategies potentially only applicable to operating crewmembers. For example, a passenger on an airplane is not required to meet the same health or fitness standards as pilots or flight attendants, as they do not significantly contribute to the safety of a flight (although see also Chapter 2.6 in this book for a discussion of the responsibility of passengers for some aspects of travel, such as survivability). In the case of space travel, however, there will likely be at least minimum health standards required of all passengers in order to safely tolerate the additional (to normal flight) physical and psychological stressors of spaceflight.

As technology continues to develop, spacecraft may be autonomously piloted, with ground crews responsible for flight safety. In this instance, fatigue management to ensure vigilant attention in these ground crews will be paramount. Fatigue has been highlighted as an under-researched risk to current remotely piloted aircraft operations, especially given that the primary task of monitoring (as opposed to operating a vehicle) is particularly sensitive to fatigue (Nesthus et al., 2021). Therefore, as the industry changes, future controls may need to be adapted from current fatigue management approaches and applied to meet new challenges.

6.3.5 CONCLUSIONS

There are several factors to consider when attempting to manage fatigue in space transport. Many of the factors contributing to sleep loss and circadian misalignment on Earth translate to and are potentially exacerbated in space, for example, irregular schedules and inadequate sleeping environments. In addition, constraints unique to space travel such as microgravity, isolation and confinement, and non-24-hour light-dark cycles, present new challenges for fatigue management. The diversity of current and future missions in terms of duration, vehicle design, mission goals, crew size, and light-dark cycle length, will require a range of countermeasures and strategies in order to manage fatigue based on specific challenges. Fatigue management in this area of transportation is especially critical given the potentially catastrophic consequences of a fatigue-related error.

SUMMARY POINTS FOR PRACTITIONERS

- Many of the fatigue risks in space are common to Earth, for example, reduced sleep due to noise, light, temperature, and circadian misalignment, which in turn is due to inappropriate light exposure and irregular shift patterns.
- There are several unique fatigue risks associated with space transport, including the as-yet undetermined influence of microgravity, the impact of isolation and confinement on psychosocial health, exposure to non-24-hour light-dark cycles, and the potential erratic changes to work schedules as dictated by mission goals.
- Countermeasures such as improved sleeping quarters, strategic exposure to light, and scheduling tools have been used to manage fatigue in current spaceflight missions and more research is underway to optimise these interventions.
- The advent of commercial spaceflight provides the opportunity for a more diverse population of space travellers. Current fatigue management tools may need to be adapted to manage fatigue in this new era of space transport.

REFERENCES

Barger, L. K., Flynn-Evans, E. E., Kubey, A., Walsh, L., Ronda, J. M., Wang, W., Wright, K. P., Jr., & Czeisler, C. A. (2014a). Prevalence of sleep deficiency and use of hypnotic drugs in astronauts before, during, and after spaceflight: An observational study. *The Lancet Neurology,* **13,** 904–912.

Barger, L. K., Sullivan, J. P., Vincent, A. S., Fiedler, E. R., Mckenna, L. M., Flynn-Evans, E. E., Gilliland, K., Sipes, W. E., Smith, P. H., Brainard, G. C., & Lockley, S. W. (2012).

Learning to live on a Mars day: Fatigue countermeasures during the Phoenix Mars Lander mission. *Sleep, 35,* 1423–1435.

Barger, L. K., Wright Jr, K. P., Burke, T. M., Chinoy, E. D., Ronda, J. M., Lockley, S. W., & Czeisler, C. A. (2014b). Sleep and cognitive function of crewmembers and mission controllers working 24-h shifts during a simulated 105-day spaceflight mission. *Acta Astronautica, 93,* 230–242.

Basner, M., Dinges, D. F., Mollicone, D., Ecker, A., Jones, C. W., Hyder, E. C., Di Antonio, A., Savelev, I., Kan, K., Goel, N., Morukov, B. V., & Sutton, J. P. (2013). Mars 520-d mission simulation reveals protracted crew hypokinesis and alterations of sleep duration and timing. *Proceedings of the National Academy of Sciences, 110,* 2635–2640.

Basner, M., Dinges, D. F., Mollicone, D. J., Savelev, I., Ecker, A. J., Di Antonio, A., Jones, C. W., Hyder, E. C., Kan, K., Morukov, B. V., & Sutton, J. P. (2014). Psychological and behavioral changes during confinement in a 520-day simulated interplanetary mission to Mars. *PLoS One, 9,* e93298.

Basner, M., Müller, U., & Elmenhorst, E. M. (2011). Single and combined effects of air, road, and rail traffic noise on sleep and recuperation. *Sleep, 34,* 11–23.

Beard, B. L. (2020). Characterization of International Space Station crew members' workload contributing to fatigue, sleep disruption and circadian de-synchronization. Report No. NASA/TM-20205006969. Moffett Field, CA: NASA Ames Research Center.

Begault, D. R. (2018). Assessment and mitigation of the effects of noise on habitability in deep space environments: report on non-auditory effects of noise. Report No. NASA/TM-2018-219748. Moffett Field, CA: NASA Ames Research Center.

Brainard, G. C., Barger, L. K., Soler, R. R., & Hanifin, J. P. (2016). The development of lighting countermeasures for sleep disruption and circadian misalignment during spaceflight. *Current Opinion in Pulmonary Medicine, 22,* 535–544.

Brainard, G. C., Coyle, W., Ayers, M., Kemp, J., Warfield, B., Maida, J., Bowen, C., Bernecker, C., Lockley, S. W., & Hanifin, J. P. (2013). Solid-state lighting for the International Space Station: Tests of visual performance and melatonin regulation. *Acta Astronautica, 92,* 21–28.

Broyan, J., Welsh, D., & Cady, S. (2010). International space station crew quarters ventilation and acoustic design implementation. Report No. AIAA 2010-6018. In *40th International Conference on Environmental Systems.*

Buysse, D. J., Monk, T. H., Carrier, J., & Begley. (2005). Circadian patterns of sleep, sleepiness, and performance in older and younger adults. *Sleep, 28,* 1365–1376.

Caddick, Z. A., Gregory, K., Arsintescu, L., & Flynn-Evans, E. E. (2018). A review of the environmental parameters necessary for an optimal sleep environment. *Building and Environment, 132,* 11–20.

Christensen, J. M., & Talbot, J. M. (1986). A review of the psychological aspects of space flight. *Aviation, Space, and Environmental Medicine, 57,* 203–212.

Cohen, E., & Spector, S. (eds.) (2019). *Space tourism: The elusive dream.* Bingley, UK: Emerald Publishing Limited.

Cranford, N., & Turner, J. L. (2021) Step 3, Artemis: Moon Missions as an astronaut testbed for Mars [Online]. National Aeronautics and Space Administration. Available at: www.nasa.gov/feature/step-3-artemis-moon-missions-as-an-astronaut-testbed-for-mars [Accessed 10 Dec 2021].

Czeisler, C. A., Chiasera, A. J., & Duffy, J. F. (1991). Research on sleep, circadian rhythms and aging: Applications to manned spaceflight. *Experimental Gerontology, 26,* 217–232.

Czeisler, C. A., Duffy, J. F., Shanahan, T. L., Brown, E. N., Mitchell, J. F., Rimmer, D. W., Ronda, J. M., Silva, E. J., Allan, J. S., & Emens, J. S. (1999). Stability, precision, and near-24-hour period of the human circadian pacemaker. *Science, 284,* 2177–2181.

Deroshia, C. W., Colletti, L. C., & Mallis, M. M. (2008). The effects of the Mars Exploration Rovers (MER) work schedule regime on locomotor activity circadian rhythms, sleep and fatigue. Report No. NASA/TM-2008-214560. Moffett Field, CA: NASA Ames Research Center.

Dijk, D. J., Neri, D. F., Wyatt, J. K., Ronda, J. M., Riel, E., Ritz-De Cecco, A., Hughes, R. J., Elliott, A. R., Prisk, G. K., West, J. B., & Czeisler, C. A. (2001). Sleep, performance, circadian rhythms, and light-dark cycles during two space shuttle flights. *American Journal of Physiology-Regulatory, Integrative and Comparative Physiology*, **281**, R1647–R1664.

Dinges, D. F., Basner, M., Ecker, A. J., Baskin, P., & Johnston, S. L. (2019). Effects of zolpidem and zaleplon on cognitive performance after emergent morning awakenings at Tmax: A randomized placebo-controlled trial. *Sleep*, **42**, zsy258.

Ellis, S. R. (2000). Collision in space. *Ergonomics in Design*, **8**, 4–9.

Flynn-Evans, E. E., Barger, L. K., Kubey, A. A., Sullivan, J. P., & Czeisler, C. A. (2016a). Circadian misalignment affects sleep and medication use before and during spaceflight. *Npj Microgravity*, **2**, 15019.

Flynn-Evans, E. E., Caddick, Z. A., Gregory, K., & Center, J. S. (2016b). Sleep environment recommendations for future spaceflight vehicles. In: Stanton N., Landry S., Di Bucchianico G., & Vallicelli A. (eds). *Advances in human aspects of transportation. advances in intelligent systems and computing, vol 484*. Cham: Springer.

Flynn-Evans, E. E., Kirkley, C., Young, M., Bathurst, N., Gregory, K., Vogelpohl, V., End, A., Hillenius, S., Pecena, Y., & Marquez, J. J. (2020). Changes in performance and bio-mathematical model performance predictions during 45 days of sleep restriction in a simulated space mission. *Scientific Reports*, **10**, 15594.

Frost, J. D., Jr., Shumate, W. H., Salamy, J. G., & Booher, C. R. (1976). Sleep monitoring: The second manned Skylab mission. *Aviation, Space, and Environmental Medicine*, **47**, 372–382.

Gronfier, C., Wright, K. P., Kronauer, R. E., & Czeisler, C. A. (2007). Entrainment of the human circadian pacemaker to longer-than-24-h days. *Proceedings of the National Academy of Sciences*, **104**, 9081–9086.

Gundel, A., Nalishiti, V., Reucher, E., Vejvoda, M., & Zulley, J. (1993). Sleep and circadian rhythm during a short space mission. *The Clinical Investigator*, **71**, 718–724.

Gundel, A., Polyakov, V. V., & Zulley, J. (1997). The alteration of human sleep and circadian rhythms during spaceflight. *Journal of Sleep Research*, **6**, 1–8.

Guo, J. H., Qu, W. M., Chen, S. G., Chen, X. P., Lv, K., Huang, Z. L., & Wu, Y. L. (2014). Keeping the right time in space: Importance of circadian clock and sleep for physiology and performance of astronauts. *Military Medical Research*, **1**, 23.

Kanas, N. (1985). Psychosocial factors affecting simulated and actual space missions. *Aviation, Space, and Environmental Medicine*, **56**, 806–811.

Kanas, N. (1990). Psychological, psychiatric, and interpersonal aspects of long-duration space missions. *Journal of Spacecraft and Rockets*, **27**, 457–463.

Kawasaki, A., Wisniewski, S., Healey, B., Pattyn, N., Kunz, D., Basner, M., & Münch, M. (2018). Impact of long-term daylight deprivation on retinal light sensitivity, circadian rhythms and sleep during the Antarctic winter. *Scientific Reports*, **8**, 1–12.

Mairesse, O., Macdonald-Nethercott, E., Neu, D., Tellez, H. F., Dessy, E., Neyt, X., Meeusen, R., & Pattyn, N. (2019). Preparing for Mars: Human sleep and performance during a 13 month stay in Antarctica. *Sleep*, **42**, zsy206.

Mallis, M. M., & Deroshia, C. (2005). Circadian rhythms, sleep, and performance in space. *Aviation, Space, and Environmental Medicine*, **76**, B94–B107.

Marquez, J. J., Edwards, T., Karasinski, J. A., Lee, C. N., Shyr, M. C., Miller, C. L., & Brandt, S. L. (2021). Human performance of novice schedulers for complex spaceflight operations timelines. *Human Factors*. DOI:10.1177/00187208211058913.

Maryatt, B. (2019). Improvements to on-orbit sleeping accommodations. In *49th International Conference on Environmental Systems*. Boston, Massachusetts.

Maryatt, B., Van Wie, M., & Clark, T. (2018). Recommendations for next generation crew quarters.. *48th International Conference on Environmental Systems*. Albuquerque, NM, 8–12 July.

Monk, T. H., Buysse, D. J., Billy, B. D., & Degrazia, J. M. (2004). Using nine 2-h delays to achieve a 6-h advance disrupts sleep, alertness, and circadian rhythm. *Aviation, Space, and Environmental Medicine*, **75**, 1049–1057.

Monk, T. H., Buysse, D. J., Billy, B. D., Kennedy, K. S., & Willrich, L. M. (1998). Sleep and circadian rhythms in four orbiting astronauts. *Journal of Biological Rhythms*, **13**, 188–201.

Monk, T. H., Kennedy, K. S., Rose, L. R., & Linenger, J. M. (2001). Decreased human circadian pacemaker influence after 100 days in space: A case study. *Psychosomatic Medicine*, **63**, 881–885.

Morphew, E. (2001). Psychological and human factors in long duration spaceflight. *McGill Journal of Medicine*, **6**, 74–80.

Najjar, R. P., Wolf, L., Taillard, J., Schlangen, L. J., Salam, A., Cajochen, C., & Gronfier, C. (2014). Chronic artificial blue-enriched white light is an effective countermeasure to delayed circadian phase and neurobehavioral decrements. *PloS one*, **9**, e102827.

NASA Technical Standard. (1995). NASA Manned Systems Integration Standards: Volume 1, Section 5, Natural and Induced Environments. Report No. STD-3000.

Nesthus, T., Fercho, K., Durham, J., Mofle, T., Nesmith, B., & Hu, P. (2021). Summary final report for Unmanned Aircraft Systems in Air Carrier Operations: UAS operator fatigue. Report No. DOT/FAA/AM-21/16. Washington DC: Federal Aviation Administration.

Nicholson, A. N. (1972). Sleep patterns in the aerospace environment. *Journal of the Royal Society of Medicine*, **65**, 192–194.

Palinkas, L. A. (1992). Going to extremes: The cultural context of stress, illness and coping in Antarctica. *Social Science & Medicine*, **35**, 651–664.

Palinkas, L. A., & Suedfeld, P. (2008). Psychological effects of polar expeditions. *The Lancet*, **371**, 153–163.

Putcha, L., Berens, K. L., Marshburn, T. H., Ortega, H. J., & Billica, R. D. (1999). Pharmaceutical use by U.S. astronauts on space shuttle missions. *Aviation, Space, and Environmental Medicine*, **70**, 705–708.

Roberts, T. G. (2021). International Astronaut Database [Online]. Aerospace Security. Available at: https://aerospace.csis.org/data/international-astronaut-database/ [Accessed 20 Dec 2021].

Roulette, J. (2021). More than 600 human beings have now been to space [Online]. *The New York Times*. Available: www.nytimes.com/2021/11/10/science/600-astronauts-space.html [Accessed 10 Dec 2021].

Sandal, G. M., Vaernes, R., & Ursin, H. (1995). Interpersonal relations during simulated space missions. *Aviation, Space, and Environmental Medicine*, **66**, 617–624.

Santy, P. A., Faulk, D. M., & Davis, J. R. (1994). Strategies for the preflight circadian shifting of Space Shuttle crews. *Journal of Clinical Pharmacology*, **34**, 535–542.

Santy, P. A., Kapanka, H., Davis, J. R., & Stewart, D. F. (1988). Analysis of sleep on Shuttle missions. *Aviation, Space, and Environmental Medicine*, **59**, 1094–1097.

Scheer, F. A., Wright Jr, K. P., Kronauer, R. E., & Czeisler, C. A. (2007). Plasticity of the intrinsic period of the human circadian timing system. *PloS One*, **2**, e721.

Shelat, S., Karasinski, J., Flynn-Evans, E., & Marquez, J. (2022). Evaluation of user experience of self-scheduling software for astronauts: Defining a satisfaction baseline. *Proceedings of the 24th international conference on Human-Computer Interaction, 26 June–1 July, 2022 (virtual).*

Stoilova, I., Zdravev, T., & Yanev, T. (2000). Evaluation of sleep in space flight. *Comptes Rendus de l'Academi Bulgare des Sciences, 53,* 59–62.

Whitson, P. A., Putcha, L., Chen, Y. M., & Baker, E. (1995). Melatonin and cortisol assessment of circadian shifts in astronauts before flight. *Journal of Pineal Research, 18,* 141–147.

Wotring, V. E. (2015). Medication use by U.S. crewmembers on the International Space Station. *The FASEB Journal, 29,* 4417–4423.

Wotring, V. E., & Smith, L. K. (2020). Dose tracker application for collecting medication use data from International Space Station crew. *Aerospace Medicine and Human Performance, 91,* 41–45.

6.4 The Future of Fatigue Management

Strategies, Policies, and Societal Expectations

Mark R. Rosekind[1], Erin E. Flynn-Evans[2], and Kevin B. Gregory[2]

[1]Department of Health Policy and Management, Johns Hopkins University, Baltimore, MD, USA
[2]Fatigue Countermeasures Laboratory, NASA Ames Research Center, Moffett Field, CA, USA

CONTENTS

6.4.1 INTRODUCTION

The requirements for global, 24/7 transportation operations create significant challenges to the human operators central to maintaining a safe, productive system. In every transportation mode, basic human physiological requirements for sleep and circadian stability can be disrupted by diverse, dynamic, around-the-clock operational needs. For example, in these operational environments, humans can confront limited sleep opportunities, working across time zones, changing shift schedules, night-time operations, no or adverse fatigue management policies, short call-outs (communications to report for duty), insufficient sleep recovery, minimal training on sleep and circadian factors underlying safety and health risks, and poor human-centred design. As discussed throughout this book, sleep and circadian disruption create known risks to safety, performance, and health.

Societal needs for the transportation of people and goods, safety, security, food, water, energy, health, and sustainability continue to expand. In the foreseeable future, humans will have continuing critical and central roles in developing, providing, and maintaining operations to meet these needs globally. Technology offers new opportunities to supplement and complement human resources, but even human monitoring of automated systems is known to present vigilance and response challenges for the operators. Acknowledging these many challenges presents an opportunity to implement fatigue management efforts that can reduce risk and enhance safety throughout transportation. Managing human fatigue in future around-the-clock, global transportation operations can be a model for providing safe, effective, and efficient societal mobility.

This chapter explores issues and opportunities, and proposes a road map with specific actions to pursue future fatigue management. Specifically, these opportunities will be examined within three areas: Strategies, policies, and societal expectations. Strategies address fatigue risk management systems (FRMS), education, wearables and other new technology, proactive and predictive data analysis, and learning from incidents and accidents. Policies examine governmental regulations versus organisational policies, elements of effective policies and regulations, and preparing for new technologies and operational demands. Societal expectations explore societal versus individual risk/benefit considerations, cost/benefit issues, and global perspectives. Throughout this chapter there are 16 specific **opportunity/actions** (Table 6.4.1) that are identified to translate the discussion into a road map for enhancing future fatigue management in transportation.

6.4.2 STRATEGIES

6.4.2.1 THE FUTURE OF FATIGUE RISK MANAGEMENT SYSTEMS

FRMS (see also Chapter 4.1) are currently the prevalent process for managing fatigue in safety-sensitive transportation operations within organisations. While FRMS are intended to adapt as information and operations change, there are opportunities to enhance and expand the FRMS process for future operations in areas of fatigue education, technology integration, data collection, and incident investigations.

The Future of Fatigue Education

Although fatigue education has always been a core element of FRMS, there is a critical need to expand educational opportunities that target individuals, organisations, and our society with tailored information. Basic fatigue education that includes information on the causes, consequences, and countermeasures for fatigue should be foundational to any fatigue education training programme (Avers et al., 2009). However, a strategic, tailored, and targeted approach to education in a transportation organisation (or company) can provide more actionable information to operators and managers that aligns with specific fatigue challenges they face. As technology evolves and as new issues emerge, operators should be provided with up-to-date information on how to adapt to the changing nature of operations.

Fatigue Education for Individuals

Currently, there are no standards for what should be included in fatigue education or how such training should be deployed within an organisation. Programmes range from brief, generic, in-person, or online training sessions to multi-day workshops and frequent hands-on sessions with trained personnel (Barger et al., 2018; Smith & Wallace, 2016; Steffen et al., 2015). The frequency of training required to ensure information retention also needs to be established. The content of such programmes is similarly diverse, with most providing information on sleep, circadian rhythms, and work hours, but with fewer providing information on managing issues such as commuting, workload, and family/social life. In aggregate, fatigue education sessions have been shown to be effective in increasing off-duty sleep and on-duty alertness, while reducing fatigue and related symptoms, but diversity in approaches, and individual and workplace factors, make it challenging to deploy fatigue education relevant to everyone in a given organisation (Avers et al., 2009; Barger et al., 2018; Sprajcer et al., 2021). **Opportunity/action #1: Develop consensus standards for content, frequency, evaluation, and updating of fatigue education programmes.**

Beyond generalised fatigue education, information tailored to the unique challenges faced by individuals in a given workplace can offer more operationally specific and relevant training. There should be core information that is common across fatigue education training, along with the information that should be specific to the nature of the organisation (e.g., trucking, rail, and aviation) and to the individual's role in the workplace (e.g., line operators, schedulers, dispatch, and management). The tailored information could be gathered from annual surveys, or information extracted from a fatigue-reporting system or potentially from wearable fatigue detection tools. Understanding relevant organisational and individual factors is critical to the implementation of an effective fatigue education programme. **Opportunity/action #2: Develop models of tailored elements to incorporate in fatigue education programmes.**

Fatigue education should also evolve in response to changing technology. Major advancements, such as aircraft that fly longer, the introduction of sophisticated automation capabilities in road vehicles, and sensing technologies such as positive train control in rail operations, all have the potential to interact with and modify how human operators engage with systems when fatigued. For example, when active driving tasks in road vehicles are managed by the vehicle rather than by the driver (an objective of self-driving capabilities), latent driver sleepiness can be unmasked that may compromise response speed in takeover or emergency situations (Flynn-Evans et al., 2021). The influence of technology innovations on fatigue may not be fully understood at this time but should be acknowledged in training and monitored closely.

Opportunity/action #3: Create a system to monitor technology advancements relevant to fatigue management.

Fatigue Education for Organisations

Given the need for robust and dynamic fatigue education in safety-sensitive transportation organisations, it is critical that organisations maintain the proficiency of those involved in providing fatigue education. The responsibility for delivering company fatigue education programs often resides among individuals in an organisation's safety department, who may not have an extensive background in fatigue science. As a result, these individuals must be provided with ongoing training to support their role within the organisation. However, there are currently limited and disparate opportunities for such "train-the-trainer" training. Historically, some government organisations have provided formal annual fatigue education training for distinct domains, such as aviation, to support this process (Rosekind et al., 2001). Unfortunately, such training opportunities have been inconsistently funded, creating an unreliable environment for ongoing training. Similarly, some professional societies, sleep, and safety organisations have created web-based or in-person training opportunities for fatigue education programmes. These programmes have typically been broad in scope and may not provide trainers with the skills needed to develop bespoke fatigue education within their organisations. **Opportunity/action #4: Develop reliable, ongoing "train-the-trainer" training opportunities that cover issues specific to operational domains and that are continuously updated.**

Eventually, fatigue education must be integrated within an organisation's safety culture. While some stand-alone fatigue education sessions have yielded positive effects months to years after a single training session (Gander et al., 2005), others have failed to realise any lasting benefits (Arora et al., 2007). Therefore, once dedicated fatigue training has been deployed to a population, additional ongoing training opportunities must be embedded within the workplace culture to maintain collective knowledge and visibility. For example, topical fatigue education information should be regularly included in safety newsletters and briefings, and updates should be provided when operational changes occur and when adopting new policies (e.g., napping). Providing such targeted information offers timely, actionable information for the workforce, while also keeping fatigue education prominent in the safety culture of an organisation. **Opportunity/action #5: Implement specific plans that integrate fatigue education into organisational safety culture in an ongoing manner.**

Fatigue Education for Society

The societal demand for a rested, alert, and safe workforce depends on communal knowledge regarding the benefits of sleep and the risks associated with sleep loss. The value that a society places on sleep health can be informed by how fatigue risk management is communicated to the public. Societal fatigue education has generally involved campaigns from government, sleep or safety organisations targeting drowsy driving or sleep disorders (Fletcher et al., 2005). However, organisations and individuals can advance societal understanding of fatigue-related issues by including information in more diverse public communications. For example, campaigns could be expanded to illustrate how customer demand for on-time delivery can, if not proactively managed by an organisation, disrupt workers' sleep and circadian rhythms, thereby affecting safety in different modes of transportation. Dissemination of fatigue-related information should be modelled after existing communications that connect issues such as weather or maintenance to safety. At the individual level, workers have an opportunity to advance public understanding of how sleep and circadian rhythms contribute to fatigue through positive peer modelling, for example, by sharing strategies for protecting sleep time as opposed to extolling sleep loss as a sign of strength. This type of multidimensional approach is necessary to change the narrative surrounding fatigue by engaging society at every level. **Opportunity/action #6: Develop a plan and resources for organisational and individual communications to the broader society on enhancing safety through fatigue management.**

6.4.2.2 WEARABLES AND NEW TECHNOLOGY

Consumer demand for technology to self-assess sleep and activity has accelerated the development of tools that can be deployed at scale for use in operational settings. There are numerous approaches that have been proposed for fatigue detection, including wearable technology that assesses sleep quantity and quality, which is then used to infer information about waking fatigue levels or performance, sometimes through the use of biomathematical models (Russell et al., 2000). Other approaches involve requiring a user to engage in frequent cognitive tests or assessment of on-the-job performance such as evaluation of lane deviations in road transport operations (Liu et al., 2009). Still other approaches involve passive monitoring of an operator's eye movements, heart rate, or other physiological proxies for fatigue (Sparrow et al., 2019). (For more on issues with fatigue detection and monitoring technology, see Chapters 1.2 and 4.6.)

There are several ways that these new technologies could transform fatigue risk management. For example, all drivers at a company could be equipped with a wearable device that provides them with information on their sleep and fatigue/performance level. This feedback could be used by individual drivers to make better decisions about sleep, thereby reducing fatigue. While on the job, based on their individual information, the drivers could be provided with countermeasure recommendations, such as advice to take a nap or to consume caffeine. The data generated from the workforce as a whole could be further assessed to identify sub-optimal schedule rotations that lead to elevated fatigue. Such schedules could then be modified to reduce fatigue throughout the organisation.

Unfortunately, there is currently no technology that is evaluated and sufficiently accurate to realise this idealised use in operational settings. Indeed, the promise of introducing technology solutions to combat fatigue has been suggested for over 25 years (Dinges & Mallis, 1998), yet persistent issues have prevented progress and application. The major concern hindering the widespread use of fatigue detection technology in transportation is insufficient evaluation (Anund et al., 2015). Before a new tool can be considered for use in real-world settings, it must be clear that it is able to provide accurate measures of fatigue in a variety of operationally relevant scenarios. Providing inaccurate information to an operator has the potential to be dangerous in several ways, including by limiting trust in the system. For example, an operator who is informed by technology that they are not experiencing fatigue when, in fact, fatigue is present could continue working, thereby increasing risk. Therefore, before operational deployment, such fatigue monitoring technology must be assessed against established, accepted, gold-standard methodologies and must include a variety of scenarios (e.g., schedules, countermeasure use, sleep disorders, and individual differences). Technology development companies and government agencies must prioritise these evaluation efforts to advance the use of such devices in operations. Transportation organisations must then further evaluate devices within their workforce during actual operations to ensure that the technology is appropriate for widespread use. **Opportunity/action #7: Develop consensus methods and standards to evaluate new fatigue detection technologies and establish a central information resource for sharing results.**

Beyond the evaluated accuracy of these new technologies, there remain significant policy issues to address prior to effective implementation in real-world fatigue risk management. These issues include determining what and when data will be collected, who has access to the data, and how it will be used. Collected data must be analysed using scientific principles and accepted methods by qualified individuals in order to ensure the accuracy of findings. Data must be secured in an anonymised database to maintain trust by the workforce and to protect against disclosure of any individual's personal information. How the data is used should be pre-determined by an inclusive stakeholder group that is clearly focused on fatigue management and safety issues. An ongoing monitoring programme should be established to determine unintended consequences that may emerge, including those related to operational changes. **Opportunity/action #8: Identify relevant policy issues and develop model policies to ensure effective methods to appropriately use and protect fatigue-related data.**

6.4.2.3 PROACTIVE AND PREDICTIVE DATA ANALYSIS

As technological advances allow for the collection of objective human fatigue data at scale, such information must be integrated into proactive and predictive tools to further manage fatigue-related risk. Biomathematical models are currently used in transportation modes to design schedules that are intended to minimise fatigue during operations (Mallis et al., 2004; see also Chapter 4.3 and 4.4). However, the majority of these models are static and unable to provide predictions at an individual level (Flynn-Evans et al., 2020), limiting broader applications and tailored recommendations for specific operators. Using information gathered from new technology wearables presents an opportunity to enhance and inform biomathematical models to predict fatigue-related performance changes at both the aggregate and individual levels. In addition, such information could be integrated within other risk models, such as weather forecasting and workload modelling, to provide safety managers with a more comprehensive understanding of safety risks.

In the near term, biomathematical models could be enhanced to provide individualised scheduling and countermeasure guidance. For example, this could be accomplished by incorporating an individual's wearable or cognitive performance data into a model that dynamically adapts to refine individual-level predictions based on objective information (Ramakrishnan et al., 2015). Such enhanced models could be used to identify countermeasures for individuals who are vulnerable to sleep loss or circadian disruption-related impairment. Although these approaches have the potential to greatly improve fatigue risk management and scheduling, future models must improve predictions at the individual level (Van Dongen et al., 2007) and responses to real-world issues and scenarios such as varying patterns of light exposure and medication use (Dinges, 2004). Significantly more research and validation of these models are needed to deliver on the opportunity for such a future. **Opportunity/ action #8: Enhance modelling capabilities to reflect individual-level status and incorporate individual objective fatigue data from wearables.**

Beyond near-term opportunities, the integration of biomathematical model data into larger aggregate risk forecasting is a long-term goal. The use of these enhanced biomathematical models in future operations could take multiple forms. First, fatigue data gathered from operational environments could be analysed by model developers to refine models to inform operational-specific schedule design (Paul et al., 2020). Such an approach could provide better aggregate predictions improving scheduling by incorporating diverse factors into predictions. For example, if pilots flying a specific long-haul operation were found to preferentially sleep relative to local night-time at the destination (i.e., a circadian misaligned state), then predictive schedule modelling could account for performance relative to that sub-optimal sleep timing. This information could then be incorporated into models, thereby improving the accuracy of predictions regarding subsequent pilot fatigue. These data could then be fused with other risk prediction data, such as weather, air traffic, and maintenance history to provide a dispatcher or scheduler with a more complete aggregate risk overview for a given flight operation. This would provide in-time information to initiate operational changes if needed to manage overall operational safety risks. The development of such a risk model would be transformative as it would allow for proactive assessment of many factors that could interact to increase risks of an incident or accident, creating the opportunity to manage these identified risks and enhance system safety. However, current modelling capabilities and technology are not yet sufficient for the development of such a risk dashboard. Realising this vision will require continued efforts to develop accurate and validated modelling, standardised data architecture and processing, and easy to interpret data visualisations or scores to help operational decision-makers assess risk. Each of these requirements will involve extensive research and validation to yield actionable predictions. **Opportunity/ action #9: Pursue research and validation to produce an aggregate risk model that incorporates relevant objective fatigue data.**

6.4.2.4 LEARNING FROM INCIDENTS AND ACCIDENTS

Given the dynamic, complex nature of 24/7 transport operations, it is difficult to imagine how fatigue related to human operators will ever be eliminated. As a result, incidents and accidents attributable to fatigue will continue to occur and offer a critical opportunity to provide lessons that can prevent future occurrences. Transportation crashes and incidents must be investigated to determine whether fatigue was causal or contributory and what recommendations can lead to new strategies that minimise or eliminate future fatigue-related risks. National governmental safety boards, such as the US National Transportation Safety Board (NTSB), typically evaluate major transportation disasters and provide formal recommendations to any organisation that could prevent a reoccurrence and enhance future safety. These recommendations can be made to regulators, local and national governments, safety or standards organisations, companies, or any group that can reduce risks identified in an investigation. The recommendations can address broad areas for improvement, such as regulations, policies, procedures, education and training, technology issues, and human-centred design (Marcus & Rosekind, 2017). Fatigue has been identified as a factor in crashes across all modes of transportation, with the first NTSB fatigue probable cause in aviation identified over 25 years ago (NTSB, 1994; Rosekind et al., 1994). An NTSB study of all major investigations over a 12-year period identified that 20% had either a probable cause, contributing factor or finding that involved fatigue (Marcus & Rosekind, 2017). Organisations should establish their own incident response and investigation procedures to evaluate crashes, incidents, and near-misses as ways to identify and mitigate identified fatigue sources. Thorough evaluation of such incidents and accidents, followed by implementation of recommendations, is an important objective for future fatigue management.

Initially, organisations should formalise incident response and investigation procedures to be conducted by a cross-functional group with relevant expertise and independence. Chapters 2.4 and 2.5 in this book describe established Investigation Board procedures including data collection, analysis, and interpretation that can be models for an organisation. It is critical to ensure that investigators are knowledgeable regarding the scientific foundations of fatigue, understand how fatigue can contribute to an incident, assess fatigue factors in a consistent and systematic manner, and are sufficiently funded to enable a thorough review. For example, many people mistakenly believe that a fatigue-related accident occurs only when someone has fallen asleep during operations. While this does occur, in reality, fatigue leads to unstable cognitive performance, which can be causal or contributory to an incident or accident (Lim & Dinges, 2008). This cognitive performance impairment can result in degraded or impaired vigilance, reaction times, decision-making, situational awareness, and more. These cognitive impairments arise from sleep deficiency (e.g., not getting enough sleep on a regular basis or staying awake too long), circadian disruption (e.g., working during biological night), or sleep inertia (e.g., performing immediately upon waking from sleep). Therefore, investigation of incidents should include an evaluation of sleep history, timing, environment, work schedules, and factors such as sleep disorders and medication use. National accident investigation agencies have established best practices for assessing fatigue that should be adopted for use investigating incidents by transportation organisations (Rudin-Brown & Rosberg, 2021; Price & Coury, 2015). These investigation procedures have been in use for a long time and continue to evolve by incorporating the latest science and technology. **Opportunity/action #10: Implement cross-functional, independent incident response/investigation procedures.**

Beyond investigating the role of fatigue in transportation incidents and crashes, it is critical that lessons learnt be translated into recommendations that are subsequently implemented to ensure that the same fatigue-related incidents do not reoccur.

Implementing some recommendations may be straightforward, directly under company control, and completed quickly, while others may involve regulatory change, complex policy determinations, and long-term commitments. Maintaining a strong FRMS that includes a robust incident response and investigation component provides companies with another effective tool to address identified, known fatigue risks. Broader recommendation implementation, for example, that involving regulatory change, will be more complex and involve longer timelines. For example, a review of accident investigations in US transportation found that 16% of recommendations made to aviation regulators were open and had an unacceptable resolution (Marcus & Rosekind, 2017). Basically, this means that 16% of NTSB aviation recommendations made to aviation regulators to address fatigue had no action or an unacceptable action taken by the recipients. This represents a potential target for legislative reform, whereby fatigue recommendations issued by national accident investigation boards would be prioritised in an effort to promote safety. NTSB findings, probable cause determinations, identified contributing factors, and recommendations represent costly lessons learnt that must lead to change and reduced risk.

These are highly visible and tragic events that become lost opportunities if they are not used to enhance transportation safety. Investigating, which is a reactive process, can lead to proactive measures that prevent tragic fatigue-related transportation crashes from occurring in the future. **Opportunity/action #11: Implement and track all investigation recommendations.**

6.4.3 POLICIES

6.4.3.1 GOVERNMENTAL REGULATIONS VS ORGANISATIONAL POLICIES

Generally, policies relevant to fatigue management can be considered in two ways: government regulations or organisational policies. Government regulations can be created through a variety of mechanisms at the national, state, and local levels with the distinction of being law. This establishes a legal requirement that can be enforced through a variety of authorities. Depending on the level of government, establishing regulations is often a lengthy, rigorous process. Creating the regulation may require a significant amount of research data, identifying specific outcomes or performance criteria, cost/benefit analyses, public comment periods, and subsequent review and revisions prior to publishing a final rule. At the national level, this process can take years with specific timelines related to the particular agency that promulgates the regulation. Once established, it is likely that the law will be in place for a long time, hence the thorough process. Depending on the regulatory agency, a variety of enforcement authorities are typically available to ensure the regulation is followed.

While companies are required to comply with regulations, organisational policies can be created that supplement or complement regulations. Though company policies do not have the legal authority of regulations, they can be enforced through other mechanisms available at a company level. Even in the absence of a regulatory requirement, a company can establish fatigue management policies to address known safety risks associated with transportation operations. For example, company policies could address complex scheduling factors, establish a napping programme or provide an anonymous fatigue reporting system. Company policies can offer a more flexible and timely solution to managing fatigue than regulatory schemes. They also should be directly connected to the education programme provided at the company, such as policies supporting breaks, nap opportunities, and strategic caffeine use. It is likely that the most effective fatigue management systems will incorporate both governmental regulatory and company policy approaches.

6.4.3.2 ELEMENTS OF EFFECTIVE POLICIES AND REGULATIONS

Based on long-standing sleep and circadian science there are policy and regulatory elements that would be considered foundational for effective regulations and policies (Dinges et al., 1996; Flight Safety Foundation, 1997; Flight Safety Foundation and National Business Aviation Association, 2014). However, while there are fatigue-related regulations and policies in place across modes, controlled studies with accepted objective methods evaluating the effectiveness of these approaches are almost non-existent (Rosekind et al., 2006; Lamp et al., 2019; Sprajcer et al., 2021). Given the diversity and complexity of operational schedules and requirements, it would be useful to have outcome data examining the effectiveness of representative regulations and policies, including consideration of unintended consequences.

An extensive scientific literature on sleep and circadian rhythms has been acknowledged and incorporated into current regulations and policies in many countries. For example, international principles and guidelines for duty/rest scheduling in commercial aviation were published in 1996, extended to business aviation in 1997, and updated in 2014 (Dinges et al., 1996; Flight Safety Foundation, 1997; Flight Safety Foundation and National Business Aviation Association, 2014). These publications provide foundational scientific information translated into operational guidance for these flight environments. A few generic, representative examples of how the science is translated into operational use illustrate aspects of effective regulations and policies. Clearly, these are only a few selected examples.

On average, human adults physiologically require about 8 hours of sleep. Generally, this translates to a minimum 8-hour uninterrupted sleep opportunity within a scheduled off-duty period. Total scheduled off duty periods should therefore be longer than the sleep opportunity to provide time for commuting to/from sleep location, meals, and other personal needs. Over time, sleep loss builds into a sleep debt and providing one- or two-night sleep recovery opportunities can be needed to zero-out this debt. Extended periods of wakefulness, greater than 16 hours, can engender cognitive performance decrements equivalent to chronic sleep loss and alcohol impairment (Dawson & Reid, 1997; Arendt et al., 2001). Therefore, limiting duty period length and consecutive duties can address some fatigue risks. Perhaps the most complex physiological challenge is posed by the 24-hour cycle of the internal circadian clock that controls physiological and behavioural rhythms, programmed for a 16-hour period of wakefulness during daylight and 8-hours sleep during the dark of night. Any operational factor that disrupts this circadian stability, such as night work and day sleep, crossing time zones or changing work/sleep start and end times can disrupt sleep and create fatigue-related cognitive performance impairments.

These are a just few representative examples of how scientific research can guide operational scheduling regulations and policies to address known fatigue risks. Other opportunities beyond scheduling can also be incorporated into regulations or policies to reduce risks. For example, FRMS, countermeasures such as napping and activity breaks, sleep disorders information and screening, anonymous fatigue reporting, and education/training programmes can be formalised within regulatory and policy schemes focused on fatigue management. **Opportunity/action #12: Identify and incorporate relevant sleep and circadian scientific elements into regulatory and policy efforts.**

6.4.4 PREPARING FOR NEW TECHNOLOGIES AND OPERATIONAL DEMANDS

The predictability and consistency of established regulations and policies provide an important foundation for long-term fatigue management in operational settings. However, as new technological innovations become available and operational demand evolves to reflect new technology or societal needs, parallel changes in regulations and policies may be needed. Incorporating mechanisms for nimble and flexible approaches to fatigue management that can reflect evolving technology and demands will ensure that regulations and policies remain relevant. These approaches could include regulatory requirements for review, evaluation, and potential revision within a specific timeframe (e.g., after 1 year, after 5 years). Company policies could have a similar review process to ensure opportunities to update and incorporate the latest science or reflect new technology or operational demands. **Opportunity/action #13: Implement mechanisms to ensure regulations and policies remain flexible and reflect the latest fatigue science, technology, and operational demands.**

6.4.5 SOCIETAL EXPECTATIONS

Perhaps worthy of its own chapter or book (see also Chapter 3.5), societal expectations about fatigue management are rarely discussed, studied, or addressed in the context of safety in our society. The few thoughts here, and mostly questions, are intended to provoke consideration, research, and future actions that may provide another mechanism to address future fatigue management.

6.4.5.1 SOCIETAL VS INDIVIDUAL RISK/BENEFIT CONSIDERATIONS

There are obvious safety risks related to fatigue in transportation: Lives lost and injuries—often occurring in milliseconds during operations. How do individuals evaluate the benefits that offset these individual risks? Is it economics (e.g., shift differential) or work/life flexibility? Are these risks well understood by the individuals confronting them? How are societal risks assessed, understood, and communicated?

Major societal transportation disasters demand world attention in their moment but are the lessons learnt incorporated into ongoing fatigue risk management? **Opportunity/ action #14: Pursue research examining the societal versus individual risk/ benefits of fatigue management.**

6.4.5.2 Cost/Benefit Issues

There are estimates of the societal economic costs associated with fatigue with an occasional focus on transportation (Walsh, 2004; Leger, 1994; Kessler et al., 2011). There are also data examining productivity costs linked to fatigue, including sleep disorders, and individual-related costs to companies (Rosekind et al., 2010; Ricci et al., 2007). The obvious assumption is that, by reducing or eliminating these fatigue-related risks, lives and costs are saved. However, it would be useful to have more data on these benefits. While costs associated with fatigue have received the most attention, quantifying the benefits (broadly defined) would provide greater justification for undertaking fatigue management efforts. Often a company will have a specific dollar amount with clear and quantified costs for implementing a fatigue management programme, but the benefits are usually less quantified in terms of cost savings, prevention, or optimising performance/productivity. **Opportunity/action #15: Conduct research to further quantify the individual, organisational, and societal benefits of fatigue management.**

6.4.5.3 Global Perspectives

The fatigue risks and challenges portrayed in this book are confronted by every transportation operation and system in the world. Obviously, there are differences by world regions, modes, and other factors, but human-centred transportation will continue to confront fatigue challenges. While there have been international meetings to exchange research findings and engage in policy discussions, there remain significant opportunities to consider coordinated global actions that would advance future fatigue management for our societal transportation needs. One aviation example would be through the International Civil Aviation Organisation (ICAO) where fatigue working groups on data, operations, and regulations could advance fatigue management efforts for the global aviation community. **Opportunity/action #16: Pursue global fatigue management actions related to safety, productivity, and policy, including areas for collaboration.**

6.4.6 CONCLUSIONS

Globally, humans will continue to have critical and central roles in developing, providing, and maintaining safe transportation operations. Managing human fatigue can be a model for providing safe, effective, and efficient societal mobility. Future fatigue management can be advanced through actions that enhance strategies, policies, and societal expectations with the 16 specific opportunities/actions (Table 6.4.1) identified in this chapter.

TABLE 6.4.1
Opportunities and Actions to Enhance Future Fatigue Management in Transportation

#1	Develop consensus standards for content, frequency, evaluation, and updating of fatigue education programmes.
#2	Develop models of tailored elements to incorporate in fatigue education programmes.
#3	Create a system to monitor technology advancements relevant to fatigue management.
#4	Develop reliable, ongoing "train-the-trainer" training opportunities that cover issues specific to operational domains and that are continuously updated.
#5	Implement specific plans that integrate fatigue education into organisational safety culture in an ongoing manner.
#6	Develop a plan and resources for organisational and individual communications to the broader society on enhancing safety through fatigue management.
#7	Develop consensus methods and standards to evaluate new fatigue detection technologies and establish a central information resource for sharing results.
#8	Enhance modelling capabilities to reflect individual-level status and incorporate individual objective fatigue data from wearables.
#9	Pursue research and validation to produce an aggregate risk model that incorporates relevant objective fatigue data.
#10	Implement cross-functional, independent incident response/investigation procedures.
#11	Implement and track all investigation recommendations.
#12	Identify and incorporate relevant sleep and circadian scientific elements into regulatory and policy efforts.
#13	Implement mechanisms to ensure that regulations and policies remain flexible and reflect the latest fatigue science, technology, and operational demands.
#14	Pursue research examining the societal versus individual risk/benefits of fatigue management.
#15	Conduct research to further quantify the individual, organisational, and societal benefits of fatigue management.
#16	Pursue global fatigue management actions related to safety, productivity, and policy, including areas for collaboration.

SUMMARY POINTS FOR PRACTITIONERS

- Education remains foundational to effective fatigue management; therefore, ensure that programmes are updated frequently, tailored to the operational setting, and implemented into the organisational safety culture.
- Establish a cross-functional incident response team with appropriate expertise in fatigue science, track fatigue-related recommendations, and confirm their ongoing implementation.
- Monitor and evaluate technology advancements relevant to fatigue management, incorporate validated technology where relevant, and ensure appropriate confidentiality practices are followed.
- Pursue modelling capabilities that reflect individual-level status to incorporate individual objective fatigue data from wearables.

- Implement fatigue science-based policies that support education programme elements and conduct ongoing policy reviews and updates to ensure relevance and flexibility.

REFERENCES

Anund, A., Fors, C., Kecklund, G., Leeuwen, W. v., & Åkerstedt, T. (2015). *Countermeasures for fatigue in transportation: A review of existing methods for drivers on road, rail, sea and in aviation.* (Report No. VTI rapport 852A). Swedish National Road and Transport Research Institute. www.diva-portal.org/smash/get/diva2:807456/FULLTEXT01.pdf

Arnedt, J. T., Wilde, G. J., Munt, P. W., & MacLean, A. W. (2001). How do prolonged wakefulness and alcohol compare in the decrements they produce on a simulated driving task? *Accident Analysis & Prevention, 33*(3), 337–344.

Arora, V. M., Georgitis, E., Woodruff, J. N., Humphrey, H. J., & Meltzer, D. (2007). Improving sleep hygiene of medical interns: Can the sleep, alertness, and fatigue education in residency program help? *Archives of Internal Medicine, 167*(16), 1738–1744.

Avers, K. E., Hauck, E. L., Blackwell, L. V., & Nesthus, T. E. (2009). *Flight attendant fatigue. Part 6: Fatigue countermeasure training and potential benefits.* (Report No. DOT/FAA/AM-09/20). Civil Aerospace Medical Institute. https://apps.dtic.mil/sti/pdfs/ADA510457.pdf

Barger, L. K., Runyon, M. S., Renn, M. L., Moore, C. G., Weiss, P. M., Condle, J. P.,... . Sequeira, D. J. (2018). Effect of fatigue training on safety, fatigue, and sleep in emergency medical services personnel and other shift workers: A systematic review and meta-analysis. *Prehospital Emergency Care, 22*(sup1), 58–68.

Dawson, D., & Reid, K. (1997). Fatigue, alcohol and performance impairment. *Nature, 388*(6639), 235–235.

Dinges, D., & Mallis, M. (1998). *Managing fatigue by drowsiness detection: Can technological promises be realized?* International Conference on Fatigue and Transportation, 3rd, 1998, Fremantle, Western Australia. https://trid.trb.org/view/539294

Dinges, D. F. (2004). Critical research issues in development of biomathematical models of fatigue and performance. *Aviation, Space, and Environmental Medicine, 75*(3), A181–A191.

Dinges, D. F., Graeber, R. C., Rosekind, M. R., & Samel, A. (1996). *Principles and guidelines for duty and rest scheduling in commercial aviation.* (Report No. TM 110404). NASA Ames Research Center. https://ntrs.nasa.gov/api/citations/19990063635/downloads/19990063635.pdf

Fletcher, A., McCulloch, K., Baulk, S. D., & Dawson, D. (2005). Countermeasures to driver fatigue: A review of public awareness campaigns and legal approaches. *Australian and New Zealand Journal of Public Health, 29*(5), 471–476.

Flight Safety Foundation. (1997). Principles and guidelines for duty and rest scheduling in corporate and business aviation. *Flight Safety Digest, 16*(1). Flight Safety Foundation. https://flightsafety.org/fsd/fsd_feb97.pdf

Flight Safety Foundation and National Business Aviation Association. (2014). *Duty/rest guidelines for business aviation.* https://flightsafety.org/wp-content/uploads/2016/09/DutyRest2014_final1.pdf

Flynn-Evans, E. E., Kirkley, C., Young, M., Bathurst, N., Gregory, K., Vogelpohl, V.,... . Marquez, J. J. (2020). Changes in performance and bio-mathematical model performance predictions during 45 days of sleep restriction in a simulated space mission. *Scientific Reports, 10*(1), 15594. https://doi.org/10.1038/s41598-020-71929-4

Flynn-Evans, E. E., Wong, L. R., Kuriyagawa, Y., Gowda, N., Cravalho, P. F., Pradhan, S.,.... . Wilaiprasitporn, T. (2021). Supervision of a self-driving vehicle unmasks latent sleepiness relative to manually controlled driving. *Scientific Reports*, *11*(1), 1–13.

Gander, P. H., Marshall, N. S., Bolger, W., & Girling, I. (2005). An evaluation of driver training as a fatigue countermeasure. *Transportation Research Part F: Traffic Psychology and Behaviour*, *8*(1), 47–58.

Kessler, R. C., Berglund, P. A., Coulouvrat, C., Hajak, G., Roth, T., Shahly, V.,.... . Walsh, J. K. (2011). Insomnia and the performance of US workers: Results from the America Insomnia Survey. *Sleep*, *34*(9), 1161–1171.

Lamp, A., Chen, J. M., McCullough, D., & Belenky, G. (2019). Equal to or better than: The application of statistical non-inferiority to fatigue risk management. *Accident Analysis & Prevention*, *126*, 184–190.

Leger, D. (1994). The cost of sleep-related accidents: A report for the National Commission on Sleep Disorders Research. *Sleep*, *17*(1), 84–93.

Lim, J., & Dinges, D. F. (2008). Sleep deprivation and vigilant attention. *Annals of the New York Academy of Sciences*, *1129*(1), 305–322.

Liu, C. C., Hosking, S. G., & Lenné, M. G. (2009). Predicting driver drowsiness using vehicle measures: Recent insights and future challenges. *Journal of Safety Research*, *40*(4), 239–245.

Mallis, M. M., Mejdal, S., Nguyen, T. T., & Dinges, D. F. (2004). Summary of the key features of seven biomathematical models of human fatigue and performance. *Aviation, Space, and Environmental Medicine*, *75*(3), A4–A14.

Marcus, J. H., & Rosekind, M. R. (2017). Fatigue in transportation: NTSB investigations and safety recommendations. *Injury Prevention*, *23*(4), 232–238.

National Transportation Safety Board (NTSB). (1994). *Uncontrolled collision with terrain American International Airways Flight 808, Douglas DC-8-61, N814CK, U.S. Naval Air Station, Guantanamo Bay, Cuba, August 18, 1993*. (Report No. 199417). NTSB, Washington, DC. https://ntrl.ntis.gov/NTRL/dashboard/searchResults/titleDetail/PB9 4910406.xhtml

Paul, M. A., Hursh, S. R., & Love, R. J. (2020). The importance of validating sleep behavior models for fatigue management software in military aviation. *Military Medicine*, *185*(11–12), e1986–e1991.

Price, J. M., & Coury, B. G. (2015). A method for applying fatigue science to accident investigation. *Reviews of Human Factors and Ergonomics*, *10*(1), 79–114.

Ramakrishnan, S., Lu, W., Laxminarayan, S., Wesensten, N. J., Rupp, T. L., Balkin, T. J., & Reifman, J. (2015). Can a mathematical model predict an individual's trait-like response to both total and partial sleep loss? *Journal of Sleep Research*, *24*(3), 262–269.

Ricci, J. A., Chee, E., Lorandeau, A. L., & Berger, J. (2007). Fatigue in the US workforce: Prevalence and implications for lost productive work time. *Journal of Occupational and Environmental Medicine*, 1–10.

Rosekind, M. R., Gander, P. H., Connell, L. J., & Co, E. L. (2001). *Crew factors in flight operations X: Alertness management in flight operations*. (Report No. DOT/FAA/AR-01-01). NASA Ames Research Center. https://ntrs.nasa.gov/api/citations/20020078410/downloads/20020078410.pdf

Rosekind, M. R., Gregory, K. B., & Mallis, M. M. (2006). Alertness management in aviation operations: Enhancing performance and sleep. *Aviation, Space, and Environmental Medicine*, *77*(12), 1256–1265.

Rosekind, M. R., Gregory, K. B., Mallis, M. M., Brandt, S. L., Seal, B., & Lerner, D. (2010). The cost of poor sleep: Workplace productivity loss and associated costs. *Journal of Occupational and Environmental Medicine*, 91–98.

Rosekind, M. R., Gregory, K. B., Miller, D. L., Co, E. L., Lebacqz, J. V., & Statler, I. C. (1994). *Analysis of crew fatigue in AIA Guantanamo Bay Aviation Accident*. (Report No. 20010114272). NASA Ames Research Center.

Rudin-Brown, C. M., & Rosberg, A. (2021). Applying principles of fatigue science to accident investigation: Transportation Safety Board of Canada (TSB) fatigue investigation methodology. *Chronobiology International, 38*(2), 296–300.

Russell, C., Caldwell, J., Arand, D., Myers, L., Wubbels, P., & Downs, H. (2000). Validation of the fatigue science readiband actigraph and associated sleep/wake classification algorithms. *Arch LLC*.

Smith, K. C., & Wallace, D. P. (2016). Improving the sleep of children's hospital employees through an email-based sleep wellness program. *Clinical Practice in Pediatric Psychology, 4*(3), 291.

Sparrow, A. R., LaJambe, C. M., & Van Dongen, H. P. (2019). Drowsiness measures for commercial motor vehicle operations. *Accident Analysis & Prevention, 126*, 146–159.

Sprajcer, M., Thomas, M. J., Sargent, C., Crowther, M. E., Boivin, D. B., Wong, I. S., ... Dawson, D. (2021). How effective are fatigue risk management systems (FRMS)? A review. *Accident Analysis & Prevention*, 106398.

Steffen, M. W., Hazelton, A. C., Moore, W. R., Jenkins, S. M., Clark, M. M., & Hagen, P. T. (2015). Improving sleep. *Journal of Occupational and Environmental Medicine, 57*(1), 1–5.

Van Dongen, H. P., Mott, C. G., Huang, J.-K., Mollicone, D. J., McKenzie, F. D., & Dinges, D. F. (2007). Optimization of biomathematical model predictions for cognitive performance impairment in individuals: Accounting for unknown traits and uncertain states in homeostatic and circadian processes. *Sleep, 30*(9), 1129–1143.

Walsh, J. K. (2004). Clinical and socioeconomic correlates of insomnia. *Journal of Clinical Psychiatry, 65*(8), 13–19.

Index

For Product Safety Concerns and Information please contact our EU
representative GPSR@taylorandfrancis.com
Taylor & Francis Verlag GmbH, Kaufingerstraße 24, 80331 München, Germany